MIDWIFERY & WOMEN'S HEALTH NURSE PRACTITIONER CERTIFICATION REVIEW GUIDE

Second Edition

Edited by

Beth M. Kelsey, EdD, WHNP-BC

Assistant Professor
School of Nursing
Ball State University
Muncie, Indiana

Board of Directors
National Association of Nurse Practitioners in Women's Health (NPWH)
Washington, DC

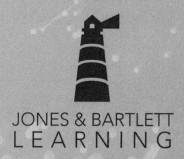

JONES & BARTLETT
LEARNING

World Headquarters

Jones & Bartlett Learning
40 Tall Pine Drive
Sudbury, MA 01776
978-443-5000
info@jblearning.com
www.jblearning.com

Jones & Bartlett Learning
Canada
6339 Ormindale Way
Mississauga, Ontario L5V 1J2
Canada

Jones and Bartlett Learning
International
Barb House, Barb Mews
London W6 7PA
United Kingdom

Jones & Bartlett Learning books and products are available through most bookstores and online booksellers. To contact Jones & Bartlett Learning directly, call 800-832-0034, fax 978-443-8000, or visit our website, www.jblearning.com.

Substantial discounts on bulk quantities of Jones & Bartlett Learning publications are available to corporations, professional associations, and other qualified organizations. For details and specific discount information, contact the special sales department at Jones & Bartlett Learning via the above contact information or send an email to specialsales@jblearning.com.

The authors, editor, and publisher have made every effort to provide accurate information. However, they are not responsible for errors, omissions, or for any outcomes related to the use of the contents of this book and take no responsibility for the use of the products and procedures described. Treatments and side effects described in this book may not be applicable to all people; likewise, some people may require a dose or experience a side effect that is not described herein. Drugs and medical devices are discussed that may have limited availability controlled by the Food and Drug Administration (FDA) for use only in a research study or clinical trial. Research, clinical practice, and government regulations often change the accepted standard in this field. When consideration is being given to use of any drug in the clinical setting, the health care provider or reader is responsible for determining FDA status of the drug, reading the package insert, and reviewing prescribing information for the most up-to-date recommendations on dose, precautions, and contraindications, and determining the appropriate usage for the product. This is especially important in the case of drugs that are new or seldom used.

Production Credits

Publisher: Kevin Sullivan
Acquisitions Editor: Amy Sibley
Associate Editor: Patricia Donnelly
Editorial Assistant: Rachel Shuster
Production Editor: Amanda Clerkin
Associate Marketing Manager: Katie Hennessy

V.P., Manufacturing and Inventory Control: Therese Connell
Composition: DataStream Content Solutions, LLC
Cover Design: Scott Moden
Cover Image: © Hocusfocus/Dreamstime.com
Printing and Binding: Courier Kendallville, Inc.
Cover Printing: Courier Kendallville, Inc.

To order this product, use ISBN: 978-0-7637-1500-0

Library of Congress Cataloging-in-Publication Data
Midwifery & women's health nurse practitioner certification review guide / [edited by] Beth M. Kelsey.—2nd ed.
        p. ; cm.
    Rev. ed. of: Midwifery/women's health nurse practitioner certification review guide. c2004.
    Includes bibliographical references and index.
    ISBN 978-0-7637-7417-2 (pbk.)
    1. Nurse practitioners—Examinations, questions, etc.   2. Midwives Examinations, questions, etc.   3. Gynecologic nursing—Examinations, questions, etc.   4. Maternity nursing—Examinations, questions, etc.   5. Women—Diseases—Examinations, questions, etc.   6. Women—Health and hygiene—Examinations, questions, etc.   I. Kelsey, Beth.
II. Midwifery/women's health nurse practitioner certification review guide.
    [DNLM: 1. Midwifery—Examination Questions.   2. Genital Diseases, Female—nursing—Examination Questions.
3. Nurse Midwives—Examination Questions.   4. Nurse Practitioners—Examination Questions.   5. Pregnancy Complications—nursing—Examination Questions.   6. Women's Health—Examination Questions.   WY 18.2 M6288 2011]
    RT82.8.M53 2011
    610.73092—dc22
                                                                                                    2010018003

6048

Printed in the United States of America
14 13 12   10 9 8 7 6 5 4 3 2

Contents

Chapter 8

**Nongynecological Disorders/
    Problems   245**

*Sandra K. Pfantz
Beth M. Kelsey
Mary C. Knutson*

Chapter 9

**Advanced Practice Nursing and
    Midwifery: Role Development, Trends,
    and Issues   337**

Patricia Burkhardt

Preface

A comprehensive review essential for those preparing to take the midwifery (AMBC) or women's health nurse practitioner certification (NCC) examinations. The *Midwifery & Women's Health Nurse Practitioner Certification Review Guide* was developed for both of these nursing specialties because of the many commonalities they share that enhance the delivery of care to women during their life span. Experts in the field of women's health as well as midwifery combined their expertise and wisdom to provide an invaluable resource that will not only assist women's health nurse practitioners and midwives in their pursuit of success on their respective certification examinations, but assist them in their delivery of care in the practice setting. In addition, multiple resources have been utilized to ensure the integrity of this text so that it is representative of the kinds of questions that may be encountered by both specialties during the examination process.

Although the birthing process itself may not fall within the realm of the women's health nurse practitioner practice, the knowledge of the process will add a valuable component which can only improve the quality of the care provided by the nurse practitioner. An acute awareness of the childbearing process and its implications throughout a woman's life span can only improve the outcome of care delivered.

Many nurses preparing for certification examinations find that reviewing an extensive body of scientific knowledge requires a very difficult search of many sources that must be synthesized to provide a review base for the examination. The purpose of this review guide is to provide a succinct, yet comprehensive review of the core material.

The book has been organized to provide the reader with test-taking and study strategies first. This is an imperative prerequisite for success in the certification examination arena.

This chapter is followed by chapters on General Health Assessment and Health Promotion, Women's Health, Pregnancy, Midwifery Care of Newborn, Intrapartum and Postpartum, Gynecological Disorders/Problems, and Nongynecological Disorders. The final chapter addresses professional issues that directly impact the midwife and nurse practitioner, including nursing research, roles, ethical issues, health policy/legislative issues, and legal aspects of practice.

Following each chapter are test questions, which are intended to serve as an introduction to the testing arena. These questions are representative of those found on the examinations. A bibliography is included at the completion of each chapter for those who need a more in depth discussion of the subject matter.

The editor and contributing authors are certified nurse practitioners and certified nurse midwives. They have designed this book to assist potential examinees to prepare for success in the certification examination process as well as improve the examinee's knowledge in the practice setting.

It is assumed that the reader of this review guide has completed a course of study in either a women's health nurse practitioner or midwifery program. It is not intended to be a basic learning tool.

Contributors

Penelope Morrison Bosarge, MSN, RNC, WHNP
Women's Health Nurse Practitioner
Coordinator Women's Health Care Nurse Practitioner
Program
University of Alabama, Birmingham
School of Nursing
Birmingham, Alabama

Patricia Burkhardt, DrPH, CNM
Nurse Midwife
Associate Clinical Professor
Midwifery Program
Division of Nursing
New York University
New York, New York

Beth M. Kelsey, EdD, WHNP-BC
Women's Health Nurse Practitioner
Assistant Professor
School of Nursing
Ball State University
Muncie, Indiana

Mary C. Knutson, MN, RNC, ANP
Adult Nurse Practitioner
Nurse Consultant
Alaska Department Health & Social Services
Anchorage, Alaska

Anthony A. Lathrop, MSN, CNM, RDMS
Perinatal Nurse–Midwife
Maternal–Fetal Medicine
Northern Illinois Regional Perinatal Center
Rockford Memorial Hospital
Rockford, Illinois

Anne A. Moore, MSN, RNC, WHNP, FAANP
Women's Health Nurse Practitioner
Professor
School of Nursing
Vanderbilt University
Nashville, Tennessee

Sandra K. Pfantz, DrPH, APRN
Adult Nurse Practitioner
Associate Professor
School of Nursing
St. Xavier University
Department of Family Medicine
University of Illinois at Chicago
Chicago, Illinois

Susan P. Shannon, MS, CNM, RNC
Nurse Midwife
Director, Women's and Infant Services
Sharon Hospital
Sharon, Connecticut
California State University, Los Angeles

Instructions for Using the Online Access Code Card

Enclosed within this review guide you will find a printed "access code card" containing an access code providing you access to the new online interactive testing program, JB TestPrep. This program will help you prepare for certification exams, such as the American Nurse Credentialing Center's (ANCC's) certification exam to become a certified nurse practitioner. The online program includes the same multiple choice questions that are printed in this study guide. You can choose a "practice exam" that allows you to see feedback on your response immediately, or a "final exam," which hides your results until you have completed all the questions in the exam. Your overall score on the questions you have answered is also compiled. Here are the instructions on how to access JB TestPrep, the Online Interactive Testing Program:

1. Find the printed access code card bound in to this book.
2. Go to www.JBLearning.com/usecode.
3. Enter in your 10-digit access code, which you can find by scratching off the protective coating on the access code card.
4. Follow the instructions on each screen to set up your account profile and password. Please note: Only select a course coordinator if you have been instructed to do so by an institution or an instructor.
5. Contact Jones & Bartlett Learning technical support if you have any questions:
   Call 800-832-0034
   Visit www.jblearning.com and select "Tech Support"
   Email info@jblearning.com

Test-Taking Strategies and Techniques

We all respond to testing situations in different ways. What separates the successful test taker from the unsuccessful one is knowing how to prepare for and take a test. Preparing yourself to be a successful test taker is as important as studying for the test. Each person needs to assess and develop their own test-taking strategies and skills. The primary goal of this chapter is to assist potential examinees in knowing how to study for and take a test.

◘ STRATEGY #1: KNOW YOURSELF

When faced with an examination, do you feel threatened, experience butterflies or sweaty palms, or have trouble keeping your mind focused on studying or on the test questions? These common symptoms of test anxiety plague many of us, but can be used advantageously if understood and handled correctly (Divine & Kylen, 1979). Over the years of test taking, each of us has developed certain testing behaviors, some of which are beneficial, while others present obstacles to successful test taking. You can take control of the test-taking situation by identifying the undesirable behaviors, maintaining the desirable ones, and developing skills to improve test performance.

◘ STRATEGY #2: DEVELOP YOUR THINKING SKILLS

Understanding Thought Processes

In order to improve your thinking skills and subsequent test performance, it is best to understand the types of thinking as well as the techniques to enhance the thought process. Everyone has a personal learning style, but we all must proceed through the same process to think.

Thinking occurs on two levels—the lower level of memory and comprehension and the higher level of application and analysis (ABP, 1989). Memory is the ability to recall facts. Without adequate retrieval of facts, progression through the higher levels of thinking cannot occur easily. Comprehension is the ability to understand memorized facts. To be effective, comprehension skills must allow the person to translate recalled information from one context to another. Application, or the process of using information to know why it occurs, is a higher form of learning. Effective application relies on the use of understood memorized facts to verify intended action. Analysis is the ability to use abstract or logical forms of thought to show relationships and to distinguish the cause and effect between the variables in a situation.

As applied to testing situations, the thought process from memory to analysis occurs quite quickly. Some examination items are designed to test memory and comprehension, while others test application and analysis. An example of a memory question is as follows:

Clients' initial response to learning that they have a terminal illness is generally:

a) Depression
b) Bargaining
c) *Denial*
d) Anger

To answer this question correctly, the individual has to retrieve a memorized fact. Understanding the fact, knowing why it is important or analyzing what should be done in this situation is not needed. An example of a question that tests comprehension is as follows:

> Shortly after having been informed that she is in the terminal stages of breast cancer, Mrs. Jones begins to talk about her plans to travel with her husband when he retires in two years. The nurse should know that:
>
> a) The diagnosis could be wrong and Mrs. Jones may not be dying.
> b) *Mrs. Jones is probably responding to the news by using the defense mechanism of denial.*
> c) Mrs. Jones is clearly delusional.
> d) Mrs. Jones is not responding in the way most clients would.

In order to answer this question correctly, an individual must retrieve the fact that denial is often the first response to learning about a terminal illness and that Mrs. Jones' behavior is indicative of denial.

In a higher level of thinking examination question, individuals must be able to recall a fact, understand that fact in the context of the question and apply this understanding to explaining why one answer is correct after analyzing the answer choices as they relate to the situation (Sides & Cailles, 1989). An example of an application analysis question is as follows:

> Mr. Smith has just learned that he has an inoperable brain tumor. His comment when the nurse speaks to him later is, "This can't possibly be true. Mistakes are made in hospitals all the time. They might have mixed up my test results." The nurse's most appropriate response would be to:
>
> a) Refer Mr. Smith for a psychiatric consultation
> b) *Neither agree nor disagree with Mr. Smith's comment*
> c) Confront Mr. Smith with his denial
> d) Agree with Mr. Smith that mistakes can happen and tell him you will see about getting repeat tests

To answer this question correctly, the individual must recall the fact that denial is often the initial response to learning about a terminal illness; understand that Mr. Smith's response in this case is evidence of the normal use of denial; apply this knowledge to each option, understanding why it may or may not be correct; and analyze each option for what action is most appropriate for this situation. Application/analysis questions require the examinee to use logical rationale, which demonstrates the ability to analyze a relationship, based on a well-defined principle or fact. Problem-solving ability becomes important as the examinee must think through each question option, deciding its relevance and importance to the situation of the question.

Building Your Thinking Skills

Effective memorization is the cornerstone to learning and building thinking skills (Olney, 1989). We have all experienced "memory power outages" at some time, due in part to trying to memorize too much, too fast, too ineffectively. Developing skills to improve memorization is important to increasing the effectiveness of your thinking and subsequent test performance.

Technique #1

Quantity is *not* quality, so concentrate on learning important content. For example, it is important to know the various pharmacologic agents appropriate for the management of chronic obstructive pulmonary disease (COPD), not the specific dosages for each medication.

Technique #2

Memory from repetition, or saying something over and over again to remember it usually fades. Developing memory skills that trigger retrieval of needed facts is more useful. Such skills are as follows:

Acronyms
These are mental crutches that facilitate recall. Some are already established such as PERRL (pupils equal, round, reactive to light), or PAT (paroxysmal atrial tachycardia). Developing your own acronyms can be particularly useful since they are your own word association arrangements in a singular word. Nonsense words or funny, unusual ones are often more useful since they attract your attention.

Acrostics
This mental tool arranges words into catchy phrases. The first letter of each word stands for something that is recalled as the phrase is said. Your own acrostics are most valuable in triggering recall of learned information since they are your individual situation associations. An example of an acrostic is as follows:

> **K**issing **P**atty **P**roduces **A**ffection stands for the four types of nonverbal messages: **K**inesics, **P**aralanguage, **P**roxemics, and **A**ppearance.

ABCs
This technique facilitates information retrieval by using the alphabet as a crutch. Each letter stands for a symptom, which when put together creates a picture of the clinical presentation of the disease. For example, the characteristics of the disease and symptoms of osteoarthritis using the ABC technique are as follows:

a) Aching or pain
b) Being stiff on awakening
c) Crepitus
d) Deterioration of articular cartilage
e) Enlargements of distal interphalangeal joints
f) Formation of new bone at joint surface

g) Granulation inflammatory tissue

h) Heberden's nodes

One Letter

Recall is enhanced by emphasizing a single letter. The major symptoms of schizophrenia are often remembered as follows:

Affect (flat)

Autism

Auditory hallucinations

Imaging

This technique can be used in two ways. The first is to develop a nickname for a clinical problem that when said produces a mental picture. For example, "a wan, wheezy pursed lip" might be used to visualize a patient with pulmonary emphysema who is thin, emaciated, experiencing dyspnea, with a hyperinflated chest, who has an elongated expiratory breathing phase. A second form of imaging is to visualize a specific patient while you are trying to understand or solve a clinical problem when studying or answering a question. For example, imagine an elderly man who is experiencing an acute asthma attack. You are trying to analyze the situation and place him in a position that maximizes respiratory effort. In your mind you visualize him in various positions of side lying, angular and forward, imaging what will happen to the man in each position. A second form of imaging is to visualize a specific situation while you are trying to answer a question. For example, if you are trying to remember how to describe active listening or physical attending skills, see yourself in a comfortable environment, facing the other person, with open posture and eye contact.

Rhymes, Music, and Links

The absurd is easier to remember than the most common. Rhymes, music, or links can add absurdity and humor to learning and remembering (Olney, 1989). These retrieval tools are developed by the individual for specific content. For example, making up a rhyme about diabetes may be helpful in remembering the predominant female incidence, origin of disease, primary symptoms, and management, as illustrated by:

There once was a woman

whose beta cells failed.

She grew quite thirsty

and her glucose levels sailed.

Her lack of insulin caused her to

increase her intake,

And her increased urinary output

was certainly not fake.

So she learned to watch her diet

and administer injections

That kept her healthy, happy

and free of complications.

Words that rhyme can also be used to jog the memory about important characteristics of phenomena. For example, the stages of group therapy can be remembered and characterized by the following, according to Tuckman (1965):

Forming

Storming

Norming

Performing

Setting content to music is sometimes useful for remembering. Melodies that are repetitious jog the memory by the ups and downs of the notes and the rhythm of the music.

Links connect key words from the content by using them in a story. An example given by Olney (1989) for remembering the parts of an eye is: IRIS watched a PUPIL through the LENS of a RED TIN telescope while eating CORN-EA on the cob.

Additional memory aids may also include the use of color or drawing for improving recall. Use different colored pens or paper to accentuate the material being learned. For example, highlight or make notes in blue for content about respiratory problems and in red for cardiovascular content. Drawing assists with visualizing content as well. This is particularly helpful for remembering the pathophysiology of the specific health problem.

The important thing to remember about remembering is to use good recall techniques.

Technique #3

Improving higher-level thinking skills involves exercising the application and analysis of memorized fact. Small group review is particularly useful for enhancing these high level skills. It allows verbalization of thought processes and receipt of input about content and thought process from others (Sides & Cailles, 1989). Individuals not only hear how they think, but how others think as well. This interaction allows individuals to identify flaws in their thought process as well as to strengthen their positive points.

Taking practice tests is also helpful in developing application/analysis thinking skills. These tests permit the individual to analyze thinking patterns as well as the cause-and-effect relationships between the question and its options. The problem-solving skills needed to answer application/analysis questions are tested, giving the individual more experience through practice (Dickenson-Hazard, 1990).

◘ STRATEGY #3: KNOW THE CONTENT

Your ability to study is directly influenced by organization and concentration (Dickenson-Hazard, 1990). If effort is spent on both of these aspects of exam preparation, examination success can be increased.

Preparation for Studying: Getting Organized

Study habits are developed early in our educational experiences. Some of our habits enhance learning, although others do not. To increase study effectiveness, organization of study materials and time is essential. Organization decreases frustration, allows for easy resumption of study, and increases concentrated study time.

Technique #1

Create your own study space. Select a study area that is yours alone, free from distractions, comfortable and well lighted. The ventilation and room temperature should be comfortable since a cold room makes it difficult to concentrate and a warm room may make you sleepy (Burkle & Marshak, 1989). All your study materials should be left in your study space. The basic premise of a study space is that it facilitates a mind set that you are there to study. When you interrupt study, it is best to leave your materials just as they are. Do not close books or put away notes as you will just have to relocate them, wasting your study time, when you do resume study.

Technique #2

Define and organize the content. From the test giver, secure an outline or the content parameters that are to be examined. If the test giver's outline is sketchy, develop a more detailed one for yourself using the recommended text as a guideline. Next, identify your available study resources: class notes, old exams, handouts, textbooks, review courses, or study groups. For national standardized exams, such as initial licensing or certification, it is best to identify one or two study resources that cover the content being tested and stick to them. Attempting to review all available resources is not only mind boggling, but increases anxiety and frustration as well. Make your selections and stay with them.

Technique #3

Conduct a content assessment. Use a simple rating scale such as the following:

  1 = requires no review
  2 = requires minimal review
  3 = requires intensive review
  4 = start from the beginning

Read through the content outline and rate each content area (Dickenson-Hazard, 1990). **Table 1-1** provides a sample exam content assessment. Be honest with your assessment. It is far better to recognize your content weaknesses when you can study and remedy them, rather than thinking during the exam how you wished you had studied more. Likewise with content strengths: if you know the material, do not waste time studying it.

■ **Table 1-1**   Sample Content Assessment

Exam Content: Theories & Skills	
Category: Provided by Test Giver	**Rating: Provided by Examinee**
Group dynamics	2
Group process	2
Behavior modification	3
Crisis intervention	1
Reality therapy	4
Communication process	3
Interviewing skills	3
Self-care	4
Decision making	1
Legal/ethical issues	2
Cognitive techniques	2
Mental status evaluation	3
Problem solving	3
Community resources evaluation	3
Nursing process	3
Nursing theory	2
Role theory	3
Change theory	2
Communication theories	2
Organizational theory	2
Research design	2
Research evaluation	2
Research application	2
Team building	3
Conflict management	2
Teaching/learning skills	3
Supervisory skills	3
Observation skills	3
Evaluation skills	2
Nursing diagnosis	3
DSM IV	3
Grief and loss theory	3
Death and dying	2
Stress management theory	2
Stress management skills	4
Family dynamics	2
Assertiveness training skills	3
Motivation skills	4

Houseman, C. (Ed.). (1998). *Psychiatric certification review guide for the generalist and clinical specialist in adult, child, and adolescent psychiatric and mental health nursing* (2nd ed.). Sudbury, MA: Jones and Bartlett.

■ **Table 1-2** Sample Study Plan

Goal: Achieve a passing grade on the certification exam. Time available: 2 Months		
Objective	**Activity**	**Date Accomplished**
Understand elements of milieu therapy	Read section in Chapter 2	Feb. 5 & 6, 1 hour each day
	Read notes from review class and combine with notes taken from text	Feb. 7, 1 hour
	Review combined notes and sample test questions	Feb. 8, 1 hour
Master social/cultural/ethnic factors	Read section in Chapter 2—take notes on chapter content	Feb. 9 & 10, 1 hour each day
	Read notes from review class and combine with notes taken from text	Feb. 11, 1 hour
	Review combined notes and sample test questions	Feb. 12, 1 hour
Know material contained in Code for Nurses with Interpretive Statements	Read ANA Publication—Take notes on content	Feb. 13 & 14, 1 hour each day

Houseman, C. (Ed.). (1998). *Psychiatric certification review guide for the generalist and clinical specialist in adult, child, and adolescent psychiatric and mental health nursing* (2nd ed.). Sudbury, MA: Jones and Bartlett.

Technique #4

Develop a study plan. Coordinate the content that needs to be studied with the time available (Sides & Cailles, 1989). Prioritize your study needs, starting with weak areas first. Allow for a general review at the end of the study plan. Lastly, establish an overall goal for yourself—something that will motivate you when it is brought to mind.

Table 1-2 illustrates a study plan developed on the basis of the exam content assessment in Table 1-1. Conducting an assessment and developing a study plan should require no more than 50 minutes. It is a wise investment of time with potential payoffs of reduced study stress and enhanced exam success.

Technique #5

Begin now and use your time wisely. The smart test taker begins the study process early (Olney, 1989). Sit down, conduct the content assessment and develop a study plan as soon as you know about the exam. Do not procrastinate!

Getting Down To Business: The Actual Studying

There is no better way to prepare for an examination than individual study (Dickenson-Hazard, 1989). The responsibility to achieve the goal you set for this exam lies with you alone. The means you employ to achieve this goal do vary and should begin with identifying your peak study times and using techniques to maximize them.

Technique #1

Study in short bursts. Each of us have our own biologic clock that dictates when we are at our peak during the day. If you are a morning person, you are generally active and alert early in the day, slowing down and becoming drowsy by evening. If you are an evening person, you do not completely wake up until late morning and hit your peak in the afternoon and evening. Each person generally has several peaks during the day. It is best to study during those times when your alertness is at its peak (Dickenson-Hazard, 1990).

During our concentration peaks, there are mini-peaks, or bursts of alertness (Olney, 1989). These alertness peaks of a concentration peak occur because levels of concentration are at their highest during the first part and last part of a study period. These bursts can vary from 10 minutes to 1 hour depending on the extent of concentration. If studying is sustained for 1 hour there are only two mini peaks; one at the beginning and one at the end. There are eight mini-peaks if that same hour is divided into 4, 10-minute intervals. Hence it is more helpful to study in short bursts (Olney, 1989). More can be learned in less time.

Technique #2

Cramming can be useful. Since concentration ability is highly variable, some individuals can sustain their mini-peaks for 15, 20, or even 30 minutes at a time.

Pushing your concentration beyond its peak is fruitless and verges on cramming, which in general is a poor study technique. There are, however, times when cramming, a short-term memory tool, is useful. Short-term memory generally is at its best in the morning. A quick review or cram of content in the morning can be useful the day of the exam (Olney, 1989). Most studying, however, is best accomplished in the afternoon or evening when long-term memory functions at its peak.

Technique #3

Give your brain breaks. Regular times during study to rest and absorb the content are needed by the brain. The best approach to breaks is to plan them and give yourself a conscious break (Dickenson-Hazard, 1990). This approach eliminates the "day dreaming" or "wandering thought" approach to breaks that many of us use. It is better to get up, leave the study area and do something non-study related for longer breaks. For shorter breaks of 5 minutes or so, leave your desk, gaze out the window or do some stretching exercises. When your brain says to give it a rest, accommodate it! You will learn more with less stress.

Technique #4

Study the correct content. It is easy for all of us to become bogged down in the detail of the content we are studying. However, it is best to focus on the major concepts or the "state of the art" content. Leave the details, the suppositions and the experience at the door of your study area. Concentrate on the major textbook facts and concepts that revolve around the subject matter being tested.

Technique #5

Fit your studying to the test type. The best way to prepare for an objective test is to study facts, particularly anything printed in italics or bold. Memory enhancing techniques are particularly useful when preparing for an objective test. If preparing for an essay test, study generalities, examples, and concepts. Application techniques are helpful when studying for this type of an exam (Burkle & Marshak, 1989).

Technique #6

Use your study plan wisely. Your study plan is meant to be a guide, not a rigid schedule. You should take your time with studying. Do not rush through the content just to remain on schedule. Occasionally study plans need revision. If you take more or less time than planned, readjust the plan for the time gained or lost. The plan can guide you, but you must go at your own pace.

Technique #7

Actively study. Being an active participant in study rather than trying to absorb the printed word is also helpful. Ways to be active include: taking notes on the content as you study; constructing questions and answering them; taking practice tests; or discussing the content with yourself. Also, using your individual study quirks is encouraged. Some people stand, others walk around and some play background music. Whatever helps you to concentrate and study better, you should use.

Technique #8

Use study aids. Although there is no substitute for individual studying, several resources, if available, are useful in facilitating learning. Review courses are an excellent means for organizing or summarizing your individual study. They generally provide the content parameters and the major concepts of the content that you need to know. Review courses also provide an opportunity to clarify not-well-understood content, as well as to review known material (Dickenson-Hazard, 1990). Study guides are useful for organizing study. They provide detail on the content that is important to the exam. Study groups are an excellent resource for summarizing and refining content. They provide an opportunity for thinking through your knowledge base, with the advantage of hearing another person's point of view. Each of these study aids increases understanding of content and when used correctly, increases effectiveness of knowledge application.

Technique #9

Know when to quit. It is best to stop studying when your concentration ebbs. It is unproductive and frustrating to force yourself to study. It is far better to rest or unwind, then resume at a later point in the day. Avoid studying outside your morning or afternoon concentration peaks and focus your study energy on your right time of day or evening.

◘ STRATEGY #4: BECOME TEST-WISE

Most nursing examinations are composed of multiple-choice questions (MCQs). This type of question requires the examinee to select the best response(s) for a specific circumstance or condition. Successful test taking is dependent not only on content knowledge but on test-taking skill as well. If you are unable to impart your knowledge through the vehicle used for its conveyance, i.e., the MCQ, your test-taking success is in jeopardy.

Technique #1

Recognize the purpose of a test question. Most test questions are developed to examine knowledge at two separate levels: memory and application. A memory question requires the examinee to recall and comprehend facts from their knowledge base while an application question requires the examinee to use and apply the knowledge (ABP, 1989). Memory questions test recall, but application questions test synthesis and problem-solving skills. When taking a test you need to be aware of whether you are being asked a fact or to use that fact.

Technique #2

Recognize the components of a test question. Multiple choice questions may include the basic components of a background statement, a stem and a list of options. The background statement presents information that facilitates the examinee in answering the question. The stem asks or states the intent of the question. The options are four to five possible responses to the question. The correct option is called the *keyed response* and all other options are called *distractors* (ABP, 1989). Knowing the components of a test question helps you sift through the information presented and focus on the question's intent (see **Table 1-3**).

Technique #3

Recognize the item types. Basically two styles of MCQs are used for examinations. One requires the examinee to select the one best answer; the other requires selection of multiple correct answers. Among the one-best-answer styles there are three types. The A type requires the selection of the best response among those offered. The B type requires the examinee to match the options with the appropriate statement. The X type asks the examinee to respond either true or false to each option (ABP, 1989). **Most standardized tests, such as those used for nursing licensure and certification, are composed of four or five option-A type questions.**

Technique #4

Practice, practice, practice. Taking practice tests can improve performance. Although they can assist in evaluation of your knowledge, their primary benefit is to assist you with test-taking skills. You should use them to evaluate your thinking process, your ability to read, understand and interpret questions, and your skills in completing the mechanics of the test.

Exam resources, including sample questions for the American Nurses Credentialing Center (ANCC) certification exams, are available online at: http://www.nursecredentialing.org/Certification/ExamResources.aspx.

◘ STRATEGY #5: APPLY BASIC RULES OF TEST TAKING

Technique #1

Follow your regular routine the night before a test. Eat familiar foods. Avoid the temptation to cram all night. Go to bed at your regular time (Nugent and Vitale, 1997).

Technique #2

Be prepared for exam day. It is important to familiarize yourself with the test site, the building, the parking, and travel route prior to the exam day. If you must travel, arrive early to allow time for this familiarization. It is helpful to make a list of things you need on the exam day: pencils, admission card, watch, and a few pieces of hard candy as a quick energy source. On exam day allow yourself plenty of time to arrive at the site. Wear comfortable clothes and have a good breakfast that morning.

■ **Table 1-3**   Anatomy of a Test Question

Background statement	A woman brings her 65-year old mother in to see a clinical nurse specialist because she is concerned that it is now a month since her mother was widowed, and she continues to be tearful when talking about the loss and wants to visit the grave regularly.
Stem	Which of the following initial approaches would most likely result in compliance with your nursing recommendations?
Options	a. Three or four short questions followed by a request to a psychiatrist to prescribe an antidepressant b. Immediate reassurance only c. *Careful listening and open-ended questions* d. Referring the mother to a support group

Houseman, C. (Ed.). (1998). *Psychiatric certification review guide for the generalist and clinical specialist in adult, child, and adolescent psychiatric and mental health nursing* (2nd ed.). Sudbury, MA: Jones and Bartlett.

Technique #3

Understand all the directions for the test. Know if the test has a penalty for guessing or if you should attempt every question (Nugent and Vitale, 1997).

Technique #4

Read the directions carefully. An exam may have several types of questions. Be on the lookout for changing item types and be sure you understand the directions on how you are to answer before you begin reading the question.

Technique #5

Use time wisely and effectively. Allow no more than 1 minute per question. Skip difficult questions and return to them later or make an educated guess.

Technique #6

Read and consider all options. Be systematic and use problem-solving techniques. Relate options to the question and balance them against each other.

Technique #7

Check your answers. Reconsider your answers, especially those in which you made an educated guess. You may have gained information from subsequent questions that is helpful in answering previous questions or may be less anxious and more objective by the end of the test.

◘ SOME DOS & DON'TS TO REMEMBER

- Do identify key words in the stem before looking at options.
- Do confine your thinking to the information provided.
- Do eliminate wrong answers and focus on the one or two most likely correct responses.
- Do guess; generally there is no penalty (loss of extra points) for having done so—true for ANCC exams.
- Don't spend too much time on any one question—it is a timed examination.
- Don't second-guess—your first response is likely the best response.
  - If you tend to second-guess your responses, only review questions that you could not answer on the first pass through the exam—computer-based exams allow you to mark questions that you may want to address later in the exam.
- Don't change an answer without a good reason, such as having misread the question.

Considerations for computerized examinations:

All ANCC certification examinations are computer-based exams.

- Be sure that you have completed all information needed to register for the exam.
- Bring a photo ID—If a letter of authorization is needed, have it with you.
- If you are easily distracted by sound, consider using earplugs (these may be available at the testing center; check before using your own).
- Personal items such as books, laptop computers, iPods, cellular telephones, food or drink are not allowed during testing, secure these items elsewhere.
- Arrive 30 minutes before the appointed testing time.
- If you are not comfortable taking exams using a computer, consider taking a practice exam usually available at the examination site.
- Use computer-based practice exams, particularly if you are unfamiliar with this testing format. Sample online questions for each ANCC certification exam are available at: http://www.nursecredentialing. org/Certification/ExamResources.aspx.
- Know what to do if you experience any electronic or other difficulties during the examination. In addition to addressing the issue at the test site, you should also notify the certifying board (inform ANCC about problems during exam using the post-test survey).

◘ STRATEGY #6: PSYCH YOURSELF UP: TAKING TESTS IS STRESSFUL

Although a little stress can be productive, too much can incapacitate you in your studying and test taking (Divine & Kylen, 1979). For persons with severe test anxiety, interventions such as cognitive therapy, systematic desensitization, study skills counseling and biofeedback have all been used with some success (Spielberger, 1995). Techniques derived from these approaches can influence the results achieved by changing attitudes and approaches to test taking and thereby reducing anxiety. Psyching yourself up can have a positive effect and make examinations a nonanxiety-laden experience (Dickenson-Hazard, 1990). The following techniques are based on the principles of successful test taking as presented by Sides & Cailles (1989). Incorporation of these techniques can improve response and performance in examination situations.

Technique #1

Adopt an "I can" attitude. Believing you can succeed is the key to success. Self-belief inspires and gives you the power to achieve your goals. Without a success attitude, the road to your goal is much harder. We all stand an equal chance of success in this world. It is those who believe they can who achieve it. This "I can" attitude must permeate all your efforts in test taking, from studying to improving your skills, to actually writing the test.

Technique #2

Take control. By identifying your goal, deciding how to accomplish it and developing a plan for achieving it, you take control. Do not leave your success to chance; control it through action and attitude.

Technique #3

Think positively. Examinations are generally based on a standard that is the same for all individuals. Everyone can potentially pass. Performance is influenced not only by knowledge and skill but by attitude as well. Those individuals who regard an exam as an opportunity or challenge will be more successful.

Technique #4

Project a positive self-fulfilling prophecy. While preparing for an examination, project thoughts of the positive outcomes you will experience when you succeed. Self-talk is self-fulfilling. Expect success, not failure, for yourself.

Technique #5

Feel good about yourself. Without feeling a sense of positive self-worth, passing an examination is difficult. Recognize your professional contributions and give yourself credit for your accomplishments. Think "I will pass," not "I suppose I can."

Technique #6

Know yourself. Focus exam preparation and test taking on your strengths. Try to alter your weaknesses instead of becoming hung up on them. If you tend to overanalyze, study and read test questions at face value. If you are a speed demon when taking a test, slow down and read more carefully.

Technique #7

Failure is a possibility. We all have failed at something at some point in our lives. Rather than dwelling on the failure, making excuses and believing you will fail again, recognize your mistakes and remedy them. Failure is a time to begin again; use it as a motivator to do better. It is not the end of the world unless you allow it to be. It is best to deal with the failure and move on, otherwise it interferes with your success.

Technique #8

Persevere, persevere, persevere! Endurance must underlie all your efforts. Call forth those reserve energies when you have had all you think you can take. Rely upon yourself and your support systems to help you maintain a sense of direction and keep your goal in the forefront.

Technique #9

Motivation is muscle. Most individuals are motivated by fear or desire. The fear in an exam situation may be one of failure, the unknown or discovery of imperfection. Put your fear into perspective; realize you are not the only one with fear and that all have an equal opportunity for success. Develop strategies to reduce fear and use fear to your advantage by improving the imperfections. Desire is a powerful motivator, and you should keep the rewards of your desire foremost in your mind. Whatever motivates you, use it to make you successful. Reward yourself during your exam preparation and once the exam has been completed. You alone hold the key to success; use what you have wisely.

◘ SUMMARY

This chapter has provided concepts, strategies and techniques for improving study and test-taking skills. Your first task in improvement is to know yourself: how you study and how you take a test. You should use your strengths and remedy the weaknesses. Next you need to develop your thinking skills. Work on techniques to improve memory and reasoning. Now you need to organize your study and concentrate on using your strengths and these new and improved skills to be successful. Create a study space, develop a plan of action, then implement that plan during your periods of peak concentration. Before taking the exam, be sure you understand the components of a test question, can identify key words and phrases and have practiced. Apply the test-taking rules during the exam process. Finally, believe in yourself, your knowledge, and your talent. Believing you can accomplish your goal facilitates the fact that you will.

◘ BIBLIOGRAPHY

American Board of Pediatrics. (1989). *Developing questions and critiques.* Unpublished material.

Burke, M. M., & Walsh, M. B. (1992). *Gerontologic nursing.* St. Louis: Mosby Year Book.

Burkle, C. A., & Marshak, D. (1989). *Study program: Level 1*. Reston, VA: National Association of Secondary School Principals.

Conaway, D. C., Miller, M. D., & West, G. R. (1988). *Geriatrics*. St. Louis: Mosby Year Book.

Dickenson-Hazard, N. (1989). Making the grade as a test taker. *Pediatric Nursing, 15,* 302–304.

Dickenson-Hazard, N. (1989). Anatomy of a test question. *Pediatric Nursing, 15,* 395–399.

Dickenson-Hazard, N. (1990). The psychology of successful test taking. *Pediatric Nursing, 16,* 66–67.

Dickenson-Hazard, N. (1990). Study smart. *Pediatric Nursing, 16,* 314–316.

Dickenson-Hazard, N. (1990). Study effectiveness: Are you 10 a.m. or p.m. scholar? *Pediatric Nursing, 16,* 419–420.

Dickenson-Hazard, N. (1990). Develop your thinking skills for improved test taking. *Pediatric Nursing, 16,* 480–481.

Divine, J. H., & Kylen, D. W. (1979). *How to beat test anxiety*. New York: Barrons Educational Series, Inc.

Millman, J., & Pauk, W. (1969). *How to take tests*. New York: McGraw-Hill Book Co.

Millonig, V. L. (Ed.). (1994). *The adult nurse practitioner certification review guide* (rev. ed). Potomac, MD: Health Leadership Associates.

Nugent, P. M., & Vitale, B. A. (1997). *Test success: Test-taking techniques for beginning nursing students*. Philadelphia, PA: F. A. Davis Co.

Olney, C. W. (1989). *Where there's a will, there's an A*. New Jersey: Chesterbrook Educational Publishers.

Sides, M., & Cailles, N. B. (1989). *Nurse's guide to successful test taking*. Philadelphia, PA: J. B. Lippincott Co.

Sides, M., & Korchek, N. (1998). *Nurse's guide to successful test taking: Learning strategies for nurses* (3rd ed.). Philadelphia, PA: Lippincott-Raven.

Sides, M., & Korchek, N. (1994). *Nurse's guide to successful test taking* (2nd ed.). Philadelphia, PA: J. B. Lippincott.

Spielberger, C. D., & Vagg, P. R. (1995). *Test anxiety: Theory, assessment, and treatment*. Washington, DC: Taylor and Francis.

2

General Health Assessment and Health Promotion

Beth M. Kelsey

◘ HEALTH HISTORY

- Purpose and correlation to physical examination
  1. Begins the client–clinician relationship
  2. Identifies the client's main concerns
  3. Provides information for risk assessment and health promotion
  4. Provides focus for physical examination and diagnostic/screening tests
  5. Provides information about cultural variations in health beliefs and practices

- Components of the health history
  1. Reason for visit/chief complaint—brief statement in client's own words of reason for seeking health care
  2. Presenting problem/illness—chronological account of problem(s) for which client is seeking care
     a. Description of principle symptoms should include
        OLDCARTS mnemonic:
        (1) *O*nset
        (2) *L*ocation
        (3) *D*uration
        (4) *C*haracteristics
        (5) *A*ggravating/Associated factors
        (6) *R*elieving factors
        (7) *T*emporal factors
        (8) *S*everity
     b. Include pertinent negatives in symptom descriptions
     c. Describe impact of illness/problem on client's usual lifestyle
     d. Summarize current health status and health promotion/disease prevention needs if client has no presenting problem
  3. Past health history
     a. General state of health as client perceives it
     b. Childhood illnesses
     c. Major adult illnesses
     e. Psychiatric illnesses
     f. Accidents/injuries
     g. Surgeries/other hospitalizations
     h. Blood transfusions—dates and number of units
  4. Current health status
     a. Current medications—prescription, over-the-counter, herbal
     b. Allergies—name of allergen, type of reaction
     c. Tobacco, alcohol, illicit drugs—type, amount, frequency
     d. Nutrition—24-hour diet recall, recent weight changes, eating disorders, special diet
     e. Screening tests—dates and results
     f. Immunizations—dates
     g. Sleep patterns
     h. Exercise/leisure activities
     i. Environmental hazards
     j. Use of safety measures—safety belts, smoke detectors
     k. Disabilities—functional assessment if indicated

5. Family health history—provide information about possible genetic, familial and environmental associations with client's health
   a. Age and health or age and cause of death of immediate family members—parents, siblings, children, spouse/significant other
   b. Specific conditions to ask about include—heart disease, hypertension, stroke, diabetes, cancer, epilepsy, kidney disease, thyroid disease, asthma, arthritis, blood diseases, tuberculosis, alcoholism, allergies, congenital anomalies, mental illness
   c. Indicate if client is adopted and/or does not know family health history
6. Psychosocial/cultural health history
   a. Living situation
   b. Support system
   c. Stressors (including violence)
   d. Typical day
   e. Religious beliefs
   f. Outlook on present and future
   g. Special issues to address with adolescent clients include (*HEADSS*) *H*ome, *E*ducation, *A*ctivities, *D*rugs, *S*ex, *S*uicide
   h. Cultural assessment considerations
      (1) Cultural/ethnic identification—place of birth, length of time in country
      (2) Communication—language spoken, use of nonverbal communication, use of silence
      (3) Space—degree of comfort with distance between self and other, degree of comfort with touching by another
      (4) Social organization—family structure and roles, influence of religion
      (5) Time—past, present or future oriented, view of time—clock-oriented or social-oriented
      (6) Environmental control—internal or external locus of control, belief in supernatural forces
7. Obstetric history—may include in separate section, past health history or review of systems—includes all pregnancies regardless of outcome
   a. Gravidity—total number of pregnancies including a current pregnancy
   b. Parity—total number of pregnancies reaching 20 weeks or greater gestation
      (1) Include term, preterm, and stillbirth deliveries
      (2) Include length of each pregnancy, type of delivery, weight and sex of infant, length of labor, complications during prenatal, intrapartum, or postpartum periods, infant complications, cause of stillbirth if known
   c. Abortions—spontaneous and induced
   d. GTPAL—*G*ravida, *T*erm, *P*reterm, *A*bortion, *L*iving children is a commonly used method of obstetric history notation
   e. Any infertility evaluation and treatment
8. Menstrual history—may include in separate section or in review of systems
   a. Age at menarche, regularity, frequency, duration, and amount of bleeding
   b. Date of last normal menstrual period
   c. Use of pads, tampons, douching
   d. Abnormal uterine bleeding
   e. Premenstrual symptoms
   f. Dysmenorrhea
   g. Perimenopausal symptoms
   h. Age at menopause, use of hormone therapy, postmenopausal bleeding
9. Sexual history/contraceptive use—may include in separate section, under current health status, or in review of systems
   a. Age at first sexual intercourse—consensual/nonconsensual
   b. History of sexual abuse or sexual assault
   c. Sexual orientation
   d. Current sexual relationship(s)
      (1) Frequency of sexual intercourse
      (2) Satisfaction or concerns with sexual relationship(s)
      (3) Dyspareunia, orgasmic or libido problems
   e. Sexually transmitted disease (STD)/human immunodeficiency virus (HIV) risk assessment
      (1) Total number of sexual partners and number in past 3 months
      (2) Types of sexual contact—vaginal, oral, and/or anal
      (3) Use of condoms or other barrier methods
      (4) Previous history of sexually transmitted infections
      (5) Use of injection drugs or sex with partner who has used injection drugs
      (6) Sex while drunk, stoned, or high
      (7) Previous testing for HIV
   f. Current and future desire for pregnancy
   g. Contraceptive use
      (1) Establish if pregnancy is not a concern—hysterectomy, not sexually active, only sexually active with females, menopausal
      (2) Current method, length of time used, satisfaction, problems or concerns
      (3) Previous methods used, when, length of time used, satisfaction, problems or concerns, reason for discontinuation

10. Review of systems—used to assess common symptoms for each major body system to avoid missing any potential or existing problems—special focus for women's reproductive health includes:
    a. Endocrine—menses, breasts, pregnancy, thyroid, menopause
    b. Genitourinary
       (1) In utero exposure to diethylstilbestrol (DES) if born before 1971
       (2) Uterine or ovarian problems
       (3) History or symptoms of STD or pelvic infection
       (4) History or symptoms of vaginal infections
       (5) History of abnormal Pap tests—date, abnormality, treatment
       (6) History or symptoms of urinary tract infection
       (7) Symptoms of urinary incontinence
11. Concluding question—is there anything else I need to know about your health in order to provide you with the best health care?

- Risk factor identification
  1. Consider prevalence (existing level of disease) and incidence (rate of new disease) in general population and in your client population
  2. Determine risks specific to client related to the following:
     a. Gender
     b. Age
     c. Ethnic or racial background
     d. Family history
     e. Environmental exposures
     f. Lifestyle
     g. Geographic area
     h. Inadequate preventive health care

- Problem-oriented medical record—organized sequence of recording information using SOAP format
  1. SOAP format
     a. S—subjective information obtained during history
     b. O—objective information obtained through physical examination and laboratory/diagnostic test results
     c. A—assessment of objective and subjective data to determine a diagnosis with rationale or a prioritized differential diagnosis
     d. P—plan to include diagnostic tests, therapeutic treatment regimen, client education, referrals and date for reevaluation
  2. Problem list—list each identified existing or potential problem and indicate both onset and a resolution date
  3. Progress notes—use SOAP format for information documented at follow-up visits

PHYSICAL EXAMINATION (GENERAL SCREENING EXAMINATION)

- Purpose and correlation to health history
  1. Begins laying on of hands—diagnostic and therapeutic
  2. Findings may indicate need for further health history information
  3. Takes into account normal physical variations of different age and racial/ethnic groups

- Techniques of examination
  1. Inspection—observation using sight and smell
     a. Takes place throughout the history and physical examination
     b. Includes general survey and body-system–specific observations
  2. Auscultation—use of hearing usually with stethoscope to listen to sounds produced by the body
     a. Diaphragm best for high-pitched sounds, e.g., S_1, S_2 heart sounds
     b. Bell best for low-pitched sounds, e.g., large blood vessels
  3. Percussion—use of light, brisk tapping on body surfaces to produce vibrations in relation to density of underlying tissue and/or to elicit tenderness
     a. Provides information about size, shape, location and density of underlying organs or tissue
     b. Percussion sounds are distinguished by intensity (soft–loud), pitch (high–low), and quality
     c. Tympany—loud, high-pitched, drum-like sound, e.g., gastric bubble, gas-filled bowel
     d. Hyperresonance—very loud, low-pitched, boom-like sound, e.g., lungs with emphysema
     e. Resonance—loud, low-pitched, hollow sound, e.g., healthy lungs
     f. Dull—soft-to-moderate, moderate-pitched, thud-like sound, e.g., liver, heart
     g. Flat—soft, high-pitched sound, very dull, e.g., muscle, bone
  4. Palpation—use of hands and fingers to gather information about body tissues and organs through touch
     a. Finger pads, palmar surface of fingers, ulnar surface of fingers/hands, and dorsal surface of hands are used
     b. Light palpation—about 1 cm in depth, used to identify muscular resistance, areas of tenderness and large masses or areas of distention

c. Deep palpation—about 4 cm in depth, used to delineate organs and to identify less obvious masses

- Screening examination
  1. General appearance—posture, dress, grooming, personal hygiene, body or breath odors, facial expression
  2. Anthropometric measurements
     a. Height and weight
     b. Body mass index (BMI) provides measurement of total body fat; weight (kg)/height (m²); tables available to calculate BMI based on the individual's height and weight
        (1) Underweight—BMI less than 18.5
        (2) Normal weight—BMI 18.5 to 24.9
        (3) Overweight—BMI 25 to 29.9
        (4) Obesity—BMI 30 to 39.9
        (5) Extreme obesity—BMI 40 or greater
     c. Waist circumference
        (1) Provides measurement of abdominal fat as an independent prediction of risk for type 2 diabetes, dyslipidemia, hypertension, and cardiovascular disease in individuals with BMI between 25 and 39.9 (overweight and obesity)
        (2) Has little added value in disease risk prediction in individuals with BMI 40 or greater (extreme obesity)
        (3) Measure with horizontal mark at uppermost lateral border of right iliac crest and cross with vertical mark at midaxillary line; place tape measure at the cross and measure in horizontal plane around abdomen while standing
        (4) In adult female increased relative risk is indicated at greater than 35 in (88 cm)
  3. Skin, hair and nails
     a. Skin—color, texture, temperature, turgor, moisture, lesions
     b. Hair—color, distribution, quantity, texture
     c. Nails—color, shape, thickness
     d. Skin lesion characteristics—size, shape, color, texture, elevation, exudate, location, and distribution
        (1) Primary lesions—occur as an initial, spontaneous reaction to an internal or external stimulus (macule, papule, pustule, vesicle, wheal)
        (2) Secondary lesions—result from later evolution or trauma to a primary lesion (ulcer, fissure, crust, scar)
     e. ABCDEs of malignant melanoma—*A*symmetry, *B*orders irregular, *C*olor blue/black or variegated, *D*iameter greater than 6 mm, *E*levation

  4. Head, eyes, ears, nose and throat
     a. Head and neck
        (1) Skull and scalp—no masses or tenderness
        (2) Facial features—symmetrical and in proportion
        (3) Trachea—midline
        (4) Thyroid—palpable with no masses or tenderness, rises symmetrically with swallowing
        (5) Neck—full range of motion (ROM) without pain
        (6) Lymph nodes
           (a) Preauricular, postauricular, occipital, tonsillar, submandibular, submental, superficial cervical, posterior and deep cervical chains, supraclavicular
           (b) Normal findings—less than 1 cm in size, nontender, mobile, soft, and discrete
     b. Eyes
        (1) Visual acuity
           (a) Snellen chart for central vision; normal 20/20
           (b) Rosenbaum card or newspaper for near vision
           (c) Impaired near vision—presbyopia
           (d) Impaired far vision—myopia
        (2) Peripheral vision—estimated with visual fields by confrontation test
        (3) External eye structures—eyebrows equal; lids without lag or ptosis; lacrimal apparatus without exudate, swelling or excess tearing; conjunctiva clear with small blood vessels and no exudate; sclera white or buff colored
        (4) Eyeball structures
           (a) Cornea and lenses—no opacities or lesions
           (b) Pupils—*P*upils *E*qual, *R*ound, *R*eact to *L*ight and *A*ccommodate (PERRLA)
        (5) Extraocular muscle (EOM) function—symmetrical movement through the six cardinal fields of gaze without lid lag or nystagmus
        (6) Ophthalmoscopic examination—red reflex present with no clouding or opacities; optic disc yellow to pink color with distinct margins; arterioles light red and two-thirds of the diameter of veins with bright light reflex; veins dark red and larger than arterioles with no light reflex; no venous tapering at the arteriole-venous crossings

c. Ears
   (1) Hearing evaluation
      (a) Whispered voice—able to hear softly whispered words in each ear at 1 to 2 feet
      (b) Weber test—tests for lateralization of sound through bone conduction; normally hear sound equally in both ears
      (c) Rinne test—compares bone and air conduction of sound; normally air conducted (AC) sound is heard for twice as long as bone conducted (BC) sound (AC:BC = 2:1)
      (d) Weber and Rinne tests help in differentiating conductive and sensorineural hearing loss
   (2) External ears—symmetrical, no inflammation, lesions, nodules, or drainage
   (3) Tragus tenderness may indicate otitis externa; mastoid process tenderness may indicate otitis media
   (4) Otoscopic examination
      (a) External canal—no discharge, inflammation, lesions or foreign bodies; varied amount, color, and consistency of cerumen
      (b) Tympanic membrane—intact, pearly gray, translucent, with cone of light at 5:00 to 7:00; umbo and handle of malleus visible; no bulging or retraction
d. Nose and sinuses
   (1) Nasal mucosa pinkish red; septum midline
   (2) Frontal and maxillary sinuses nontender
e. Mouth and oropharynx
   (1) Mouth—lips, gums, tongue, mucous membranes all pink, moist, without lesions or inflammation; teeth—none missing, free from caries or breakage
   (2) Oropharynx—tonsils; posterior wall of pharynx without lesions or inflammation

5. Respiratory system
  a. Chest symmetrical, anterior/posterior diameter less than transverse diameter; respiratory rate 16 to 20 breaths per minute; rhythm regular; no rib retraction or use of accessory muscles; no cyanosis or clubbing of fingers
  b. Anterior and posterior respiratory expansion—symmetrical movement when client inhales deeply

  c. Tactile fremitus—decreased with emphysema, asthma, pleural effusion; increased with lobar pneumonia, pulmonary edema
  d. Percussion—resonant throughout lung fields
  e. Auscultation—vesicular over most of lung fields; bronchovesicular near main bronchus and bronchial over trachea
   (1) Adventitious sounds—crackles (intermittent, nonmusical, brief sound); rhonchi (low-pitched, snoring quality); wheezes (high-pitched, shrill quality); pleural friction rub (grating or creaking sound)
   (2) Transmitted voice sounds/vocal resonance—normally voice sounds are muffled or indistinct; bronchophony, egophony, whispered pectoriloquy indicate fluid or a solid mass in lungs

6. Cardiovascular system
  a. Blood pressure—less than 120/80 mm Hg and pulse 60 to 90 beats per minute (bpm), regular, not bounding or thready
  b. Heart
   (1) Apical impulse—4th to 5th left intercostal space (ICS) medial to the midclavicular (MCL) line, no lifts or thrills
   (2) Auscultation at 2nd right ICS, 2nd, 3rd, 4th, 5th left ICS at the sternal border and 5th left ICS at the MCL
      (a) Assess rate and rhythm
      (b) Identify S_1 and S_2 at each site—S_1 heard best at apex, S_2 heard best at base
      (c) Identify extra heart sounds at each site
         i. Physiologic split S_2—may normally be heard during inspiration
         ii. Fixed split S_2—heard in inspiration and expiration; may be heard with atrial septal defect or right ventricular failure
         iii. Increased S_3—early diastole, low-pitched; may be normal in children, young adults, and in late pregnancy; not normal in older adults
         iv. Increased S_4—late diastole, low-pitched, may be normal in well trained athletes and older adults; heard with aortic stenosis and hypertensive heart disease
         v. Murmurs—systolic murmur may be physiologic (pregnancy) or pathologic

(diseased valves); diastolic murmur usually indicates valvular disease

   a) Note timing, duration, pitch, intensity, pattern, quality, location, radiation, respiratory phase variations
   b) Murmur of mitral stenosis—early/late diastole, low-pitched, grade I to IV; heard loudest at apex without radiation; no respiratory phase variation
   vi. Clicks and snaps—heard with heart valve abnormalities
   vii. Pericardial friction rub—grating sound heard throughout cardiac cycle; heard with pericarditis

c. Neck vessels
   (1) No jugular venous distention
   (2) Carotid arteries—strong, symmetrical, no bruits

d. Extremities (peripheral arteries)
   (1) No erythema, pallor or cyanosis, no edema or varicosities; skin warm; capillary refill time less than 2 seconds; normal hair distribution; no muscle atrophy
   (2) Pulses strong and symmetrical—brachial, radial, femoral, dorsalis pedis, posterior tibial
   (3) Lymph nodes less than 1 cm, non-tender, mobile, soft and discrete—axillary, epitrochlear, inguinal

7. Abdomen
   a. Symmetrical, no lesions or masses; no visible pulsations or peristalsis
   b. Active bowel sounds; no vascular bruits or friction rubs
   c. No guarding, tenderness or masses on palpation
   d. Liver border—edge smooth, sharp, non-tender; no more than 2 cm below right costal margin
   e. Spleen and kidneys—usually not palpable
   f. Aorta—slightly left of midline in upper abdomen; less than 3 cm width
   g. Percussion—tympany is predominant tone; dullness over organs or any masses
   h. Liver span—normally 6 to 12 cm at the right MCL
   i. Splenic dullness—6th to 10th ICS just posterior to midaxillary line on left side
   j. No tenderness on fist percussion over the costovertebral angle; costovertebral angle

tenderness (CVAT) may indicate kidney problem

8. Musculoskeletal system
   a. No gross deformities; body aligned; extremities symmetrical; normal spinal curvature; no involuntary movements
   b. Muscle mass and strength equal bilaterally; full range of motion without pain
   c. No inflammation, nodules, swelling, crepitus, or tenderness of joints

9. Neurologic system
   a. Cranial nerves (CN)—CN II through XII routinely tested, CN I tested if abnormality is suspected
      (1) CN I (olfactory)—test ability to identify familiar odors
      (2) CN II (optic)—test visual acuity, peripheral vision, and inspect optic discs
      (3) CN III, IV, VI (oculomotor, trochlear, abducens)—observe for PERRLA, EOM function, and ptosis
      (4) CN V (trigeminal)—palpate strength of temporal and masseter muscles, test for sharp/dull and light touch sensation on forehead, cheeks, and chin
      (5) CN VII (facial)—observe for any weakness, asymmetry, or abnormal movements of face
      (6) CN VIII (acoustic)—assess auditory acuity; perform Weber and Rinne tests
      (7) CN IX (glossopharyngeal) and CN X (vagus)—observe ability to swallow; symmetry of movement of soft palate and uvula when client says "ah"; gag reflex; any abnormal voice quality
      (8) CN XI (spinal accessory)—observe and palpate strength and symmetry of trapezius and sternocleidomastoid muscles
      (9) CN XII (hypoglossal)—observe tongue for any deviation, asymmetry, or abnormal movement
   b. Cerebellar function—smooth coordinated gait, able to walk heel to toe, balance maintained with eyes closed (Romberg test); rapid rhythmic alternating movements smooth and coordinated
   c. Sensory function—able to identify superficial pain and touch; able to identify vibration on bony prominences and passive position change of fingers and toes; normal response to discriminatory sensation tests; all findings symmetrical
   d. Deep tendon reflexes—brisk and symmetrical (biceps, brachioradialis, triceps, patellar, Achilles)

10. Mental status
    a. Physical appearance and behavior—well groomed, emotional status appropriate to situation; makes eye contact; posture erect
    b. Cognitive abilities—alert and oriented, able to reason; recent and remote memory intact; able to follow directions
    c. Emotional stability—no signs of depression or anxiety; logical thought processes, no perceptual disturbances
    d. Speech and language skills—normal voice quality and articulation, coherent, able to follow simple instructions
    e. Mini Mental Status Examination (MMSE)—standardized screening tool used for mental status assessment
    f. Depression screening tools—Beck Depression Inventory, Zung Self-Rating Depression Scale, Geriatric Depression Scale

- Detailed reproductive examination
  1. Breasts
     a. The female breast extends from the second to the sixth ribs and from the sternal border to the midaxillary line
     b. Inspect breasts with client in sitting position and hands pushing against hips; view breasts from all sides to assess for symmetry and skin changes
        (1) Tanner sexual maturity rating in adolescent
        (2) Skin—smooth, color uniform, no erythema, masses, retraction, dimpling or thickening
        (3) Symmetry—breast shape or contour is symmetrical; some difference in size of breasts and areola is common and usually normal
        (4) Nipples—pointing in same direction; no retraction or discharge, no scaling; long-standing nipple inversion is usually normal variation
     c. Palpate axillary, supraclavicular, infraclavicular lymph nodes with patient in sitting position and arms relaxed at sides
     d. Palpate breasts with client lying down, arm above head, small pillow under shoulder/lower back on side being examined if needed to provide even breast tissue distribution
        (1) Include entire area from midaxillary line, across inframammary ridge and fifth/sixth rib, up lateral edge of sternum, across clavicle, back to midaxillary line
        (2) Palpate using finger pads of middle three fingers with overlapping dime

shaped circular motions in a vertical strip pattern over entire area including nipples; do not squeeze nipples unless client indicates they have spontaneous nipple discharge
        (3) Palpate each area of breast tissue using three levels of pressure—light, medium, and deep
        (4) Follow same procedures for client with implants as correctly placed implants are located behind breast tissue
        (5) Include palpation of chest wall, skin, and incision area in client with mastectomy
        (6) Breast tissue—consistency varies from soft fat to firmer glandular tissue, physiologic nodularity may be present, there may be a firm ridge of compressed tissue under lower edge of breasts
        (7) Describe any palpable mass or lymph nodes in terms of location according to clock face as examiner faces client—size, shape, mobility, consistency, delimitation, and tenderness
        (8) Describe any nipple discharge in terms of whether spontaneous/not spontaneous, bilateral/unilateral, single or multiple ducts, color, and consistency
  2. Pelvic examination
     a. Positioning—client lying supine with head and shoulders elevated, lithotomy position, buttocks extending slightly beyond edge of table, draped from midabdomen to knees, drape depressed between knees to allow eye contact
     b. Inspection and palpation of external structures—mons pubis, labia majora and minora, clitoris, urethral meatus, vaginal introitus, paraurethral (Skene) glands, Bartholin glands, perineum
        (1) Tanner sexual maturity rating in adolescent
        (2) Mons pubis—pubic hair inverted triangular pattern, skin smooth with uniform color
        (3) Labia majora—may be gaping or closed and dry or moist, tissue soft and homogenous, covered with hair in postpubertal female
        (4) Labia minora—moist and dark pink, tissue soft and homogenous
        (5) Clitoris—approximately 2 cm or less in length and 0.5 cm in diameter
        (6) Urethral meatus—irregular opening or slit

(7) Vaginal introitus—thin vertical slit or large orifice, irregular edges from hymenal remnants, moist

(8) Skene and Bartholin glands—opening of Skene glands just posterior to and below urethral meatus, opening of Bartholin glands located posteriorly on each side of vaginal orifice and not usually visible

(9) Perineum—consists of tissue between introitus and anus, smooth, may have episiotomy scar

(10) Note presence of any abnormal hair distribution, discoloration, erythema, swelling, atrophy, lesions, masses, discharge, malodor, fistulas, tenderness

c. Pelvic floor muscles—form supportive sling for pelvic contents and functional sphincters for vagina, urethra, and rectum, able to constrict introitus around examining finger, no anterior or posterior bulging of vaginal walls, incontinence, or protrusion of cervix or uterus when client bears down

d. Inspection of internal structures

(1) Vaginal walls—pink, rugated, homogenous, may have thin, clear/cloudy, odorless discharge

(2) Cervix—midline, smooth, round, pink, about 2.5 cm diameter, protrudes 1–3 cm into vagina; points posteriorly with anteverted uterus, anteriorly with retroverted uterus, horizontally with midposition uterus; nabothian cysts may be present; os small and round (nulliparous), may be oval, slit-like, or stellate if parous; may have area of darker red epithelial tissue around os if squamocolumnar junction is on ectocervix

(3) Note presence of discoloration, erythema, swelling, atrophy, friable tissue, lesions, masses, discharge that is profuse, malodorous, thick, curdy or frothy, gray, green or yellow, adherent to vaginal walls

e. Palpation of internal structures

(1) Vaginal walls—smooth, nontender

(2) Cervix—smooth, firm, mobile, nontender, about 2.5 cm diameter, protrudes 1–3 cm into vagina

(3) Uterus—smooth, rounded contour, firm, mobile, nontender; 5.5 to 8 cm long and pear shaped in nulliparous female, may be 2 to 3 cm larger in parous female; position anteverted, anteflexed, midplane, retroverted, or retroflexed

(4) Adnexa—fallopian tubes nonpalpable; ovaries ovoid, smooth, firm, mobile, slightly tender; size during reproductive years 3 cm × 2 cm × 1 cm

(5) Note presence of enlargements, masses, irregular surfaces, consistency other than firm, deviation of positions, immobility, tenderness

f. Rectovaginal examination

(1) Purpose—palpate retroverted uterus; screen for colorectal cancer in females 50 years of age and older; assess pelvic pathology

(2) Repeat the maneuvers of the bimanual examination with index finger in vagina and middle finger in rectum

(3) Rectum—smooth, nontender without masses; firm anal sphincter tone

(4) Rectovaginal septum—smooth, intact, nontender, without masses

• Infection control

1. Prevention of contamination

a. Clean work surface for each client

b. Prepare equipment/supplies prior to examination

c. Conduct pelvic examination with attention to preventing contamination of equipment such as examination lights and lubricant containers

2. Standard precautions

a. Foundation for preventing infection transmission during patient care

b. Transmission of infectious agents requires three elements—source or reservoir for infectious agent; susceptible host with portal of entry receptive to the agent; mode of transmission from source of infectious agent to susceptible host

c. Use applies to blood, all body fluids, secretions and excretions (except sweat), nonintact skin, and mucous membranes

d. Wash hands immediately after gloves are removed, between patient contacts, and when otherwise indicated

e. Wear gloves when probability may exist of contact with blood, body fluids, secretions, excretions, mucous membranes, nonintact skin, and contaminated materials

f. Use mask, eye protection, face shield, gown as needed to protect skin and mucous membranes during procedures likely to generate splashes or sprays of blood, body fluids, secretions, or excretions

g. Routinely clean and disinfect environmental surfaces including frequently touched surfaces in patient care areas

h. Adequately clean, disinfect, or sterilize reusable equipment

i. Use proper disposal for contaminated single-use items

j. Dispose of needles and other sharp items in proper puncture resistant containers; do not recap, bend or break used needles; if recapping required use one-handed scoop technique

k. Use mouthpiece, resuscitation bag, other ventilation devices for patient resuscitation

◘ NONGYNECOLOGICAL DIAGNOSTIC STUDIES/LABORATORY TESTS

- Complete blood count (CBC) with differential
  1. RBC count—measurement of red blood cells per cubic millimeter of blood
     a. Normal findings (adult female)—4.2 to 5.4 million/mm^3
     b. Low values—hemorrhage, hemolysis, dietary deficiencies, hemoglobinopathies, bone marrow failure, chronic illness, medications
     c. High values—dehydration, diseases causing chronic hypoxia such as congenital heart disease, polycythemia vera, medications
  2. Hematocrit (Hct)/Hemoglobin (Hgb)—rapid indirect measurement of RBC count
     a. Hct—percentage of total blood volume that is made up of RBCs
        (1) Normal findings (nonpregnant adult female)—37 to 47%
        (2) Normal findings (pregnant adult female)—33% or greater in first and third trimesters, 32% or greater in second trimester
     b. Hgb—measurement of total hemoglobin (which carries oxygen) in the blood
        (1) Normal findings (nonpregnant adult female)—12 to 16 g/dL
        (2) Normal findings (pregnant adult female)—11 g/dL or greater in first and third trimesters, 10.5 g/dL or greater in second trimester
     c. Low values—anemia, hemoglobinopathies, cirrhosis, hemorrhage, dietary deficiency, bone marrow failure, renal disease, chronic illness, some cancers
     d. High values—erythrocytosis, polycythemia vera, severe dehydration, severe chronic obstructive pulmonary disease

  e. Heavy smokers and individuals living at higher elevations may also have higher Hgb levels
  3. Red blood cell indices—provides information about size, weight, and Hgb concentration of RBCs; useful in classifying anemias
     a. Mean corpuscular volume (MCV)—average volume or size of a single RBC
        (1) Normal finding—80 to 95 mm^3, normocytic
        (2) Microcytic/abnormally small—seen with iron deficiency anemia and thalassemia
        (3) Macrocytic/abnormally large—seen with megaloblastic anemias such as vitamin B$_{12}$ deficiency and folic acid deficiency
     b. Mean corpuscular hemoglobin (MCH)—average amount or weight of Hgb within an RBC
        (1) Normal finding—27 to 31 pg/cell
        (2) Causes for abnormalities same as with MCV
     c. Mean corpuscular hemoglobin concentration (MCHC)—average concentration or percentage of Hgb within a single RBC
        (1) Normal finding—32 to 36 g/dL, normochromic
        (2) Decreased concentration or hypochromic—seen with iron deficiency anemia and thalassemia
  4. White blood cell (WBC) count with differential—provides information useful in evaluating individual with infection, neoplasm, allergy, or immunosuppression
     a. Normal finding for total WBC (adult)—5000 to 10,000/mm^3
     b. Increased WBC count—seen with infection, trauma, inflammation, some malignancies, dehydration
     c. Decreased WBC count—seen with some drug toxicities, bone marrow failure, overwhelming infections, immunosuppression
     d. May be elevated in late pregnancy and during labor
     e. Neutrophils—increased with acute bacterial infections and trauma; increased immature forms (band or stab cells) referred to as a "shift to left," seen with ongoing acute bacterial infection
     f. Basophils and eosinophils—increased with allergic reactions and parasitic infections; not increased with bacterial or viral infection
     g. Lymphocytes and monocytes—increased with chronic bacterial and acute viral infections

5. Peripheral blood smear—microscopic examination of smear of peripheral blood to examine RBCs, platelets, and leukocytes
6. Platelet count—used to evaluate abnormal bleeding or blood clotting
   a. Normal finding (adult)—150,000 to 400,000/mm^3
   b. Low count (thrombocytopenia)—hypersplenism, hemorrhage, leukemia, cancer chemotherapy, infection
   c. High count (thrombocytosis)—some malignant disorders, polycythemia vera, rheumatoid arthritis

- Urinalysis—dipstick and/or microscopic evaluation of urine
  1. Includes evaluation of appearance, color, odor, pH, protein, specific gravity, leukocyte esterase, nitrites, ketones, crystals, casts, glucose, WBCs, and RBCs
  2. Obtain midstream clean catch specimen so culture can be performed if urinalysis indicates infection
  3. Normal findings
     a. No nitrites, ketones, crystals, casts, or glucose
     b. Clear, amber yellow, aromatic
     c. pH 4.6 to 8.0
     d. Protein 0 to 8 mg/dL
     e. Specific gravity (adult)—1.005 to 1.030
     f. Leukocyte esterase negative
     g. WBCs 0 to 4 per high power field (HPF)
     h. RBCs at 2 or less

- Blood glucose—used for diagnosis and evaluation of diabetes mellitus
  1. Fasting glucose
     a. No caloric intake for at least 8 hours
     b. Normal finding (adult)—less than 100 mg/dL
     c. Impaired fasting glucose—100 to 125 mg/dL
     d. Diagnostic for diabetes—126 mg/dL or greater
  2. Two-hour postload glucose during oral glucose tolerance test (OGTT)
     a. Sample obtained 2 hours after a glucose load containing the equivalent of 75 g of glucose dissolved in water
     b. Normal finding—less than 140 mg/dL
     c. Impaired glucose tolerance—140 mg/dL to 199 mg/dL
     d. Diagnostic for diabetes—200 mg/dL or greater
  3. American Diabetes Association (ADA) criteria for the diagnosis of diabetes mellitus

     a. Symptoms of diabetes plus random non-fasting glucose concentration of 200 mg/dL or greater
     b. Fasting glucose of 126 mg/dL or greater
     c. 2-hour post glucose 200 mg/dL or greater
     d. Repeat testing on a subsequent day to confirm diagnosis
     e. ADA recommends using fasting glucose rather than OGTT for screening
  4. HbA$_{1c}$ or A$_{1c}$
     a. Not presently recommended for the diagnosis of diabetes
     b. Gold standard for measurement of long-term (previous 60–90 days) glycemic control in individuals with diabetes
     c. Reliable tool for evaluating need for drug therapy and monitoring effectiveness of therapy
     d. Good diabetic control—less than 7%

- Blood urea nitrogen (BUN) and creatinine—used in evaluation of renal function
  1. BUN—indirect measure of renal and liver function
     a. Normal finding (adult)—10 to 20 mg/dL
     b. Increased levels—hypovolemia, dehydration, reduced cardiac function, gastrointestinal bleeding, starvation, sepsis, renal disease
     c. Decreased levels—liver failure, malnutrition, nephrotic syndrome
  2. Serum creatinine—indirect measure of renal function
     a. Normal finding (adult female)—0.5 to 1.1 mg/dL
     b. Increased levels—renal disorders, dehydration
     c. Decreased levels—debilitation and decreased muscle mass

- Lipid profile—determines risk for coronary heart disease and evaluation of hyperlipoproteinemia
  1. Includes total cholesterol, triglycerides, high density lipoproteins (HDL), and low density lipoproteins (LDL)
  2. Fast for 12 to 14 hours prior to obtaining sample
  3. Total cholesterol normal level (adult)—less than 200 mg/dL; may be elevated in pregnancy
  4. Triglycerides normal finding (adult female)—35 to 135 mg/dL; may be elevated in pregnancy
  5. HDL—removes cholesterol from peripheral tissues and transports to liver for excretion
     a. Normal level (adult)— 40 mg/dL or greater
     b. Low levels associated with increased risk for heart and peripheral vascular disease

6. LDL—cholesterol carried by LDL can be deposited into peripheral tissues
   a. Normal finding (adult)—less than 130 mg/dL
   b. High levels associated with increased risk for heart and peripheral vascular disease

- Thyroid function studies
  1. Thyroid stimulating hormone (TSH)—used to diagnose hyperthyroidism, primary hypothyroidism, differentiate primary from secondary hypothyroidism, and to monitor thyroid replacement or suppression therapy
     a. Normal finding (adult)— 0.4 to 4.7 mU/mL
     b. Increased levels—seen with primary hypothyroidism and thyroiditis
     c. Decreased levels—seen with secondary hypothyroidism, hyperthyroidism; suppressive doses of thyroid medication
     d. Debate on lowering upper limit of normal to 3.0 mU/mL to detect mild thyroid disease
  2. Free thyroxine (FT_4)—used in diagnosis of thyroid disease
     a. Normal finding (adult female)—0.58 to 1.64 ng/dL
     b. Increased levels—hyperthyroidism and acute thyroiditis
     c. Decreased levels—hypothyroidism
  3. Total thyroxine (T_4)
     a. Normal finding (adult female)—4.5 to 12.0 µg/dL
     b. Measurement affected by increases in thyroxine-binding globulin (TBG)
     c. Causes for increased TBG include pregnancy, oral contraceptive use, and estrogen therapy

- Blood type and Rh factor—used to determine blood type prior to donating or receiving blood and to determine blood type in pregnant women
  1. Blood types are grouped according to presence or absence of antigens A, B, and Rh on RBCs
  2. Individual without a particular antigen may develop antibodies to that antigen if exposed through blood transfusion or fetal-maternal blood mixing
  3. Blood type O negative (universal donor because no antigens on RBCs), AB positive (universal recipient because no antibodies to react to transfused blood)

- Infectious disease screening
  1. Rubella (German measles)
     a. Hemagglutination inhibition (HAI) test—used to detect immunity to rubella and diagnose rubella infection
        (1) Titer of 1:10 or greater indicates immunity to rubella
        (2) High titers (1:64 or greater) may indicate current rubella infection
     b. Rubella IgM antibody titer—used if pregnant woman has a rash suspected to be from rubella; if titer is positive recent infection has occurred; IgM antibodies appear 1 to 2 days after onset of rash and disappear 5 to 6 weeks after infection
  2. HIV tests—used for diagnosis of human immunodeficiency virus infection
     a. Sensitive screening tests—enzyme immunoassay (EIA) or rapid test
     b. Reactive screening tests must be confirmed by supplemental test—Western blot or immunofluorescence assay (IFA)
     c. HIV antibody detectable in 95% of individuals within 6 months of infection
     d. Polymerase chain reaction (PCR)—used to confirm indeterminate Western blot results or negative results in persons with suspected HIV infection
     e. HIV plasma ribonucleic acid (RNA) testing may be used if suspect recent HIV infection before development of immune response; positive HIV RNA testing should be confirmed with subsequent antibody testing to document seroconversion
  3. Hepatitis B (HBV) tests
     a. Hepatitis B surface antigen (HBsAg)—rises before onset of clinical symptoms, peaks during first week of symptoms and returns to normal by time jaundice subsides
        (1) Indicates active HBV infection—individual is infectious
        (2) Individual is considered a carrier if HBsAg persists
     b. Hepatitis B surface antibody (HBsAb)—appears 4 weeks after disappearance of surface antigen
        (1) Indicates end of acute infectious phase and signifies immunity to subsequent infection
        (2) Also used to denote immunity after administration of hepatitis B vaccine
  4. Tuberculosis—purified protein derivative (PPD) test
     a. Usually positive within 6 weeks after infection
     b. Does not indicate whether infection is active or dormant
     c. Centers for Disease Control and Prevention (CDC) definition of positive PPD

(1) High risk population 5 mm induration or greater

(2) Moderate risk population 10 mm induration or greater

(3) General population 15 mm induration or greater

   d. Once positive reaction, usually persists for life

   e. False negatives may result from incorrect administration (must be intradermal) or immunosuppression

   f. False positive may result if individual had prior immunization with bacillus of Calmette and Guerin (BCG) vaccine

   g. PPD test is contraindicated if history of BCG vaccination or active TB since severe local reaction can occur

- Sickle cell screening (Sickle Cell Prep, Sickledex)—used to screen for sickle cell disease and trait
  1. Positive test—presence of Hgb S indicates sickle cell disease or trait
  2. Hgb electrophoresis is definitive test to be performed if screening test is positive; identifies Hgb type and quantity

- Liver function studies
  1. Bilirubin
     a. Normal findings (adult)—total bilirubin 0.3 to 1.0 mg/dL; direct (conjugated) bilirubin 0.1 to 0.3 mg/dL; indirect (unconjugated) bilirubin 0.2 to 0.8 mg/dL
     b. Elevated direct bilirubin level—occurs with gallstones and obstruction of extrahepatic duct
     c. Elevated indirect bilirubin level—seen with hepatocellular dysfunction (hepatitis, cirrhosis) and hemolytic anemias
  2. Albumin
     a. Normal finding (adult)—3.5 to 5.0 g/dL
     b. Increased levels—dehydration
     c. Decreased levels—seen with liver disease, malabsorption syndromes, nephropathies, severe burns, malnutrition, and inflammatory disease
  3. Liver enzymes
     a. Alkaline phosphatase (ALP)
        (1) Normal finding—30 to 120 U/L
        (2) Elevated levels—liver disease, bone disease, and myocardial infarction
     b. Aspartate aminotransferase (AST), alanine aminotransferase (ALT), lactic dehydrogenase (LDH), and 5′ nucleotidase
        (1) Normal findings—AST 0–35 U/L, ALT 4–36 U/L, LDH 100–190 U/L
        (2) Useful in differentiating cause for ALP elevation

   c. Gamma-glutamyl transpeptidase (GGT)
      (1) Normal finding—8–38 U/L
      (2) Elevated levels with liver disease, myocardial infarction, pancreatic disease, and heavy or chronic alcohol use

- Stool for occult blood
  1. Annual screen for individuals over 50 years of age and for evaluation of gastrointestinal conditions that may cause gastrointestinal (GI) bleeding
  2. Positive test—may indicate GI cancer or polyps; peptic ulcer disease; inflammatory or ischemic bowel disease; GI trauma; bleeding caused by medications
  3. Several interfering factors can cause false positives or negatives
     a. Red meat and some raw fruits/vegetables if consumed within 3 days prior or during the test period can result in false positive
     b. Large amounts of vitamin C consumed within 3 days prior to or during the test period can result in false negative
  4. Positive test requires further evaluation with sigmoidoscopy, colonoscopy, or barium enema

◘ HEALTH MAINTENANCE AND RISK FACTOR IDENTIFICATION

- Nutrition
  1. Evaluation of nutritional status
     a. Anthropometric measurements—height, weight, BMI, waist circumference
     b. General appearance—skin, hair, muscle mass
     c. Biochemical measurements—Hgb/Hct, lipid analysis, serum albumin, serum glucose, serum folate
     d. 24-hour diet recall or 3 to 4 day food diary
     e. Use of vitamin, mineral, and herbal supplements
  2. Dietary Guidelines for Americans (US Department of Health and Human Services [USDHHS], 2005)
     a. Eat a variety of nutrient-dense foods from the basic food groups
     b. Balance the food you eat with physical activity to maintain or improve weight
     c. Eat a good variety of two and one half cups of vegetables and two cups of fruit each day (reference 2000 calories intake)
     d. Eat six ounces of grains with at least one half whole grain products each day
     e. Eat three cups of fat-free or low-fat milk or equivalent milk products each day

f. Eat five and one half ounces of meat and beans choosing low fat lean meats, more fish, beans, peas, nuts and seeds

g. Choose a diet low in fat (20 to 35% of calories), saturated fats (< 10% of calories), trans fats as low as possible, and cholesterol (300 mg or less/day)

h. Choose and prepare foods and beverages with little added sugar

i. Choose a diet moderate in salt and sodium (< 2300 mg/day—approximately one teaspoon of salt)

j. Drink alcoholic beverages only in moderation (no more than one drink daily for women); one drink = 12 ounce of beer, 5 ounces of wine, 1.5 ounces of hard liquor

3. Calcium and vitamin D requirements for women

  a. National Institute of Health/National Institute of Arthritis and Musculoskeletal and Skin Diseases (NIAMS) (2009)

    (1) 14 to 18 years of age—1300 mg/day of calcium; same amount if pregnant or lactating

    (2) 19 to 50 years of age—1000 mg/day of calcium, same amount if pregnant or lactating

    (3) 51 years of age and older—1200 mg/day of calcium

    (4) Adults—400 to 600 IU/day of vitamin D

  b. National Osteoporosis Foundation (2008)

    (1) Adults under age 50—1000 mg/day of calcium; 400 to 800 IU/day of vitamin D

    (2) Adults age 50 and over—1200 mg/day of calcium; 800 to 1000 IU of vitamin D

  c. Sources of calcium—milk, yogurt, soybeans, tofu, canned sardines and salmon with edible bones, cheese, fortified cereals and orange juice, supplements

  d. Sources of vitamin D—fortified milk, egg yolks, saltwater fish, liver, supplements, regular exposure to direct sunlight without sunscreen

4. Folate requirements for women of childbearing age

  a. 0.4 mg folic acid/day

  b. Women of childbearing age who have had an infant with neural tube defect or who have seizure disorders or insulin dependent diabetes may benefit from a higher dose of 4 mg folic acid/day starting 1 month before trying to become pregnant

  c. Sources—dried beans, leafy green vegetables, citrus fruits and juices, fortified cereals; most multivitamins contain 0.4 mg folic acid

5. Iron requirements for nonpregnant women

  a. 14 to 18 years of age—15 mg/dL each day

  b. 19 to 50 years of age—18 mg/dL each day

  c. 51 years of age or older—8 mg/dL each day

  d. Sources—meat, fish, poultry, fortified cereals, dried fruits, dark green vegetables, supplements

6. Special concerns

  a. Eating disorders—see section on Lifestyle/Family Alterations in Nongynecological Disorders chapter

  b. Vegetarians—plan diet to avoid deficiencies in protein, calcium, iron, vitamin B_{12}, and vitamin D

  c. Older adults—consider effects of chronic illness, medications, isolation, decrease in ability to taste and smell, limited income

- Physical activity

1. There is strong evidence that regular physical activity lowers risk for heart disease, stroke, high blood pressure, adverse lipid profile, type 2 diabetes, metabolic syndrome, colon and breast cancers; prevents weight gain and promotes weight loss; improves cardiovascular and muscular fitness; reduces depression; improves cognitive function in older adults.

2. Sixty percent of Americans are not regularly physically active and 25% report no physical activity at all.

3. Physical Activity Guidelines for Americans (USDHHS, 2008)

  a. Engage in at least 150 minutes of moderate intensity or 75 minutes of vigorous intensity aerobic physical activity each week; performed for at least 10 minutes per episode; spread throughout the week

  b. Moderate intensity exercise achieves 50 to 69% of maximum heart rate—maximum average heart rate equals 220 minus age

  c. Examples of aerobic physical activity—brisk walking, running, bicycling, jumping rope, swimming

  d. Engage in muscle strengthening activities of moderate or high intensity involving all major muscle groups 2 or more days each week

  e. Examples of muscle strengthening activities—weight lifting, exercises with elastic bands or use of body weight (push-ups, tree climbing) for resistance

  f. Include bone strengthening activity in exercise regimen—running, brisk walking, weight training, tennis, dancing

- Routine screening recommendations

1. Breast self-examination (BSE)

a. American Cancer Society (ACS)—beginning in their 20s, inform of benefits and limitations of BSE and provide instruction for women who choose to do BSE; it is acceptable for women to choose not to do BSE or to do BSE irregularly

b. American College of Obstetricians and Gynecologists (ACOG)—adult women should perform BSE monthly

2. Clinical breast examination
   a. ACS—every 3 years from age 20 to 39 years
   b. American College of Obstetricians and Gynecologists (ACOG) periodic evaluation, yearly or as appropriate for women older than age 18 years
   c. ACS and ACOG—yearly clinical breast examination for women age 40 and older

3. Mammogram
   a. ACS—yearly beginning at age 40 years
   b. ACOG—every 1–2 years from age 40–49 years, then yearly

4. Magnetic Resonance Imaging (MRI)
   a. ACS and ACOG—not recommended for routine breast cancer screening in women with average risk (< 15% lifetime risk)
   b. ACS—combination of yearly mammogram and MRI for women at high risk (> 20% lifetime risk) starting at 30 years of age
   c. ACS—discuss risk and benefits of combined yearly mammogram and MRI for women at moderately increased risk (15 to 20%)
   d. ACOG—combination of yearly mammogram and MRI in women with BRCA gene mutation beginning at age 25 or younger based on earliest age of onset in family
   e. Risk assessment tools—BRCAPRO, Claus model, Tyrer-Cuzick model

5. Pap test
   a. ACS—begin approximately 3 years after woman begins having vaginal intercourse but not later than 21 years of age
   b. ACOG—begin at age 21 years
   c. ACS—perform yearly if using conventional pap smear or every 2 years if using liquid-based test
   d. ACOG—perform every 2 years for women between ages 21 years to 29 years
   e. ACS and ACOG—for women age 30 and older who have had 3 consecutive satisfactory normal Pap tests, screening may be done every 3 years unless history of in utero DES exposure, HIV infection or immunosuppression
   f. ACOG—for women age 30 and older with combination of negative Pap test and negative HPV test perform Pap tests no more than every 3 years

6. Chlamydia screening—CDC—yearly screening for all sexually active females 25 years of age or younger

7. Blood Pressure—National High Blood Pressure Education Program (NHBPEP) of the National Heart, Lung and Blood Institute (NHLBI)—at least every 2 years for adults

8. Cholesterol
   a. Third Report of the National Cholesterol Education Program (NCEP) Expert Panel on Detection, Evaluation, and Treatment of High Blood Cholesterol in Adults (Adult Treatment Panel III or ATP III)—Recommendations for Cholesterol Screening (2001)
      (1) Fasting lipid profile (total cholesterol, LDL, HDL, triglycerides) once every 5 years beginning at age 20 years
      (2) Total cholesterol
         (a) Desirable level—less than 200 mg/dL
         (b) Borderline high—200 to 239 mg/dL
         (c) High—240 mg/dL or greater
      (3) LDL
         (a) Optimal level—less than 100 mg/dL
         (b) Near optimal/above optimal—100 to 129 mg/dL
         (c) Borderline high—130 to 159 mg/dL
         (d) High—160 to 189 mg/dL
         (e) Very high—190 mg/dL or greater
      (4) HDL
         (a) Low—less than 40 mg/dL (considered a risk for CHD)
         (b) High—60 mg/dL or greater (protective against CHD)
      (5) Triglycerides
         (a) Normal—less than 150 mg/dL
         (b) Borderline high—150 to 199 mg/dL
         (c) High—200 mg/dL or greater
   b. CHD risk factors for women include being 55 years of age or older, family history of premature CHD (male relative < 55 years, female relative < 65), cigarette smoking, hypertension, HDL at less than 40 mg/dL, diabetes mellitus
   c. Desirable cholesterol is less than 200 mg/dL, HDL 60 mg/dL or greater, LDL at less than 130 mg/dL

9. Fecal occult blood test—ACS and ACOG yearly beginning at age 50

10. Sigmoidoscopy
    a. ACS and ACOG—every 5 years beginning at age 50 (or colonoscopy every 10 years or double contrast barium enema every 5 years)
    b. More frequent testing and starting at younger age for those with risk factors including inflammatory bowel disease and personal or family history of colonic polyps or colon cancer
11. Plasma glucose—American Diabetic Association recommendations
    a. Fasting plasma glucose every 3 years starting at age 45
    b. More frequent testing and starting at younger age for those with risk factors including blood pressure higher than 140/90 mm Hg; diabetes in first-degree relative; African American, Asian, Hispanic, Native American; obesity at 120% or greater of desirable weight or BMI at 27 or higher; history of gestational diabetes or baby weighing more than 9 pounds at birth; HDL at less than 40 mg/dL or triglyceride level at 250 mg/dL or greater
12. Thyroid function
    a. United States Prevention Task Force (USPTF)—routine screening for thyroid function is not warranted in asymptomatic individuals
    b. ACOG—TSH periodically for women with an autoimmune condition or strong family history of thyroid disease
13. Tuberculosis
    a. Centers for Disease Control and Prevention (CDC) and ACOG—perform on all individuals at high risk
    b. See section on Respiratory Disorders in Nongynecological Disorders chapter for more information on tuberculosis and risk factors
14. Vision—American Academy of Ophthalmology recommendations for screening for visual acuity and glaucoma by an ophthalmologist
    a. Every 3 to 5 years for African Americans age 20 to 39
    b. Every 2 to 4 years for individuals age 40 to 64 and every 1 to 2 years beginning at age 65 regardless of race
    c. Yearly for diabetic individuals regardless of age
15. Dental—American Dental Association recommends that adults should have routine dental care and preventive services including oral cancer screening at least once every year
16. Bone mineral density (BMD)—National Osteoporosis Foundation (NOF) recommendations

    a. Screen all women 65 years of age or older for osteoporosis/osteopenia with BMD test
    b. Screen postmenopausal women less than 65 years of age with risk factors

- Immunizations
    1. Hepatitis B
       a. Effective in 95% of cases in preventing hepatitis B virus (HBV) infection
       b. High-risk groups for whom HBV vaccination is recommended include, but are not limited to, individuals who have multiple sex partners; are household contacts or sex partners of those with HBV infection; are injection drug users; are healthcare workers or are otherwise at occupational risk; inmates of long-term correctional institutions
       c. Three-dose series with the second and third doses at 1 and 6 months after the first dose
    2. Influenza
       a. Recommended for all individuals who want to reduce likelihood of getting influenza or spreading it to others
       b. Recommended yearly for all individuals age 50 years and older
       c. Recommended yearly for younger individuals with pulmonary, cardiovascular, or other chronic medical disorders and those who may transmit influenza to individuals at increased risk
       d. Recommended for all women who will be in the second or third trimesters of pregnancy during the influenza season; administration of influenza vaccine is considered safe at any stage of pregnancy
       e. Trivalent inactivated influenza vaccine (TIV) given IM in one dose
       f. Live attenuated influenza vaccine (LAIV) given intranasally—only use for healthy, nonpregnant individuals younger than 50 years of age
    3. Pneumococcus
       a. Recommended one time for all immunocompetent individuals age 65 and older
       b. Recommended for individuals 64 years of age or younger who have chronic illness, functional or anatomic asplenia, immunocompromising conditions, organ or bone marrow transplant recipients, and those whose living conditions place them at high risk for pneumonia
       c. A single revaccination 5 or more years after the initial vaccination is recommended for individuals who received the vaccine

5 or more years previously and were less than 65 years old at the time of the vaccination; individuals with functional or anatomic asplenia, organ or bone marrow transplant recipients; and immunocompromised individuals

4. Rubella
   a. Recommended for all nonpregnant women of childbearing age who lack documented evidence of immunity or prior immunization after 12 months of age
   b. Contraindications—pregnancy (advise not to become pregnant for 4 weeks after vaccination); immunocompromised individuals except those who are HIV positive; hypersensitivity to neomycin
   c. May be given to breastfeeding women

5. Tetanus and diphtheria
   a. Tetanus-diphtheria (Td) vaccine series should be completed
   b. Booster vaccination every 10 years for adults
   c. May be given in pregnancy if indicated in second or third trimester

6. Varicella
   a. Recommended for all adolescents and adults who have not had chickenpox, given in two doses 4 to 8 weeks apart
   b. Contraindications—pregnancy (advise not to become pregnant for 4 weeks after vaccination), history of anaphylactic reaction to neomycin, immunocompromised individuals

7. Zoster (shingles)—one time dose recommended for all individuals 60 years of age or older regardless of previous history of herpes zoster (shingles) or chickenpox

8. Hepatitis A
   a. Recommended for individuals who live in or are traveling to countries with high levels of Hepatitis A infection; intravenous drug users; those with occupational exposure risks; food handlers; and individuals with chronic liver disease or clotting factor disorders
   b. Two doses at least 6 months apart
   c. Combination hepatitis A and hepatitis B vaccine given in three doses with second dose 1 month after first dose and third dose 6 months after first dose

9. Human papilloma virus (HPV)
   a. Recommended as routine vaccination for females 11 to 12 years of age; may be given as young as 9 years of age
   b. Three doses with second dose 2 months after first dose and third dose 6 months after first dose

   c. Recommended as a catch-up vaccination for females 13 to 26 years of age who did not receive it when younger

10. Meningococcal
    a. Recommended for all individuals 11–18 years of age; college freshmen living in dormitories; individuals with anatomic or functional asplenia; individuals traveling to regions where meningococcal disease is hyperendemic or epidemic
    b. One-time dose

11. Immunizations during pregnancy
    a. Live attenuated-virus vaccines should *not* be given during pregnancy
    b. Inactivated virus vaccines, bacterial vaccines, toxoids, and tetanus immunoglobulin may be given if indicated

- Smoking cessation
  1. Overall, 17.4% of adult women currently smoke cigarettes (CDC data from 2007).
  2. In women of reproductive age, 22.4% currently smoke cigarettes (CDC data from 2006).
  3. Of female high school students, 19.4% currently smoke cigarettes (CDC data from 2007).
  4. Smoking cessation interventions should be individualized in relation to the smoker's physical and psychological dependence and the stage of readiness for change.
  5. Behavior modification strategies—provide self-help materials and/or refer to a smoking cessation class.
  6. Pharmacologic aids
     a. Nicotine replacement therapy (gum, patches, inhalers, nasal spray, lozenges)—help to reduce the physical withdrawal symptoms that occur with smoking cessation.
        (1) Major side-effects—local skin reactions with patch; mouth and throat irritation with gum, lozenge, and inhaler; nasal irritation with spray; headache; dizziness; nausea
        (2) Contraindications—serious cardiac arrhythmias, severe angina, recent myocardial infarction, concurrent smoking, pregnancy category D
        (3) Client education
            (a) Individual must stop smoking before initiating nicotine replacement therapy
            (b) Provide specific instructions for the chosen route of delivery
     b. Bupropion hydrochloride sustained release tablets—reduces cravings smokers experience; exact manner of action unknown; probably acts on brain pathways

involved in nicotine addiction and withdrawal
  (1) Major side effects—insomnia, dry mouth, nausea, skin rash
  (2) Contraindications—seizure disorder, eating disorder, use of an MAO inhibitor, concomitant use of other forms of bupropion
  (3) Pregnancy category B; not recommended during breastfeeding
  (4) Client education
      (a) Individual should initiate medication 1 to 2 weeks before smoking cessation
      (b) Recommended duration of therapy is up to 6 months
  c. Varenicline tablets—reduces withdrawal symptoms; blocks effect of nicotine if individual resumes smoking; nicotinic acetylcholine receptor partial agonist
      (1) Major side-effects—nausea, changes in dreaming, constipation, gas, vomiting, neuropsychiatric symptoms
      (2) Contraindications—precautions with psychiatric disorders and renal impairment
      (3) Pregnancy category C; not recommended during breastfeeding
      (4) Client education
          (a) Individual should initiate medication 1 week before smoking cessation
          (b) Concomitant use of nicotine replacement may increase side effects
          (c) Discontinue medication and report any agitation, depression, and suicidal ideation.

- Safety—Address use of seat belts, safety helmets, smoke alarms, occupational safety, and other injury prevention

- Sexuality
  1. Sexual history—see section on Health History in this chapter
  2. PLISSIT model used by clinicians who are not sex therapists or psychiatrists/psychologists to address sexual concerns and to make appropriate referrals—*P*ermission giving, *L*imited *I*nformation giving, *S*pecific *S*uggestions, *I*ntensive *T*herapy
  3. Sexual practices
     a. Sexuality includes a wide range of behaviors—sexual intercourse, fantasy, self-stimulation, noncoital pleasuring, erotic stimuli other than touch, communication about needs and desires
     b. Sexual lifestyle—bisexuality, heterosexuality, homosexuality, long-term monogamy, serial monogamy, multiple partners, celibacy
  4. Sexual response cycle
     a. Masters and Johnson (four phases)—excitement (arousal), plateau, orgasm, resolution
     b. Kaplan (three phases)—desire, excitement, orgasm
     c. Basson (nonlinear model)—demonstrates that emotional intimacy, sexual stimuli, and relationship satisfaction affect female sexual response
  5. Female sexual dysfunction
     a. Etiology may include relationship factors, medical conditions, medication side effects, psychological factors, sexual abuse history
     b. Must cause personal distress to be considered a sexual dysfunction
     c. May be persistent or recurrent, lifelong or acquired, generalized or situational
     d. Assessment—thorough health history, focused sexual and gynecological history, complete physical examination, focused gynecological examination
     e. Management—PLISSIT model for education, counseling, referral; treatment of related medical problems; change in medications
     f. Classification of female sexual dysfunction
        (1) Hypoactive sexual desire disorder—hypoactive sexual desire; sexual aversion disorder
        (2) Sexual arousal disorder—inability to attain or maintain sufficient sexual excitement; may have lack of lubrication or feeling of erotic genital sensations
        (3) Sexual orgasmic disorder—difficulty, delay in, or absence of orgasm following sufficient stimulation and arousal
        (4) Sexual pain disorders
            (a) Dyspareunia—genital pain associated with sexual intercourse
            (b) Vaginismus—involuntary contraction of musculature of the outer third of the vagina that interferes with vaginal penetration
            (c) Noncoital sexual pain disorder—genital pain induced by noncoital sexual stimulation; e.g., endometriosis, vestibulitis, genital mutilation or trauma

6. Male sexual dysfunction
   a. Erectile disorder—inability to obtain or maintain an adequate erection suitable for sexual activity; factors may include performance anxiety, neurologic and vascular disorders, diabetes, hormonal deficiency, alcoholism, medications
   b. Premature ejaculation—inability to delay ejaculation to a point that is mutually desirable for both partners; factors may include sexual inexperience and anxiety

◘ PRECONCEPTION CARE

- Historical factors linking birth defects and certain drugs
  1. Thalidomide
  2. Radiation exposure
  3. DES

- Goals of preconception care
  1. Assistance in preventing unintended pregnancies
  2. Identification of risk factors that could affect reproductive outcomes
  3. Identification and management of medical conditions that could be affected by pregnancy or could affect reproductive outcomes, e.g., diabetes
  4. Initiation of education and desired preventive interventions prior to conception

- Timing of preconception care—integrate into well-woman visits for all reproductive-age women

- Components of preconception care
  1. Assessment—family history, medical/surgical history, infectious disease history, obstetric history, environmental history, cultural health beliefs/practices, psychosocial history including violence, nutrition assessment, paternal health history
  2. Education/counseling and interventions
     a. Health promotion/disease prevention/risk reduction
        (1) Rubella, varicella and hepatitis B vaccinations if needed
        (2) Nutrition counseling for weight loss or gain as needed
        (3) Smoking cessation
        (4) Discontinuation of alcohol use
        (5) Treatment for substance abuse/addiction
        (6) Limit environmental/occupational exposures that may be teratogenic
        (7) Folic acid supplementation
        (8) Optimal glucose control for diabetics
        (9) Dietary management for phenylketonuria
        (10) STD testing and treatment as indicated
        (11) HIV counseling and testing as indicated
        (12) Medication changes as needed to avoid teratogens such as some antiseizure medications
     b. Resources/referrals
        (1) Genetic testing and counseling as indicated—repeated spontaneous abortions, ethnic background that is high risk for autosomal recessive disorder, previous infant with congenital anomaly, age 35 or older
        (2) Dietary counseling
        (3) Substance abuse treatment
        (4) Domestic violence resources

◘ PARENTING

- Definitions
  1. Parent(s)—the person or persons responsible for a child's care and long-term welfare
  2. Infant–parent attachment—process by which parent and infant develop an affectionate, reciprocal relationship that endures over time

- Conditions promoting attachment
  1. Parental emotional well-being and ability to trust
  2. Social support system
  3. Competent level of communication and caregiving skills
  4. Proximity with the infant

- Risk factors for abuse or neglect
  1. Immaturity of parent(s)—adolescent parents at high risk
  2. Isolation/lack of support system
  3. Parent rejected or abused as child
  4. Emotional instability
  5. Lack of knowledge about development and care of children
  6. Low self-esteem
  7. Stressful situations—spousal abuse, poverty, unemployment

- Anticipatory guidance (birth to 1 year)
  1. Growth and development
     a. Physical growth—height and weight
     b. Motor development—early reflexive responses, gross and fine motor skills
     c. Cognitive development—sensorimotor and language

    d.   Psychosocial development—temperament, emotional development, attachment

2. Immunization schedule and health maintenance visits
3. Nutritional needs—nutritional requirements, introduction of solid foods, weaning
4. Safety promotion/injury prevention—Shaken Baby Syndrome, use of infant car seats, accident prevention, prevention of abduction

◘ AGING

- Definition
  1. Aging—process of growing older, regardless of chronologic age
  2. Senescence—mental and physical decline associated with the aging process

- Etiology/Incidence
  1. Theories of aging—biologic, sociologic, and developmental
  2. By the year 2030, 25% of Americans will be older than 65 years
  3. Poverty—elderly women living alone or in ethnic minorities tend to be poorer than elderly men; they are more likely to have only public healthcare coverage or no insurance
  4. Elder abuse and neglect—approximately 4% of elderly individuals are victims of abuse each year

- Signs and symptoms
  1. Dry skin, pruritus, delayed wound healing
  2. Decreased visual and hearing acuity
  3. Decreased taste and smell sensations
  4. Decreased exercise tolerance
  5. Decreased muscle strength
  6. Changes in sleep-wake cycle
  7. Cognitive and memory changes

- Differential diagnosis—other medical conditions that may account for signs and symptoms
  1. Hypothyroidism
  2. Glaucoma, cataracts
  3. Chronic cardiac and pulmonary disorders
  4. Depression
  5. Alzheimer's disease

- Physical findings
  1. Anthropometric—percentage of total body fat increases, waist-to-hip ratio increases, height may decrease due to thinning of cartilage between vertebrae and changes in posture (kyphosis)

2. Skin—skin thinner and less elastic, thinning and graying of hair, increase in benign skin lesions, thick, ridged nails
3. Head, eyes, ears, nose, throat (HEENT)
   a. Arcus senilis—opaque ring at margins of cornea with decreased tear production
   b. Increased cerumen, increased hair in ear canals
   c. Dry buccal mucosa with atrophy of salivary glands; decreased taste sensation
4. Respiratory—rib cage less mobile, increased anterior–posterior (AP) diameter
5. Cardiovascular/peripheral vascular—slower heart rate, increase in systolic BP, may have carotid bruits, peripheral vessels distended and tortuous
6. Breasts—size and elasticity decrease
7. Abdomen—decreased muscle tone, may have less pain with abdominal pathology
8. Musculoskeletal—decrease in muscle mass, kyphosis
9. Neurologic—slower reaction time, may have decreased response to pain stimuli
10. Reproductive organs—sparse pubic hair, smaller labia, shorter, narrow vaginal canal with thin, smooth vaginal walls, shorter cervix, smaller uterus and atrophy of the ovaries

- Diagnostic tests and findings
  1. Most laboratory values not significantly changed by aging in the absence of disease process
  2. Decreased glucose tolerance common in older people—fasting glucose levels increase after age 50
  3. Mammography—American Cancer Society (ACS) and American College of Obstetricians and Gynecologists (ACOG) do not currently recommend a cut-off point for screening related to age

- Management—ACOG periodic (yearly or as appropriate) health examination recommendations for women 65 years of age and older include:
  1. Health history to include health status update, dietary assessment, physical activity, substance abuse, medications, abuse/neglect, sexual practices
  2. Physical examination—height and weight; blood pressure; examination of oral cavity, thyroid, heart, lungs, breasts, abdomen, and skin; pelvic and rectovaginal examination; other as indicated
  3. Laboratory/diagnostic procedures—dipstick urinalysis, mammography, and fecal occult blood test every year, cholesterol every 3 to 5 years, Pap test every 1 to 3 years,

sigmoidoscopy every 5 years or colonoscopy every 10 years, TSH every 3 to 5 years
4. Other screening tests—visual acuity/glaucoma and hearing
5. Counseling—sexuality, diet, exercise, psychosocial concerns, cardiovascular risk factors, hormone replacement therapy, injury prevention
6. Immunizations—Td booster every 10 years, influenza vaccination annually, pneumococcal vaccination once, zoster (shingles) vaccination once
7. Pharmacologic considerations
   a. Age-related decreases in hepatic metabolism and renal elimination, changes in body fat distribution, and central nervous system changes may have an impact on drug absorption, distribution, metabolism and excretion
   b. Polypharmacy—increased risk for adverse reactions, drug interactions, noncompliance, and increased cost with use of multiple medications

◘ PHARMACOLOGY

Pharmacokinetics

- Absorption
  1. Movement of drug from site of entry into the body
  2. Affected by cell membranes, blood flow, drug solubility, pH, drug concentration, dosage form
  3. Bioavailability—percentage of active drug that is absorbed and available to the target tissue

- Distribution
  1. Movement of drug throughout body via circulatory system
  2. Affected by permeability of capillaries and cardiac function
  3. Plasma protein binding—drugs may attach to proteins (mainly albumin) in the blood; only unbound drug is active; as free drug is excreted more of drug is released from binding to replace what is lost; competition for binding sites by different drugs and hypoalbuminemia can affect amount of free drug that is available
  4. Blood-brain barrier and placental barrier affect drug distribution

- Metabolism
  1. Chemical inactivation of drug by conversion to a more water soluble compound that can be excreted from the body
  2. Chemical alterations are produced by microsomal enzymes mainly in the liver

3. Hepatic first pass effect—orally administered drug goes from GI tract through portal system to liver before going to the general circulation; some metabolism of drug may occur as it is taken up by hepatic microsomal enzymes

- Excretion
  1. Removal of drug from body via the kidneys, intestines, sweat and salivary glands, lungs, or mammary glands
  2. Urinary excretion—glomerular filtration, active tubular secretion, and partial reabsorption
  3. Enterohepatic recirculation—some fat soluble drugs may be reabsorbed into the bloodstream from the intestines and returned to the liver

Pharmacodynamics (Study of Mechanism of Drug Action on Living Tissue)

- Drug effects produced by
  1. Drug-receptor interaction
  2. Drug-enzyme interaction
  3. Nonspecific drug interaction

- Affinity—propensity of a drug to bind itself to a given receptor site

- Efficacy—ability to initiate biologic activity as a result of such binding

- Drug–response relationship
  1. Plasma level profile—plasma concentration of a drug and therapeutic effectiveness over a course of time; dependent on rates of absorption, distribution, metabolism, and excretion
  2. Biologic half-life—time required to reduce by one half the amount of unchanged drug that is in the body at the time equilibrium is established

Adverse Reactions

- Predictable—may occur related to
  1. Age
  2. Body mass
  3. Gender
  4. Pathologic state
  5. Circadian rhythm
  6. Genetic factors
  7. Psychologic factors

- Unpredictable types include:
  1. Drug allergy
  2. Idiosyncrasy
  3. Tolerance
  4. Drug dependence

- Iatrogenic responses include:
  1. Blood dyscrasias
  2. Hepatic toxicity
  3. Renal damage
  4. Teratogenic effects
  5. Dermatologic effects

Drug Interactions

- Antagonism—combined effect of two drugs is less than the sum of the drugs acting separately

- Summation—combined effect of two drugs equals the sum of the individual effects of each drug

- Synergism—combined effect of two drugs is greater than the sum of each drug acting independently

- Potentiation—one drug increases the effect of the other drug

Drug Contraindications

- Allergies, medical conditions, concurrent use of another drug, age, pregnancy, lactation may be drug contraindications

- Food and Drug Administration (FDA) Pregnancy Safety Classifications
  1. Category A—studies indicate no risk to fetus
  2. Category B—studies indicate no risk in animal fetus; information in pregnant women unavailable
  3. Category C—adverse effects reported in animal fetus; information in pregnant women is unavailable
  4. Category D—possible fetal risk in humans reported; in selected cases potential benefits may outweigh risks for use of drug
  5. Category X—fetal abnormalities reported and positive evidence of fetal risk in humans is available; these drugs should not be used in pregnancy

Client Education

- Purpose of drug, mechanism of action, effectiveness

- Benefits and risks

- Dosage and administration

- Major side-effects/adverse reactions

- Plan for follow-up

◘ QUESTIONS

Select the best answer.

1. A 17-year-old client presents at the clinic with the following reason for seeking care. "I have been sick for 3 days. I feel sick to my stomach and have diarrhea." Which of the following would be most appropriate to document as her reason for visit/chief complaint?

   a. Flu-like symptoms
   b. Gastrointestinal distress
   c. "I feel sick to my stomach and have diarrhea"
   d. Possible pregnancy, needs further evaluation

2. Which of the following would be considered a subjective assessment finding to be placed in the S section of SOAP format charting?

   a. Motile trichomonads
   b. Mucopurulent discharge
   c. Trichomoniasis vaginitis
   d. Vaginal itching

3. Which of the following includes a pertinent negative that needs to be documented?

   a. 16-year-old female who has never been sexually active; no history of STDs
   b. 25-year-old female with abdominal pain; no nausea, vomiting, or diarrhea
   c. 40-year-old female with depression; past history of suicidal attempt
   d. 60-year-old female with stress incontinence; no breast mass or nipple discharge

4. Appropriate information to include in the review of systems section of the health history would include:

   a. Alert, cooperative, well groomed
   b. Had measles and chicken pox as a child
   c. Occasional loss of urine with coughing
   d. Walks 2 miles a day for exercise

5. Which of the following would most appropriately be documented in the A section of SOAP charting format?

   a. Breast self-examination instructions provided
   b. Positive urine pregnancy test
   c. Client states she would like to quit smoking
   d. Mucopurulent cervicitis

6. The bell of the stethoscope should be used when listening for:

   a. Bowel sounds
   b. Carotid bruits
   c. Lung sounds
   d. S_1 and S_2 heart sounds

7. Evaluation of extraocular muscle movement (EOM) includes:

   a. Ophthalmoscopic examination
   b. PERRLA evaluation
   c. Six cardinal fields of gaze
   d. Visual fields by confrontation

8. Which of the following constitutes a normal Weber test?

   a. Able to hear whispered words at 1 to 2 feet
   b. Air conduction longer than bone conduction
   c. Lateralization of sound to the ear being tested
   d. Sound heard equally in both ears

9. When auscultating lung sounds, the normal finding over most of the lung fields is:

   a. Bronchial
   b. Resonant
   c. Tympanic
   d. Vesicular

10. Increased tactile fremitus would be an expected finding with:

    a. Asthma
    b. Emphysema
    c. Lobar pneumonia
    d. Pleural effusion

11. The sound heard over the cardiac area if there is pericarditis is mostly likely to be a/an:

    a. Diastolic murmur
    b. Fixed split S_2
    c. Friction rub
    d. Increased S_4

12. Which of the following is an abnormal abdominal examination finding in an adult?

    a. Abdominal aorta 2.5 cm in width
    b. Liver border nonpalpable
    c. Liver span 8 cm at the right MCL
    d. Splenic dullness at the left anterior axillary line

13. One of the cranial nerves for which you would test both motor and sensory function is:

    a. CN II—optic nerve
    b. CN V—trigeminal nerve
    c. CN X—vagus nerve
    d. CN XI—spinal accessory nerve

14. A client with an Hgb of 10.2 g/dL and an RBC indices indicating both microcytosis and hypochromia most likely has:

    a. Folic acid deficiency
    b. Iron deficiency

   c. Severe dehydration
   d. Vitamin B_{12} deficiency

15. A client with an increased WBC count related to infectious hepatitis would most likely have an elevated level of:

    a. Basophils
    b. Eosinophils
    c. Lymphocytes
    d. Neutrophils

16. Expected thyroid function test findings with primary hypothyroidism include:

    a. Decreased TSH and decreased FT_4
    b. Decreased TSH and increased FT_4
    c. Increased TSH and decreased FT_4
    d. Increased TSH and increased FT_4

17. A pregnant woman presents with a recent-onset rash. Which of the following laboratory results would be reassuring that this is not likely rubella?

    a. HAI titer of 1:10 at her initial visit 1 month earlier
    b. HAI titer of 1:128 at the current visit
    c. Increased IgG antibody levels at the current visit
    d. Increased IgM antibody levels at the current visit

18. A client who had hepatitis B 6 months ago currently has no symptoms but has a positive test for HbsAg. This most likely indicates that she:

    a. Has immunity to future infection
    b. Has persistent active infection
    c. Is a chronic carrier of hepatitis B
    d. Is in the early stage of reinfection

19. A false negative TB test may be the result of:

    a. Dormant infection
    b. Immunosuppression
    c. Intradermal injection
    d. Prior BCG vaccination

20. An individual with cholecystitis would most likely have a/an:

    a. Decreased alkaline phosphatase
    b. Decreased indirect bilirubin
    c. Increased albumin level
    d. Increased direct bilirubin

21. Measuring waist circumference is most appropriate when the client's BMI places her in which of the following categories:

    a. Underweight
    b. Normal weight

   c. Overweight

   d. Extreme Obesity

22. A 58-year-old woman who is not on estrogen therapy gets an average daily dietary calcium intake of 500 mg. According to National Institute of Health recommendations, she should be advised to take a daily supplement of at least:

   a. 500 mg

   b. 700 mg

   c. 1000 mg

   d. 1500 mg

23. A 53-year-old woman is at the clinic for her annual examination. She had the following tests 1 year ago—fecal occult blood test and sigmoidoscopy. Three years ago she had a normal lipid profile and fasting blood glucose. She has never had a TSH level. If she has no relevant risk factors she should have the following tests done or ordered at her current visit:

   a. Lipid profile, fasting blood glucose, and fecal occult blood test

   b. Lipid profile, TSH, and sigmoidoscopy

   c. Fasting blood glucose and fecal occult blood test

   d. Fasting blood glucose, fecal occult blood test, and TSH

24. Appropriate management for a 45-year-old white woman who has no diabetes risk factors and no symptoms of diabetes with a fasting glucose of 130 mg/dL would include:

   a. Inform client she has impaired glucose tolerance

   b. Order HbA_{1c} level

   c. Repeat glucose testing on another day

   d. Repeat glucose screening in 3 years

25. Which of the following pharmacokinetic changes could decrease the effect of a medication?

   a. Decrease in plasma protein binding

   b. Increase in hepatic first pass effect

   c. Increase in enterohepatic recirculation

   d. Increase in bioavailability

26. "One plus one equals three" best describes which of the following drug interactions?

   a. Antagonism

   b. Potentiation

   c. Summation

   d. Synergism

27. Tests for cerebellar function include:

   a. Deep tendon reflex evaluation

   b. Short-term memory evaluation

   c. Discriminatory sensation tests

   d. Romberg test for balance

28. A healthy 70-year-old female is at the clinic in November for her annual examination. She had influenza vaccination 1 year ago. She had a pneumococcal vaccination and a tetanus booster vaccination 10 years ago. What vaccinations should be given at the current visit?

   a. Influenza only

   b. Influenza and pneumococcal

   c. Influenza and tetanus booster

   d. Influenza, pneumococcal, and tetanus booster

29. Client education concerning the use of bupropion hydrochloride for smoking cessation should include:

   a. Discontinue smoking prior to initiation of this medication

   b. The medication should not be used for more than 8 weeks

   c. Initiate the medication at least 1 week prior to smoking cessation

   d. Side-effects may include drowsiness and weight gain

30. Which of the following statements regarding influenza vaccination during pregnancy is true?

   a. Influenza vaccination should only be given if the woman has health problems placing her at high risk for complications with influenza

   b. Influenza vaccination may be safely given in any trimester of pregnancy

   c. Intranasal influenza vaccine is recommended for pregnant women to reduce chances for side-effects

   d. Influenza vaccination is contraindicated during pregnancy

31. The drug category in which adverse effects have been reported in an animal fetus and information in pregnant women is unavailable is:

   a. Category B

   b. Category C

   c. Category D

   d. Category X

32. Which of the following heart sounds may be a normal finding for a woman in the third trimester of pregnancy?

   a. Diastolic murmur

   b. Fixed split S_2

   c. S_3

   d. S_4

33. Pelvic findings on examination of a 22-year-old nulliparous woman are uterus 7 cm in length and ovaries 3 cm × 2 cm × 1 cm. These findings are consistent with:

    a. Enlarged uterus and enlarged ovaries
    b. Enlarged ovaries and normal size uterus
    c. Enlarged uterus and normal size ovaries
    d. Normal size uterus and normal size ovaries

34. A laboratory test finding of increased immature neutrophils (shift to the left) is consistent with a/an:

    a. Acute bacterial infection
    b. Acute viral infection
    c. Allergic reaction
    d. Chronic bacterial infection

35. An elderly woman has had gastroenteritis with vomiting and diarrhea for the past 3 days. Her mucous membranes appear dry, and she says she has not urinated yet today. Expected laboratory test findings related directly to her current condition might include:

    a. Decreased urine specific gravity
    b. Decreased hematocrit
    c. Increased blood glucose
    d. Increased blood urea nitrogen

36. The blood type in which an individual has no antigens on their RBCs is:

    a. AB+
    b. AB−
    c. O+
    d. O−

37. A woman who describes finding her partner sexually attractive but is not able to maintain sufficient sexual excitement and lubrication during sexual activity has:

    a. Hypoactive sexual desire disorder
    b. Sexual arousal disorder
    c. Sexual orgasmic disorder
    d. Vaginismus

38. Authorities recommend that African Americans begin regular screening at an earlier age than the general population recommendations for:

    a. Breast cancer
    b. Colon cancer
    c. Diabetes
    d. Thyroid disease

39. The second and third doses of the human papilloma virus (HPV) vaccination should be given:

    a. 1 month and 3 months after the initial dose
    b. 2 months and 3 months after the initial dose

    c. 2 months and 6 months after the initial dose
    d. 3 months and 12 months after the initial dose

40. Which of the following vaccinations should *not* be given to an individual who is immunocompromised?

    a. Hepatitis A
    b. Pneumococcal
    c. Rubella
    d. Varicella

41. An abnormal finding on ophthalmoscopic examination would be:

    a. Arterioles smaller than veins
    b. Optic disk that is yellow
    c. Presence of a red reflex
    d. Tapering of the veins

42. When examining the cervix of a 20-year-old female, you note that most of the cervix is pink but there is a small ring of dark red tissue surrounding the os. This is most likely:

    a. An endocervical polyp
    b. Due to cervical dysplasia
    c. Due to cervical infection
    d. The squamocolumnar junction

43. The laboratory test that is done for definitive diagnosis of sickle cell disease is:

    a. Hgb electrophoresis
    b. Peripheral blood smear
    c. RBC indices
    d. Sickle cell preparation

44. A woman who is currently pregnant, has had two full-term deliveries and one abortion would be considered:

    a. Gravida 2 Para 2
    b. Gravida 3 Para 2
    c. Gravida 3 Para 3
    d. Gravida 4 Para 2

45. The best position for palpating the axilla is with the woman:

    a. Lying down with her arm above the head on the side you are examining
    b. Lying down with her arm at her side on the side you are examining
    c. Sitting up with her arm raised above her head on the side you are examining
    d. Sitting up with her arm down on the side you are examining

46. Which of the following would be considered a positive PPD result?

    a. General population—5 mm induration
    b. General population—10 mm induration
    c. Moderate-risk population—5 mm induration
    d. High-risk population—5 mm induration

47. Abnormal findings on a urinalysis would include:

    a. pH 5.0
    b. Specific gravity 1.5
    c. WBCs 3 per HPF
    d. Protein 4 mg/dL

48. Which of the following types of vaccines should *not* be given during pregnancy?

    a. Bacterial vaccines
    b. Inactivated virus vaccines
    c. Live attenuated virus vaccines
    d. Immunoglobulins

49. Which of the components of the PLISSIT model would best describe instructing a couple on the use of water soluble lubrication for dyspareunia caused by vaginal dryness?

    a. Permission giving
    b. Limited information
    c. Specific instructions
    d. Intensive therapy

50. Good dietary sources for folic acid include:

    a. Chicken
    b. Dried beans
    c. Egg yolks
    d. Milk

51. Expected physical findings with aging include:

    a. Decrease in total body fat
    b. Increase in benign skin lesions
    c. Increase in heart rate
    d. Increased response to pain stimuli

52. Which of the following would *not* be an expected pelvic examination finding in a 70-year-old woman?

    a. Narrow vaginal canal
    b. Palpable ovaries
    c. Small uterus
    d. Thin vaginal walls

ANSWERS

1. c	27. d
2. d	28. d
3. b	29. c
4. c	30. b
5. d	31. b
6. b	32. c
7. c	33. d
8. d	34. a
9. d	35. d
10. c	36. d
11. c	37. b
12. d	38. c
13. b	39. c
14. b	40. d
15. c	41. d
16. c	42. d
17. a	43. a
18. c	44. d
19. b	45. d
20. d	46. d
21. c	47. b
22. b	48. c
23. c	49. c
24. c	50. b
25. b	51. b
26. d	52. b

BIBLIOGRAPHY

American Cancer Society. (2009). *Can breast cancer be found early?* Retrieved on July 10, 2009 from www.cancer.org.

American College of Obstetricians and Gynecologists. (2009). Routine screening for hereditary breast and ovarian cancer recommended. *ACOG News Release*, March 20, 2009.

American College of Obstetricians and Gynecologists. (2009). Cervical cytology screening. *ACOG Practice Bulletin, 109*, 1–12.

American Diabetes Association. (2009). Position statement: Diagnosis and classification of diabetes mellitus. *Diabetes Care, 32* (suppl 1), S62–S67.

Association of Reproductive Health Professionals. (2005). Women's sexual health in midlife and beyond. *ARHP Clinical Proceedings, May 2005*, 3–27.

Bickley, L. (2009). *Bates' guide to physical examination and history taking* (10th ed.). Philadelphia, PA: Lippincott, Williams, & Wilkins.

Branson, B., Handsfield, H., Lampe, M., Janssen, R. et al. (2006). Revised recommendations for HIV testing of adults, adolescents, and pregnant women in healthcare settings. *MMWR, 55*(RR14), 1–17.

Centers for Disease Control (CDC). (2008). Smoking prevalence among women of reproductive age, United States—2006. *MMWR, 57*(31), 849–852.

Centers for Disease Control (CDC). (2008). Cigarette smoking among high school students, United States—1991–2007. *MMWR, 57*(25), 689–691.

Chernecky, C., & Berger, B. (2008). *Laboratory tests and diagnostic procedures* (5th ed.). St. Louis: Saunders Elsevier.

Ferri, F. (2009). *Ferri's clinical advisor 2009: Instant diagnosis and treatment.* Philadelphia, PA: Mosby Elsevier.

Giger, J., & Davidhizer, R. (2004). *Transcultural nursing assessment and intervention* (4th ed.). St. Louis: Mosby, Inc.

Hackley, B., Kriebs, J., & Rousseau, M. (2007). *Primary care of women: A guide for midwives and women's health providers.* Sudbury, MA: Jones and Bartlett.

National Cholesterol Education Program. (2001). *Third report of the expert panel on detection, evaluation, and treatment of high blood cholesterol in adults (adult treatment panel III).* Bethesda, MD: National Heart, Lungs and Blood Institute.

National Heart, Lung, and Blood Institute (NHLBI). (2008). *How are overweight and obesity diagnosed.* Retrieved on April 11, 2010 from www.nhlbi.nih.gov/health/dci/Diseases/obe/obe_diagnosis.html.

National Heart, Lung, and Blood Institute (NHLBI). (2003). *The seventh report of the Joint National Committee on Prevention, Detection, Evaluation, and Treatment of High Blood Pressure.* Washington, DC: National Institute of Health.

National Institute of Arthritis, Musculoskeletal, and Skin Diseases. (2009). *Nutrition and bone health.* Washington, DC: National Institute of Health.

National Osteoporosis Foundation. (2008). *Clinician's guide to prevention and treatment of osteoporosis.* Washington, DC: National Osteoporosis Foundation.

Saslow, D., Boetes, C., Burke, W., Harms, M. et al. (2007). American Cancer Society guidelines for breast cancer screening with MRI as an adjunct to mammography. *CA Cancer Journal for Clinicians, 57,* 75–89.

Saslow, D., Hannan, J., Osuch, J. et al. (2004). Clinical breast examination: Practical recommendations for optimizing performance and reporting. *CA Cancer Journal for Clinicians, 54,* 327–344.

Saslow, D., Runowicz, C., Solomon, D. et al. (2002). American Cancer Society guidelines for the early detection of cervical neoplasia and cancer. *CA Cancer Journal for Clinicians, 52*(6), 342–362.

Seidel, H., Ball, J., Dains, J., & Benedict, G. (2006). *Mosby's guide to physical examination* (6th ed.). St. Louis: Mosby, Inc.

Siegel, J., Rhinehart, E., Jackson, M., Chiarello, L., & Healthcare Infection Control Practices Advisory Committee (2007). *2007 guideline for isolation precautions: Preventing transmission of infectious agents in healthcare settings.*

Smith, R., Cokkinides, V., & Brawley, O. (2008). Cancer screening in the United States: A review of current American Cancer Society guidelines and cancer screening issues. *CA Cancer Journal for Clinicians, 58,* 161–179.

Smith, R., Saslow, D., Sawyer, K. et al. (2003). American Cancer Society guidelines for breast cancer screening: Update 2003. *CA Cancer Journal for Clinicians, 53*(3), 141–169.

Tharpe, N., & Farley, C. (2009). *Clinical practice guidelines for midwifery and women's health* (3rd ed.). Sudbury, MA: Jones and Bartlett.

The Advisory Committee on Immunization Practices. (2009). *Recommended adult immunization schedule United States.* Atlanta: Department of Health and Human Services—Centers for Disease Control and Prevention.

US Department of Health and Human Services. (2008). *Physical activity guidelines for Americans.* Washington, DC: USDHHS.

US Department of Health and Human Services. (2005). *Dietary guidelines for Americans.* Washington, DC: USDHHS.

Varney, H., Kriebs, J., & Gegor, C. (2004). *Varney's midwifery* (4th ed.). Sudbury, MA: Jones and Bartlett.

Wynne, A., Woo, T., & Olyaei, A. (2007). *Pharmacotherapeutics for nurse practitioner prescribers* (2nd ed.). Philadelphia, PA: F. A. Davis.

3

Women's Health

Beth M. Kelsey

Anne A. Moore

◘ GYNECOLOGY (NORMAL)

- Anatomy and physiology of reproductive organs
  1. Breast—located on anterior chest; a modified sweat/mammary gland responsible for lactation
     a. Body—composed of lobes, lobules, and alveoli
        (1) Lobes—15 to 20 each breast; forms circle ending in Tail of Spence; located in the upper outer quadrant of each breast terminating in the axillary area
        (2) Lobules—extend from lobes terminating in alveoli; network of ducts extend from lobules forming lactiferous sinuses that direct milk toward nipple; interlobule breast tissue composed of fat
        (3) Alveoli—located at terminus of lobules; responsible for milk production
        (4) Unique proliferation occurs under influence of estrogen during puberty
     b. Nipple—composed of pigmented erectile tissue, areola, and Montgomery's glands; terminus into which lactiferous sinuses secrete milk
        (1) Areola—circular pigmented area that surrounds the nipple
        (2) Montgomery's glands—sebaceous glands that circle the nipple located within the areola
  2. External genitalia—composed of the vulva and its associated structures

  a. Vulva—visible external structures bordered by symphysis pubis anteriorly, buttocks posteriorly, and thighs laterally; develops as a secondary sex characteristic under the influence of estrogen during puberty
     (1) Mons pubis—fatty tissue prominence overlying symphysis pubis, covered by coarse hair inverted in a triangular pattern
     (2) Labia majora—two longitudinal folds of adipose tissue extending from the mons pubis downward enclosing four structures:
        (a) Labia minora—thin folds inside/parallel to the labia majora; forms prepuce anteriorly, encloses the vestibule, and terminates in the fourchette
        (b) Clitoris—small erectile body of tissue; abundant supply of sensory nerve endings; rich vascular supply; important for female sexual response
        (c) Vestibule—contains urethral/vaginal openings, hymen, Skene's glands, Bartholin's glands
        (d) Perineum—located between the fourchette anteriorly and the anus posteriorly
  b. Pelvic musculature—consists of perineal muscles and pelvic floor muscles
     (1) Perineal muscles

(a) Bulbocavernosus—surrounds vagina acting as weak sphincter
(b) Ischiovernosus—surrounds clitoris; responsible for clitoral erection
(c) Superficial/deep transverse perineal muscles—converge with urethral sphincter
(d) External anal sphincter
(2) Pelvic floor muscles
(a) Levator ani—pubococcygeus, iliococcygeus, and ischiococcygeus muscles
(b) Pubococcygeus—pubovaginalis, puborectalis, and pubococcygeus proper
3. Internal pelvic structures—develop primarily as a result of stimulation by estrogen initiated during puberty; structures reach their adult size/appearance by approximately age 16
a. Vagina—muscular/membranous canal that connects the external genitalia to the uterus
(1) Length—approximately 7 cm anterior, 10 cm posterior
(2) Stratified squamous epithelium
(3) Rugae—corrugated sidewalls; allows for distention during coitus and childbirth
(4) pH—acidic due to prevalence of lactobacilli; due to influence of estrogen initiated during puberty
b. Uterus—pear shaped organ that is composed of the following:
(1) Cervix—round, firm terminus to the uterus that protrudes into the vagina
(a) Os—opening in cervix that provides access to the uterine cavity; external os is proximal to the vagina, internal os is proximal to the uterine cavity
(b) Squamocolumnar junction—juncture of the squamous epithelium covering the cervical body (portio) and the columnar epithelium lining the endocervix
(c) Transformation zone—site of original squamocolumnar junction (established during gestation) and the current site; area where squamous metaplasia occurs
(d) Squamous metaplasia—process whereby columnar cells of the endocervix are replaced by mature squamous epithelium

(2) Uterine body—extends upward from cervix and lies in the pelvic cavity; contains cavity or potential space that can accommodate pregnancy
(a) Located between bladder and rectum
(b) Averages 8 cm in length, 5 cm in width, 3 cm in thickness
(c) Composed externally of thick myometrial muscles (myometrium)
(d) Composed internally of columnar epithelium (endometrium); shed during menstruation
(e) Fundus—top portion where fallopian tubes insert
(f) Isthmus (lower uterine segment)—immediately superior to cervix
(g) Corpus—main body
c. Fallopian tubes—ciliated oviducts that transport ova from the ovaries to the uterus
(1) Length—approximately 10 cm
(2) Interstitial portion—within uterus
(3) Isthmus—main body
(4) Ampulla—adjacent to the ovary; receives ova at ovulation
(5) Fimbriated ends/Infundibulum
d. Ovary—pair of endocrine organs located at the end of fallopian tube
(1) Responsible for secretion of steroid hormones—estrogen/progesterone
(2) Approximately 3 cm × 2 cm × 1 cm
(3) Cyclic release of ovum

• Puberty/Adolescence—adolescence defined means "to grow up"; puberty denotes the biology of adolescence, beginning around age 9 and culminating in development of regular menstrual cycles
1. Hormonal changes—begin as hypothalamic-pituitary-ovarian axis matures
a. Gonadotropin-releasing hormone (GnRH)—released from hypothalamus
b. Gonadotropins—follicle stimulating hormone (FSH) and luteinizing hormone (LH) released from anterior pituitary gland in response to GnRH
c. Estrogen—primarily released by ovary in response to FSH; results in development of secondary sex characteristics and ultimately in menstruation
2. Physical changes—tanner staging–physical characteristics of breast/pubic hair development/distribution that delineate progressive advancement of physiologic maturity

a. Growth spurt—girls may grow from 6 to 11 cm taller; greatest height velocity occurs around age 12 or just prior to onset of menses

b. Thelarche—breast development; begins with breast budding around age 9, progresses to conical shape followed by fully developed breast with round contour around age 17

c. Adrenarche—growth of pubic and axillary hair; results from secretion of adrenal androgens; usually starts after breast development begins

d. Menstruation—results from shedding of estrogen primed endometrium; average age is 12.5 years following peak height velocity

3. Psychosocial/cultural changes
   a. Developmental tasks
      (1) Establish independence—struggle with authority vs autonomy
      (2) Experimentation—means of achieving cognitive development
      (3) Develop self-esteem
      (4) Establish peer relationships
   b. Cognitive development
      (1) Progression from concrete operational thinking (7 to 12 years) to formal logical operations (12 years and older)
      (2) True logical thought and manipulation of abstract concepts emerge from 12 to 16 years

- Reproductive years
  1. Effect of hormones
     a. Estrogen—steroid hormone responsible for development of secondary sex characteristics; produced by ovarian follicles, adrenal cortex, corpus luteum; predominant in follicular phase of menstrual cycle
        (1) Estradiol—most potent; derived from ovarian follicles, particularly dominant follicle; primary estrogen of reproductive age
        (2) Estrone—estrogen of menopause; converted from androstenedione produced by adrenal gland and ovarian stroma
        (3) Estriol—least potent; estrogen of pregnancy; derived from conversion of estrone and estradiol in liver, uterus, placenta, and fetal adrenal gland
        (4) Breasts develop fully to round adult contour—development/growth of ductal system, lobular, alveolar growth
        (5) External genitalia
            (a) Mons and labia majora increase in size
            (b) Clitoris enlarges
        (6) Internal pelvic structures
            (a) Vagina lengthens to approximately 10 cm; pH less than 4.5; rugae appear
            (b) Uterus—proliferative endometrium; thin, clear cervical mucus
            (c) Ovaries—follicular development; approximately 3 cm long, 2 cm wide, and 1 cm thick
     b. Progesterone—steroid hormone produced by ovarian corpus luteum and conversion of adrenal pregnenolone/pregnenolone sulfate; luteal phase of menstrual cycle
        (1) Uterus—secretory endometrium; thickens cervical mucus
        (2) Ovary—supplied by corpus luteum; level of 3 ng/mL or greater indicates ovulation
        (3) Breast—subcutaneous fluid retention
     c. Prostaglandin—20-carbon molecules derived from arachidonic acid through action of prostaglandin synthetase enzymes
        (1) Increased production by the uterus as with primary dysmenorrhea
        (2) Increases uterine activity resulting in ischemia
     d. Follicle stimulating hormone—gonadotropin; released by anterior pituitary gland in response to GnRH from hypothalamus
        (1) Ovary—stimulates follicular growth
        (2) Positive/negative feedback from ovarian hormones determines level
     e. Luteinizing hormone—gonadotropin, released by anterior pituitary gland in response to GnRH from hypothalamus
        (1) "Surge" responsible for physical act of ovulation
        (2) Induces steroidogenesis and increases synthesis of androgens by the internal cells of ovary
        (3) Promotes follicular atresia in nondominant follicles
        (4) Promotes final growth of graafian follicle
        (5) Promotes luteinization of granulosa cells
     f. Prolactin—anterior pituitary gland hormone
        (1) Progressive release during pregnancy
        (2) Stimulates synthesis of milk proteins in mammary tissue
        (3) Stimulates epithelial growth in breast during pregnancy

g. Gonadotropin-releasing hormone (GnRH)—released from hypothalamus
  (1) Stimulates anterior pituitary gland to release FSH/LH
  (2) Pulsatile release
h. Adrenal hormones—adrenal cortex
  (1) Cortisol—metabolizes proteins, carbohydrates, fats
  (2) Aldosterone—regulates sodium and potassium; decreases sodium/increases potassium secretion by kidney
  (3) Androstenedione—converted to estrone in adipose tissue
  (4) Testosterone—can be converted to estradiol

2. Menstrual cycle—timed from beginning of one menstrual bleed to beginning of consecutive bleed; average 28 days plus or minus 2 days; duration 4 to 6 days plus or minus 2 days; volume average 40 cc
  a. Ovarian cycle—defined by ovarian changes
    (1) Follicular phase
      (a) Begins day 1 menses
      (b) Variable length (time frame)
      (c) Increased FSH/LH
      (d) Increased E_2 from dominant follicle
      (e) Decreased FSH
      (f) LH surge (peak 10 to 12 hours before ovulation)
      (g) Thin cervical mucus
    (2) Ovulation
      (a) Prostaglandins and proteolytic enzymes break down the follicular wall
      (b) Follicle ruptures releasing oocyte
      (c) Occurs 32–44 hours after LH surge begins
      (d) Maximal production of thin, stretchy, cervical mucus (spinnbarkeit—refers to ability of cervical mucus to be "stretched" between examining fingers; increased stretch equals increased influence of estrogen)
      (e) Peak sexual desire
      (f) Increase in basal body temperature (BBT) of 0.2 to 0.5°F
    (3) Luteal phase
      (a) Begins after ovulation occurs
      (b) Approximately 14 days plus or minus 2 days in length
      (c) Corpus luteum (CL) formed from ruptured follicle; secretes progesterone—peak 7 to 8 days postovulation
      (d) Thickened cervical mucus
      (e) Maintained increase in BBT
      (f) If no pregnancy, CL regresses and progesterone decreases
      (g) Ends with onset menses
  b. Uterine cycle—defined by endometrial changes
    (1) Proliferative phase—estrogen influence
      (a) Endometrium grows/thickens
      (b) Lasts approximately 10 days from end of menses to ovulation
    (2) Secretory phase—progesterone influence
      (a) Average 12 to 16 days
      (b) From ovulation to menses
      (c) Endometrial hypertrophy
      (d) Increased vascularity
      (e) Favorable for implantation of fertilized ovum
    (3) Menstruation—declining progesterone from CL
      (a) Endometrium undergoes involution, necrosis, sloughing
      (b) 3 to 6 days average

3. Breast health
  a. Breast self-examination (BSE)
    (1) American Cancer Society (ACS)—beginning in their 20s, inform of benefits and limitations of BSE and provide instruction for women who choose to do BSE; it is acceptable for women to choose not to do BSE or to do BSE irregularly
    (2) American College of Obstetricians and Gynecologists (ACOG)—adult women should perform BSE monthly
    (3) Studies indicate breast self-examination alone does not reduce number of cancer deaths; it should not be used in place of clinical breast examination and mammography (National Cancer Institute)
    (4) Inspection—in front of mirror
      (a) Hands pressed on hips
      (b) Observe for symmetry, dimpling, contour
    (5) Palpation
      (a) In upright position with arm slightly raised, palpate the underarm area on each side
      (b) Reclining with pillow under shoulder; arm raised
      (c) Pads of three middle fingers used, overlapping dime sized circular motions at three levels of pressure over entire area of both breasts

(d) Use vertical up and down pattern across entire chest wall; clavicle to inframammary fold, sternum to posterior axillary line

b. Screening mammography
   (1) Age 40 to 50
      (a) American Cancer Society (ACS)—annual screening
      (b) National Cancer Institute (NCI)—screening every 1 to 2 years/consult with provider
      (c) Strong family history (maternal grandmother, mother, sister) may warrant earlier/more frequent screening
   (2) Older than age 50—annual screening
   (3) Dense breast tissue in younger women limits reliability
   (4) 10 to 15% false negative rate for detection of malignancies

c. BRCA1/BRCA2-breast cancer gene testing
   (1) 5 to 10% of breast cancer is hereditary
   (2) Women with mutated BRCA1 gene have 80% risk of breast cancer by age 65
   (3) Indicated if
      (a) Strong family history—first/second generation female relatives
      (b) Ashkenazic Jewish descent
   (4) Not cost effective as general screening

d. Clinical breast examination—see General Health Assessment/Health Promotion chapter for detailed information

4. Psychosocial/cultural factors
   a. Menstruation
      (1) Viewed as unclean by some cultures
      (2) Intercourse may be prohibited with any vaginal bleeding
      (3) View of individual influenced by family/community/society
   b. Growth/development
      (1) Influenced by culture/ethnicity
      (2) Influenced by nutritional status
   c. Health promotion behaviors—prioritized by culture/society/socioeconomic conditions

• Menopause
   1. Definitions
      a. Menopause—cessation of menses; average age in US is 51 years; genetically predetermined; confirmed after 12 consecutive months without a period
      b. Climacteric—term used to describe the physiologic changes associated with the change from reproductive to nonreproductive status; 2–8 years before menopause until 1 year after last period
      c. Perimenopause—another term for climacteric
      d. Postmenopause—phase of life following menopause
      e. Premature menopause (premature ovarian failure)—cessation of menses before age 40

   2. Physiology
      a. As climacteric begins, the rhythmic ovarian and endometrial responses of the menstrual cycle decline and eventually stop
      b. Number of responsive follicles decreases with resultant decreased production of estradiol throughout climacteric
      c. With decreasing estradiol, FSH levels increase
      d. At the end of the climacteric, ovary contains no follicles and endometrium atrophies so that reproductive capability is terminated
      e. After menopause, estrone becomes principal estrogen
      f. Estrone produced through aromatization of androstenedione; androstenedione is an androgen produced by adrenal cortex and ovarian stroma; converted to estrone in peripheral fat cells
      g. After menopause, both FSH and LH levels are elevated
      h. Generally rely on cessation of menses, hypoestrogenic symptoms, age, and consistently elevated FSH for diagnosis of menopause

   3. Laboratory findings
      a. FSH—greater than 40 mIU/mL
      b. LH—3-fold elevation after menopause (20–100 mIU/mL)
      c. Estradiol—less than 20 pg/mL

   4. Possible menstrual changes in climacteric
      a. No change
      b. Oligomenorrhea/Polymenorrhea—cycles shorter or longer than usual
      c. Hypomenorrhea/Hypermenorrhea—bleeding lighter/shorter or heavier/longer than usual
      d. Metrorrhagia—irregular intervals, amount variable

   5. Physical changes
      a. Reproductive organs
         (1) Labia—decrease in subcutaneous fat and tissue elasticity
         (2) Vagina

(a) Thinning of epithelium; decreased rugae, increase in pH of greater than or equal to 5.0

(b) May have pruritus, leukorrhea, friability, increased susceptibility to infection

(c) May have dyspareunia

(3) Cervix—decrease in size, os may become flush with vaginal walls, may become stenotic

(4) Uterus and ovaries—decrease in size and weight; ovaries usually not palpable

b. Urinary tract

(1) Decreased muscle tone—urethra and trigone area of bladder

(2) Atrophic changes in urethra and periurethral tissue—stress incontinence may occur

(3) Hypoestrogenic effects in trigone area; lowered sensory threshold to void—sensory urge incontinence may occur

(4) Urinary urgency, frequency, and dysuria due to atrophic changes in urethra and periurethral tissue

c. Breasts—reduction in size and flattened appearance; decrease in glandular tissue

d. Skin

(1) Thinning/decreased activity of sebaceous and sweat glands

(2) Hyperpigmentation/hypopigmentation

(3) Scalp, pubic, and axillary hair becomes thinner and drier

e. Bone integrity

(1) Increased bone loss associated with decrease in estrogen

(2) See section on Osteoporosis in Nongynecological Problems chapter for more information

6. Vasomotor symptoms—hot flashes

a. Observed in 75% of women during climacteric

b. Mechanism responsible not known; gonadotropin-related effect on the central thermoregulatory function of the hypothalamus (measurable increase in body surface heat and decrease in core temperature)

c. Sudden feeling of warmth followed by visible redness of upper body and face

d. May be associated with profuse sweating and palpitations

e. May awaken during the night, leading to insomnia, sleep disturbance, cognitive (memory), and affective (anxiety) disorders with loss of REM sleep

f. Generally cease within 2–3 years after menopause

7. Cardiovascular system effects

a. Lipid levels—increase in low-density lipoproteins (LDL), very low-density lipoproteins (VLDL), and triglycerides, possible decrease in high-density lipoproteins (HDL)

b. Regulation of clotting processes—increase in certain fibrinolytic and procoagulation factors

c. Vasoactive substances—increase in endothelin and decrease in angiotensin converting enzyme (vasoconstrictors), increase in nitric oxide and decrease in prostacyclin (vasodilators)

d. Extent of impact of decreased estrogen levels on cardiovascular disease not definitively established

8. Alterations in mood

a. Majority of women do not have psychological problems attributable to menopause

b. Depression in menopause often related to history of previous depression

c. Depression/irritability may be related to sleep disturbances caused by hot flashes

d. Perceived health shown to be a major factor related to depression in perimenopausal women; individual characteristics and self-perception appear to be important determinants of each woman's experience of the climacteric

e. More research is needed to establish hormonal influences on mood changes that occur during the perimenopause

9. Cognitive function

a. Memory impairment may be indirectly related to decreased estrogen secondary to hot flashes and sleep disturbance

b. WHIMS trial—risk of dementia increased in healthy women aged 65 to 79 years using estrogen or estrogen with progesterone therapy

c. Unclear how estrogen or estrogen with progesterone therapy impacts cognitive function in younger menopausal women

10. Sexuality

a. Diminished genital sensation, less vaginal expansion, and decreased vasocongestion may cause some changes in orgasm experience—increased time to reach orgasm, shorter duration of orgasm, decreased strength of orgasmic contractions

b. Freedom from fear of pregnancy, freedom from contraceptives, and increased privacy as children leave home may increase sexual enjoyment

c. Dyspareunia, loss of partner, medications, and chronic illness may affect sexual desire and activity

11. Health assessment/Health promotion
    a. Health history
       (1) Family and personal history—focus on risks for cancer, heart disease, osteoporosis
       (2) High-risk behavior evaluation—smoking, alcohol, drugs, STD/HIV risks
       (3) Menstrual history—focus on irregular bleeding problems
       (4) Nutrition and exercise assessment
       (5) Psychosocial assessment—sexuality, stressors, support system, domestic violence
    b. Physical assessment
       (1) Blood pressure
       (2) Height and weight
       (3) BMI
       (4) Complete physical examination
    c. Screening tests
       (1) Pap test every 1–3 years (ACOG, ACS, North American Menopause Society [NAMS])
       (2) Rectal examination and stool for occult blood annually beginning age 50 (ACS, NAMS)
       (3) Sigmoidoscopy age 50 and then every 3–5 years or colonoscopy every 10 years, or double contrast barium enema every 5–10 years (ACS, NAMS)
       (4) Mammography every year starting at age 40 (ACS, NAMS)
       (5) Cholesterol with HDL every 5 years beginning at age 20; more frequent and additional lipid tests as needed (National Cholesterol Education Program [NCEP] of the National Heart, Lung, and Blood Institute)
       (6) Plasma glucose every 3 years if age 45 years or older and for younger women with risk factors (American Diabetic Association, NAMS)
       (7) Thyroid function/TSH every 3–5 years for age 65 years and older; begin screening earlier if presence of autoimmune condition or strong family history of thyroid disease (ACOG)
       (8) Hearing screening for 65 years and older
       (9) Screening for visual acuity and glaucoma by ophthalmologist every 2–4 years from age 40–64 and every 1–2 years beginning at age 65; earlier and more frequent screening if risk factors are present (American Academy of Ophthalmology)
       (10) Other as determined by risk factors
    d. Immunizations—see section on immunizations in General Health Assessment and Health Promotion chapter
    e. Counseling and education
       (1) High-risk behaviors
       (2) Nutrition—see section on nutrition in General Health Assessment and Health Promotion chapter
       (3) Self-examination—breasts, skin, vulva
       (4) Physical activity—see section on physical activity in General Health Assessment and Health Promotion chapter
       (6) Injury prevention—seat belts, safety helmets for bike riding, smoke detectors, fall prevention
       (7) Sexuality
       (8) Management of menopausal symptoms
       (9) Benefits and risks of hormone therapy (HT)
       (10) Health maintenance checkup schedule
    f. Contraception for women over 40
       (1) Continue contraception until FSH level indicates no longer fertile or no menses for 1 year
       (2) Options
           (a) Combination (estrogen-progestin) contraception
               i. Safe option for nonsmoking, nonobese, healthy perimenopausal women
               ii. Noncontraceptive benefits may be especially attractive to the perimenopausal woman—relief of vasomotor symptoms, menstrual regulation
           (b) Progestin-only contraception also safe option
           (c) Approaches used in deciding when to discontinue hormonal contraception include reaching age 55 (90% of women have reached menopause by this age) vs two FSH levels while off of hormonal contraception and using a nonhormonal contraceptive
           (d) Intrauterine contraception (IUC)
               i. Long lasting, effective contraceptive option
               ii. Levonorgestrel IUS (LNG IUS) may also be therapeutic for

perimenopausal women with heavy bleeding

    (e) Barrier methods are acceptable options

    (f) Sterilization—most prevalent contraceptive method among married women in the US

    (g) Fertility awareness methods less effective during perimenopause with irregular menstrual cycles

12. Hormone therapy (HT)

  a. Indications

    (1) Relief of menopausal symptoms related to estrogen deficiency—vasomotor instability, vulvar/vaginal atrophy

    (2) Prevention of osteoporosis

  b. Other potential benefits—reduction in risk for colon cancer

  c. Contraindications

    (1) Thromboembolic disorders or thrombophlebitis

    (2) Known or suspected breast cancer

    (3) Estrogen dependent cancer

    (4) Liver dysfunction or disease

    (5) Undiagnosed abnormal uterine bleeding

    (6) Known or suspected pregnancy

  d. Potential risks

    (1) Endometrial hyperplasia/cancer

    (2) Breast cancer

      (a) Relationship with HT inconclusive

      (b) Possible small, but significant increase of breast cancer with long-term HT

    (3) Gallbladder disease

    (4) Thromboembolic disorders

  e. Assessment prior to initiation of HT

    (1) Health history with attention to specific contraindications and precautions

    (2) General physical examination, gynecological examination with Pap test, breast examination, mammogram

    (3) Base decisions concerning HT use on woman's symptoms, treatment goals, benefit-risk analysis

  f. Routine follow-up after HT initiation

    (1) Reevaluate in 3 months—assess therapeutic effectiveness and any problems

    (2) Annual follow-up thereafter if no problems

      (a) Evaluate continuing need for HT and discontinue as appropriate

      (b) Consider nonhormonal drugs for osteoporosis prevention if long-term therapy needed

  g. Regimen options

    (1) 0.625 mg conjugated estrogen or equivalent is dosage shown to prevent osteoporosis in 90% of postmenopausal women

    (2) 10–14 days each month of 10 mg of medroxyprogesterone acetate (MPA) or equivalent or daily doses of 2.5–5.0 mg recommended for prevention of endometrial hyperplasia

    (3) Continuous-combined regimen

      (a) Estrogen and progestin every day

      (b) Lower cumulative dose of progestin than with cyclic regimens

      (c) May have unpredictable bleeding

      (d) After several months endometrium atrophies and amenorrhea usually results

      (e) No estrogen-free period during which vasomotor symptoms can occur

    (4) Continuous-cyclic regimen

      (a) Estrogen every day

      (b) Progestin added 10 to 14 days each month

      (c) No estrogen-free period during which vasomotor symptoms can occur

      (d) Withdrawal bleeding when progestin withdrawn each month

    (5) Cyclic regimen

      (a) Estrogen days 1 to 25

      (b) Progestin added last 10 to 14 days

      (c) Followed by 3 to 6 days of no therapy

      (d) Withdrawal bleeding when progestin withdrawn each month

    (6) Continuous unopposed estrogen—for woman without uterus

  h. Types of estrogen—17β estradiol, estradiol acetate, conjugated estrogen, esterified estrogen, estropipate (estrone), estriol (plant based)

  i. Types of progesterone/progestin—medroxyprogesterone acetate, norethindrone, norethindrone acetate, norgestrel, micronized progesterone (plant based)

  j. Routes of administration

    (1) Oral

      (a) Estrogen, progestin or combination

      (b) First-pass metabolism determines bioavailability

      (c) Increased HDL

      (d) Increased triglycerides

    (2) Transdermal patches

(a) Estrogen and progestin or estrogen only

(b) Can use with continuous-cyclic regimen or continuous-combined regimen

(c) No significant impact on HDL or triglycerides

(d) May have less adverse effects on gallbladder and coagulation factors than oral estrogen

(3) Vaginal estrogen creams

(a) Treatment of vulvar and vaginal atrophy

(b) May use initially with oral estrogen to get more immediate relief

(c) Will not provide relief from vasomotor symptoms

(d) Some systemic absorption possible

(e) Need cyclic progestin with intact uterus

(4) Estrogen vaginal ring (Estring)

(a) Little or no systemic absorption

(b) Approved for treatment of vulvar/vaginal atrophy

(c) Will not relieve vasomotor symptoms

(d) 90 days duration

(e) Do not need cyclic progestin

(5) Estrogen vaginal ring (Femring)

(a) Systemic absorption

(b) Approved for treatment of vasomotor symptoms and vulvar/vaginal atrophy

(c) 90 days duration

(d) Requires added progestin if have intact uterus

(6) Topical sprays, gels, and emulsions—17β-estradiol

(a) Systemic absorption

(b) No significant impact on HDL or triglycerides

(c) May have less adverse effects on gallbladder and coagulation factors than oral estrogen

(d) Need cyclic progestin with intact uterus

(e) Topical progesterone preparations may not provide sufficient endometrial protection

k. Progestin-only may be used if estrogen is contraindicated

(1) Effective in relieving vasomotor symptoms; may have a positive impact on calcium balance

(2) Not effective in relief of vulvovaginal symptoms; may have adverse effect on lipid metabolism

l. Testosterone may be added if extreme vasomotor symptoms not relieved by estrogen alone; oral, transdermal, injections, subcutaneous implants

(1) May be especially useful after surgical menopause

(2) May increase energy level, feeling of well being, libido

(3) Side-effects—acne, hirsutism, clitoromegaly

(4) Does not appear to have negative lipid effect but more studies needed

m. Bioidentical hormones

(1) Hormones chemically identical to hormones produced by women during their reproductive years—17β-estradiol, estrone, estradiol, progesterone, testosterone

(2) Bioidentical hormone therapy (BHT) provides one or more of these hormones as active ingredients

(3) 17β-estradiol is available in several FDA-approved ET products in oral, transdermal, transcutaneous, and vaginal preparations

(4) One FDA-approved bioidentical progesterone product is available in oral form

(5) Custom compounded BHT uses commercially available hormones with the type and amount prescribed by the clinician

(6) Custom compounded BHT products are *not* FDA approved; there is no evidence that they are safer than conventional HT; the same contraindications apply to their use

(7) No evidence that saliva testing is effective for customizing hormone dosing regimens

n. Side-effects of HT

(1) Breast tenderness—estrogen or progestin (usually subsides after first few weeks)

(2) Nausea—estrogen (relieved if taken at mealtime or bedtime)

(3) Skin irritation with transdermal patches

(4) Fluid retention and bloating—estrogen or progestin

(5) Alterations in mood—estrogen or progestin

o. Management of side-effects may include:

(1) Lowering dose

    (2) Altering route of administration

    (3) Changing to different formulation

  p. Management of bleeding during HT

    (1) Continuous–cyclic regimen—usually experience some uterine bleeding; starts last few days of progestin administration or during hormone-free days; earlier bleeding, heavy or persistent bleeding may indicate endometrial hyperplasia and warrants endometrial evaluation

    (2) Continuous–combined regimen—erratic spotting and light bleeding of 1 to 5 days duration in first year; endometrial biopsy if bleeding heavier or longer than usual

13. Nonhormonal management of vasomotor symptoms

  a. Antidepressants (SSRI, SNRI), gabapentin, clonidine—not FDA approved for this purpose

  b. Avoiding caffeine, alcohol, cigarettes, spicy foods, and big meals

  c. Regular, moderate exercise—may also help alleviate insomnia

  d. Wearing layers and natural fibers

  e. Sleeping in a cool room

  f. Keeping a thermos of ice water available

  g. Stress management and relaxation techniques

  h. Vitamin E—anecdotal reports of relief, placebo-controlled studies not supportive

  i. Soy foods and isoflavine supplements

14. Nonhormonal management of vulvovaginal symptoms

  a. Water soluble lubricants

  b. Regular sexual activity

  c. Noncoital methods of sexual expression—massage, mutual masturbation if penetration is painful

◘ DIAGNOSTIC STUDIES AND LABORATORY TESTS

- Pap test
  1. Purpose—a screening technique
     a. Increases detection and treatment of precancerous and early cancerous lesions of the uterine cervix
     b. Decreases morbidity and mortality from invasive cervical cancer
  2. Schedule
     a. ACS—begin approximately 3 years after woman begins having vaginal intercourse but not later than 21 years of age
     b. ACOG—begin at 21 years of age
     c. ACS—yearly if using conventional pap smear or every 2 years if using liquid-based test
     d. ACOG—every 2 years from 21 to 29 years of age regardless of type of test used
     e. ACS and ACOG—for women age 30 and older who have had three consecutive satisfactory normal pap tests, screening may be done every 3 years unless history of in utero DES exposure, HIV infection, or immunosuppression
     f. ACOG—for women age 30 and older with combination of negative pap test and negative HPV test, perform Pap tests no more than every 3 years
  3. Procedure
     a. Instruct patient to avoid douching, intercourse, and use of vaginal creams for 48 hours prior to Pap test screening
     b. Midcycle sampling is ideal (avoid when vaginal bleeding present)
     c. Speculum may be lubricated with water prior to insertion
     d. Entire squamocolumnar junction must be sampled with spatula/broom to avoid false negative related to sampling technique
     e. Endocervical sampling must be obtained with broom/cytobrush
     f. Rapid fixation with cytologic fixative is essential to avoid air-drying artifact unless specimen is transferred to aqueous solution

- Wet mounts (preparations)
  1. Purpose—to detect organisms responsible for symptoms of vulvar, vaginal, cervical, and uterine infections through microscopic evaluation of vaginal discharge
  2. Procedure
     a. Obtain specimen from vaginal sidewalls
     b. Prepare initial slide with saline to detect clue cells, epithelial cells, RBC, WBC, trichomonads, yeast hyphae, and spores
     c. Second specimen can be prepared with KOH to facilitate visualization of yeast buds and pseudohyphae
     d. Addition of KOH may also be used to detect presence of amines (whiff test)

- Colposcopy
  1. Purpose—to allow inspection of vagina and cervix using a binocular microscope; detects lesions/abnormalities that may be biopsied for histologic examination
  2. Procedure

a. Careful, thorough inspection with colposcope
b. Swab cervix/vagina; apply dilute acetic acid to cervix/vagina
c. Areas of abnormality identified
    (1) Aceto white areas
    (2) Vascular patterns
        (a) Punctuation
        (b) Mosaicism
        (c) "Corkscrew" vessels
d. Biopsy
    (1) Identify squamous cell lesions indicated by Pap test screen
    (2) Apply silver nitrate/monsels if biopsy sites continue to bleed
e. Endocervical curretage
    (1) Indicated for glandular abnormalities indicated by Pap test
    (2) 360-degree sample of endocervical canal

- Pregnancy test
  1. Purpose—to detect human chorionic gonadotropin (hCG) in blood/urine; qualitative determines positive or negative test for pregnancy; quantitative measures amount of hCG to ascertain gestational age; serial results determine viability/growth of conceptus
  2. Procedure for urine tests
     a. Obtain first morning specimen if possible as it will be most concentrated
     b. Assess client for use of drugs that may cause false positive results, e.g., anticonvulsants, hypnotics, tranquilizers
     c. Assess urine for blood or protein if false positive suspected
  3. Beta subunit radioimmunoassay (RIA)—serum; quantitative; reliable at 7 days postconception; no cross-reactivity with other hormones
  4. Enzyme-linked immunosorbent assay (ELISA)—immunometric test—urine or serum; qualitative; quantitative—serum only; reliable at 7 to 10 days postconception; no cross-reactivity with other hormones
  5. Agglutination inhibition test—urine; qualitative only; reliable at 14 to 21 days postconception; cross-reactivity with FSH, LH, TSH possible with some tests

- Ultrasound
  1. Purpose—use of high-frequency sound waves to evaluate internal organs/ structure for diagnostic purposes
     a. Distinguish between solid and cystic abdominal/breast or pelvic masses

b. Confirm viability and location of gestation/products of conception
c. Determine endometrial thickness
d. Evaluate size/location of uterine myomas
e. Evaluate adnexal masses/fullness
    (1) Ectopic pregnancy
    (2) Ovarian cysts—serial evaluation
f. Predict ovulation—infertility evaluation
g. Evaluate fetal growth
h. Detect fetal anomalies/abnormalities
  2. Procedure
     a. For transabdominal pelvic ultrasound, patient instructed to have full bladder
     b. Transvaginal ultrasound does not require full bladder
     c. Transducer is passed over tissue to be examined; breast, abdomen, pelvis

- Mammogram
  1. Purpose—radiographic examination of the breast to determine presence of small cancerous, precancerous, and benign lesions
  2. Equipment—mammograms should be performed at a site accredited by the American College of Radiology Mammography Accreditation Program to ensure low-dose, accurate equipment, and trained professional staff
  3. Procedure
     a. Instructions to avoid use of any underarm deodorant spray or powder prior to procedure
     b. Typically two views taken of each breast for screening mammogram
     c. Results explained clearly and follow-up planned accordingly
  4. Diagnostic mammography
     a. Performed if suspicious lesion found on clinical or self-breast examination
     b. Targets a specific area with multiple views
  5. Referral and/or biopsy recommended on any clinically suspicious lesion regardless of mammography results

- Biopsy
  1. Endometrial
     a. Purpose—to determine endometrial status, identify infection, inflammation, hyperplasia, and malignancies in the endometrium
        (1) Evaluation of abnormal uterine bleeding
            (a) Perimenopausal
            (b) Postmenopausal
        (2) Rule out/confirm endometritis
        (3) Infertility evaluation
            (a) "Date" the endometrium

(b) Confirm/rule out luteal phase defect

b. Procedure

(1) Bimanual examination—determine uterine position and size

(2) Local anesthesia may be injected/applied at site for tenaculum attachment

(3) Attach tenaculum to stabilize cervix/provide traction

(4) Paracervical block may be used

(5) Gently pass pipelle through cervix

(6) Withdraw stilette/aspirate with syringe while rotating pipelle

(7) Transfer contents of pipelle/syringe into fixative

(8) Remove tenaculum—control bleeding

(a) Silver nitrate

(b) Monsel's solution

2. Cervical—see colposcopy

3. Breast

a. Purpose—fine needle biopsy to determine whether breast mass found on examination or through imaging contains benign or malignant cells

b. Procedure

(1) Area identified and local anesthetic injected superficially

(2) 21-gauge needle attached to syringe inserted directly into area

(3) Negative pressure applied through aspiration with syringe

(4) Contents placed in specimen container/slide with fixative

4. Vulvar

a. Purpose—sample areas of vulva that appear abnormal for diagnostic purposes

b. Procedure

(1) Area identified and local anesthetic injected

(2) Punch biopsy instrument used in rotating motion to remove sample

(3) Specimen placed in histologic solution

(4) Bleeding controlled with silver nitrate/Monsel's solution

- Screening tests for sexually transmitted diseases (STD)

1. *Chlamydia trachomatis*

a. Tissue culture—endocervix, urethra, rectum, pharynx

b. Nucleic acid amplification test (NAAT)—test recommended by CDC; includes option of testing with urine sample

c. Other nonculture tests—direct fluorescent antibody (DFA), enzyme immunoassay (EIA), DNA probe

2. *Neisseria gonorrhoeae* (GC)

a. Culture—cervix, urethra, rectum, pharynx; plated on Thayer-Martin/other medium

b. Nonculture tests—NAAT, EIA, DNA probe

3. *Treponema pallidum* (syphilis)

a. Dark field microscopy examination and direct fluorescent antibody tests of lesion exudate or tissue are definitive methods of diagnosing early syphilis

b. Serology—provides for presumptive diagnosis

(1) Nontreponemal tests

(a) Venereal Disease Research Laboratories (VDRL)

(b) Rapid plasma reagin (RPR)

(c) Become positive 1 to 2 weeks past chancre

(d) Reported as nonreactive or reactive

(e) Reactive test also reported quantitatively as titer

(f) Nonspecific

(g) False positives associated with mononucleosis, collagen vascular disease, and some other medical conditions; usually see low titer 1:8

(h) Reactive nontreponemal tests must be confirmed with a treponemal test

(i) Titers are also used for follow up after treatment

(j) Nontreponemal tests usually become nonreactive with time after treatment

(2) Treponemal tests

(a) Fluorescent treponemal antibody absorption test (FTA-ABS)

(b) Treponema pallidum immobilization test (TPI)

(c) Reported as positive or negative; not quantitative

(d) Specific

(e) Treponemal tests usually remain positive indefinitely after treatment

4. Genital herpes simplex

a. Tissue culture of lesion

(1) Gold standard test

(2) Sensitivity varies with stage of infection—highest if sample of vesicular lesion

b. Other tests available—DNA probe testing, direct fluorescent antibody/enzyme assay, polymerase chain reaction (PCR)

c. Type-specific serologic tests—serum; detect presence of HSV-1 and HSV-2 antibodies; may take 4 to 12 weeks for seroconversion; useful if history suggestive of HSV but no current lesions, negative culture of lesions but suspect HSV infection, partner with known HSV infection, or patient with HIV infection

d. Cytologic tests—Pap test and Tzanck preparation are insensitive and nonspecific; should not be relied on for diagnosis

5. Human papillomavirus (HPV)
   a. *Condyloma acuminata* (genital warts)
      (1) Generally diagnosed by inspection
      (2) Punch biopsy—rarely needed unless uncertain of lesion
   b. Cervical/flat condyloma/HPV
      (1) Inspection by colposcopy after acetic acid stain application
      (2) Cervical cytology (Pap test)
      (3) Viral DNA testing
6. Chancroid—culture/DNA probe
7. Trichomoniasis
   a. Microscopic evaluation of vaginal secretions with saline wet mount
      (1) Motile, flagellated protozoa
      (2) Greater than 10 WBC/high power field
   b. Vaginal pH greater than 4.5
8. Hepatitis B (HBV)
   a. Serologic testing
   b. Hepatitis B surface antigen (HBsAg)—seen with active infection; carrier state
   c. Hepatitis B surface antibody (HBsAb)—seen with convalescence, indicates immunity to HBV
   d. Hepatitis B core antibody (HBcAb)—indicates past infection; chronic hepatitis
   e. Hepatitis B e-antigen (HBeAg)—seen with acute infection; indicates infectivity
   f. Hepatitis B e-antibody (HBeAb)—seen with convalescence; indicates decreased infectivity
9. Human immunodeficiency virus (HIV)
   a. Sensitive screening tests—enzyme immunoassay (EIA) or rapid test; 99% sensitivity at longer than 12 weeks postexposure
   b. Reactive screening tests must be confirmed by supplemental tests that are highly specific—Western blot or immunofluorescence assay (IFA); HIV antibody detectable in 95% of individuals within 6 months of infection

- Serum hormonal levels
  1. Purpose—to evaluate and monitor treatment of infertility; to assist in differential diagnosis of gonadal dysfunction; to assist in diagnosis of certain neoplasms

2. Estradiol—pg/mL
   a. Follicular phase—20 to 150
   b. Midcycle—150 to 750
   c. Luteal phase—30 to 450
   d. Postmenopause—20 or less
3. Follicle stimulating hormone—mIU/mL
   a. Follicular phase—5 to 25
   b. Midcycle—20 to 30
   b. Luteal phase—5 to 25
   c. Postmenopause—40 to 250
4. Luteinizing hormone—mIU/mL
   a. Follicular phase—5 to 25
   b. Midcycle—75 to 150
   c. Luteal phase—5 to 40
   d. Postmenopause—30 to 200
5. Progesterone—ng/mL
   a. Follicular phase—less than 2
   b. Luteal phase—2 to 20
   c. Postmenopause—less than 0.2

- Laparoscopy
  1. Purpose—to provide direct visualization of internal reproductive organs for diagnosis and treatment of certain conditions
     a. Provides for inspection of internal reproductive organs
     b. Diagnostic for endometriosis
     c. Assists in diagnosis of
        (1) Pelvic pain
        (2) Infertility
        (3) Ectopic pregnancy
        (4) Ovarian cysts/neoplasia
        (5) Uterine fibroids
        (6) Pelvic adhesions
     d. Therapeutic uses
        (1) Tubal ligation
        (2) Appendectomy
        (3) Infertility procedures—harvesting ova for IVF or GIFT procedure
        (4) Lyse adhesions
        (5) Laser/fulguration of endometrial implants
  2. Procedure
     a. General anesthesia administered
     b. Incision into peritoneal cavity
     c. CO_2 instilled—approximately 3 liters
        (1) Distends abdominal cavity
        (2) Allows visibility of organs
     d. Second small incision made; laparoscope inserted—facilitates inspection
     e. Additional incision made to facilitate instrumentation if procedure performed
     f. Patient may experience abdominal/referred shoulder pain following procedure related to CO_2 instillation

- Bone density testing/Bone densitometry
  1. Purpose—diagnosis and monitoring treatment of osteoporosis
  2. Procedure for DEXA scan—most-used technique
     a. Patient lies supine while imager passes over body
     b. Process takes about 10 to 15 minutes
     c. Computer calculates density of patient's bones
  3. Image/regions scanned
     a. Hip
     b. Spine
     c. Wrist/forearm
     d. Heel
  4. Dual energy x-ray absorptiometry (DEXA)
     a. Multiple sites—femoral neck and lumbar spine most common; also finger, forearm, heel; hip BMD is best predictor of hip fractures and predicts fractures at other sites
     b. Most-utilized method
     c. Low radiation
  5. Quantitative computerized tomography
     a. Spine and forearm
     b. Greater radiation exposure
     c. Expensive
  6. Single x-ray absorptiometry (SXA)—heel
  7. Quantitative ultrasound—tibia or heel
  8. Assessment (T-score)—bone density compared to a young normal adult
     a. Normal—BMD within 1 standard deviation (SD) of young normal adult; T-score above –1
     b. Osteopenia—BMD between 1 and 2.5 SD below that of young normal adult; T-score between –1 and –2.5
     c. Osteoporosis—BMD 2.5 SD or more below that of young normal adult; T-score at or below –2.5

◻ FERTILITY CONTROL

- Combination oral contraceptives (COC)
  1. Description—pill taken daily for contraception or for specific noncontraceptive benefits; combination of estrogen and progestin
     a. Monophasic pills—deliver constant amount of estrogen/progestin throughout cycle
     b. Multiphasic pills—vary amount of estrogen and/or progestin delivered throughout cycle
     c. Patterns of use—monthly cycling (21/7), shortened pill-free interval, extended cycle
  2. Mechanism of action
     a. Estrogen—inhibits ovulation through suppression of FSH, alters cellular structure of endometrium; stabilizes endometrium; potentiates progestin
        (1) Ethinyl estradiol (E_2)—most prevalent synthetic estrogen in COC
        (2) Mestranol—weaker estrogen; utilized in older COC formulations
     b. Progestin—inhibits ovulation through suppression of LH; produces atrophic endometrium; thickens cervical mucus; decreases ovum transport through fallopian tube; may inhibit capacitation of sperm
        (1) Norethindrone
        (2) Norethindrone acetate
        (3) Norgestrel
        (4) Levonorgestrel
        (5) Ethynodiol diacetate
        (6) Norgestimate
        (7) Desogestrel
        (8) Gestodene (not available in US)
        (9) Drosperinone
  3. Effectiveness/First year failure rate
     a. Perfect use—0.1%
     b. Typical use—5%
  4. Advantages
     a. Ease of use
     b. Reversible
     c. Effective
     d. May reduce incidence of/afford protection against
        (1) Acne
        (2) Dysmenorrhea
        (3) Pelvic inflammatory disease
        (4) Ectopic pregnancy
        (5) Endometriosis
        (6) Anemia
        (7) Osteoporosis
        (8) Benign breast disease
        (9) Functional ovarian cysts
        (10) Ovarian cancer; endometrial cancer
        (11) Atherogenesis
        (12) Rheumatoid arthritis
        (13) Migraine headaches
        (14) Premenstrual syndrome
        (15) May be used as emergency contraception
  5. Disadvantages/side-effects
     a. Does not prevent transmission of STD/HIV
     b. Requires user compliance/daily dosing schedule
     c. Side-effects may include:
        (1) Estrogenic effects
           (a) Nausea
           (b) Increased breast size
           (c) Cyclic weight gain
           (d) Leukorrhea
           (e) Cervical eversion/ectopy

(f) Hypertension

(g) Increased cholesterol concentration in gallbladder bile

(h) Growth of leiomyomata

(i) Telangiectasia

(j) Chloasma

(k) Hepatocellular adenomas/cancer (rare)

(l) Cerebrovascular accidents

(m) Thromboembolic complications including pulmonary emboli

(n) Stimulation of breast neoplasia

(2) Progestogenic side-effects (alone or in combination with estrogen)

(a) Breast tenderness

(b) Headaches

(c) Hypertension

(d) Decreased libido

(3) Androgenic effects

(a) Increased appetite/weight gain

(b) Depression, fatigue

(c) Acne, oily skin

(d) Increased breast tenderness/size

(e) Increased LDL cholesterol

(f) Decreased HDL cholesterol

(g) Decreased carbohydrate tolerance/increased insulin resistance

(h) Pruritus

6. Contraindications (Centers for Disease Control and Prevention [CDC] recommendations)

a. Individual characteristics or known pre-existing medical/pathologic condition affecting eligibility for use of a contraceptive method classified under one of four categories (CDC, 2010)

(1) Category 1—condition for which there is no restriction on use of the method

(2) Category 2—condition where advantages of using method generally outweigh theoretical or proven risks

(3) Category 3—condition where theoretical or proven risks usually outweigh advantages of using method

(4) Category 4—condition that represents an unacceptable health risk if method is used

b. Category 4 for COC use—do not use method if following conditions exist:

(1) Smoker 35 year of age or older, 15 or more cigarettes/day

(2) Multiple risk factors for arterial cardiovascular disease

(3) Hypertension ($\geq 160/\geq 100$) or hypertension with vascular disease

(4) Acute deep vein thrombosis (DVT) or pulmonary embolism (PE)

(5) History of DVT or PE and one or more risk factors for recurrence

(6) Major surgery with prolonged immobilization

(7) Known thrombogenic mutations

(8) History of or current ischemic heart disease, stroke, complicated valvular heart disease

(9) Migraine headaches with aura at any age; migraine headache at 35 years of age or older with/without aura

(10) Breast cancer within past 5 years

(11) Diabetes with nephropathy, retinopathy, neuropathy, other vascular disease; or longer than 20 years duration

(12) Active viral hepatitis, severe cirrhosis, hepatocellular adenoma, malignant hepatoma

(13) Systemic lupus erythematosus (SLE) with positive or unknown antiphospholipid antibodies

(14) Peripartum cardiomyopathy—normal or mildly impaired cardiac function and less than 6 months postpartum; moderately or severely impaired cardiac function

(15) Solid organ transplantation with complications

c. Category 3 for COC use—use of the method not generally recommended for the following conditions unless other more appropriate methods are not available or acceptable:

(1) Breastfeeding and less than 1 month postpartum

(2) Less than 21 days postpartum if not breastfeeding

(3) Smoker 35 year of age or older, less than 15 cigarettes/day

(4) Hypertension—adequately controlled or 140–159/90–99

(5) Known hyperlipidemia—consider type, severity, and other cardiovascular risk factors

(6) Migraine headache without aura and less than 35 years of age that starts or worsens with COC use

(7) History of breast cancer with no evidence of disease for 5 years

(8) Symptomatic gallbladder disease; history of cholestasis related to past COC use

(9) Mild cirrhosis

(10) History of bariatric surgery with malabsorptive procedure

(11) History of DVT or PE with no risk factors for recurrence

(12) Peripartum cardiomyopathy with normal or mildly impaired cardiac function and 6 or more months postpartum

(13) Moderate or severe inflammatory bowel disease with associated risks for DVT or PE

7. Management
   a. Health assessment prior to initiation of method
     (1) Elicit information from thorough history concerning any contraindications/risk to use of COCs
     (2) Pelvic examination/Pap test not required prior to initiating COC unless other indications
     (3) Blood pressure
     (4) Clinical breast examination if 20 years of age or older recommended
     (5) Mammogram if age 40 or older
   b. Health assessment at follow-up visits
     (1) Patients may be assessed yearly if no risk factors
     (2) Patients with risk factors may be seen at 3 to 6 month intervals
   c. Special considerations
     (1) Drug interactions—drugs that may decrease the effectiveness of COC include:
       (a) Rifampin
       (b) Lamotrigine
       (c) Phenobarbital
       (d) Phenytoin
       (e) Topirimate
       (f) Carbamazepine
       (g) Primidone
       (h) Saint John's Wort
       (i) Some antiretroviral drugs
     (2) Drug interactions—COC may potentiate effect of some drugs
       (a) Benzodiazepines
       (b) Anti-inflammatory corticosteroids
       (c) Bronchodilators
     (3) Management of breakthrough bleeding/spotting
       (a) Common side-effect of first 3 months of use
       (b) Reinforce to take pills daily at the same time
       (c) Change to 30–35 mcg estrogen if on 20 mcg COC
       (d) Change to COC with different progestin
       (e) If problem persists consider another cause for bleeding, e.g., infection, polyps
     (4) Management of absence of withdrawal bleeding

       (a) Occurs in about 5% of women after several years of COC use
       (b) Rule out pregnancy
       (c) No intervention required if woman is okay with no menses
       (d) Change to 30–35 mcg estrogen if on 20 mcg COC
       (e) Add supplemental estrogen to regimen for first 3 weeks of one cycle

8. Instructions for use
   a. General instructions
     (1) Quick start—reasonably certain not pregnant, take first pill on day of office visit; backup method for 7 days
     (2) First day start—take first pill on first day of menses; no backup method needed
     (3) Sunday start—take first pill on first Sunday after menses starts; use backup method for 7 days
     (4) Pill taken at approximately same time each day
     (5) If nausea occurs, pill can be taken with meals or at bedtime
     (6) Backup method (condoms) used if efficacy/absorbency compromised by severe vomiting/diarrhea
     (7) Condom use for prevention of STD/HIV
   b. Missed pills
     (1) If one or two pills missed, take one active pill as soon as remembered and next pill taken at normal time, no backup method needed; consider emergency contraception (EC) if pills missed in first week and sexual intercourse was unprotected
     (2) If three or more pills missed in weeks 1 or 2, take two pills on day remembered and then resume one pill each day; use backup method for 7 days; consider emergency contraception (EC) if pills missed in first week and sexual intercourse was unprotected
     (3) If three or more pills missed in week 3 (of traditional 4-week pack); finish active pills of current pack; do not take placebo pills; start new pack next day
   c. Warning signs (ACHES)
     (1) *A*bdominal pain (severe)
     (2) *C*hest pain (sharp, severe, shortness of breath)
     (3) *H*eadache (severe, dizziness, unilateral)
     (4) *E*ye problems (scotoma, blurred vision, blind spots)
     (5) *S*evere leg pain (calf or thigh)

- Progestin-only pills (POP)
  1. Description—pill taken daily for purposes of contraception; comprised of synthetic progestins in lower doses than those used in combination oral contraceptive pills
  2. Mechanism of action
     a. Inhibits ovulation through suppression of FSH and LH
     b. Produces atrophic endometrium
     c. Thickens cervical mucus
     d. Slows ovum transport through fallopian tube
     e. May inhibit sperm capacitation
  3. Effectiveness/First year failure rate
     a. Perfect use—0.5%
     b. Typical use—5%
  4. Advantages
     a. Ease of use
     b. Reversible
     c. Effective
     d. Contains no estrogen for women in whom it is contraindicated or who cannot tolerate estrogenic side-effects
     e. Can be used during lactation
  5. Disadvantages and side-effects
     a. Effectiveness may be compromised by drug interactions due to low-dose formulation
        (1) Rifampin
        (2) Phenobarbital
        (3) Phenytoin
        (4) Primidone
        (5) Carbamazepine
        (6) Griseofulvin
     b. Decreased availability/increased expense compared to COC
     c. Strict daily dosing schedule
     d. Possible side-effects include:
        (1) Increased incidence of functional follicular cysts
        (2) Menstrual cycle irregularities
        (3) Mastalgia
        (4) Depression
     e. No protection against STD/HIV
  6. Contraindications (CDC recommendations)
     a. Category 4 for POP use—do not use method if breast cancer within past 5 years
     b. Category 3 for POP use—use of the method not generally recommended for the following conditions unless other more appropriate methods are not available or acceptable:
        (1) History of breast cancer with no evidence of disease for 5 years
        (2) Severe cirrhosis, benign hepatocellular adenoma, malignant hepatoma
        (3) History of bariatric surgery with malabsorptive procedure
        (4) Ischemic heart disease or stroke occurring while on POP
        (5) Migraine with aura at any age that starts or worsens with POP use
        (6) SLE and positive or unknown antiphospholipid antibodies
        (7) Taking ritonivar-boosted protease inhibitors as part of HIV/AIDS treatment; some anticonvulsants; rifampin or rifabutin
  7. Management
     a. Health assessment prior to initiation of method—refer to COC section
     b. Health assessment at follow-up visits—refer to COC section
     c. Special considerations—ectopic pregnancy more likely if pregnancy occurs
  8. Instructions for using the method
     a. General instruction
        (1) Pills started on cycle day 1 (first day of menses)
        (2) Pill taken at same time each day every day; no placebo/off week
        (3) If more than 3 hours late taking pill, backup method should be used for 48 hours
     b. Warning signs
        (1) Severe low abdominal pain
        (2) No bleeding after series of regular cycles
        (3) Severe headache

- Transdermal contraceptive system
  1. Description—patch applied to skin; delivers continuous daily systemic dose of progestin (norelgestromin) and estrogen (ethinyl estradiol), new patch applied each week for 3 weeks followed by 1 week without patch to induce withdrawal bleeding
  2. Mechanism of action—same as COC
  3. Effectiveness/First year failure rate
     a. Perfect use—0.99%
     b. Typical use—1.24%
  4. Advantages
     a. Ease of use—no daily dosing regimen
     b. Reversible
     c. Effective
     d. Good menstrual cycle control
  5. Disadvantages and side-effects
     a. Does not prevent transmission of STD/HIV
     b. Skin irritation at application site
     c. Other side-effects similar to those of COC
  6. Contraindications (CDC recommendations)—same as with COC except history of bariatric surgery not relevant

7. Management
   a. Health assessment prior to initiation— same as with COC
   b. Health assessment at follow-up visits— same as with COC
   c. Special considerations
      (1) May be less effective in women who weigh 90 kg (198 pounds) or more
      (2) Probably same drug interactions as with COC
8. Instructions for using the method
   a. Quick start—reasonably certain not pregnant, apply patch on day of office visit or when convenient; backup method for 7 days
   b. First day start—apply patch on first day of menses; no backup method needed
   c. Sunday start—apply patch on first Sunday after menses starts; use backup method for 7 days
   d. Patch applied to buttocks, abdomen, upper torso front or back (excluding breasts), upper outer arm
   e. New patch applied on same day each week for total of 3 weeks
   f. Patch not worn on week 4; withdrawal bleeding will occur
   g. Use of condoms considered for STD/HIV prevention
   h. New patch applied if current patch partially or completely pulls away from skin
   i. Healthcare provider contacted if warning signs occur—same as COC warning signs

- Combination injectable contraceptives (Lunelle)— no longer available in US; available in other countries
  1. Description—intramuscular injection administered every 28 to 30 days for contraception; combination of estrogen (estradiol cypionate) and progestin (medroxy-progesterone acetate)
  2. Mechanism of action—same as COC
  3. Effectiveness/First year failure rate
     a. Perfect use—0.3%
     b. Typical use—0.3%
  4. Advantages
     a. Ease of use—no daily dosing regimen
     b. Reversible
     c. Effective
     d. Good menstrual cycle control
  5. Disadvantages and side-effects
     a. Does not prevent transmission of STD/HIV
     b. Side-effects similar to those of COC
  6. Contraindications (WHO recommendations)— same as with COC; not included in CDC recommendation

7. Management
   a. Health assessment prior to initiation— same as with COC
   b. Health assessment at follow-up visits
      (1) Requires injection every 28 to 30 days
      (2) Assess for side-effects/problems
   c. Special considerations
      (1) If more than 33 days between injections, increased risk for pregnancy
      (2) Probably same drug interactions as with COC
8. Instructions for using the method
   a. Administer injection intramuscularly in deltoid, anterior thigh, gluteal muscle
   b. Administer first injection within 5 days of start of menstrual period
   c. Administer new injection every 28 to 30 days (33 days at most)
   d. May have bleeding 2 to 3 weeks after first injection
   e. Then regular bleeding pattern occurring 22 to 25 days after each injection
   f. Use backup method of contraception if late for injection
   g. Consider use of condoms for STD/HIV prevention
   h. Healthcare provider contacted if warning signs occur—same as COC warning signs

- Contraceptive vaginal ring (NuvaRing)
  1. Description—soft, malleable, clear plastic ring; delivers continuous, systemic dose of estrogen (ethinyl estradiol) and progestin (etonogestrel); worn in vagina for 3 weeks followed by 1 week without ring to induce withdrawal bleeding
  2. Mechanism of action—same as COC
  3. Effectiveness/First year failure rate
     a. Perfect use—0.3%
     b. Typical use—2%
  4. Advantages
     a. Ease of use—no daily dosing regimen
     b. Reversible
     c. Effective
     d. Good menstrual cycle control
  5. Disadvantages and side-effects
     a. Does not prevent transmission of STD/HIV
     b. Side-effects similar to those of COC
     c. Vaginal discharge/vaginal irritation
  6. Contraindications (CDC recommendations)— same as with COC except history of bariatric surgery not relevant
  7. Management
     a. Health assessment prior to initiation— same as with COC

b. Health assessment at follow-up visits—
same as with COC

c. Special considerations—probably same
drug interactions as with COC

8. Instructions for using the method

    a. Quick start—reasonably certain not preg-
nant, insert ring on day of office visit or
when convenient; backup method for 7
days

    b. First day start—insert ring on first day of
menses; no backup method needed

    c. Days 2 to 5 of menstrual cycle—insert ring
and use backup method for 7 days

    d. Hands washed before inserting

    e. Ring folded and gently inserted into
vagina

    f. Exact position of ring in vagina is not
important

    g. Ring left in vagina for 3 weeks then
removed

    h. New ring inserted in 7 days

    i. If ring is expelled or removed for 3 hours
or more, backup method used for next 7
days after ring is reinserted in vagina

    j. If ring is left in vagina for more than 3
weeks but less than 4 weeks, it should be
removed; new ring inserted after 1 week
ring-free period

    k. If ring is left in vagina more than 4 weeks,
it may not protect from pregnancy;
backup method used until new ring in vagina for 7 days

    l. Use of condoms considered for STD/HIV
prevention

    m. Healthcare provider contacted if warning
signs occur—same as COC warning signs

- Progestin-only injectable contraception (Depo-
Provera DMPA)

    1. Description—intramuscular or subcutaneous,
injectable progestin administered in 3-month
intervals for contraception

    2. Mechanism of action

        a. Inhibits ovulation through suppression of
FSH and LH

        b. Produces atrophic endometrium

        c. Thickens cervical mucus

        d. Slows ovum transport through fallopian
tube

        e. May inhibit sperm capacitation

    3. Effectiveness/First year failure rate

        a. Perfect use—0.3%

        b. Typical use—0.3%

    4. Advantages

        a. Ease of use

        b. Effective

        c. Long-term contraceptive option

d. Does not require compliance with daily/
event regimen

e. Does not have drug interaction profile

f. Results in absence of menstrual bleeding
in up to 50% of women by end of first year
of use (four injections); by end of second
year, 70% are amenorrheic

g. Contains no estrogen for women in whom
it is contraindicated or who cannot toler-
ate estrogenic side-effects

h. Can be used during lactation

i. May decrease the following

    (1) Intravascular sickling in patients with
sickle cell disease

    (2) Incidence of seizures in affected
individuals

5. Disadvantages/side-effects

    a. Menstrual cycle irregularities

    b. Mastalgia

    c. Depression

    d. No protection against STD/HIV

    e. Not immediately reversible—requires 3
months to be eliminated

    f. Requires routine 3-month injection
schedule

    g. Weight gain

        (1) Average 5.4 pounds first year

        (2) 13.8 pounds after 4 years

    h. 6 to 12 month delayed return to fertility in
some women

    i. Decreased bone density in long-term
(greater than 5 years) user—returned to
normal following discontinuance

    j. May decrease HDL cholesterol

6. Contraindications (CDC recommendations)

    a. Category 4 for DMPA use—do not use
method if breast cancer within past 5
years

    b. Category 3 for DMPA use—use of the
method not generally recommended for
the following conditions unless other
more appropriate methods are not available or acceptable:

        (1) Multiple risk factors for arterial car-
diovascular disease

        (2) Hypertension ($\geq$160/100) or with vas-
cular disease

        (3) Current/history of ischemic heart dis-
ease or stroke

        (4) Migraine with aura at any age that
starts or worsens with DMPA use

        (5) History of breast cancer with no evi-
dence of disease for 5 years

        (6) Unexplained vaginal bleeding before
evaluation

        (7) Diabetes with nephropathy, retinopa-
thy, neuropathy, other vascular disease; or longer than 20 years duration

(8) Severe cirrhosis, benign hepatocellular adenoma, malignant hepatoma

(9) SLE with positive or unknown antiphospholipid antibodies

(10) SLE with severe thrombocytopenia—initiation category 3, continuation category 2

(11) Rheumatoid arthritis or long-term corticosteroid therapy with history of or risk factors for nontraumatic fractures

7. Management

  a. Health assessment prior to initiation of method

    (1) Refer to COC section

    (2) Include relevant health history

    (3) Baseline weight assessment

  b. Health assessment at follow-up visits

    (1) Return every 3 months for injection

    (2) Determine bleeding pattern—hematocrit/hemoglobin if excessive

    (3) Assess for side-effects/problems

    (4) Weight

  c. Special considerations

    (1) May have added benefits for women with

      (a) Seizure disorder—some data indicate decrease in frequency of grand mal seizures; seizure medication has no impact on DMPA efficacy

      (b) Sickle cell disease—some data indicate association with reduction in frequency of sickle cell crises

    (2) No adverse effect on milk volume after established and may enhance milk production in lactating woman

8. Instructions for using the method

  a. Explain importance of adherence to 3-month injection schedule—contraceptive efficacy maintained for 14 weeks after injection

  b. Administer first injection within first 5 days of menstrual period; no backup method needed

  c. If irregular menses, rule out pregnancy—menstrual/coital history and pregnancy test; use backup method for 7 days after injection

  d. Counsel patients regarding possibility of irregular bleeding; use of backup contraception if more than 3 months between injections; use of condoms for STD/HIV prevention

  e. Procedure for injection

    (1) IM formulation—deep intramuscular injection in deltoid or gluteal muscle;

SC formulation—anterior thigh or abdominal wall

(2) Do not massage injection site (alters absorption/efficacy)

(3) Observe patient for 20 minutes following first injection to rule out allergic reaction

  f. Warning signs

    (1) Frequent intense headache

    (2) Heavy, irregular bleeding

    (3) Depression

    (4) Abdominal pain (severe)

    (5) Signs of infection at injection site (prolonged redness, bleeding, pain, discharge)

- Progestin-only implants

1. Etonogestrel implant (Implanon)

  a. Description—long-term (3 years) contraceptive; single rod-shaped implant placed subdermally inner side of upper arm; provides low dose sustained release of the progestin etonogestrel

  b. Mechanism of action

    (1) Suppresses LH—ovulation inhibited in almost all users

    (2) Produces atrophic endometrium

    (3) Thickens cervical mucus

  c. Effectiveness/First year failure rate

    (1) Perfect use—0.01%

    (2) Typical use—0.01%

    (3) Unknown if overweight/obesity may reduce efficacy

  d. Advantages

    (1) Ease of use

    (2) Effective

    (3) Reversible—most users ovulate within 6 weeks after removal

    (4) Contains no estrogen for women with contraindications to estrogen or who cannot tolerate estrogenic side-effects

    (5) Can be used during lactation

    (6) Affords long-term contraception (3 years)

  e. Disadvantages and side-effects

    (1) Requires clinician insertion and removal, removal requires minor surgical procedure

    (2) Specific information on drug interactions is not available, very low dose progestin, potential for reduced efficacy with same drugs as listed for POP

    (3) Pain, bruising, infection (potential) at insertion site

    (4) Irregular, prolonged, more frequent uterine bleeding especially in first few months; may have amenorrhea

(5) No protection against STD/HIV

(6) Implant may be visible

(7) Possible side-effects include

    (a) Increased incidence of functional ovarian cysts

    (b) Headache

    (c) Emotional lability

    (d) Breast tenderness

    (e) Loss of libido

    (f) Vaginal secretion changes—dryness, leukorrhea

    (g) Acne

f. Contraindications (CDC recommendations)

(1) Category 4 for etonogestrel implant use—do not use method if breast cancer within past 5 years

(2) Category 3 for use etonogestrel implant—use of the method not generally recommended for the following conditions unless other more appropriate methods are not available or acceptable:

    (a) Ischemic heart disease or stroke occurring while using method

    (b) Migraine headaches with aura at any age if starts or worsens after implant insertion

    (c) Unexplained vaginal bleeding before evaluation

    (d) History of breast cancer with no evidence of disease for 5 years

    (e) Severe cirrhosis, benign hepatocellular adenoma, malignant hepatoma

    (f) SLE with positive or unknown antiphospholipid antibodies

g. Management

(1) Health assessment prior to initiation of method—same as COC

(2) Health assessment at follow-up visits

    (a) Return 1 month after insertion to assess site

    (b) Routine annual visits

h. Instructions for using the method

(1) Discuss possible bleeding changes prior to insertion

(2) Inform patient must be replaced every 3 years for effective contraception

(3) Insert within days 1 to 5 of menses; no backup method needed

(4) If irregular menses, rule out pregnancy with menstrual and coital history and pregnancy test

(5) If inserted other than days 1 to 5 of menses, use backup method for 7 days

(6) Discuss use of condoms for STD prevention

(7) Warning signs to report

    (a) Abdominal pain (severe)

    (b) Arm pain or signs of infection

    (c) Heavy vaginal bleeding

    (d) Missed menses after period of regularity

    (e) Onset of severe headaches

2. Levonorgestrel implant (Norplant)—not currently available in US, although some women may still have these implants; long-term (5 years) contraceptive system of six rod-shaped implants placed subdermally in inner upper arm; provides low dose sustained release of progestin levonorgestrel

- Emergency contraception

1. Definition—method used to prevent conception after unprotected coitus; involves use of either hormone-containing pills—levonogestrel alone (Plan B or generic), or combination of ethinyl estradiol and norgestrel or levonorgestrel (COC), or copper-containing intrauterine contraception (IUC)

2. Mechanism of action

a. Emergency contraception pill (ECP)

(1) Inhibits or delays ovulation

(2) May alter sperm/ova transport

(3) Will not disrupt an established pregnancy—minimal endometrial effect

b. Copper-containing IUC

(1) Prevents fertilization (regular use)

(2) Interferes with implantation

3. Effectiveness

a. ECP

(1) Depends on preexisting fertility

(2) Reduces risk of pregnancy by at least 75%

b. Copper-containing IUC—reduces risk of pregnancy by more than 99%

4. Advantages

a. Provides means of emergency contraception in event of any of the following:

(1) Unplanned intercourse

(2) Method failure—condom breaks/leaks; IUC expelled; cap/diaphragm dislodged/improperly placed

(3) Missed COC pills at beginning of pack

(4) Late for contraceptive injection

(5) ECP may be provided with instructions for use for women using any contraceptive method

b. Can provide continuous contraception (IUC)

5. Disadvantages and side-effects

a. ECP

(1) Nausea/vomiting—less common with levonorgestrel-only (Plan B or generic)
(2) Change in next menses
b. Copper-containing IUC
(1) Irregular, heavy bleeding
(2) Uterine cramping/abdominal pain
(3) Refer to section on IUC
6. Precautions and risks
a. Contraindications (CDC recommendations) for ECP—no category 3 or 4 contraindications
b. Contraindications (CDC recommendations) for copper-containing IUC—see IUC section
7. Management
a. Health assessment prior to initiation of method
(1) Health history—menstrual, first episode of unprotected sex in cycle to determine if need pregnancy test, last episode of unprotected sex to assure within time frame for emergency contraception
(2) Urine pregnancy test if episode of unprotected sex more than 1 week ago
(3) If using IUC—see IUC section for required history and examination
(4) Discuss/provide ongoing contraception
b. Health assessment at follow-up visits
(1) Pregnancy test if no menses within 3 weeks
(2) Routine follow-up for ongoing contraception
8. Instructions for using the method
a. ECP
(1) Begin first dose as soon as possible after unprotected sex and within 120 hours for maximum effectiveness
(2) If vomiting within 2 hours, provide with anti-emetic to take 1 hour before a repeated dose of ECP
(3) Inform client that ECP will not provide any ongoing protection from pregnancy
(4) Provide with contraception of choice—resume current method or begin new method immediately; wait until next day to start or restart oral contraceptives to prevent nausea/vomiting
(5) Levonorgestrel-only (Plan B or generic)
(a) One dose of 1.5 mg levonorgestrel—one pill (Plan B) or two pills (generic)
(b) Available OTC if 17 years of age or older
(c) Available as prescription for females younger than 17 years of age
(6) COC
(a) Two doses of 100 to 120 mcg ethinyl estradiol + 0.50 to 0.60 mg levonorgestrel or norgestrel 12 hours apart
(b) May be 5-, 4-, or 2-pill regimen depending on brand used
(c) Caution regarding correct pills to use in triphasic pack
b. Copper-containing IUC
(1) Can be inserted up to 5 days after unprotected sex
(2) No evidence that progestin-containing IUC offers effective emergency contraception

- Intrauterine contraception (IUC)
1. Description—device placed in uterus for purpose of long-acting contraception
a. Copper T 380A
(1) "T" shaped plastic device with copper wrapped around both vertical stem and horizontal arms
(2) Effective for 10 years
b. Levonorgestrel Intrauterine System (LNG IUS)
(1) "T" shaped plastic frame with steroid reservoir in vertical stem that contains levonorgestrel
(2) 20 mcg of levonorgestrel released daily into uterine cavity
(3) Effective for 5 years
2. Mechanism of action
a. Copper T 380A
(1) Copper may inhibit sperm capacitation
(2) Alters tubal/uterine transport of ovum
(3) Enzymatic influence on endometrium
b. LNG IUS—progestin influence
(1) Thickens cervical mucus
(2) Produces atrophic endometrium
(3) Slows ovum transport through tube
(4) Inhibits sperm motility and function
3. Effectiveness/First year failure rate
a. Perfect use
(1) Copper T—0.6%
(2) LNG IUS—0.71%
b. Typical use
(1) Copper T—0.8%
(2) LNG IUS—0.71%
4. Advantages
a. Ease of use
b. Not coitally dependent
c. Effective
d. Reversible

    e.   Cost-effective (if used longer than 1 year)

    f.   LNG IUS can decrease blood loss during menses

    g.   Effective choice for women who cannot use estrogen-containing methods

    h.   Can be used during lactation

5.   Disadvantages and side-effects

    a.   Altered menstrual bleeding patterns

        (1) Increased amount and length of menstrual bleeding—Copper T; first few months of LNG IUS

        (2) Increased dysmenorrhea—Copper T

        (3) Absence of bleeding—LNG IUS

    b.   Risk of PID—increased risk first 20 days following insertion

    c.   Risk of spontaneous expulsion

        (1) May go undetected by the woman

        (2) More likely at time of menses

6.   Contraindications (CDC recommendations)

    a.   Category 4 for IUC use—do not use method if following conditions exist:

        (1) Known/suspected pregnancy

        (2) Postpartum or postabortion sepsis

        (3) Unexplained vaginal bleeding prior to insertion and before evaluation

        (4) Gestational trophoblastic disease with persistently elevated hCG levels or malignant disease

        (5) Cervical cancer prior to insertion and awaiting treatment

        (6) Current breast cancer within past 5 years—LNG IUS only

        (7) Any uterine anatomical abnormalities distorting uterine cavity incompatible with IUC insertion

        (8) Current PID, purulent cervicitis, chlamydia, or gonorrhea—initiation but not continuation

        (9) Endometrial cancer—initiation but not continuation

      (10) Known pelvic tuberculosis—initiation but not continuation

    b.   Category 3 for IUC use—use of the method not generally recommended for the following conditions unless other more appropriate methods are not available or acceptable:

        (1) Ischemic heart disease occurring after insertion—LNG IUS only

        (2) Migraine headache with aura starting after insertion—LNG IUS only

        (3) Gestational trophoblastic disease with decreasing or undetectable hCG levels

        (4) History of breast cancer with no evidence of disease for 5 years—LNG IUS only

        (5) High likelihood of exposure to chlamydia or gonorrhea—initiation but not continuation

        (6) AIDS—unless clinically well on antiretroviral therapy—initiation but not continuation

        (7) Severe cirrhosis, benign hepatocellular adenoma, or malignant hepatoma—LNG IUS only

        (8) SLE with positive or unknown antiphospholipid antibodies—LNG IUS only

        (9) SLE with severe thrombocytopenia—initiation of Copper T IUC only

      (10) Solid organ transplantation with complications—initiation but not continuation

      (11) Pelvic tuberculosis—continuation

7.   Management

    a.   Health assessment prior to initiation of method

        (1) History to include

            (a) STD/PID, vaginitis symptoms

            (b) STD risk factors

            (c) HIV status/exposure

            (d) Pap test history of abnormal results

            (e) Heavy menses/anemia

            (f) Menstrual history

        (2) Physical examination to include

            (a) Speculum examination to assess for possible vaginal/cervical infection

            (b) Pap test (if none within past year)

            (c) Cervical cultures/wet prep (if history/physical examination indicates)

            (d) Bimanual examination—contour, size, consistency, mobility, position of uterus

            (e) Hgb/Hct if history of anemia

    b.   Health assessment at follow-up visits

        (1) Speculum examination at first menses after insertion—check for IUD strings

        (2) Assessment for any signs/symptoms of pelvic infection

        (3) Hgb/Hct if excessive bleeding

    c.   Special considerations

        (1) Timing of insertion

            (a) Not necessary to wait for menses if evidence that patient is not pregnant

            (b) May be inserted within 48 hours after delivery (vaginal and cesarean)

            (c) May be inserted 4 or more weeks postpartum

(d) Insertion after 48 hours and before 4 weeks postpartum is associated with increased risk of uterine perforation

(e) May be inserted immediately following first or second trimester abortion

(2) Menstrual abnormalities (spotting, bleeding)

(a) Nonsteroidal anti-inflammatory drugs (NSAID) may reduce bleeding if initiated at start of menses

(b) Hgb/Hct if excessive or prolonged bleeding

   i. Ferrous sulfate for 2 months if Hgb less than 11.5 g—repeat Hgb/Hct at 3 months

   ii. Remove IUC if Hgb less than 9 g—repeat Hgb/Hct 1 month

(c) Assess for endometritis/PID if bleeding associated with pain

   i. Tests for chlamydia, gonorrhea, and bacterial vaginosis

   ii. Uterine tenderness

   iii. Treat with antibiotics appropriate for PID if suspicious

(d) Persistent bleeding requires further evaluation

(e) Remove IUC if patient desires and provide alternative contraception; may consider switch to LNG IUS if having excessive bleeding with CU 380T and wants to continue IUC as method

(3) Cramping and pain

(a) If severe—rule out perforation

(b) If mild—NSAID/other analgesic or remove IUC

(c) May indicate infection, pregnancy

(4) Expulsion—2 to 10% within first year

(a) Symptoms—cramping, spotting, dyspareunia, lengthening of string

(b) Partial expulsion

   i. Remove IUC

   ii. Rule out pregnancy/infection

   iii. Replace IUC if patient desires

   iv. Doxycycline for 5 to 7 days

(c) Complete expulsion

   i. Pregnancy test

   ii. Replace IUC if patient desires

(5) Pregnancy

(a) Spontaneous abortion (SAB)

   i. Remove IUC

   ii. Doxycycline/ampicillin for 7 days

   iii. Ferrous sulfate if anemic/heavy bleeding

(b) Patient requests abortion—remove IUC and refer

(c) Patient wants to continue pregnancy—visible strings

   i. Advise concerning risk for spontaneous abortion—decreased risk with IUC removal early in pregnancy

   ii. Gently remove IUC

   iii. Warning about possible ectopic

(d) Patients wants to continue pregnancy—no visible strings

   i. Advise concerning risk for spontaneous abortion

   ii. Ultrasound to determine if IUC present

   iii. Monitor for intrauterine infection throughout pregnancy and retrieve IUC at delivery

   iv. If intrauterine infection occurs refer for evacuation of uterus

(6) Perforation, embedding

(a) Perforation occurs 1 in 1,000 insertions

   i. May/may not be associated with severe pain at time of insertion

   ii. U/S to determine location—may require laproscopic removal

   iii. If protrusion through cervix, can be removed in office with local anesthetic

(b) Embedding

   i. Can remove IUC from uterus with forceps if visualized

   ii. May need to be removed with dilatation and curretage (D&C)

(7) PID

(a) Most IUC related PID occurs within the first 20 days after insertion

(b) No evidence supporting the use of prophylactic antibiotics to reduce post insertion infection

(c) Treat PID with appropriate antibiotics

(d) Not necessary to remove IUC unless has current high risk for STI

(8) Actinomyces-like organisms on Pap test

(a) Pap test does not diagnose actinomycosis infection

(b) Actinomyces is normal female genital tract organism

(c) Pelvic actinomycosis is very rare but serious infection

(d) Asymptomatic—inform IUC user, no treatment necessary

(e) Symptomatic—endometritis

    i. Treat with antibiotics—sensitive to penicillin and several other antibiotics

    ii. Remove IUC—actinomyces organism preferentially grows on foreign bodies

8. Instructions for using the method

  a. Check IUD strings

    (1) After each menses

    (2) If increased cramping

    (3) If absent—use backup birth control and notify healthcare provider

    (4) If longer

      (a) May be in process of expulsion

      (b) Use backup birth control and notify healthcare provider

  b. Signs of infection—notify healthcare provider if

    (1) Pelvic pain

    (2) Vaginal discharge

    (3) Unexplained vaginal bleeding

  c. Monitor menses—notify provider if any of the following:

    (1) Heavy, irregular bleeding

    (2) Missed menses—may have amenorrhea with LNG IUS

    (3) Increased cramping

  d. Warning signs (PAINS)

    (1) *P*eriod late/missed; abnormal spotting or bleeding

    (2) *A*bdominal pain

    (3) *I*nfection—vaginal discharge

    (4) *N*ot feeling well—fever, aches, chills

    (5) *S*tring missing, shorter or longer

- Vaginal spermicides
1. Description—cream, foam, suppository, tablet, film, gel, or other preparation that destroys sperm when placed in vagina
2. Mechanism of action
  a. Nonoxynol-9 or octoxynol-9 is active ingredient
  b. Destroys sperm cell membrane
3. Effectiveness/First year failure rate
  a. Perfect use—6%
  b. Typical use—21% to 28%
4. Advantages
  a. Accessible
  b. Inexpensive
  c. Readily available backup method
  d. No systemic effects

5. Disadvantages and side-effects
  a. Coitally dependent
  b. Does not protect against STD/HIV
  c. Potential for allergy/sensitivity/irritation
  d. Must follow instructions for effective use
6. Precautions and risks
  a. Individuals with skin sensitivities may want to test/avoid use
  b. Individual must be capable of following instructions for use
  c. Vaginal abnormalities (septa, prolapse) may preclude use
7. Management
  a. No health assessment needed prior to initiation of method
  b. Special considerations
    (1) Encourage use of spermicide with condom for increased effectiveness
    (2) Frequent use of spermicides (more than two times a day) associated with vulvovaginal epithelium disruption and theoretically could increase susceptibility to HIV infection
    (3) CDC category 3 for women who have HIV/AIDS
8. Instructions for using method
  a. Spermicide used with each act of intercourse
  b. All instructions read carefully
  c. Spermicide left in place (no douching) for 6 hours following last intercourse
  d. Instructions should be followed regarding how long prior to intercourse the spermicide may be inserted—if too much time has lapsed, pregnancy may occur
  e. Spermicide placed deep within vagina
  f. Adequate time should be allowed for spermicide to dissolve (if film, tablets, or suppositories)
  g. With foam use—canister should be shaken well, as directed, prior to filling applicator

- Male condom
1. Description—latex/polyurethane/natural membranous sleeve placed over erect penis prior to intercourse to prevent transmission of semen/sperm into vaginal vault
2. Mechanism of action—barrier; prevents transmission of semen/sperm into vagina
3. Effectiveness/First year failure rate
  a. Perfect use—3%
  b. Typical use—14%
4. Advantages
  a. Accessible
  b. Cost-effective
  c. Prevents transmission of STD (except membrane condoms)

    d. Active involvement of male partner

    e. Prevents allergic reaction to semen

    f. Arrests development of antisperm antibodies in infertility patients

    g. May help prevent premature ejaculation

    h. Does not require visit to healthcare provider

5. Disadvantages and side-effects

    a. Decreased penile sensitivity

    b. Interrupts act of love making

    c. Not appropriate for men with erectile dysfunction

    d. Requires active involvement of male partner

    e. Possibility of condom rupture

6. Contraindications

    a. Latex allergy (male or female partner)—use polyurethane

    b. Spermicide allergy (if condoms lubricated with spermicide)

7. Management

    a. No health assessment needed prior to initiation of method

    b. Special considerations

      (1) Membrane condoms may not protect against STD/HIV

      (2) Petroleum/oil based lubricants may decrease effectiveness of latex condoms (okay for polyurethane condom)

8. Instructions for using method

    a. New condom used with each act of intercourse

    b. Use water soluble lubricants with latex condoms—KY jelly, Astroglide, Replens, Lubrin

    c. Condom unrolled over penis completely (to the base)

    d. Penis withdrawn from vagina soon after ejaculation—condom secured at base of penis to prevent spillage

    e. If condom slips/breaks

      (1) Before ejaculation—apply new condom

      (2) After ejaculation—consider emergency contraception

- Female condom

1. Description—polyurethane sheath placed in the vagina that acts as a barrier to prevent direct contact with seminal fluid during intercourse

2. Mechanism of action—barrier, protects vagina/vulva from direct contact with penis/seminal fluid

3. Effectiveness/First year failure rate

    a. Perfect use—5%

    b. Typical use—21%

4. Advantages

    a. Prevents transmission of STD

      (1) Decreases risk of cervical dysplasia/neoplasia related to HPV

      (2) Decreases risk of PID and sequelae due to decreased transmission of GC and chlamydia

    b. Does not require use of spermicide

    c. Accessible

    d. Controlled by the woman

    e. Does not require visit to healthcare provider

5. Disadvantages and side-effects

    a. Coitally dependent

    b. Noisy

    c. May be aesthetically unappealing

    d. Expensive

6. Precautions and risks

    a. Must be properly inserted/positioned

    b. Polyurethane allergy

7. Management

    a. No health assessment needed prior to initiation of method

    b. Special considerations—women with vaginal abnormalities should not use this method

8. Instructions for using the method

    a. Pouch held with open end down—inner ring should be at bottom of pouch

    b. Inner ring squeezed together and inner ring and pouch inserted into vagina

    c. Inner ring pushed deep into vagina

    d. Outer ring should rest outside vulva

    e. Condom removed immediately after intercourse

    f. Outer ring squeezed together and twisted to prevent spillage

    g. Discard the whole condom

    h. New condom used with each act of intercourse

    i. Male condom should not be used when using female condom—may adhere together causing dislodgement

- Diaphragm

1. Description—reusable latex dome that covers anterior vaginal wall, including cervix; spermicide placed in dome covers cervix affording increased contraceptive protection; types include:

    a. Flat spring

      (1) Good for women with firm vaginal tone

      (2) Gentle spring strength

    b. Coil spring

      (1) Good for women with average vaginal tone

(2) Firm spring strength
c. Arcing spring
    (1) Good for women with lax vaginal tone
    (2) Firm spring strength
d. Wide seal
    (1) Good for women with average/lax vaginal tone
    (2) Available as arcing or coil spring
2. Mechanism of action
    a. Barrier—prevents direct cervical contact with seminal fluid
    b. Spermicide—nonoxynol-9/octoxynol-9 destroys sperm cell membrane
3. Effectiveness/First year failure rate
    a. Perfect use—6%
    b. Typical use—20%
4. Advantages
    a. Cost effective—may be used for 1 to 2 years
    b. Affords some protection against STDs—possible decreased incidence of PID
    c. No systemic effects
5. Disadvantages and side-effects
    a. Requires sizing by trained clinician and instructions in use
    b. May have sensitivity to latex/spermicide
    c. Increased risk of bacterial vaginosis and UTI
        (1) Due to increased colonization with *E coli*
        (2) Related to use of spermicide
        (3) Mechanical irritation/compression against urethra
    d. Does not afford absolute protection from STD/HIV
    e. Risk of toxic shock—2 to 3/100,000 per year
6. Contraindications (CDC recommendations)
    a. Category 4 for diaphragm use
        (1) Allergy to latex; does not apply to non-latex diaphragms
        (2) High risk for HIV—related to concerns about frequent spermicide use disrupting vaginal epithelium rather than diaphragm
    b. Category 3 for diaphragm use—use of method not generally recommended for the following conditions unless other more appropriate methods are not available or acceptable:
        (1) History of toxic shock syndrome
        (2) HIV/AIDS—related to concerns about frequent spermicide use disrupting vaginal epithelium rather than diaphragm
7. Management
    a. Health assessment prior to initiation of method
        (1) Health history to determine if special circumstances or contraindications
        (2) Vaginal examination to determine any abnormal anatomy that may preclude proper fit and retention—prolapse, cystocele, rectocele, vaginal septum
        (3) Proper fit by trained professional—determine appropriate size and type for woman's anatomy
    b. Health assessment at follow-up visits—recheck fit following childbirth or if patient gains/loses 15 pounds or more
8. Instructions for using the method
    a. General instructions (patient)
        (1) Insert just prior to intercourse or up to 6 hours before
        (2) Coat inner dome with 1 tablespoon of spermicide
        (3) Pinch sides of diaphragm and insert fully into vagina
            (a) Tuck anterior rim behind symphysis
            (b) Be certain that dome covers cervix
        (4) If repeated intercourse, insert another application of spermicide in vagina; do not remove diaphragm
        (5) Leave diaphragm in place for at least 6 hours following last intercourse
        (6) Do not leave in place for more than 24 hours
        (7) After each use wash and store diaphragm in clean, cool, dark environment
        (8) Do not use with oil-based lubricants or vaginal medications
        (9) Replace diaphragm yearly
        (10) Assess for holes/tears periodically by filling with water and inspecting for leaks
        (11) Consider emergency contraception if diaphragm is dislodged during or less than 6 hours after sex
    b. Warning signs (toxic shock)
        (1) High fever
        (2) Nausea, vomiting, diarrhea
        (3) Syncope, weakness
        (4) Joint/muscle aches
        (5) Rash resembling sunburn

- Cervical cap (FemCap)
    1. Description—reusable silicone cap, fits over cervix providing barrier contraception; spermicide placed in dome affords additional contraceptive efficacy; three sizes—22 mm, 26 mm, 30 mm
    2. Mechanism of action
        a. Barrier—prevents direct cervical contact with seminal fluid

b. Spermicide—nonoxynol-9/octoxynol-9 destroys sperm cell membrane

3. Effectiveness/First year failure rate
   a. Perfect use
      (1) Parous women—26%
      (2) Nulliparous women—9%
   b. Typical use
      (1) Parous women—40%
      (2) Nulliparous women—20%

4. Advantages
   a. Cost-effective—may be used for 1 to 2 years
   b. Affords some protection against STDs
   c. Possible decreased incidence of PID
   d. Possible decreased incidence of cervical dysplasia/neoplasia
   e. No systemic effects
   f. May be left in place for 48 hours
   g. Does not require insertion of more spermicide with repeat intercourse
   h. Does not increase incidence of bladder infection

5. Disadvantages and side-effects
   a. Requires trained clinician for sizing
   b. Sensitivity to silicone/spermicide
   c. Does not afford absolute protection against STD/HIV
   d. Not every woman can be fitted appropriately
   e. May become dislodged during intercourse

6. Contraindications (CDC recommendations)
   a. Category 4 for cervical cap use—high risk for HIV—related to concerns about frequent spermicide use disrupting vaginal epithelium rather than the cervical cap
   b. Category 3 for cervical cap use—use of method not generally recommended for the following conditions unless other more appropriate methods are not available or acceptable:
      (1) HIV/AIDS—related to concerns about frequent spermicide use disrupting vaginal epithelium rather than the cervical cap
      (2) History of toxic shock syndrome

7. Management
   a. Health assessment prior to initiation of method
      (1) Pap test within past year
      (2) Visualization of cervix to rule out abnormalities
         (a) Extensive lacerations
         (b) Cervicitis
         (c) Asymmetry
      (3) Palpation of cervix
         (a) Length
         (b) Position
         (c) Circumference

b. Health assessment at follow-up visits—re-evaluate cap fit especially if patient complains of dislodgement during intercourse
   c. Special considerations
      (1) Do not use less than 6 weeks postpartum, immediate postabortion, or during menses
      (2) Not all women can achieve a good cervical cap fit
         (a) Cervix too short
         (b) Cap sizes not appropriate
      (3) Efficacy significantly decreased in parous women

8. Instructions for using method
   a. Insert cap at least 30 minutes prior to intercourse to create suction
   b. Fill one third of cap with spermicide
   c. Compress rim prior to insertion
   d. Advance into vagina so rim can slide over cervix
   e. Check that cap covers cervix
   f. Not necessary to reinsert spermicide with repeated intercourse
   g. Leave in place for at least 6 hours and no more than 48 hours after sex
   h. Warning signs (toxic shock)—refer to diaphragm section

- Lea's shield
  1. Description—reusable oval-shaped silicone device fits over cervix and part of upper vagina providing barrier contraception; airflow valve lets air between cervix and shield escape, creating a seal between shield and vagina; flexible ring used to help with removal; spermicide placed inside device affords additional contraceptive efficacy; one size
  2. Mechanism of action
     a. Barrier—prevents direct cervical contact with seminal fluid
     b. Spermicide—nonoxynol-9/octoxynol-9 destroys sperm cell membrane
  3. Effectiveness/First year failure rate
     a. Perfect use—8%
     b. Typical use—no information
  4. Advantages
     a. No fitting required—one size fits all
     b. Reusable—good for about 6 months
     c. No systemic effects
     d. May afford some protection against some STDs
  5. Disadvantages and side-effects
     a. Prescription required
     b. Increased risk of bacterial vaginosis and UTI
     c. Does not afford absolute protection from STD/HIV

d. Potential risk of toxic shock—same as with diaphragm
e. May have sensitivity to silicone or spermicide
6. Contraindications (CDC recommendations not specifically provided)—considered same as for diaphragm and cervical cap
7. Management
   a. No health assessment needed prior to initiation of method
   b. Special considerations
      (1) Abnormal vaginal anatomy—prolapse, cystocele, rectocele may prevent proper placement
      (2) Do not use if delivery within past 6 weeks, recent abortion, or vaginal bleeding
8. Instructions for using the method
   a. Apply spermicide around rim of shield
   b. Fold shield and insert as high in vagina as possible
   c. Check that cervix is covered by shield
   d. Leave in place for 6 hours following intercourse
   e. Use additional spermicide in vagina if repeat intercourse
   f. Do not leave in place more than 40 hours
   g. Consider emergency contraception if shield becomes dislodged during intercourse
      (1) After use wash with soap and water and air dry
      (2) Replace every 6 months
      (3) Warning signs (toxic shock)—see Diaphragm section

- Contraceptive sponge
  1. Description—small pillow-shaped polyurethane sponge containing 1 g of nonoxynol-9 spermicide, concave side fits over cervix, polyester loop facilitates removal, one size
  2. Mechanism of action
     a. Barrier—prevents direct cervical contact with seminal fluid
     b. Spermicide—nonoxynol-9 destroys sperm cell membrane
  3. Effectiveness/First Year Failure Rate
     a. Perfect use
        (1) Nulliparous—9%
        (2) Parous—20%
     b. Typical use
        (1) Nulliparous—16%
        (2) Parous—32%
  4. Advantages
     a. No prescription required
     b. No systemic effects

c. May be used with male condom for additional contraceptive and STD protection
5. Disadvantages and side-effects
   a. Does not afford absolute protection form STD/HIV
   b. Significant decrease in efficacy for parous women versus nulliparous woman
   c. Potential risk of toxic shock—same as with diaphragm
   d. May have sensitivity to polyurethane or spermicide
6. Contraindications (CDC recommendations not specifically provided)—consider same as for diaphragm and cervical cap
7. Management
   a. No health assessment needed prior to initiation of method
   b. Special considerations
      (1) Abnormal vaginal anatomy—prolapse, cystocele, rectocele may prevent proper placement
      (2) Do not use if delivery within past 6 weeks, recent abortion, or vaginal bleeding
8. Instructions for using the method
   a. Moisten sponge with tap water prior to use
   b. Insert deep into vagina
   c. Check to be sure cervix is covered by sponge
   d. Leave in place for at least 6 hours after last intercourse
   e. If repeated intercourse no additional spermicide needed
   f. Do not wear the sponge for more than 24 to 30 hours
   g. Discard sponge after use

- Fertility awareness methods
  1. Description—method of contraception using abstinence during estimated fertile period based on all or some of the following methods
     a. Menstrual cycle pattern (calendar method)
     b. Basal body temperature (BBT)—determines ovulation
     c. Evaluation of cervical mucus (ovulation/Billings method)—determines ovulation
     d. Sympto-thermal method—combines BBT with evaluation of cervical mucus and cervical position/consistency
     e. Standard days method—consider self fertile days 8 through 19 of each menstrual cycle
  2. Mechanism of action—intercourse is avoided during fertile period
     a. Ovum remains fertile for 24 hours

b. Sperm viability approximately 72 hours
c. Most pregnancies occur when intercourse occurs before ovulation

3. Effectiveness/First year failure rate
    a. Perfect use
        (1) Calendar method—9%
        (2) BBT—2%
        (3) Ovulation method—3%
        (4) Sympto-thermal—2%
        (5) Standard days method—5%
    b. Typical use for all methods—25%

4. Advantages
    a. Minimal cost
    b. Natural
        (1) No systemic effects
        (2) No localized side-effects, e.g., latex allergy
    c. Can be utilized for contraception and conception planning

5. Disadvantages and side-effects
    a. Requires motivation from both partners
    b. Requires periodic abstinence
    c. No protection against STD/HIV

6. Precautions and risks
    a. Not reliable for women with the following conditions:
        (1) Irregular menses (consider sympto-thermal and ovulation methods)
        (2) Perimenopausal
        (3) Recently postpartum
        (4) Have had recent menarche
    b. Not a suitable method for
        (1) Women who cannot accurately evaluate their fertile period
            (a) Inability to use/read thermometer
            (b) Inability to understand cervical mucus/changes
            (c) Inability to time intercourse based on calendar evaluation
        (2) Couples unwilling to abstain during fertile time period
        (3) If nonconsensual coitus is likely to occur

7. Management
    a. Health assessment prior to initiation of method
        (1) History to reflect pattern of menses
        (2) Evaluation of client's willingness/ability to check cervical mucus/consistency/position
    b. Health assessment at follow-up visits—BBT/sympto-thermal chart evaluation
    c. Special considerations—combination of fertility awareness methods more effective than single method

8. Instructions for using the method
    a. Calendar method
        (1) Keep record of menstrual cycle intervals for several months
        (2) From the shortest cycle length, subtract 18 days—this determines first fertile day
        (3) From the longest cycle length, subtract 11 days—this determines last fertile day
        (4) Use these numbers to determine days of abstinence for every cycle
    b. Basal body temperature (BBT) method
        (1) Take temperature each morning before rising
            (a) BBT thermometer
            (b) Temperature can be oral, vaginal, or rectal (maintain same route)
        (2) Record on BBT chart
        (3) Temperature increase of 0.4°F or higher at ovulation—remains elevated for at least 3 days
        (4) Abstain from intercourse until 3-day temperature increase occurs
    c. Ovulation method
        (1) Inspect cervical mucus/secretions on underwear, toilet tissue with fingers, beginning day after menses
        (2) Determine consistency—elastic, slippery, wet by touch indicates pre-ovulatory
            (a) Amount increases; becomes thinner and more elastic around time of ovulation
            (b) After ovulation, mucus becomes thick, tacky, and cloudy
        (3) Abstain from intercourse during "wet days" at onset of increased, slippery, thin mucus discharge until 4 days past the peak day (last day of clear, stretchy, slippery secretions)
        (4) Abstain from intercourse during menses due to inability to assess mucus
    d. Sympto-thermal method—combines ovulation, BBT, and assessment of consistency/position of cervix in vagina
        (1) Uses cervical assessment method and BBT
        (2) Ovulatory pain "mittelschmertz" may be indicator
        (3) Abstain until latter of two methods indicates "safe" time
    e. Standard days method
        (1) Abstain from intercourse days 8 through 19 of each menstrual cycle
        (2) CycleBeads are color coded string of beads to help woman keep track of cycle days

- Lactational amenorrhea method
  1. Description—method of contraception for women who are breastfeeding without supplementation or with minimal supplementation and have not had a postpartum menstrual cycle
  2. Mechanism of action—high prolactin
     a. FSH normal; LH decreased—no ovarian follicular development
     b. Inhibits pulsatile GnRH
     c. Results in anovulation
  3. Effectiveness/First year failure rate
     a. Perfect use—0.5% to 1.5% (if amenorrheic)
     b. Typical use—data not available
  4. Advantages
     a. Temporary
     b. No cost
     c. Highly effective until infant nutritional requirements mandate supplementation (approximately 6 months)
     d. Not coitally dependent
     e. Advantageous for infant
        (1) Nutritional
        (2) Bonding
     f. Requires no devices
     g. Minimal systemic effects
  5. Disadvantages and side-effects
     a. Woman must breastfeed completely or with minimal supplementation—may lead to exhaustion
     b. Decreased estrogen due to absence of follicular development
        (1) Atrophic vaginitis
        (2) Decreased vaginal lubrication
        (3) Dyspareunia
     c. Affords no protection against STD/HIV
  6. Precautions and risks
     a. Efficacy decreases with resumption of menses
     b. Must breastfeed completely or with minimal supplementation
  7. Management
     a. No health assessment needed prior to initiation of method
     b. Special considerations—should not use vaginal estrogen cream to treat atrophic vaginitis
        (1) Absorption can inhibit milk production
        (2) Recommend use of vaginal lubricants
  8. Instructions for using the method
     a. Minimal or no supplementation should be used
     b. Alternative contraceptive method should be considered when any of the following occur
        (1) Menses
        (2) Regular supplementation is being used
        (3) Long periods without breastfeeding
        (4) Baby is 6 months old
     c. Ovulation may occur before onset of menses

- Coitus interruptus (withdrawal)
  1. Description—contraceptive method whereby male withdraws penis from vagina prior to ejaculation
  2. Mechanism of action—no contact between sperm and ovum
  3. Effectiveness/First year failure rate
     a. Perfect use—4%
     b. Typical use—19%
  4. Advantages
     a. Requires no devices
     b. No systemic effects
     c. No expense
     d. May result in decreased transmission of HIV (man to woman)
  5. Disadvantages and side-effects
     a. Requires self-control on part of male partner
     b. Requires ability to predict time of ejaculation
     c. Does not afford protection from STD
  6. Precautions and risks—should not be used by men with premature ejaculatory disorder
  7. Management
     a. No health assessment needed prior to initiation of method
     b. Special considerations
        (1) In itself, preejaculatory fluid contains no sperm
        (2) If multiple acts of coitus occur, efficacy is decreased as subsequent preejaculatory fluid may have "carry over" sperm from previous ejaculation
  8. Instructions for using the method
     a. Male partner should void prior to intercourse
     b. Penis is withdrawn prior to ejaculation—ejaculation occurs away from vaginal area
     c. Repeated orgasms may result in presence of sperm in preejaculatory fluid

- Abstinence
  1. Description—contraception based on abstaining from penile–vaginal or penile–rectal contact
  2. Mechanism of action—no possibility of conception as genital contact does not occur
  3. Effectiveness/First year failure rate

a. Perfect use—0%

b. Typical use—data not available

4. Advantages

    a. No cost

    b. No side-effects

    c. Protection against sexually transmitted diseases

5. Disadvantages—requires motivation and acceptance by both partners

6. Precautions and risks—couples should refrain from alcohol/drug use to "stay in control"

7. Management—no health assessment needed prior to initiation of method

8. Instructions for using the method

    a. Avoid any penile–vaginal/rectal contact

    b. Consider alternative means of intimacy/ sexual expression, e.g., mutual masturbation

    c. Avoid alcohol or drug use; may affect commitment to method

- Female sterilization

1. Description—permanent contraception for woman achieved through surgical means; commonly performed on outpatient basis or postpartum prior to discharge

2. Mechanism of action

    a. Fallopian tubes are obstructed to prevent union of sperm and ovum

    b. Transabdominal—laparoscopy or mini-laparoscopy approach; general or local anesthesia

        (1) Surgical ligation—Pomeroy procedure

        (2) Surgical ligation and attachment to uterine body—Irving procedure

        (3) Electrocauterization

        (4) Section of tube excised

            (a) Pritchard procedure

            (b) Fimbriectomy

        (5) Occluded—compressed with silastic band (Falope Ring) or clip (Filshie)

    c. Transcervical (Essure)

        (1) Micro-insert device inserted in tubes transcervically through hysteroscope

        (2) Office procedure with local anesthesia

3. Effectiveness/First year failure rate

    a. Perfect use—0.5%

    b. Typical use—0.5%

4. Advantages

    a. Affords permanent contraception

    b. Highly effective

    c. Cost-effective over long term

    d. Not coitally dependent

5. Disadvantages and side-effects

    a. Invasive surgical procedure requiring anesthesia

b. Reversal is difficult, expensive and, often, unsuccessful

c. No protection against STD/HIV

d. Initially expensive

6. Precautions and risks

    a. Surgical procedure

        (1) Operative complications—bladder/ uterine/intestinal injury may occur

        (2) Anesthetic complications—death (rare)

    b. Wound infection

    c. If pregnancy occurs following procedure, increased risk of ectopic

7. Management

    a. Health assessment prior to initiation of method

        (1) Assess if patient candidate for surgery

        (2) Assess psychological readiness for permanent contraceptive method

    b. Health assessment at follow-up visits— assess for signs/symptoms of infection

        (1) Fever

        (2) Wound tenderness

        (3) Wound drainage

        (4) Abdominal pain

    c. Special considerations

        (1) Consent form signed in advance

        (2) Patient should be advised procedure is irreversible

8. Instructions for using the method

    a. Nothing by mouth at least 8 hours prior to procedure

    b. Need transportation assistance from hospital/clinic to home

    c. Rest for at least 24 hours recommended following procedure

    d. Light lifting only for 1 week

    e. No coitus for 1 week

    f. Continue another method of contraception for 3 months after Essure insertion

    g. Confirm correct placement and tubal occlusion with hysterosalpingogram 3 months after Essure insertion

    h. Warning signs (notify healthcare provider)

        (1) Fever greater than 100°F

        (2) Severe pain

        (3) Drainage from incision

        (4) Dizziness/fainting/vertigo

- Male sterilization

1. Description—permanent contraception involving occlusion of vas deferens, preventing transmission of sperm through semen

    a. Surgical resection—surgical incision made in scrotum; vas deferens is resected

b. Occlusion—surgical incision made in scrotum; vas deferens is divided and fulgurated/tied/cauterized

c. No scalpel—ring forceps secures vas deferens; dissecting forceps punctures skin of scrotum; vas deferens lifted out and occluded

2. Mechanism of action—sperm not present in ejaculate

3. Effectiveness/First year failure rate
   a. Perfect use—0.10%
   b. Typical use—0.15%

4. Advantages
   a. Cost-effective
   b. Highly effective
   c. Affords permanent contraception
   d. Not coitally dependent
   e. No systemic effects/artificial devices

5. Disadvantages and side-effects
   a. Initial expense
   b. Should be considered irreversible
   c. Invasive surgical procedure
   d. No protection against STD/HIV

6. Precautions and risks
   a. Surgical procedure
   b. Wound infection

7. Management
   a. Health assessment prior to initiation of procedure—assess psychological readiness for permanent contraceptive method
   b. Health assessment at follow-up visits—assess for signs/symptoms of infection
      (1) Fever
      (2) Wound tenderness
      (3) Wound drainage
      (4) Swelling
   c. Special considerations
      (1) Relationship between vasectomy and prostate cancer unclear
         (a) Study data conflicting
         (b) Prostate screening postvasectomy is same as for men in general population
      (2) Procedure does not confer immediate sterility—up to 20 ejaculations will contain sperm

8. Instructions for using the method
   a. Rest recommended for approximately 48 hours following procedure
   b. Apply ice pack to scrotum for minimum of 4 hours after procedure
   c. Avoid lifting/exercise for minimum of 1 week
   d. Keep area dry for 48 hours
   e. Abstain from intercourse for 48 hours
   f. Continue using other contraception until minimum of 20 ejaculations/

12 weeks; obtain semen analysis to confirm azoospermia

g. Warning signs
   (1) Fever greater than 100°F
   (2) Increasing pain
   (3) Increasing swelling/tension on stitches
   (4) Bleeding/drainage from incision

• Future methods
1. IUC—smaller size, frameless
   a. Less cramping
   b. Lower expulsion rates
2. Hormonal methods—lower hormone doses, improved progestins for all delivery routes
   a. Improved safety
   b. Improved bleeding patterns
3. Spermicidal agents—formulations with microbicidal properties
4. Barrier methods—designed to accommodate spermicides with microbicidal properties
5. Male hormonal options
   a. Weekly testosterone enanthate injection
   b. Testosterone implants
6. Immunocontraceptives
   a. Female—hCG vaccine; abortifacient
   b. Male—follicle stimulating hormone/luteinizing hormone releasing hormone (FSH/LHRH) vaccine

• Abortion
1. Medication abortion
   a. Mifepristone plus misoprostol
      (1) Most effective at 7 weeks' gestation or earlier
         (a) 95% effective at 7 weeks LMP or earlier
         (b) 80% effective in the ninth week LMP
      (2) Mifepristone
         (a) 19 norsteroid
         (b) Progesterone antagonist
      (3) Misoprostol—prostaglandin analogue
      (4) Method requires two clinic visits
         (a) Mifepristone orally at initial visit
         (b) Misoprostol vaginally or buccally at home 24 to 72 hours after mifepristone
         (c) 1 to 2 week follow-up appointment to assess for complete abortion
         (d) May repeat misoprostol or provide aspiration if abortion is not complete at 1 week
         (e) Aspiration abortion if pregnancy persists 2 weeks after initiation of medication abortion

b. Methotrexate plus misoprostol
   (1) 95% effective in early pregnancy
   (2) Methotrexate
      (a) Destroys trophoblastic tissue
      (b) Blocks folic acid preventing cell division
   (3) Two clinic visits
      (a) Methotrexate IM at initial visit
      (b) Misoprostol vaginally or buccally at home 3 to 7 days later
      (c) Follow-up appointment same as with mifepristone—misoprostol regimen
   (4) Avoid use of folic acid during procedure; may inhibit action of methotrexate
2. Surgical methods
   a. Vacuum aspiration (first trimester)
      (1) Suction curretage
      (2) Local anesthetic
   b. Dilation and evacuation (D&E)—can be performed up to 20 weeks' gestation
3. Pre-abortion health assessment and counseling
   a. History
      (1) LMP and menstrual history
      (2) Surgical history including gynecological surgeries
      (3) Contraceptive history
      (4) Medical history
      (5) Current medications/history of allergic responses
   b. Physical examination
      (1) Size of uterus
      (2) Note uterine/cervical position
      (3) Presence of uterine/cervical/adnexal abnormalities
         (a) Fibroids
         (b) Adnexal masses (rule out ectopic)
      (4) Laboratory tests
         (a) Pregnancy test—urine/serum
         (b) Hgb/Hct
         (c) Blood type and Rh
         (d) STD evaluation if warranted, e.g., sexual assault/patient concern
   c. Counseling
      (1) Discuss all pregnancy options
      (2) Discuss options for termination—medication, surgical
4. Postabortion health assessment and counseling
   a. Contraceptive counseling
   b. Rh immunization if patient Rh negative—give at first visit with medication abortion
   c. Prophylactic antibiotics may be given to surgical patients
      d. Tissue examined to rule out molar pregnancy
5. Potential postabortion complications
   a. Infection
   b. Retained products of conception
   c. Trauma to uterus/cervix
   d. Excessive bleeding
   e. Warning signs
      (1) Fever
      (2) Persistent/increasing lower abdominal pain
      (3) Prolonged/excessive vaginal bleeding
      (4) Purulent vaginal discharge
      (5) No return of menses within 6 weeks

◘ QUESTIONS

Select the best answer.

1. Which of the following lab values would be expected with menopause?

   a. Decreased FSH, increased LH, decreased estradiol
   b. Decreased LH, increased FSH, increased estradiol
   c. Increased FSH, increased LH, decreased estradiol
   d. Increased LH, decreased FSH, increased estradiol

2. According to the North American Menopause Society, a 45-year-old female presenting for a routine annual exam should have which of the following screening tests?

   a. Pap test, plasma glucose, thyroid function test
   b. Plasma glucose, Pap test, mammography
   c. Stool for occult blood, mammography, Pap test
   d. Thyroid function test, mammography, sigmoidoscopy

3. The most prevalent contraceptive method among married women in the United States is:

   a. Combination oral contraceptives
   b. Condoms
   c. Sterilization
   d. Withdrawal

4. A 54-year-old female with vaginal dryness causing irritation and dyspareunia has no problem with hot flashes and has a bone densitometry T score of 1.0. The best treatment for her would be:

   a. Continuous combined regimen HT
   b. Cyclic HT with added testosterone

c. Estrogen vaginal ring
d. Progestin-only therapy

5. An advantage of continuous-combined HT over continuous-cyclic HT regimens is:

a. No estrogen-free period during which vaso-motor symptoms can occur
b. Predictable withdrawal bleeding each month
c. Lower cumulative dose of progestin
d. Less negative impact on triglyceride levels

6. Which of the following women should have an endometrial biopsy/evaluation?

a. Woman on continuous-cyclic HT regimen with amenorrhea
b. Woman on continuous-cyclic HT regimen with bleeding starting last few days of progestin administration each month
c. Woman on continuous-combined HT regimen with irregular bleeding in the first year of use
d. Woman on continuous-combined HT regimen with spotting that occurs after several months of amenorrhea

7. The sebaceous glands located within the areola are called:

a. Bartholin's glands
b. Cowper's glands
c. Montgomery's glands
d. Skene's glands

8. The shift in vaginal pH that occurs during puberty is influenced by:

a. Estrogen
b. FSH
c. LH
d. Progesterone

9. A vaginal pH less than 4.5 is an expected finding:

a. In a healthy reproductive age woman
b. In a menopausal woman with atrophic vaginitis
c. In a reproductive-age woman with trichomoniasis
d. In a healthy prepubertal-age girl

10. The predominant vaginal organism responsible for normal pH in reproductive-age women is:

a. *Doderlein bacilli*
b. *Gardnerella*
c. *Haemophilus*
d. *Lactobacilli*

11. Squamous metaplasia of the cervix occurs within the:

a. Cervical os
b. Columnar epithelium
c. Squamous epithelium
d. Transformation zone

12. The portion of the uterus that is shed during menstruation is the:

a. Endometrium
b. Myometrium
c. Omentum
d. Pyometrium

13. Estrogen is released by the ovary in response to:

a. FSH
b. GnRH
c. hCG
d. LH

14. Which of the following is the least potent endogenous estrogen?

a. Estradiol
b. Estriol
c. Estrone
d. Estropipate

15. Which of the following hormones is responsible for regulating sodium and potassium by the kidneys?

a. Aldosterone
b. Androstenedione
c. Cortisol
d. DHEA

16. Which phase of the menstrual cycle is the most variable?

a. Follicular
b. Luteal
c. Ovarian
d. Secretory

17. Which hormone is dominant during the proliferative phase of the menstrual cycle?

a. Estrogen
b. LH
c. Progesterone
d. Prolactin

18. Which population is at increased risk for having a mutation of the breast cancer gene (BRCA1/2)?

a. African Americans
b. Ashkenazic Jews
c. Asians
d. Hispanics

19. The minimum conjugated estrogen dose that has been shown to prevent osteoporosis in menopausal women is:

a. 0.3 mg
b. 0.625 mg
c. 0.9 mg
d. 1.25 mg

20. A 53-year-old female who had a hysterectomy 10 years ago for dysfunctional uterine bleeding presents with complaints of severe hot flashes and night sweats for the past few months. Her lipid profile is significant for cholesterol of 220 mg/dL and triglycerides of 350 mg/dL. The most appropriate therapy for her vasomotor symptoms at this time would be:

a. Continuous-combined oral HT
b. Selective estrogen receptor modulator (raloxifene)
c. Transdermal estrogen patch
d. Vaginal estrogen cream

21. Which of the following estrogen replacement options does *not* require opposition by a progestin in a woman with an intact uterus?

a. Bioidentical oral estrogen formulation
b. Estring vaginal ring
c. Plant based (estriol) oral estrogen
d. Transdermal estrogen patch

22. Adding potassium hydroxide to a wet mount slide before viewing it under the microscope is useful in the detection of:

a. Clue cells
b. Candida pseudohyphae
c. Trichomonads
d. White blood cells

23. Which of the following statements concerning a beta subunit radioimmunoassay (RIA) pregnancy test is true?

a. It is most commonly used for qualitative hCG determination
b. It can be performed on either urine or blood
c. Cross-reaction with FSH or LH may occur during perimenopause
d. It is reliable 7 to 10 days postconception

24. The American Cancer Society recommends yearly mammogram screening beginning at age:

a. 35
b. 40
c. 45
d. 50

25. A woman who was treated for primary syphilis 1 year ago now has the following test results: VDRL nonreactive and FTA-ABS positive. These findings indicate:

a. She most likely was not adequately treated for her primary syphilis 1 year ago.
b. She has most likely become reinfected since her treatment 1 year ago.
c. She most likely has some other condition that is causing a false positive FTA-ABS.
d. She most likely was treated adequately for her syphilis and has not become reinfected.

26. When evaluating cervical mucus, the term spinn-barkeit refers to:

a. Amount
b. Cellularity
c. Clarity
d. Elasticity

27. A 24-year-old female presents to your office with a request for combination oral contraceptives. Her current medications include a bronchodilator for asthma. Management for this client should include advising her that:

a. Combination oral contraceptives are not recommended for women with asthma.
b. Combination oral contraceptives may potentiate the action of her bronchodilator.
c. She should use a backup method if using the bronchodilator several days in a row.
d. Use of progestin-only contraceptive injections may reduce her asthma attacks.

28. Which of the following contraceptive methods would be best for a woman with a seizure disorder who is taking phenytoin?

a. Combination oral contraceptives
b. Transdermal contraceptive patch
c. Progestin-only oral contraceptives
d. Progestin-only contraceptive injections

29. A client calls the clinic on Tuesday morning. She had unprotected sex Friday night and is interested in emergency contraception. Appropriate information for this client would include:

a. Emergency contraception pills are very effective for medical abortion in early pregnancy.
b. If she is not midcycle when she had sex, she does not need emergency contraception.
c. It is too late for emergency contraceptive pills, but insertion of an IUC is an option.
d. She can use emergency contraception pills even if she has had other unprotected sex since her last period.

30. The levonorgestrel-containing IUC may be a better choice than the copper-containing IUC for a woman who:

a. Has never been pregnant
b. Has dysmenorrhea
c. Is currently breastfeeding
d. Is sure she does not want more children

31. A 28-year-old female who has had an IUC for 2 years has a Pap test showing actinomycosis. She has no symptoms of infection. Appropriate management would include:

    a. Removing the IUC and repeating the Pap test in 6 months
    b. Removing the IUC, treating with doxycycline and repeating the Pap test in 1 year
    c. Keeping the IUC and repeating the Pap test in 1 year
    d. Keeping the IUC, treating with doxycycline and repeating the Pap test in 3 months

32. Which of the following diaphragms would be best for a woman with very firm vaginal tone?

    a. Arcing spring
    b. Coil spring
    c. Flat spring
    d. Wide seal

33. The type of skin lesion seen initially with toxic shock syndrome is:

    a. Diffuse sunburn-like rash
    b. Multiple vesicles on chest and extremities
    c. Petechiae on mucomembranous tissues
    d. Ulcerative lesions in genital area

34. Advantages of the cervical cap over the diaphragm include:

    a. It is has a lower failure rate.
    b. It is easier to insert.
    c. It can remain in place for 48 hours.
    d. Spermicide is not needed.

35. Which of the following statements concerning a transcervical (Essure) sterilization procedure is correct?

    a. The fallopian tubes are occluded with a silastic band.
    b. The success of reversals is higher than with other sterilization methods.
    c. It is effective within 1 to 2 weeks after the procedure.
    d. The patient needs to return for a hystosalpingogram 3 months after the procedure.

36. A woman who is undergoing a medically induced abortion using methotrexate and misoprostol should be advised to avoid which of the following during the procedure?

    a. Acetaminophen
    b. Folic acid supplements

c. Nonsteroidal anti-inflammatory drugs
d. Vitamin B_6 supplements

37. Potential disadvantages of progestin-only implants (Implanon) include:

    a. May have increased side-effects in women who are underweight
    b. May cause a significant decrease in bone mineral density
    c. May cause irregular bleeding and spotting
    d. Return to fertility after discontinuation can may take several months

38. On the average, cognitive development is completed with the formation of formal operational thought by age:

    a. 12
    b. 14
    c. 16
    d. 18

39. Which endogenous estrogen is known as the "estrogen of pregnancy"?

    a. Estradiol
    b. Estriol
    c. Estrone
    d. Estropipate

40. Increased production of _____ is associated with primary dysmenorrhea.

    a. Androstenedione
    b. Arachidonic acid
    c. Cortisol
    d. Prostaglandin

41. The optimal time each month for self-breast examination is:

    a. A few days before expected menses
    b. At approximately midcycle
    c. During the first 1 to 3 days of menses
    d. 1 to 7 days after the end of menses

42. Which of the following is *not* an FDA-approved indication for the use of hormone therapy (HT)?

    a. Prevention of cardiovascular disease
    b. Prevention of osteoporosis
    c. Relief of moderate-to-severe symptoms of vaginal atrophy
    d. Relief of moderate-to-severe vasomotor symptoms

43. Although not an approved indication, studies have indicated that HT may have the benefit of decreasing the risk for:

    a. Colon cancer
    b. Major depression

c. Osteoarthritis
d. Ovarian cancer

44. A woman who is requesting contraception and who also wants to get pregnant in 1 year should avoid using:

a. Combination oral contraceptives
b. Fertility awareness methods
c. Progestin-only oral contraceptives
d. Progestin-only contraceptive injections

45. A woman plans to use the calendar method for contraception. She has charted her menstrual cycles for several months and has noted her longest cycle to be 30 days and her shortest cycle to be 27 days. She should abstain from sexual intercourse each cycle from day ___ through day ___.

a. 9; 19
b. 10; 15
c. 11; 18
d. 12; 16

46. Which of the following statements by a client indicates she needs additional information about use of the contraceptive vaginal ring?

a. I should insert a new ring every 7 days.
b. I should expect to have regular periods while using the ring.
c. My partner can use a male condom while I am wearing the ring.
d. The exact position of the ring in the vagina is not important.

47. According to CDC initiating progestin-only contraceptive injections (DMPA) is a Category 3 when which of the following conditions exists?

a. Age 35 years or older and smoking more than 15 cigarettes daily
b. History of deep vein thrombosis or pulmonary emboli
c. Unexplained vaginal bleeding prior to evaluation
d. Use of drugs that alter liver enzymes

48. A 4-week postpartum woman who is breastfeeding presents in your office to discuss her contraceptive options. Currently she is breastfeeding on demand and is not providing any supplements. She plans to continue breastfeeding for at least 6 months. Information for this woman concerning the lactational amenorrhea method of contraception should include:

a. The expected failure rate for this method of contraception is about 20%.
b. This method is considered effective for only 3 months postpartum.

c. The woman can rely on this method as long as she is not having periods.
d. Another method of contraception should be considered when the infant begins sleeping through the night.

49. The woman in question #48 asks if she can restart birth control pills while she is still breast-feeding. The best response would be:

a. Combination oral contraceptives are contraindicated during the duration of breastfeeding.
b. All hormonal methods of contraception should be avoided while she is breastfeeding.
c. She should wait until she is having regular periods before restarting her birth control pills.
d. Progestin-only pills may be a better option for her to start at 6 weeks postpartum.

50. A woman using a diaphragm for contraception has sexual intercourse at 8:00 a.m. on Friday, at 2:00 a.m. on Saturday and again at 8:00 a.m. on Saturday. When can she safely remove her diaphragm for effective contraception while minimizing problems related to leaving the diaphragm in for extended periods of time?

a. 10:00 a.m. on Saturday
b. 2:00 p.m. on Saturday
c. 10:00 p.m. on Saturday
d. 8:00 a.m. on Sunday

51. An individual who either has active hepatitis B infection or who is a carrier would have a positive test for:

a. Hepatitis B surface antigen
b. Hepatitis B surface antibody
c. Hepatitis B e-antigen
d. Hepatitis B e-antibody

52. Which of the following statements is true concerning rapid HIV tests when compared with EIA blood test sent to a lab?

a. It may take longer after exposure for rapid HIV test to be positive.
b. Positive results of rapid HIV test are definitive, so a confirmatory test is not necessary.
c. Rapid HIV screening tests have not been FDA approved.
d. Sensitivity of both types of tests is the same.

53. A 58-year-old female has a bone densitometry test with the results of T-score –2.0. This indicates the following:

a. She has bone density that is greater than that of most women her age.

b. She has bone density that is equal to that of a young normal adult.

c. She has bone loss that is at the level for a diagnosis of osteopenia.

d. She has bone loss that is at the level for a diagnosis of osteoporosis.

54. The gold standard test for herpes simplex virus is:

a. Pap test
b. Tissue culture
c. Type-specific serologic tests
d. Tzanck test

55. The anatomical area that contains the urethral/vaginal openings, hymen, Skene's glands and Bartholin glands is called the:

a. Labia majora
b. Perineum
c. Vestibule
d. Vulva

56. Findings on a pelvic examination of a 25-year-old female include uterus 7 cm in length, right ovary 3 cm × 2 cm, and left ovary nonpalpable. These findings indicate a/an:

a. Normal uterus, normal ovaries
b. Normal uterus, enlarged right ovary
c. Enlarged uterus, normal ovaries
d. Enlarged uterus, enlarged right ovary

57. Which of the following occurs first during female puberty?

a. Beginning breast development
b. Beginning pubic hair development
c. Growth spurt
d. Menstruation

58. Which of the following structures produces gonadotropin releasing hormone (GnRH)?

a. Anterior pituitary gland
b. Hypothalamus
c. Posterior pituitary gland
d. Ovaries

59. Which of the following list of events is in the correct chronological order?

a. LH surge, ovulation, rise in BBT, thickened cervical mucus
b. Ovulation, LH surge, thickened cervical mucus, rise in BBT
c. Rise in BBT, thickened cervical mucus, ovulation, LH surge
d. Thickened cervical mucus, rise in BBT, LH surge, ovulation

60. According to CDC recommendations, which of the following would be considered a Category 4 situation for the indicated contraceptive method?

a. Levonorgestrel-containing IUC for woman with endometriosis
b. Copper-containing IUC for woman with history of breast cancer
c. Progestin-only pills for woman with past history of deep vein thrombosis
d. Vaginal contraceptive ring for woman older than 35 years of age who smokes 1 ppd

61. An advantage of the female condom is:

a. It can be used with a male condom for added protection.
b. It can be used for repeated acts of intercourse.
c. It may be used by individuals with latex allergy.
d. It has a lower failure rate than the male condom.

62. Noncontraceptive benefits of combination oral contraceptives include all of the following *except*:

a. Decrease in risk for benign breast disease
b. Decrease in risk for cervical cancer
c. Decrease in risk for endometrial cancer
d. Decrease in risk for ovarian cancer

63. For which of the contraceptive methods is there the *least* difference between the perfect use and typical use failure rates?

a. Combination oral contraceptives
b. Diaphragm
c. Intrauterine device
d. Male condom

64. A woman who weighs 200 lbs or greater may have decreased effectiveness with which of the following contraceptive methods?

a. Progestin-only injectable contraception
b. Contraceptive vaginal ring
c. Levonorgestrel intrauterine system
d. Transdermal contraceptive system

65. A woman who is taking combination oral contraceptives should be advised to use a backup method of contraception for 7 days if she:

a. Misses two pills in the second week of her pill pack
b. Misses one pill in the third week of her pill pack
c. Starts her first pack of pills on the first day of her period
d. Starts her first pack of pills using the Quick-start method

66. A 20-year-old female who is 30% overweight presents for her first Depo Provera injection. Concerns in administering Depo Provera to this woman include:

   a. She may need a larger dose than the usual 150 mg.
   b. She should return for repeat injections every 2 months.
   c. You should massage the injection site well to assure absorption.
   d. You should choose a site that assures deep IM injection.

67. Instructions for progestin-only oral contraceptive users should include:

   a. If you are more than 3 hours late taking a pill, use a backup method for 48 hours.
   b. If two pills are missed in the third week of the pack, throw away the pack and start a new one.
   c. If you miss pills in the fourth week of the pack, you do not have to use a backup method.
   d. If you miss two pills in the first week of the pack, make them up and use a backup method for 7 days.

68. A 65-year-old female currently on a cyclic HT regimen is at your office for a routine annual examination. She states she has been healthy in the last year and is having no problems with HT. On bimanual examination, a 4-cm nontender right ovary is palpated. Appropriate management would include:

   a. Discontinue HT and repeat the bimanual examination in 2 months
   b. Have her return in 1 year as this is a normal finding for a 65-year-old woman
   c. Refer her to a gynecologist for further evaluation
   d. Switch to a continuous HT regimen and reexamine her in 2 months

69. The structure in the breast that is responsible for milk production is the:

   a. Areola
   b. Alveoli
   c. Lobule
   d. Lactiferous sinus

70. The hormone that stimulates synthesis of milk is:

   a. Aldosterone
   b. Estrogen
   c. Progesterone
   d. Prolactin

71. The menopausal woman may experience some changes in sensation or the orgasmic experience during sexual activity related to:

   a. Decreased vasocongestion and decreased vaginal expansion
   b. Decreased vasocongestion and increased vaginal expansion
   c. Increased vasocongestion and decreased vaginal expansion
   d. Increased vasocongestion and increased vaginal expansion

72. Which of the following contraceptive choices should *not* be recommended for the perimenopausal woman who is having irregular menses?

   a. Combination oral contraceptives
   b. Diaphragm
   c. Fertility awareness methods
   d. LNG intrauterine system

73. Endocervical curettage is performed to evaluate abnormalities of the:

   a. Endometrial tissue
   b. Glandular epithelium
   c. Squamous epithelium
   d. Transformation zone

74. A 26-year-old female is planning to use basal body temperatures for contraception. Which of the following statements would indicate that she needs further instruction on this method?

   a. I will take my temperature the same time each day before getting out of bed.
   b. I know that I am about to ovulate when my temperature rises at least 0.4 degrees.
   c. I will need to use a special thermometer to take my basal body temperature.
   d. A rise of 0.4 degrees above my baseline for 3 days indicates it is safe to have sex.

75. The mechanism of action of mifepristone in inducing abortion is:

   a. Antiprogesterone effect on the endometrium
   b. Cervical dilatation effect
   c. Stimulatory effect on the myometrium
   d. Toxic effect on the fertilized egg

76. Instructions/information for a new user of combination oral contraceptives should include:

   a. Combination oral contraceptives may decrease the effectiveness of some antibiotics.
   b. Discontinue your pills immediately if you miss a period.

c. Start the first pack of pills on the last day of your next period.

d. Sunday starters should use a backup method for the first week of the first pack of pills.

77. The most commonly used method of determining bone density to establish a diagnosis of osteoporosis or the need for preventive treatment is:

a. Dual energy x-ray absorptiometry
b. Quantitative computerized tomography
c. Quantitative ultrasound
d. Single x-ray absorptiometry

78. Instructions for the use of nonoxynol-9 spermicide should include:

a. Place spermicide close to the opening of the vagina for maximal effectiveness.
b. Remove excess spermicide from vagina within 6 hours to reduce vaginal irritation.
c. When used with a condom, spermicide will further decrease risk for STD.
d. Frequent use of spermicide may cause vaginal changes making you more susceptible to HIV infection.

79. According to CDC recommendations, which of the following is considered to be a Category 4 condition for use of the indicated contraceptive method?

a. Use of emergency contraceptive pills by a woman who has history of deep vein thrombosis
b. Insertion of IUC in a woman with a history of PID
c. Use of combination oral contraception by a 40-year-old woman who has migraine headaches without aura
d. Use of progestin-only pills by a woman who has diabetes type 2

80. Which of the following statements concerning coitus interruptus is *not* correct:

a. It has a lower perfect use failure rate than the cervical cap.
b. It may result in a decreased risk for HIV transmission to female partner.
c. Men are typically not able to predict the timing of ejaculation.
d. There is a decreased chance for the presence of preejaculatory sperm with repeat acts of intercourse.

◘ ANSWERS

1. **c**		41. **d**
2. **b**		42. **a**
3. **c**		43. **a**
4. **c**		44. **d**
5. **c**		45. **a**
6. **d**		46. **a**
7. **c**		47. **c**
8. **a**		48. **d**
9. **a**		49. **d**
10. **d**		50. **b**
11. **d**		51. **a**
12. **a**		52. **d**
13. **a**		53. **c**
14. **b**		54. **b**
15. **a**		55. **c**
16. **a**		56. **a**
17. **a**		57. **a**
18. **b**		58. **b**
19. **b**		59. **a**
20. **c**		60. **d**
21. **b**		61. **c**
22. **b**		62. **b**
23. **d**		63. **c**
24. **b**		64. **d**
25. **d**		65. **d**
26. **d**		66. **d**
27. **b**		67. **a**
28. **d**		68. **c**
29. **d**		69. **b**
30. **b**		70. **d**
31. **c**		71. **a**
32. **c**		72. **c**
33. **a**		73. **b**
34. **c**		74. **b**
35. **d**		75. **a**
36. **b**		76. **d**
37. **c**		77. **a**
38. **c**		78. **d**
39. **b**		79. **c**
40. **d**		80. **d**

◻ BIBLIOGRAPHY

Altman, A., Moore, A., Speroff, L., and Wysocki, S. (2009). Tackling the tricky issue of bioidentical hormones. *Women's Health Care: A Practical Journal for Nurse Practitioners, 8*(7), 7–15.

American Cancer Society. (2008). *How to perform breast self examination.* Retrieved on July 2009 from http://www.cancer.org/docroot/CRI/content/CRI_2_6x_How_to_perform_a_breast_self_exam_5.asp?sitearea.

American College of Obstetricians and Gynecologists. (2009). Cervical cytology screening. *ACOG Practice Bulletin, (109),* 1–12.

Centers for Disease Control and Prevention. (2010). U.S. medical eligibility criteria for contraceptive use. *Morbidity and Mortality Weekly Report, 59*(Early Release), 1–6.

Centers for Disease Control and Prevention. (2006). Sexually transmitted diseases treatment guidelines. *Morbidity and Mortality Weekly Report, 55*(RR11), 1–100.

Chernecky, C., & Berger, B. (2008). *Laboratory tests and diagnostic procedures* (5th ed.). St. Louis: Saunders Elsevier.

Gibbs, R., Karlan, B., Haney, A., & Nygaard, I. (2008). *Danforth's obstetrics and gynecology* (10th ed.). Philadelphia, PA: Lippincott, Williams, & Wilkins.

Hackley, B., Kriebs, J., & Rousseau, M. (2007). *Primary care of women: A guide for midwives and women's health providers.* Sudbury, MA: Jones and Bartlett.

Hatcher, R., Trussell, J., Nelson, A. et al. (2007). *Contraceptive technology* (19th ed.). New York: Ardent Media, Inc.

National Osteoporosis Foundation. (2008). *Clinician's guide to prevention and treatment of osteoporosis.* Washington, DC: National Osteoporosis Foundation.

Saslow, D., Runowicz, C., Solomon, D. et al. (2002). American Cancer Society guideline for the early detection of cervical neoplasia and cancer. *CA Cancer Journal for Clinicians, 52*(6), 342–362.

Seidel, H., Ball, J., Dains, J., & Benedict, W. (2006). *Mosby's guide to physical examination* (6th ed.). St. Louis: Mosby, Inc.

Smith, R., Saslow, D., Sawyer, K. et al. (2003). American Cancer Society guidelines for breast cancer screening: Update 2003. *CA Cancer Journal for Clinicians, 53*(3), 141–169.

Tharpe, N., & Farley, C. (2009). *Clinical practice guidelines for midwifery and women's health.* Sudbury, MA: Jones and Bartlett.

The North American Menopause Society. (2007). *Menopause practice: A clinician's guide* (3rd ed.). Cleveland, OH: Author.

World Health Organization. (2009). *Medical eligibility criteria for contraceptive use* (4th ed.). Geneva, Switzerland: Author.

4

Pregnancy

Patricia Burkhardt

◻ HUMAN REPRODUCTION AND FERTILIZATION

- Process of gametogenesis
  1. Definition—Development of gametes; oogenesis or spermatogenesis
  2. Essential concepts
     a. Oogenesis—developmental process by which the mature human ovum is formed; haploid number of chromosomes
     b. Spermatogenesis—formation of mature functional spermazoa; haploid number of chromosomes
     c. Meiosis—a process of two successive cell divisions, producing cells, egg or sperm, that contain half the number of chromosomes in somatic cells
     d. Mitosis—type of cell division of somatic cells in which each daughter cell contains the same number of chromosomes as the parent cell
     e. Haploid number of chromosomes 23—possessing half the diploid or normal number of chromosomes, i.e. 46, found in somatic or body cells

- Process of fertilization
  1. Definition—union of ovum and spermatozoan; usually occurs in fallopian tubes within minutes or no more than a few hours of ovulation; most pregnancies occur when intercourse occurs 2 days before, or on day of ovulation

  2. Stages of development
     a. Zygote—a diploid cell with 46 chromosomes that results from the fertilization of the ovum by a spermatozoan
     b. Blastomeres—mitotic division of the zygote (cleavage) yields daughter cells called blastomeres
     c. Morula—the solid ball of cells formed by 16 or so blastomeres; mulberry-like ball of cells that enters the uterine cavity 3 days after fertilization
     d. Blastocyst—after the morula reaches the uterus, a fluid accumulates between blastomeres, converting the morula to a blastocyst; inner cell mass at one pole to become embryo; outer cell mass will be trophoblast
     e. Embryo—stage in prenatal development between the fertilized ovum and the fetus, i.e., between second and eighth weeks inclusive
     f. Fetus—the developing conceptus after the embryonic stage
     g. Conceptus—all tissue products of conception; embryo (fetus), fetal membranes, and placenta

- Physiology of implantation of the blastocyst
  1. Definition—blastocyst adheres to the endometrial epithelium by gently eroding between the epithelial cells of the surface endometrium; invading trophoblasts burrow into the endometrium; the blastocyst becomes encased and covered over by the endometrium

2. Implantation occurs 6–7 days after fertilization and usually in the upper, posterior wall of the uterus
3. Provides physiologic exchange between the maternal and embryonic environment prior to full placental function

☐ DEVELOPMENT OF THE PLACENTA, MEMBRANES, AND AMNIOTIC FLUID

- Essential concepts
  1. Chorion—an extra-embryonic membrane that, in early development, forms the outer wall of the blastocyst; from it develop the chorionic villi, which establish an intimate connection with the endometrium, giving rise to the placenta
  2. Chorion frondosum—the outer surface of the chorion whose villi contact the decidua basalis; the placental portion of the chorion
  3. Chorion laeve—the smooth, nonvillous portion of the chorion
  4. Syncytiotrophoblast—outer layer of cells covering the chorionic villi of the placenta that are in contact with the maternal blood or decidua
  5. Cytotrophoblast—thin inner layer of the trophoblast composed of cuboidal cell
  6. Decidua capsularias—the part of the decidua that surrounds the chorionic sac
  7. Decidua basalis—the part of the uterine decidua that unites with the chorion to form the placenta
  8. Decidua parientalis (vera)—the endometrium during pregnancy except at the site of the implanted blastocyst
  9. Amnion—the innermost fetal membrane; a thin, transparent sac that holds the fetus suspended in the liquor amnii or amniotic fluid; it grows rapidly at the expense of the extra-embryonic coelom, and by the end of the third month it fuses with the chorion, forming the amniochorionic sac, commonly called the bag of waters

- Placenta—serves as fetal lungs, liver, and kidneys until birth while growing and maintaining the conceptus in a balanced, healthful environment
  1. Anatomy
     a. Trophoblasts
     b. Chorionic villi
     c. Intervillous spaces
     d. Chorion
     e. Amnion
     f. Decidual plate
  2. Steroid and protein hormones—human trophoblasts produce more steroid and protein

hormones diverse, in greater amounts than any endocrine tissue in all of mammalian physiology
     a. Steroid hormones
        (1) Estradiol-17B
        (2) Estriol
        (3) Progesterone
        (4) Aldosterone
        (5) Deoxycorticosterone
        (6) Cortisol
     b. Protein and peptide hormones
        (1) Placental lactogen (hPL)
        (2) Chorionic gonadatropin (hCG)
        (3) Chorionic adrenocorticotropin (ACTH)
        (4) Pro-opiomelanocortin
        (5) Chorionic thyrotropin
        (6) Growth hormone variant
        (7) Parathyroid hormone-related protein (PTH-rP)
        (8) Calcitonin
        (9) Relaxin
     c. Hypothalamic-like releasing and inhibiting hormones
        (1) Thyrotropin-releasing hormone (TRH)
        (2) Gonadotropin-releasing hormone (GnRH)
        (3) Corticotropin-releasing hormone (CRH)
        (4) Somatostatin
        (5) Growth hormone-releasing hormone (GHRH)
     d. Regulation of blood flow in the placenta; maternal blood traverses the placenta randomly without preformed channels and enters the intervillous spaces in spurts propelled by the maternal arterial pressure
     e. The placental "barrier"—the placenta does not maintain absolute integrity between maternal and fetal circulations as indicated by the presence of fetal blood cells found in maternal circulation and the development of erythroblastosis fetalis

- Umbilical cord
  1. Anatomy
     a. Vessels—two arteries that carry fetal deoxygenated blood to the placenta; smaller in diameter than the vein, and one vein carrying oxygenated blood from the placenta to the fetus characterized by twisting or spiraling to minimize snarling
     b. Measurements—0.8–2 cm in diameter; average length of 55 cm with range of 30–100 cm

c. Wharton's jelly—extracellular matrix consisting of specialized connective tissue

2. Abnormalities of length—positively influenced by amniotic fluid volume and fetal mobility

a. Extremely short cord—associated with abruptio placentae or uterine inversion; the latter is rare

b. Abnormally long cord—associated with vascular occlusion by thrombi and true knots

- Amniotic fluid
  1. Production—produced by amniotic epithelium; water transfers across amnion and through fetal skin; in second trimester fetus starts to swallow, urinate and inspire amniotic fluid
  2. Volume maintenance—fetal swallowing seems to be a critical mechanism since polyhydramnios is consistently present when fetal swallowing is inhibited, but other factors contribute to volume balance
  3. Polyhydramnios—amniotic fluid index (AFI) greater than 24–25 cm
     a. Incidence—about 1% of all pregnancies
     b. Significance—two thirds are idiopathic; one third associated with fetal anomalies, maternal diabetes, or multiple gestation
     c. Etiology—central nervous system or gastrointestinal tract fetal anomalies, e.g., anencephaly, esophageal atresia
     d. Signs and symptoms—uterine size far beyond expected for gestational age (GA), difficulty auscultating fetal heart rate (FHR) and palpating fetal parts, mechanical pressure exerted by the large uterus, i.e., dyspnea, edema, heartburn, nausea
     e. Diagnosis
        (1) Physical findings—uterine enlargement associated with difficulty feeling fetal parts and auscultating fetal heartbeat
        (2) Ultrasonography (USG) differentiates from ascites or large ovarian cyst; may also identify an associated fetal anomaly
     f. Pregnancy outcome—the greater the polyhydramnios, the higher the perinatal mortality; preterm labor increases; also associated with erythroblastosis
     g. Management—treat only if symptomatic
        (1) Amniocentesis—to relieve maternal distress; will enable testing of fetal lung maturity and chromosome studies

        (2) Indomethacin—impairs production of lung liquid, increases fluid movement through fetal membranes or decreases fetal urine production

  4. Oligohydramnios—volume of amniotic fluid much less than normal
     a. Conditions associated with oligohydramnios
        (1) Fetal—almost always present with fetal urinary tract obstruction or renal agenesis
           (a) Chromosomal abnormalities
           (b) Congenital anomalies
           (c) Growth restriction
           (d) Demise
           (e) Postterm pregnancy
           (f) Ruptured membranes
        (2) Placental
           (a) Abruption
           (b) Twin-twin transfusion
        (3) Maternal
           (a) Uteroplacental insufficiency
           (b) Hypertension
           (c) Preeclampsia
           (d) Diabetes
        (4) Drugs
           (a) Prostaglandin synthesis inhibitors
           (b) Angiotensin-converting enzyme inhibitors
           (c) Idiopathic
     b. Prognosis
        (1) Early onset has poor outcome and risk of pulmonary hyperplasia greatly increased
        (2) Late pregnancy onset leads to more Cesarean sections for fetal distress
     c. Management—amnioinfusion is used most often in labor to prevent umbilical cord compression

◻ EMBRYONIC AND FETAL DEVELOPMENT

- Embryonic development—from the beginning of third week after fertilization to the end of the seventh week
  1. Fourth week—partitioning of heart begins; arm and leg buds form; amnion begins to unsheathe the body stalk that becomes the umbilical cord
  2. Sixth week—head is much larger than body; heart is completely formed; fingers and toes present
  3. All major organ systems are formed except for lungs

- Fetal development: Begins 8 weeks after fertilization; 10 weeks after onset of LMP
  1. 12 weeks—uterus palpable at the symphysis; fetus begins to make spontaneous movements
  2. 16 weeks—experienced observers can determine gender on ultrasound
  3. 20 weeks—weighs 300 g; weight now begins to increase in a linear manner
  4. 24 weeks—weighs 630 g; fat deposition begins; terminal sacs in the lungs still not completely formed
  5. 28 weeks—weighs 1100 g; papillary membrane has just disappeared from the eyes; has 90% chance of survival if otherwise normal
  6. 32–36 weeks—continues to increase weight as more subcutaneous fat accumulates

◘ DIAGNOSIS AND DATING OF PREGNANCY

- Diagnosis
  1. Signs of pregnancy
     a. Presumptive—subjective (what the woman reports)
        (1) Amenorrhea
        (2) Nausea and/or vomiting
        (3) Urinary frequency, nocturia
        (4) Fatigue
        (5) Breast tenderness, tingling, enlargement, and changes in color
        (6) Vasomotor symptoms (fainting)
        (7) Skin changes
        (8) Congestion of vaginal mucus
        (9) Maternal belief that she is pregnant
     b. Presumptive—objective (physical examination)
        (1) Continuation of elevated basal body temperature
        (2) Chadwick's sign
        (3) Appearance of Montgomery's tubercles or follicles
        (4) Expression of colostrum
        (5) Breast changes
     c. Probable
        (1) Enlargement of the abdomen
        (2) Enlargement of the uterus
        (3) Palpation of the fetal outline
        (4) Ballottement
        (5) Change in the shape of the uterus
        (6) Piskacek's sign
        (7) Hegar's sign
        (8) Goodell's sign
        (9) Palpation of Braxton Hicks contractions
        (10) Positive pregnancy test
     d. Positive
        (1) Fetal heart tones
        (2) Sonographic evidence of pregnancy
        (3) Palpation of fetal movement
  2. Differential diagnosis
     a. Pregnancy
     b. Leiomyoma
     c. Ovarian cyst
     d. Pseudocyesis

- Dating of pregnancy—determining estimated date of confinement or delivery or birth (EDC or EDD or EDB)
  1. Average duration of human pregnancy—280 days, 10 lunar months, 9 calendar months
  2. Methods to determine EDC, EDD, EDB
     a. Naegele's rule—subtract 3 months, add 7 days to the first day of the last menstrual period (LMP) then add 1 year *or* add 9 months and 7 days to the first day of the LMP
     b. Additional information is needed to more precisely set EDB, which can include:
        (1) Complete menstrual history
        (2) Contraceptive history
        (3) Sexual history
        (4) Physical examination for signs and symptoms of pregnancy
        (5) Quickening
  3. USG for gestational age determination
     a. Combination of measurements is more accurate than any one of the following measurements:
        (1) Crown rump length (CRL)
        (2) Biparietal diameter
        (3) Head circumference
        (4) Abdominal circumference
        (5) Femur length
     b. Accuracy by trimester
        (1) First trimester—CRL is accurate to 3–5 days
        (2) Second trimester—Biparietal diameter and femur length are most accurate to within 7–10 days
        (3) Third trimester—after 26 weeks all measurements are less accurate; variation in biparietal diameter and femur length is 14–21 days

◘ MATERNAL PHYSIOLOGIC ADAPTATIONS TO PREGNANCY

- Effects of pregnancy on the organs of reproduction and implications for clinical practice
  1. Uterus
     a. Nonpregnant uterus is about 70 g with a 10 mL cavity
     b. First trimester—at 6 weeks the uterus is soft, globular, and asymmetric (Piskacek's

sign); at 12 weeks it is 8–10 cm and is rising out of the pelvis

   c. Early second trimester—at 14 weeks the uterus is one quarter of the way to umbilicus; at 16 weeks it is half way to the umbilicus; 20 weeks the fundus is approximately at the umbilicus
   d. After 20 weeks, number of centimeters with tape measure equals number of weeks of gestation within 2 cm
   e. By term the uterus weighs about 1100 g with a 5-liter volume

2. Cervix
   a. Develops increased vascularity
   b. Hegar's sign is softening of the isthmus
   c. Chadwick's sign is bluish color of the cervix
   d. Goodell's sign is softening of the cervix
   e. A thick mucous plug forms secondary to glandular proliferation

3. Ovaries—corpus luteum
   a. Anovulation secondary to hormonal interruption of the feedback loop
   b. Corpus luteum persists under the influence of the hormone hCG until about 12 weeks
   c. Corpus luteum is responsible for the secretion of progesterone to maintain the endometrium and pregnancy until the placenta takes over production
   d. Ovaries also thought responsible for production of relaxin

4. Vagina
   a. Chadwick's sign—bluish color
   b. Thickening of vaginal mucosa
   c. Increase in vaginal secretions
   d. Some loosening of connective tissue in preparation for birth

5. Breasts
   a. Increase in size secondary to mammary hyperplasia
   b. Areola becomes more deeply pigmented and increased in size
   c. Colostrum may be expressed after the first several months
   d. Montgomery's follicles
   e. Vascularity increases

6. Pelvis—four pelvic types
   a. Anthropoid
      (1) 23.5% of white women and 50% of nonwhite women
      (2) Shape favors a posterior position of the fetus
      (3) Adequate for a vaginal birth due to large size
   b. Android
      (1) Commonly known as a "male" pelvis
      (2) 32.5% of white women and 15.7% of nonwhite women
      (3) Heavy heart-shaped pelvis leads to increased posterior positions, dystocia, operative births
   c. Gynecoid
      (1) Commonly known as the "female" pelvis
      (2) 41–42% of women's pelvis shapes
      (3) Good prognosis for vaginal birth
   d. Platypelloid
      (1) Rare pelvic type
      (2) Occurs in less than 3% of women
      (3) Prognosis of vaginal delivery is poor secondary to short AP diameter

- Effect of pregnancy on major body systems, with related clinical implications and patient education needs
1. Gastrointestinal
   a. Mouth and pharynx
      (1) Gingivitis is common and may result in bleeding of gums
      (2) Increased salivation
      (3) Epulis (a focal swelling of gums) may develop and resolves after the birth
      (4) Pregnancy does not increase tooth decay
   b. Esophagus
      (1) Decreased lower esophageal sphincter pressure and tone
      (2) Widening of hiatus with decreased tone
      (3) Heartburn is common
   c. Stomach
      (1) Decreased gastric emptying time
      (2) Incompetence of pyloric sphincter
      (3) Decreased gastric acidity and histamine output
   d. Large and small intestines
      (1) Decreased tone and motility
      (2) Altered enzymatic transport across villi resulting in increased absorption of vitamins
      (3) Displacement of intestines, cecum, and appendix by the enlarging uterus
   e. Gallbladder
      (1) Decreased tone
      (2) Decreased motility
   f. Liver
      (1) Altered production of liver enzymes
      (2) Altered production of plasma proteins and serum lipids
2. Genitourinary/renal
   a. Dilation of renal calyces, pelvis, and ureters resulting in increased risk of urinary tract infection

  b. Decreased bladder tone

  c. Renal blood flow increases 35–60%

  d. Decreased renal threshold for glucose, protein, water soluble vitamins, calcium, and hydrogen ions

  e. Glomerular filtration rate increases 40–50%

  f. All components of the renal-angiotensin-aldosterone system increase, resulting in retention of sodium and water, resistance of pressor effect of angiotensin II, and maintenance of normal blood pressure

3. Musculoskeletal

  a. Relaxin and progesterone affect cartilage and connective tissue

   (1) Results in a loosening of the sacroiliac joint and symphysis pubis

   (2) Encourages the development of the characteristic gait of pregnancy

  b. Lordosis

4. Respiratory

  a. Level of diaphragm rises about 4 cm because of the increase in uterine size

  b. Thoracic circumference increases by 5–6 cm and residual volume is decreased

  c. A mild respiratory alkalosis occurs due to decreased PCO_2

  d. Congestion of nasal tissues occurs

  e. Respiratory rate changes very little, but the tidal volume, minute ventilatory, and minute oxygen uptake all appreciably increase

  f. Some women experience a physiologic dyspnea, due to the increased tidal volume and lower PCO_2

5. Hematologic changes

  a. Blood volume increases 30–50% from nonpregnant levels

  b. Plasma volume expands which results in a physiologic anemia

  c. Hemoglobin averages 12.5 g/dL

  d. Some require an additional gram of iron during pregnancy

  e. Pregnancy can be considered a hypercoagulable state, since fibrinogen (Factor I), and Factors VII–X all increase during pregnancy

6. Cardiovascular system

  a. Cardiac volume increases by about 10% and peaks at about 20 weeks

  b. Resting pulse increases by 10–15 beats per minute with the peak at 28 weeks

  c. Slight cardiac shift (up and to the left) due to the enlarging uterus

  d. 90% of pregnant women develop a physiologic systolic heart murmur

  e. May have exaggerated splitting of S1, audible third sound, or soft transient diastolic murmur

  f. Cardiac output is increased

  g. Diastolic blood pressure is lower in first two trimesters due to development of new vascular beds and relaxation of peripheral tone by progesterone that results in decreased flow resistance

7. Integumentary system

  a. Vascular changes

   (1) Palmar erythema

   (2) Spider angiomas

   (3) Varicose veins and hemorrhoids

   (4) Hyperpigmentation is believed to be related to estrogens and progesterone which have a melanocyte-stimulating effect

   (5) Chloasma, freckles, nevi, and recent scars may darken

   (6) Linea nigra

   (7) Increase in sweat/sebaceous activity

   (8) Change in connective tissues resulting in striae gravidarum

  b. Hair growth

   (1) Estrogen increases the length of the anagen (growth) phase of the hair follicles

   (2) Mild hirsutism may develop in early pregnancy

8. Endocrine

  a. Pituitary

   (1) Prolactin levels are 10 times higher at term than in the nonpregnant state

   (2) Enlarges by over 100%

  b. Thyroid

   (1) Increases in size (about 13%)

   (2) Normal pregnant woman is euthyroid due to estrogen-induced increase in thyroxin binding globulin (TBG)

   (3) Thyroid-stimulating hormone (TSH) does not cross the placenta

   (4) Thyroid stimulating immunoglobulins and Thyrotropin-releasing hormone (TRH) cross the placenta

  c. Adrenal glands

   (1) Remain the same size, however, there is an increase in the zona fasciculata that produces glucocorticoid

   (2) Twofold increase in serum cortisol

  d. Pancreas

   (1) Hypertrophy and hyperplasia of the B cells

   (2) Insulin resistance as a result of the placental hormones especially hPL

9. Metabolism
   a. Weight gain during pregnancy
      (1) Recommended weight gain is 11–40 lb depending on prepregnancy body mass index (BMI)
      (2) Average weight gain is 28 lbs—1.5 lb for placenta, 2 lb for amniotic fluid, 2.5 lb for uterine growth, 3 lb for increased blood volume, 1 lb for increased breast tissue, 7.5 lb for the fetus and the remainder for maternal fat deposits
      (3) Protein metabolism is increased
      (4) Fat deposit and storage is increased to prepare for breastfeeding
      (5) Carbohydrate metabolism is altered, the blood glucose levels are 10–20% lower than prepregnant states

❑ MATERNAL PSYCHOLOGICAL/ SOCIAL CHANGES IN PREGNANCY

- Pregnancy is a time of many transitions, a woman is vulnerable, and maternal moods are labile

- First trimester (1–13 weeks)——focus on physical changes and feelings
   1. Psychological responses
      a. Ambivalence
      b. Adjustment
   2. Prenatal anticipatory guidance
      a. Normal changes of pregnancy; breast fullness, urinary frequency, nausea/vomiting, and fatigue
      b. Calculate and explain EDD and comparison with uterine size
      c. Client's and healthcare provider's expectations for visits
      d. Importance of ongoing care in pregnancy to promote well-being and prevent problems
      e. Rationale for vitamins and iron supplements
      f. Resources available for education, emergency care, etc.
      g. Discuss/review danger signs and symptoms

- Second trimester (14–26 weeks)—more aware of the fetus as a person
   1. Psychological responses
      a. Acceptance
      b. Period of radiant health
   2. Prenatal anticipatory guidance
      a. Fetal growth, movement and fetal heart tones (FHT)
      b. Personal hygiene, brassieres, vaginal discharge, etc.
      c. Infant feeding—breast and/or bottle
      d. Avoidance and alleviation of—backache, constipation, hemorrhoids, leg aches, varicosities, edema and round ligament pain
      e. Nutritional needs, diet and weight gain.
      f. Discuss/review danger signs and symptoms

- Third trimester
   1. First part (27–36 weeks)—concerned with baby's needs
      a. Psychological responses
         (1) Introversion
         (2) Period of watchful waiting
      b. Prenatal anticipatory guidance
         (1) Fetal growth and well-being
         (2) Review hygiene, clothing, body mechanics and posture, positions of comfort
         (3) Physical and emotional changes
         (4) Sexual needs/intercourse
         (5) Alleviation of backache, Braxton Hicks contractions, dyspnea, round ligament pain, leg aches or edema
         (6) Confirm infant feeding plans and discuss preparation for breastfeeding
         (7) Preparation for baby supplies and help at home
         (8) Prenatal classes/approach
         (9) Involvement of significant other
         (10) Review danger signs at each visit
         (11) If planning tubal ligation, prepare papers if required
      c. Women anticipate birth and infant care
         (1) Discuss fetal movement
         (2) Personal hygiene needs/concerns, alleviation of discomforts of pregnancy
         (3) Discuss recognition of Braxton Hicks and prodromal contractions and differentiation from true labor
         (4) Discuss labor, contractions, and labor progress and expectations of labor
         (5) Breathing and relaxation techniques; labor support options
         (6) Provisions for needs of other children, sibling issues, and care of children during hospital stay
         (7) Review signs of labor
         (8) Continue discussion of relaxation and breathing techniques; latent labor coping skills
         (9) Final home preparations
         (10) Discuss procedures particular to home/birthing center (BC), hospital—analgesia, IVs, examinations, labor

care, birthing plans, postpartum care, and supplies needed

    (11) Confirm plans for transport to the hospital, who to call, and where to go; hospitalization and process of admission

    (12) Consider birth control/family planning needs

    (13) Discuss emergency arrangements in the event of danger signs, premature rupture of membranes (PROM), bleeding, severe headache, pain, etc.

- Risk factors for psychological well-being
  1. Limited support network
  2. High levels of stress
  3. Psych/mental health issues
  4. Problem pregnancies

OVERVIEW OF ANTEPARTUM CARE

- Purpose and objectives of antepartum care—to differentiate normal and pathologic maternal-fetal alterations throughout pregnancy by employing maternal-fetal assessment methods, techniques, and parameters appropriate to the antepartum period, specifically:
  1. Application of the management process including components of history and physical examination at initial and interval visits
  2. Critical evaluation of indications and techniques for the application of therapeutics during the antepartum period
  3. Incorporation of current evidence and research in the care of women and families during the antepartum period

- Definition of the essential concepts (National Center for Health Statistics and the Centers for Disease Control and Prevention, 2003)
  1. Fertility rate—number of live births/1000 females 15–44 years of age
  2. Birth rate—number of live births per 1000 population
  3. Live birth—infant at, or sometime after birth breathes spontaneously, or shows any other sign of life
  4. Stillbirth (fetal death)—no signs of life are present at or after birth
  5. Neonatal period—28 completed days after birth
  6. Perinatal period—all births weighing 500 g or more and ending at 28 completed days after birth; when perinatal rates are based on gestational age, this is defined as 20 weeks or longer

  7. Stillbirth rate (fetal death rate)—number of stillborn infants per 1000 infants born, including live births and stillbirths
  8. Neonatal death—early neonatal death is death during the first 7 days after birth; late neonatal death is death between 7 and 28 days
  9. Neonatal mortality rate—number of neonatal deaths/1000 live births
  10. Perinatal mortality rate—number of stillbirths plus neonatal deaths per total births
  11. Infant mortality rate—number of infant deaths (first 12 months of life) per 1000 live births
  12. Maternal morbidity—illness or disease associated with childbearing
  13. Maternal mortality ratio—number of maternal deaths that result from the reproductive process/100,000 live births
  14. Abortus—fetus or embryo removed or expelled from the uterus during the first half of gestation (20 weeks or less), weighing less than 500 g
  15. Preterm infant—infant born before 37 completed weeks (259th day)
  16. Term infant—infant born after 37 completed weeks of gestation up until 42 completed weeks of gestations (260–294 days)
  17. Postterm infant—infant born anytime after completion of the 42nd week beginning with day 295
  18. Direct maternal death—death of the mother resulting from obstetrical complications of pregnancy, labor, or the puerperium; and from interventions, omissions, incorrect treatment, or a chain of events resulting from any of these factors

ANTEPARTUM VISIT

- Terminology that describes women and their pregnancies (Varney, Kriebs, & Gegor, 2004)
  1. Gravida—the number of times a woman has been pregnant
  2. Para—refers to the number of pregnancies that terminated in the birth of a fetus or fetuses that reached the point of viability, i.e., 500 g or 20 weeks' gestation
  3. Nulligravida—a woman who has never been pregnant
  4. Nullipara—a woman in her first pregnancy or who has not carried a baby to 500 g or 20 weeks
  5. Primigravida—a woman who is pregnant for the first time
  6. Primipara—a woman who had one pregnancy that ended with a birth in which the fetus reached the age of viability
  7. Multigravida—a woman pregnant two or more times

8. Multipara—has carried two or more pregnancies to viability
9. Grand multipara—has given birth seven times or more
10. TPAL numerical description of parity—four-digit system that counts all fetuses/babies born rather than pregnancies carried to viability: T = term babies ($\geq$ 37 wks or 2500 g), P = premature babies (20–36 wks; 500–2499 g), A = Abortions (any fetus born < 20 wks and 500 g), L = living children currently

- Components of the antepartum visit (initial and return)
  1. The Pregnant Patient's Bill of Rights
  2. Complete history
     a. Menstrual history
     b. Contraceptive history
     c. Obstetric history including quickening
     d. Medical/Surgical history
     e. Sexual history
     f. History or current physical, sexual, emotional abuse
     g. Medicines and/or nonallopathic healing practices
     h. Family history
     i. Genetic risk
     j. Health habits
     k. Environmental exposures
     l. Social history
     m. Exercise and nutrition history
     n. Immunizations
  3. Physical examination
     a. Height, weight, and vital signs
     b. Complete physical examination
     c. Abdominal examination
        (1) Fundal height—growth by weeks of gestation
        (2) Leopold's maneuvers—four abdominal palpation maneuvers used to determine the following fetal characteristics:
           (a) Lie
           (b) Presentation
           (c) Position
           (d) Attitude
           (e) Variety
           (f) Estimated fetal weight
        (4) Fetal heart tones—dating pregnancy and assessing fetal position; different timing using fetoscope or doptone
        (5) Bimanual examination
        (6) Uterine sizing—first trimester to determine gestational age
        (7) Clinical pelvimetry—measurement of the features of the bony pelvis with the examiner's hand

d. The pelvis—(only the true pelvis is of significance) true pelvis is bony canal through which the fetus passes that lies below the pelvic brim (linea terminalis)
   (1) Three planes of obstetric significance—inlet, midplane, and outlet
   (2) Critical diameters for evaluation of pelvic adequacy
      (a) Inlet—AP, transverse
      (b) Midplane—AP, transverse, posterior sagittal
      (c) Outlet—AP, transverse, posterior sagittal
   (3) Assessing and measuring the pelvis—clinical pelvimetry
      (a) Diagonal conjugate—extends from middle of sacral promontory to middle of lower margin of symphysis pubis; only AP diameter that can be measured clinically; should be more than 11.5 cm
      (b) Pubic arch—formed by the descending rami of pubic bones and inferior margin of symphysis pubis; angle should be at least 90 degrees
      (c) Interspinous diameter—distance between the ischial spines, normally measures 10 cm, is smallest diameter of the pelvis and defines the midplane
      (d) Ischial spines—may be prominent, encroaching or blunt; assess the sidewalls and the sacrum; best if blunt
      (e) Sacrosciatic notch—note shape and width in fingerbreadths
      (f) Side walls—side walls extend from the upper anterior angle of the sacrosciatic notch to the ischial tuberosities and are assessed as straight, convergent, or divergent; should be straight
      (g) Sacrum—assess the inclination of the sacrum, the length, and the curvature; curved is best
      (h) Intertuberous diameter—distance between the ischial tuberosities, about 11 cm

4. Laboratory studies used in the provision of antepartum care
   a. Initial visit
      (1) Blood type, Rh factor, antibody screen, CBC or hematocrit, RPR or VDRL, rubella titer, hepatitis B surface antigen (HB_sAg), urine culture/screen

(2) HIV testing should be recommended to all pregnant women with option to decline testing

(3) Gonorrhea, chlamydia, and wet prep tests as indicated by history and physical examination findings

(4) Pap test per routine recommendations

(5) PPD, Hgb electrophoresis, genetic screening tests as indicated by history and risk factors

b. Multiple marker screen—triple screen (maternal serum alphafetoprotein [MSAFP], estriol and hCG) or quad screen (MSAFP, estriol, hCG and inhibin A) at 15–22 weeks' gestation (optimal 16–18 weeks)

c. Ultrasound—may perform at approximately 18–20 weeks for gestational age and fetal structural evaluation

d. Gestational diabetes screening at 24–28 weeks—see section this chapter on Selected Obstetrical Complications—Diabetes

e. Repeat antibody screen at 26–28 weeks for Rh-negative mother

f. Repeat CBC/Hct, VDRL/RPR, Chlamydia, GC, HIV, HBsAg as indicated by history, physical examination findings, and risk factors in third trimester

g. Group B streptococcus (GBS) screening at 35–37 weeks—vaginal introitus and rectal specimens

h. Some other laboratory studies that might be indicated include:

(1) Amniocentesis or chorionic villus sampling(CVS)

(2) Tay-Sachs screening

(3) Maternal/paternal chromosomal studies

(4) Chest radiographs

(5) Blood chemistry (SMA 6 & 12, or Chem 7 & 20)

(6) Thyroid studies

(7) Toxoplasmosis testing

(8) Cytomegalovirus (CMV)

(9) HSV cultures or antibody testing

(10) ANA

(11) Antiphospholipid antibodies

(12) Serum iron studies

(13) Blood glucose studies (3-hour GTT, FBS, 2-hour postprandial, and hemoglobin A1c)

5. Subsequent (interval) prenatal visits—frequency of

a. Every 4 weeks to 28 or 32 weeks

b. From 28 or 32 weeks to 36 weeks every 2 weeks

c. Weekly visits from 36 weeks to 41 weeks

d. Some prefer biweekly visits 41 weeks to delivery

e. Schedule more frequent visits as appropriate; some providers recommend fewer prenatal visits if there are no problems

6. Content of prenatal revisits

a. History

b. Physical examination—blood pressure, urine dipstick, weight, FHT, fundal height

c. Anticipatory management

d. Anticipatory guidance

e. Health education and counseling

f. Appropriate screening

- Prenatal risk factors

1. History

a. Genetic factors

(1) Maternal age at or older than 35

(2) Previous child with a chromosome abnormality

(3) Family history of birth defects or mental retardation

(4) Ethnic/racial origins

(a) African—sickle cell disease

(b) Mediterranean or East Asian—B thalassemia

(c) Jewish—Tay-Sachs disease

b. Multiple pregnancy losses/previous stillbirth

c. Psychological/mental health disorders

d. History of IUGR

e. Preterm birth(s)

2. Current pregnancy

a. Abnormal multiple marker screening

b. Exposure to possible teratogens

(1) Radiation

(2) Alcohol/medications/other substances

(3) Occupational exposures

(4) Infections

(a) Toxoplasmosis

(b) Rubella

(c) CMV

(d) Syphilis

c. Intrauterine Growth Retardation (IUGR)

d. Oligohydramnios/polyhydramnios

e. Diabetes

(1) Pregestational

(2) Gestational

(3) Insulin dependent

f. Hypertension

(1) Chronic

(2) Gestational

g. Preeclampsia/eclampsia

h. Multiple gestation

i. PROM

j. Post dates

k. Decreased fetal movement
l. Rh isoimmunization

◻ COMMON DISCOMFORTS OF PREGNANCY AND COMFORT MEASURES

- Nausea and vomiting of pregnancy (most common in first trimester)
  1. Small frequent meals, no restriction on the kind of food nor how often
  2. Discontinue prenatal vitamins with iron until nausea and vomiting resolved; continue folic acid
  3. Raspberry tea or peppermint tea, carbonated beverages, hard candy
  4. Acupressure, including sea bands for wrists
  5. Ginger 1 g per day in divided doses
  6. Pyridoxine (Vitamin B_6) 25 mg bid or tid orally
  7. Doxylamine 12.5 mg bid or qid with pyridoxine orally
  8. Metoclopramide 5 to 10 mg g q6–8h orally
  9. Promethazine 25 mg q4h per rectal suppository

- Breast tenderness
  1. Good support brassiere
  2. Careful lovemaking
  3. Reassurance that it will soon pass

- Backache
  1. Consider musculoskeletal strain, sciatica, sacroiliac joint problem, preterm labor, urinary tract infection
  2. Nonpathologic—related to normal changes in pregnancy
     a. Massage
     b. Application of ice or heat
     c. Hydrotherapy
     d. Pelvic rock
     e. Good body mechanics
     f. Pillow in lumbar area when sitting, or between legs when lying on side
     g. Pregnancy support harness or girdle
     h. Good support brassiere
     i. Supportive low-heeled shoes
  3. Sacroiliac joint problems
     a. Teach appropriate exercises
     b. Nonelastic sacroiliac belt
     c. Trochanteric belt worn below the abdomen at the femoral heads to increase joint stability

- Fatigue
  1. Reassurance that this is a normal first trimester problem and will pass
  2. Mild exercise and good nutrition

  3. Decrease activities and plan rest periods
  4. Decrease fluid intake in evening to decrease nocturia

- Heartburn
  1. Small frequent meals
  2. Decrease amount of fluids taken with meals; drink fluids between meals
  3. Papaya (may recommend fresh, dried, juice, or enzymes)
  4. Elevate head of bed 10–30 degrees
  5. Slippery Elm Bark throat lozenges
  6. Antacids
  7. Proton pump inhibitors and H_2 blockers—Pregnancy Category B

- Constipation
  1. Increased fluids, fiber
  2. Prune juice or warm beverage in the morning
  3. Encourage exercise
  4. Stool softeners

- Hemorrhoids
  1. Avoid constipation or straining with a bowel movement
  2. Elevate hips with pillow or knee–chest position
  3. Sitz baths
  4. Witch hazel or epsom salt compresses
  5. Reinsert hemorrhoid with lubricated finger
  6. Kegel exercises
  7. Topical anesthetics; Pregnancy Category C if combined with steroid

- Varicosities
  1. Support stockings; apply before getting out of bed
  2. Avoid wearing restrictive clothing
  3. Perineal pad if vaginal varicosities
  4. Rest periods with legs elevated; avoid crossing legs

- Leg cramps
  1. Decrease phosphate in diet; no more than two glasses of milk per day
  2. Massage affected leg
  3. Don't point toes, flex ankle to stretch calf
  4. Keep legs warm
  5. Walk, exercise
  6. Calcium tablets
  7. Magnesium tablets

- Presyncopal episodes
  1. Change positions slowly
  2. Push fluids; regular caloric/glucose intake
  3. Avoid lying flat on back; avoid prolonged standing or sitting

- Headaches
  1. Head, shoulder, and/or neck massage
  2. Acupressure
  3. Hot or cold compresses
  4. Rest
  5. Warm baths
  6. Meditation and biofeedback
  7. Aromatherapy
  8. Mild analgesic such as acetaminophen 325 mg 1–3 tablets every 4 hours as needed

- Leukorrhea
  1. Rule out vaginitis and STDs
  2. Good perineal hygiene
  3. Wear cotton crotch panties; change panties as often as necessary
  4. Unscented pantiliners
  5. Instructions to avoid douching and use of feminine sprays

- Urinary frequency
  1. Decrease fluids in evening to avoid nocturia
  2. Avoid caffeine
  3. Rule out urinary tract infection

- Insomnia
  1. Warm bath
  2. Hot drink—warm milk, chamomile tea
  3. Quiet, relaxing, minimally stimulating activities
  4. Avoid daytime napping

- Round ligament pain
  1. Rule out other causes of abdominal pain, such as appendicitis, ovarian cyst, placental separation, inguinal hernia
  2. Warm compresses, ice compresses
  3. Hydrotherapy
  4. Avoid sudden movement or twisting movements
  5. Flex knees to abdomen, pelvic tilt
  6. Support uterus with a pillow when lying down
  7. Maternity abdominal support or girdle

- Skin rash
  1. Ice
  2. Aveeno bath
  3. Diphenhydramine—25 mg orally every 4 hours as needed for itching
  4. Dermatology referral as needed

- Carpal tunnel syndrome (tingling and numbness of fingers)
  1. Good posture
  2. Lying down
  3. Rest and elevate affected hands
  4. Ice, wrist splints

  5. Mild analgesic such as acetaminophen 325 mg 1–3 tabs every 4 hours as needed

◘ NUTRITION DURING PREGNANCY

- Recommended daily allowances
  1. Calories—2,500 kcal
  2. Protein—average of 60 g/day throughout pregnancy

- Weight gain in pregnancy
  1. Body mass index (BMI) (weight/height^2)—only anthropometric measurements with documented clinical value for assessment of gestational weight gain
  2. Weight-for-height categories
     a. Underweight—BMI less than18.5
     b. Normal weight—BMI 18.5–24.9
     c. Overweight—BMI 25.0–29.9
     d. Obese—BMI 30.0 or higher
  3. Determinants of gestational weight gain
     a. Prepregnant weight—if overweight at conception more likely to gain less weight than normal-weight woman
     b. Low gestational weight gain associated with
        (1) Low family income
        (2) Black race
        (3) Young age
        (4) Unmarried status
        (5) Low educational level
     c. Multiple gestation
     d. Developing pathology—toxemia
  4. Consequences of gestational weight gain
     a. Low gestational weight gain is associated with
        (1) Growth-restricted infants
        (2) Fetal and infant mortality
     b. High gestational weight gain is associated with
        (1) Greater rate of large infant weight, which leads to
           (a) Fetopelvic disproportion
           (b) Operative delivery (forceps, vacuum, or Cesarean)
           (c) Birth trauma
           (d) Asphyxia
           (e) Mortality
        (2) Above associations are more pronounced in short women (< 157 cm or 62 in)
  5. Recommended patterns and quantity of weight gain
     a. Normal prepregnant weight—0.8–1.0 lb per week during second and third trimesters for total of 25–35 lb

b. Underweight before pregnancy—1.0–1.3 lb per week in second and third trimesters for total of 28–40 lb

c. Overweight before pregnancy—0.5–0.7 lb per week in second and third trimesters for total of 15–25 lb

d. Obese before pregnancy—0.4–0.6 lb per week in second and third trimesters for total of 11–20 lb

- Diet history—recall of fluid and solid food intake in the last 24 hours, whose purpose is to evaluate adequacy of nutrition and formulate a plan for nutrition counseling
  1. Components of diet history
     a. Qualitative components of the intake
     b. Quantitative, but only if weight is an issue
     c. Ascertain how typical the last 24-hour intake was to usual intake
  2. Components of diet counseling
     a. Diet assessment
     b. Set a weight gain goal with the woman for the pregnancy
     c. Discuss food preferences and relationship to goal
     d. Review generally or specifically at each visit, depending on results
     e. Include fetal growth as part of parameters
  3. Cultural and personal beliefs about nutrition that may modify a diet plan include:
     a. Pica—ingestion of nonfood substances, i.e., starch, clay
     b. Vegetarianism
     c. Hot and cold foods and when they can be eaten
     d. Discern eating patterns and beliefs pertinent to pregnancy in the woman's culture

◻ THE WOMAN AND HER FAMILY AND THEIR ROLE IN PREGNANCY

- Family
  1. Assessment of family size, structure and relationships
  2. Significant individuals involved in pregnancy
  3. Family roles and their relationship to family function
     a. Occupations
     b. Income levels
     c. Education levels
     d. Nationality and ethnic background
     e. Relationship status and intensity
  4. Feelings and thoughts about this pregnancy and any past pregnancies and births

- Pregnancy as essential, permanent family and life change
  1. The significance of change in relation to pregnancy
  2. Role adaptation needed to successfully cope with pregnancy
  3. Family resources to be mobilized to enable the family to cope
     a. Clear and continuous communication of information
     b. Decision making by the woman and family as indicated
     c. Family's development of an appropriate birth plan
        (1) Childbirth preparation
        (2) Breast feeding
        (3) Child-rearing classes
     d. Information regarding critical resources in birth site
        (1) Labor and birth procedures and expectations
        (2) Rooming-in
        (3) Breastfeeding support
        (4) Sibling visitation and/or presence at birth
        (5) Family visitation
        (6) Possibility of early discharge

- Perinatal loss and associated grief stages and process
  1. Factors associated with the concept of loss and grieving
     a. Perception of the individual(s) experiencing the loss of its severity
     b. Support and assistance in doing grief work
  2. Types of maternity losses
     a. Infertility
     b. Loss of a baby
        (1) Miscarriage
        (2) Abortion
        (3) Stillbirth
        (4) Adoption
     c. Loss of expectations
        (1) Premature infant
        (2) Congenital deformities
        (3) "Damaged" infant
        (4) Exclusive wife/husband relationship
  3. Stages of grief
     a. Shock, manifested by
        (1) Denial
        (2) Disbelief
        (3) Fear
        (4) Isolation
        (5) Crying
        (6) Hostility
        (7) Bitterness

        (8) Introversion
        (9) Sadness
       (10) Numbness

  b. Physical signs and symptoms
      (1) Weight loss
      (2) Insomnia
      (3) Fatigue
      (4) Restlessness
      (5) Shortness of breath
      (6) Chest pain

  c. Suffering—the reality stage
      (1) Acceptance of the reality
      (2) Adaptation
      (3) Preoccupation with lost person
      (4) Questioning of what happened and why
      (5) Feelings of fear, guilt, and anger persist

  d. Resolution—acceptance and adaptation is complete
      (1) Reinvests in other significant relationships
      (2) Moves on but remembers lost person

4. Maladaptive grief reactions
  a. Avoidance or distortion of normal grief expression
  b. Agitated depression; psychosomatic conditions
  c. Morbid attachment to possessions of deceased
  d. Persistent loss of self-esteem

5. Healthcare provider's role in helping the normal grieving process
  a. Listen
  b. Facilitate woman's expression of feelings
  c. Provide nonjudgmental environment
  d. Accept behaviors of grief

◻ TEACHING AND COUNSELING

- Principles of learning that apply to women/ families during pregnancy
  1. Factors that facilitate or impede learning
     a. Readiness of the learner; time to discuss
     b. Healthcare provider's knowledge of woman's and family's learning needs
     c. Group teaching—enhances and enriches learning
  2. Factors that critically influence teaching/ learning
     a. Alternative life styles; different cultures
     b. Disadvantaged social milieus
     c. Age and maturity—adolescents, educational level, life experience

- Principles of teaching for role of parent educator
  1. Individual teaching and counseling—topic and quantity of information need to fit the client
  2. Prioritize information provision
     a. Respond to questions or experiences of the woman
     b. Anticipatory guidance of pregnancy realities
     c. Danger signs of critical complications; drug dangers, both OTC and illegal drugs; and any other information needed for health and well-being of woman and fetus

- Childbirth education
  1. Preparation for childbearing—ultimately aids in reducing need for analgesics/anesthetics during labor
     a. Formal or informal
     b. Content to be included:
        (1) Bodily changes in pregnancy with associated reproduction anatomy
        (2) Exercises for ADL during pregnancy and for labor
        (3) Nutrition
        (4) Fetal growth and development
        (5) Substance abuse
        (6) Signs of beginning labor
        (7) Information for infant feeding decision making
        (8) Preparation for breastfeeding
        (9) Postpartal course and care
        (10) Preparation of siblings for birth
        (11) Pain coping strategies in labor
        (12) Vaginal birth after Cesarean (VBAC) versus elective repeat Cesarean section (ERCS) if previous C-section
  2. Learning needs of the breastfeeding woman
     a. Anticipatory guidance for woman with inverted nipples
     b. Principles of milk production
        (1) Caloric needs of mother
        (2) Liquid needs of mother
        (3) Mechanics of proper infant positioning and latching on
        (4) Factors that affect milk supply
  3. Learning needs for parenthood
     a. Plans for the baby's health care
     b. Needs and adaptation for the home
     c. Identification of family/social supports

- Family planning
  1. Pregnancy learning needs for postpartum contraceptive options
  2. Learning needs when considering postpartum bilateral tubal ligation

a. Expert counseling
b. Signing consent papers

- Human sexuality and pregnancy
  1. The effects of pregnancy on female and male sexual response
  2. Changes in sexual desire throughout pregnancy—impacted by hormones, energy level, relationship, body image, fears of hurting baby, cultural beliefs and practices
  3. Concept of body image—may feel awkward, clumsy, ugly, especially in late pregnancy
  4. Factors during pregnancy that may alter this image—support or lack thereof for her feelings; responses, either positive or negative, from people of importance
  5. Variations in sexual practice and their use during pregnancy
     a. Positions for intercourse—alternate positions may enhance comfort with increase in abdominal size
     b. Cunnilingus—avoid blowing into vagina to reduce risk of air embolism
     c. Fellatio
     d. Anal intercourse
  6. Sexual activity may be continued throughout a healthy pregnancy
  7. The potential relationship between orgasm and uterine contractions
     a. Contraindicated if preterm labor threatens
     b. May help initiate labor

☐ PHARMACOLOGIC CONSIDERATIONS IN THE ANTEPARTUM PERIOD

- Teratogens (derived from Greek word meaning "monster")—any agent that acts during embryonic or fetal development to produce a permanent alteration of form or function

- FDA risk factor categories for prescription drugs in pregnancy
  1. Category A—Adequate, well-controlled studies in pregnant women have not shown an increased risk of fetal abnormalities.
  2. Category B—Animal studies have revealed no evidence of harm to the fetus, however, there are no adequate and well-controlled studies in pregnant women.

  OR

  Animal studies have shown an adverse effect, but adequate and well-controlled studies in pregnant women have failed to demonstrate a risk to the fetus.

  3. Category C—Animal studies have shown an adverse effect, and there are no adequate and well-controlled studies in pregnant women.

  OR

  No animal studies have been conducted, and there are no adequate and well-controlled studies in pregnant women.
  4. Category D—Studies, adequate well-controlled or observational, in pregnant women have demonstrated a risk to the fetus. However, the benefits of therapy may outweigh the potential risk.
  5. Category X—Studies adequate, well-controlled or observational, in animals or pregnant women have demonstrated positive evidence of fetal abnormalities. The use of the product is contraindicated in women who are or may become pregnant (FDA, 2001).

- Indications and contraindications for the use of vaccinations during pregnancy
  1. Hepatitis B—high-risk women who are antigen and antibody negative can be vaccinated during pregnancy
  2. Tetanus—vaccination during pregnancy can protect at-risk newborns against neonatal tetanus; in maternal trauma, may be indicated
  3. Rubella—(German measles)—attenuated live-virus vaccine contraindicated immediately before or during pregnancy; vaccinate immediately after childbirth
  4. Varicella—attenuated live-virus vaccine (Varivax) contraindicated in pregnancy
  5. Influenza—trivalent inactivated influenza vaccine (TIV) recommended for all pregnant women during influenza season; live attenuated nasal influenza vaccine contraindicated during pregnancy

☐ TECHNIQUES USED TO ASSESS FETAL HEALTH

- Ultrasound (USG, US)
  1. Definition—method in which intermittent high-frequency sound waves are transmitted through tissues by way of a transducer placed on the abdomen or in the vagina which are then reflected off the underlying structures so that tissues, fluid, bones, fetal activity, and vessel pulsations are discernible
  2. Types of ultrasound
     a. Real-time ultrasound is the most commonly used method
     b. Transvaginal ultrasound may be used in early pregnancy
  3. Some uses for ultrasound in obstetrics
     a. Assessment of bleeding in the first trimester

b. R/O suspected ectopic pregnancy or hydatidiform mole

c. Estimated gestational age for patients with uncertain LMP

d. Evaluation of size/dates discrepancy

e. R/O suspected multiple gestations or fetal anomalies

f. Adjunct to special procedures—reproductive endocrinology procedures, CVS, amniocentesis, fetoscopy

g. Sex identification

h. Evaluation of second and third trimester bleeding

i. Evaluation of pelvic mass or uterine abnormality

j. Evaluation of placental problems, location, grade

k. Evaluation of fetal growth—macrosomia, intrauterine growth retardation (IUGR), AFI

l. Biophysical profile—AFI, fetal movements, respiratory movements, fetal tone

m. Estimation of fetal size and/or presentation

n. Rule out suspected fetal demise

- Doppler velocimetry blood flow assessment
  1. Used in tertiary settings only if utero-placental insufficiency resulting in IUGR is suspected or is present
  2. Detects velocity of blood flow through the fetal umbilical artery to the placenta and is displayed in a waveform
  3. Normal waveforms produced when the ratio of systolic to diastolic blood flow (S/D ratio) is around 3; abnormal ratio is more than 3

- Amniocentesis
  1. Amniotic fluid is aspirated from the amniotic sac and evaluated for genetic well-being or disorders, and fetal lung maturity
  2. Usually performed between 14 and 16 weeks for genetic evaluation or assessment of neural tube defects
  3. Used later in pregnancy—assessment of lung maturity; R/O amnionitis or fetal hemolytic disease (Rh or anti-D)
  4. Risks—infection, bleeding, preterm labor, PROM, fetal loss
  5. Benefits
     a. Provides early diagnosis and may decrease morbidity and mortality if elective abortion (AB) is sought
     b. May decrease psychological stress; support systems can be established prior to delivery

c. If a lethal anomaly is diagnosed and pregnancy continues, allows parents/care providers to plan, i.e. avoid a C-section

6. Special precaution—if mother is Rh negative and at risk for isoimmunization, administer RhoGAM with amniocentesis

- Chorionic villus sampling (CVS)/Chorionic villus biopsy (CVB)
  1. A sample of chorionic villi from placenta is aspirated either transabdominally or transcervically; outer trophoblastic layer is obtained because these tissues have same genetic make-up as the fetus; tissue is examined for genetic information
  2. Used for prenatal diagnosis; performed between 10 and 13 weeks
  3. Benefits
     a. Performed 3–4 weeks earlier than amniocentesis
     b. Cultures grow rapidly, resulting in early diagnosis
  4. Risks
     a. Infection, bleeding, miscarriage
     b. Risk of limb deformities (if performed before 9 weeks)
     c. Technically more difficult
     d. Contraindicated when there is a maternal blood group sensitization

- Fetal movement counting/Fetal kick counts—maternal self-report of fetal movement to assess fetal wellness
  1. Fetal movement counting (FMC)
     a. Most women are aware of fetal movement between 16 and 22 weeks' gestation; multiparas are generally aware of movement sooner than nulliparas
     b. The fetus has periods of sleep and wakefulness that change according to gestation
     c. Fetal movement is strongest between 29 and 38 weeks
     d. Fetal movement counting is a safe, simple, no-cost, noninvasive fetal assessment technique
     e. Research has demonstrated that fetal activity is a good predictor of well-being
     f. Dramatic decrease or cessation of movement is cause for concern
  2. Methods for performing FMC—adjusted to client's abilities with instructions to count fetal movements starting at 28 wks (identifiable risk present) or 34–36 weeks (low risk for uteroplacental insufficiency)
     a. Sanovsky's Protocol

(1) Count FM 30 minutes three times daily; four or more movements in a 30-minute period is reassuring

(2) If less than four movements in a 30-minute period, then continue for 1 hour

(3) Contact care provider if fewer than 10 movements or if movements become weak

b. Cardiff "Count to 10" method

(1) A chart to check off 10 fetal movements in one counting session

(2) Start at approximately the same time daily

(3) Chart how long it took to count 10 movements

(4) If fewer than 10 movements in 10 hours or amount of time to reach 10 movements increases, an NST should be performed

- Nonstress testing (NST)

1. Method to assess fetal well-being by observing the fetal heart rate response to fetal movement

2. 75% of fetuses at 28 weeks will experience heart rate accelerations in association with fetal movement

3. External electronic fetal monitoring is used to record fetal heart rate accelerations in response to fetal movement

4. Accelerations may be spontaneous or may be induced by vibro-acoustic stimulation (VAS)

5. Fetal hypoxia depresses the medullary center in the brain that controls fetal heart rate response resulting in depression of frequency or amplitude of the fetal heart rate

6. Indications for assessment of fetal well-being with NST include:

a. Decreased fetal movement

b. Postdates

c. Diabetes, hypertension, IUGR

7. Interpretation of results

a. Reactive—2 or more accelerations in fetal heart rate of 15 or more beats per minute, lasting for 15 seconds or more, within a 15 to 20-minute period

b. Nonreactive—FHR fails to demonstrate the required accelerations within a 40-minute period, requiring further evaluation

c. Unsatisfactory or inconclusive—fetal heart rate tracing that is uninterpretable or of poor quality, sometimes caused by a vigorous infant; test should be repeated (individual site protocols vary)

d. NSTs may be affected by any of the following:

(1) Fetal sleep

(2) Smoking within 30 minutes of testing

(3) Maternal intake of medications

(4) Fetal CNS anomalies

(5) Fetal hypoxia and/or acidosis

e. A nonreactive NST may be followed by a BPP, a contraction stress test, or a repeat NST

f. If indicated, NSTs should be repeated either weekly or biweekly

- Contraction stress test (CST)/Oxytocin challenge test (OCT)—assessment of fetal well-being by observing fetal heart rate response to uterine contractions

1. Physiology

a. During uterine contractions placental vessels are compressed and intervillous blood flow to the fetus is decreased

b. A fetus who is compromised or hypoxic does not have reserves

2. Method

a. Test is conducted in hospital

b. Electronic fetal monitoring (EFM); monitor the FHR response to uterine contractions

c. Contractions may be spontaneous, the result of administration of exogenous oxytocin, or from nipple stimulation

d. An acceptable test is one with 3 contractions lasting 40–60 seconds that are palpable

3. Results

a. Negative—no late or variable decelerations

b. Equivocal or suspicious—presence of nonrepetitive or nonpersistent decelerations, or long-term variability is absent

c. Positive—persistent late decelerations with 50% or more of the contractions

4. Contraindications to CST

a. Absolute—previous classical C-section or myomectomy, placenta previa, at risk for preterm labor

b. Relative—gestational age less than 37 weeks, multiple gestation

- Biophysical profile (BPP)—procedure utilizing ultrasound to evaluate five fetal variables to assess fetal risk; prospective studies have demonstrated that BPP is superior to CST as a predictor of fetal well-being or distress

1. Method

a. Test is composed of five observable variables—NST, muscle tone, breathing movements, gross body movements, and amniotic fluid volume

   b. In addition to NST, the fetus is evaluated via USG for a 30-minute time period to observe the remaining four variables

2. BPP scoring—each of the five variables is scored from 0 (abnormal) to 2 (normal); the scores for each are totaled

   a. Breathing movements—one or more episodes in 30 minutes; none = 0, present = 2

   b. Body movement—three or more discrete body or limb movements in 30 minutes; none = 0 present = 2

   c. Tone—one or more episodes of extension with return to flexion; none = 0, present = 2

   d. Qualitative amniotic fluid volume (AFV)—at least one pocket of amniotic fluid that measures at least 2 cm in 2 perpendicular planes; none = 0, present = 2

   e. Reactivity—reactive NST; nonreactive scored as 0, reactive = 2

3. Scoring interpretation criteria

   a. 8–10 is normal (in absence of oligohydramnios)

   b. 6 is equivocal, repeat testing

   c. 4 or less is considered abnormal

4. Modified BBP, NST, and amniotic fluid index—(see Postterm pregnancy section in this chapter)

- Percutaneous umbilical blood sampling (PUBS or cordocentesis)
1. Definition—process in which a needle is introduced under real-time ultrasound, through the maternal abdomen and then into the umbilical cord; blood is then aspirated or blood and/or medications are introduced into the fetus
2. Usually performed after 20 weeks
3. Used for prenatal diagnosis—Rh (anti-D) disease, fetal infections, blood factor abnormalities, chromosomal or genetic disease, fetal hypoxia assessment
4. Used to treat the fetus—fetal transfusion, administer drug therapy
5. Concerns

   a. Similar to amniocentesis and CVS procedures

   b. Must be performed by a skilled individual able to secure immediate delivery and appropriate level of neonatal care

- Methods to assess fetal lung maturity
1. Respiratory distress (RDS) is a major problem associated with preterm birth
2. Assessment of fetal lung maturity is accomplished by assessing the amniotic fluid

3. Different tests may be used to assess the factors that help prevent atelectasis
4. Prior to 39 weeks' gestation, there should be an evaluation of fetal lung maturity if labor induction or Cesarean delivery is electively scheduled to help prevent iatrogenic prematurity and respiratory distress syndrome

   a. Lecithin/sphingomyelin ratios (L/S)

     (1) Lecithin is elevated after 35 weeks

     (2) Sphingomyelin remains fairly constant

     (3) Ratio of 2:1 or greater is indicative of fetal lung maturity except in diabetes

     (4) L/S ratio may also not be accurate in hydrops fetalis and nonhypertensive glomerulonephritis

   b. Phosphatidylglycerol (PG)

     (1) Appears after 35 weeks when lungs are mature

     (2) If PG present, in combination with a favorable L/S ratio, confirms lung maturity

   c. Shake test

     (1) Amniotic fluid is shaken in a tube with saline and 95% ethanol for 15 seconds

     (2) A complete ring of bubbles on the surface is indicative of fetal lung maturity

     (3) Advantage of this procedure is it can be conducted at the bedside

     (4) Has a low false positive rate

     (5) Has a high false negative rate

   d. Foam stability test

     (1) Similar to the shake test but amniotic fluid is shaken with various amounts of 95% ethanol only

     (2) Foam formation is indicative of lung maturity

     (3) Collection of amniotic fluid

     (4) With intact membranes, fluid is obtained by amniocentesis

     (5) With ROM, fluid can be aspirated with a sterile syringe and sent for evaluation

   e. Results

     (1) L/S ratio should be above 2

     (2) If PG is present even with an L/S ratio of less than 2, the risk of respiratory distress syndrome is minimal

◘ SELECTED OBSTETRICAL COMPLICATIONS

- Abuse
1. Substance abuse

   a. Substances with known potential for abuse/addiction

     (1) Legal drugs

(a) Alcohol—17 million (6.9% of US population) report heavy drinking (5 or more drinks/occasion on 5 or more days in last 30 days)

(b) Nicotine—71 million (28.6% of US population) currently use tobacco products

(2) Illegal drugs—prevalence in 2007 was 19.9 million in US (8.0%) reporting use in past month

(a) Cocaine

(b) Hallucinogens

(c) Heroin

(d) Marijuana

(e) Nonmedical use of prescription psychotherapeutics and pain relievers

b.   Historical evolution of the concept of alcohol use in the US

(1) After WWII, dominant view linked excessive use of prescription drugs, alcohol, and use of illicit drugs with emotional instability, weak will, and poor character

(2) Jellinek's 1960 disease model for alcoholism made it a chronic, relapsing disease with a genetic component

(3) Major definition shift paved the way for the Alcoholics Anonymous approach to treatment

c.   Substance abuse in pregnancy

(1) Prevalence—Substance Abuse and Mental Health Services Administration (SAMHSA, 2009)

(a) 16.4% smoked

(b) 10.6% drank some alcohol

(c) 4.5% engaged in binge drinking

(d) 5.1% used illegal drug in past month

d.   Factors associated with increased risk for substance abuse in pregnancy include:

(1) Lack of education

(2) Low self-esteem

(3) Depression

(4) Family problems and/or family history of substance abuse

(5) Financial problems and poverty

(6) Abusive relationships

(7) Feelings of hopelessness

(8) Drug-abusing partner

e.   Maternal medical and obstetrical complications of substance abuse include:

(1) Smoking

(a) Maternal effects—preeclampsia, abruption placentae, placenta previa, spontaneous abortion, ectopic pregnancy, and premature rupture of membranes

(b) Infant effects—IUGR, premature birth, and small for gestational age

(2) Alcohol

(a) Maternal effects—spontaneous abortion and possibly some subtle neurologic problems in school-age child

(b) Infant effects—fetal alcohol syndrome (FAS), fetal alcohol effects (FAE), or alcohol-related birth defects (ARBD)

(3) Illicit drugs

(a) Effects less well known, and knowledge of long-term implications is limited

(b) Research findings confounded by social and economic factors

(c) Polydrug use further confounds the reality

(d) Maternal effects of heroin and methadone—eclampsia, placental abruption, IUGR, intrauterine death, postpartum hemorrhage, preterm labor, premature rupture of membranes

(e) Infant effects—jitteriness, hyperreflexia, restlessness, sleeplessness, poor feeding pattern, vomiting, diarrhea, shrill cry

f.   Screening

(1) Toxicology screen; most commonly done on maternal urine; more recently, meconium, infant hair sample, amniotic fluid, cord tissue

(2) History—more information gathered regarding length of time and quantity of use

(3) Combination of both

g.   Screening tools for alcohol use

(1) CAGE

C–have you felt the need to cut down on your drinking?

A–have people annoyed you by criticizing your drinking?

G–have you ever felt bad or guilty about your drinking?

E–have you ever had a drink first thing in the morning to steady your nerves or get rid of a hangover (eye-opener)

(2) TWEAK

Tolerance–how many drinks can you hold?

Worried—have close friends or relatives worried or complained about your drinking in the past year?

Eye openers—do you sometimes take a drink in the morning when you first get up?

Amnesia—has a friend or family member ever told you about things you said or did while you were drinking that you could not remember?

Cut down—do you sometimes feel the need to cut down on your drinking?

h. Management
   (1) Ideal—stop using harmful substances
   (2) Reduce quantity and types of substances used
   (3) Mobilize resources to support and encourage
   (4) Drug rehabilitation

i. Ethical considerations—who should be screened?
   (1) Universal and mandatory versus none for anyone
   (2) Screening of those with positive history or who exhibit signs of use

j. Legal implications
   (1) Mandatory reporting to child protective services
   (2) Possible loss of infant
   (3) Criminal prosecution of woman

2. Intimate partner abuse/Violence against women (VAW)
  a. Incidence of VAW—more than half of all women experience some form of abuse at some point in their lives
  b. Screening techniques for ascertaining the presence of VAW; essential questions asked during history taking include:
   (1) Have you ever been emotionally or physically abused by your partner or someone important to you?
   (2) Within the past year, have you been hit, slapped, kicked, shoved, or otherwise hurt by anyone?
   (3) Have you ever been hit, slapped, kicked, or otherwise physically hurt while you were pregnant?
  c. Definitions of VAW
   (1) Physical
     (a) Pushes, slaps, punches
     (b) Locks woman in or out of the house
     (c) Refuses to buy food
     (d) Refuses access to medical care
     (e) Destroys property or pets
     (f) Abuses children

   (2) Emotional
     (a) Engages in name calling or insults
     (b) Isolates from family and friends
     (c) Publicly humiliates
     (d) Makes all decisions
     (e) Withholds affection
   (3) Sexual
     (a) Treats women as sex objects
     (b) Forces sexual acts with self or others
     (c) Jealous anger with accusations
     (d) Withholds sex and affection
     (e) Engages in sadistic sexual acts
   (4) Financial
     (a) Withholds money
     (b) Runs up bills woman must pay
     (c) Makes all monetary decisions
     (d) Manipulates relationship through money

  d. Diagnosis of abuse
   (1) History
     (a) Depression or suicide attempts
     (b) Substance abuse
     (c) Childhood abuse (sexual or physical)
     (d) Multiple injuries
     (e) Complaints of chronic pain
     (f) Repeated spontaneous abortions (SAB), threatened abortions (TAB), and/or STD
   (2) Physical
     (a) Assessing for injuries—multiple bruises in various stages of recovery; proximal vs distal—proximal tends to be intentional; hidden injuries—breasts, abdomen, back, etc.
     (b) Treatment delays—old scars or bruises visible
     (c) Patterned injuries—with reasonable certainty can determine what kind of object caused injury, e.g., bite marks
     (d) Physical findings inconsistent with history
     (e) Genital trauma, vaginismus
     (f) Poor weight gain in pregnancy
   (3) Others
     (a) Partner appears "overprotective"
     (b) Missed appointments
  e. Effect of pregnancy on VAW
  f. Risks in pregnancy in the situation of violence/abuse, to the woman and fetus
  g. Management
   (1) Data collection
   (2) Forensic examination
   (3) Safety

(4) Counseling

(5) Acute intervention

(6) Long-term aid

(7) Referral

h. Community resources for victims of violence/abuse

i. Legal and emergency issues related to domestic violence

- First trimester bleeding
  1. Definition—bleeding occurring within the first 12 weeks of pregnancy
     a. 40% of women have some bleeding in the first trimester
     b. 80% of spontaneous abortions occur in the first 12 weeks
     c. 90% of pregnancies with bleeding will continue to term after FHT observed
  2. Differential diagnosis
     a. Implantation bleeding
     b. Threatened abortion
     c. Ectopic pregnancy
     d. Cervicitis
     e. Cervical polyps
     f. Vaginitis
     g. Trauma/Intercourse
     h. Disappearing twin
     i. Autoantibody/autoimmune disorder
  3. Diagnosis
     a. Pelvic examination
        (1) Speculum examination to visualize the cervix
        (2) Bimanual examination to assess uterus and adnexa for size and tenderness
        (3) Laboratory diagnosis
            (a) Serum hCG is positive 8–9 days after fertilization
            (b) β-hCG doubles every 48 hours with normal intra-uterine pregnancy (IUP)
            (c) β-hCG increases by only one third when an ectopic pregnancy exists
        (4) Rule of 10
            (a) β-hCG equals 100 at time of missed menses
            (b) β-hCG is 100,000 at 10 weeks (peak)
            (c) β-hCG 10,000 at term
            (d) β-hCG elimination half-life about 24 hours
            (e) 90% of ectopics have β-hCG less than 6500
  4. Treatment—depends on etiology

- Spontaneous abortion
  1. Types of abortion
     a. Spontaneous abortion—occurring without apparent cause
     b. Threatened abortion—appearance of signs and symptoms of possible loss of the fetus, i.e., vaginal bleeding with or without intermittent pain
     c. Inevitable abortion—cervix is dilating, uterus will be emptied
     d. Incomplete abortion—an abortion in which part of the products of conception has been retained in the uterus
     e. Complete abortion—all the products of conception have been expelled
     f. Missed abortion—the fetus died before completion of 20 weeks' gestation but products of conception are retained for a prolonged period of time (2 or more weeks)
     g. Habitual abortion—three or more consecutive abortions
  2. Etiology—fetal factors
     a. Abnormal development of zygote such as chromosomal abnormalities is responsible for about 60%
     b. Autosomal trisomy is the most frequently identified chromosomal anomaly, followed by Turner's syndrome
  3. Etiology—maternal factors
     a. Incidence increases with parity and/or short interconceptional period
     b. Incidence increases with maternal and paternal age
  4. Common causes of spontaneous abortion
     a. Anatomic anomalies
     b. Infections
     c. Immune factors, including autoimmune clotting disorders
     d. Endocrine effects
     e. Recreational drugs/ETOH/environmental toxins
        (1) Smoking
        (2) ETOH
        (3) Caffeine
        (4) Radiation
        (5) Cocaine
        (6) Anesthetic gasses/surgery
     f. Severe malnutrition
     g. Age of gametes
  5. Management
     a. Obtain blood type if not known
     b. Draw baseline serum β-hCG
     c. Repeat β-hCG in 48 hours
     d. Ultrasound
     e. Should be able to visualize transabdominally an IUP at hCG of 6500
     f. Should be able to visualize transvaginally an IUP at hCG of 2000

g. RhoGAM for unsensitized Rh negative women

- Inevitable or incomplete abortion
  1. Surgical D&C
  2. Chemical D&C
  3. Observant management
  4. Emotional support and anticipatory guidance

- Threatened abortion or disappearing twin
  1. Pelvic rest
  2. Emotional support and anticipatory guidance

- Ectopic pregnancy
  1. Definition—implantation of the blastocyst anywhere other than the endometrium
  2. 95% of ectopic pregnancies occur in the fallopian tube
  3. Second leading cause of maternal death in US
  4. Occurs in about 1 per 85 pregnancies; rate is highest in the 35–44 year age group
  5. Etiology
     a. STD—especially chlamydia and gonorrhea
     b. Therapeutic abortion followed by infection
     c. Endometriosis
     d. Previous pelvic surgery
     e. Failed bilateral tubal ligation
     f. Mechanical—problems with tubes such as scarring
     g. Functional—menstrual reflux, hormonal alteration of tubal motility
  6. Sites for ectopic
     a. Ampulla—78% of ectopics
     b. Isthmus—12% of ectopics
     c. Interstitial—2% of ectopics
     d. Fimbria—less than 1% of ectopics
     e. Other sites—abdominal, ovarian, and broad ligament
  7. Symptoms
     a. Amenorrhea but frequently has some vaginal spotting
     b. Lower pelvic and/or abdominal pain, which is unilateral
     c. Unilateral tender adnexal mass
     d. Some have no symptoms
  8. Clinical picture
     a. Severe abdominal pain
     b. Cervical motion tenderness
     c. Free fluid on ultrasound
     d. Cul-de-sac fullness
     e. Shoulder pain second to diaphragmatic irritation
     f. Vertigo or fainting
  9. Diagnosis
     a. Physical examination
     b. Serum β-hCG (90% of ectopics have β-hCG less than 6500; abnormal interval increases)
     c. Ultrasound
     d. Culdocentesis
     e. Laparoscopy
  10. Differential diagnosis
     a. PID
     b. Ovarian cyst
     c. Appendicitis
  11. Management
     a. Consult and transfer to medical management
     b. Tubal preservation is the goal
     c. Salpingectomy/salpingostomy/tubal resection
     d. Methotrexate
     e. RhoGAM for Rh-negative unsensitized women

- Hydatidiform mole
  1. Incidence—1:1500 to 1:2000
  2. Highest incidence at beginning and end of reproductive years with greatest incidence after age 45
  3. Symptoms
     a. Abnormal uterine bleeding
     b. Size/dates discrepancy
     c. Lack of fetal activity
     d. Hyperemesis gravidarum
     e. Gestational hypertension before 20 weeks
     f. Passage of vesicular tissue
  4. Diagnosis
     a. Ultrasound
     b. Serum β-hCG
  5. Management
     a. Uterine evacuation by suction curettage
     b. Close surveillance for persistent trophoblastic proliferation or malignant changes
     c. Recommend avoidance of pregnancy for 1 year
     d. Serial β-hCG levels every 2 weeks until normal then once a month for 6 months, then every 2 months for 1 year
     e. Chest radiograph

- Second trimester bleeding—bleeding is less common
  1. Midtrimester spontaneous abortion
     a. Etiology
        (1) May be associated with autoimmune disorders
        (2) May be related to cocaine use
        (3) May be related to anatomic or physiologic factors
  2. Incompetent cervix
     a. Symptoms

(1) Painless dilation
(2) Bloody show
(3) Spontaneous rupture of membranes
(4) Vaginal/pelvic pressure
b. Risk factors
(1) Previous midtrimester loss
(2) Cervical surgery
(3) DES
c. Treatment
(1) Consult
(2) Cervical cerclage after 12–14 weeks
(3) Success rate of 80–90%
(4) Risk of ruptured membranes or infection
(5) Monitor cervical length via transvaginal ultrasound
3. Placental anomalies
a. Low-lying placenta
(1) One third of women have low-lying placenta in first trimester
(2) Only 1% have previa in the third trimester
b. Partial abruption
(1) May resolve
(2) May reabsorb
c. Diagnosis
(1) Ultrasound
(2) Consult as needed

• Third trimester bleeding
1. Incidence—4% of all pregnancies
2. Never perform a digital vaginal examination on a woman's cervix in the presence of third trimester bleeding unless certain there is no previa!
3. Placenta previa (responsible for 20% of third trimester bleeds)
a. Definition—placenta is located over or next to the internal cervical os; may be partial (not totally covering the os), marginal (palpable at margin of os) or complete (completely covering the os)
b. Incidence
(1) From 0.4 to 0.6%
(2) Occurs in 1 of 300 pregnancies
c. Risk factors
(1) Multiparity
(2) Previous C-section or other uterine surgery
(3) Smoking
d. Signs and symptoms
(1) Primary—associated with painless vaginal bleeding
(2) Secondary—unengaged fetal presentation and/or malpresentation
(3) Sometimes bleeding is associated with contractions

e. Diagnosis
(1) History
(2) Ultrasound
f. Management
(1) Consult, in some practices may comanage
(2) Observant management until delivery
(3) If bleeding, hospitalize
(4) Tocolytic therapy may be considered
(5) May be able to deliver vaginally if bleeding is not severe and os is not completely covered
(6) If vaginal birth is considered will need double set-up for birth
(7) If complete previa, medical management and Cesarean birth
4. Placental abruption (cause of 30% of third trimester bleeds)
a. Definition—premature separation of the placenta from the uterus that may be partial or complete
b. Risk factors
(1) Hypertension—chronic or gestational
(2) Trauma
(3) Smoking
(4) Cocaine use
(5) Multiparity
(6) Uterine anomalies or tumors
c. Signs and symptoms
(1) Vaginal bleeding
(2) Uterine tenderness and rigidity
(3) Contractions or uterine irritability and/or tone
(4) Fetal tachycardia or bradycardia
d. Complications
(1) Shock
(2) Fetal compromise or death
(3) Disseminated intravascular coagulation (DIC)
e. Diagnosis
(1) Clinical evaluation
(2) Fetal monitoring
(3) Ultrasound
f. Management
(1) "Get help"
(2) Monitor clotting studies and hgb/hct, platelets
(3) Stabilize mother
(4) Effect delivery as indicated by fetal or maternal condition

• Selected problems during pregnancy
1. Birth defects or anomalies—common terms and definitions
a. Malformation—the fetus or structure is genetically abnormal, e.g., limb contracture resulting from diastrophic dysplasia

b. Deformation—a genetically normal fetus develops in an abnormal uterine environment causing structural changes, e.g., oligohydramnios causing limb contractures

c. Disruption—a genetically normal fetus suffers an insult resulting in disruption of normal development, e.g., early amnion rupture causing limb deformities

d. Syndrome—multiple abnormalities have the same cause, e.g., trisomy 18

e. Sequence—abnormalities occurred sequentially as result of one insult, e.g., oligohydramnios leading to pulmonary hypertension, limb contractures, and facial deformities

f. Association—set of abnormalities that frequently occur together but have no linked etiology

2. Genetic abnormalities

a. Critical concept definitions

(1) Phenotype—the expression of genes present in an individual, e.g., eye color, blood type, etc.

(2) Genotype—the total hereditary information present in an individual; the pair of genes for each characteristic

b. Definitions of critical patterns of inheritance

(1) Single-gene (Mendelian) disorders

(a) A mutation in a single locus or gene, in one or both members of a gene pair

(b) Incidence—0.4% by age 25; 2% during lifetime

(2) Autosomal dominant—when only one member of a gene pair determines the phenotype, e.g., BRCA 1 and 2 breast cancer

(3) Autosomal recessive—trait is expressed only when both copies of the gene are the same, e.g., cystic fibrosis, sickle cell anemia

(4) Sex-linked

(a) X-linked diseases are usually recessive, e.g., color blindness, hemophilia

(b) Y-linked diseases relate to sexual determination, cellular functions, and bone development

c. Inborn errors of metabolism—autosomal recessive disease resulting from absence of an essential enzyme causing incomplete metabolism of proteins, fats, or sugars, e.g., PKU

d. Definition of essential terms

(1) Autosome—any chromosome other than sex (X or Y) chromosomes

(2) Genome—the complete set of chromosomes or the entire genetic information present in a cell

(3) Euploidy—state of complete sets of chromosomes

(4) Aneuploidy—state of having an abnormal number of chromosomes

(5) Polyploidy—abnormal number of haploid chromosome complements

(6) Deletion—portion of a chromosome that is missing

(7) Ring chromosome—when deletions occur at both ends of the chromosome, the ends may untie to form a ring

(8) Isochromosomes—composed of either two short arms or two long arms of the chromosome fused together

e. Trisomy 21—Down syndrome, the most common, nonlethal trisomy

(1) Incidence—1 in 800–1000 newborns

(2) Etiology—almost 95% due to nondisjunction of maternal chromosome 21

(3) Signs and symptoms

(a) Marked hypotonia

(b) Tongue protrusion

(c) Small head

(d) Flattened occiput

(e) Flat nasal bridge

(f) Epicanthal folds and slanting palperbral fissures

(g) Nuchal skin fold

(h) Short, stubby fingers

(i) Single palmar crease

(j) Fifth fingers are curved inward

(k) IQ range—25–50

(4) Recurrence risk—1% until age-related risk status reached after age 35

f. Genetic counseling

(1) Goals for first step—to educate the woman and her family about testing options, indications for and implications of results

(2) Goals after abnormal screen—to inform woman of options to address the results

(3) Indications for genetic studies

(a) General screening for anomalies, e.g., neural tube defect, Trisomy 21

(b) History of birth defects or mental retardation

(c) Family history of genetic disorders

(d) Exposure to teratogens

(e) Ingestions of medications in early pregnancy known to be

teratogenic, i.e., seizure prevention drugs
        (f) Has increased likelihood due to age or ethnic roots
3. Sexually transmitted infections (Centers for Disease Control and Prevention, 2006)
    a. Definition—transmission of pathogens through sexual activities and behaviors
    b. Incidence—relatively common during pregnancy
    c. Diseases characterized by genital ulcers
        (1) Syphilis
            (a) Incidence—3.8 cases per 100,000 persons (2007)
            (b) Clinical manifestations—primary syphilis
                i. Incubation—10–90 days, usually less than 6 weeks
                ii. Primary genital lesion difficult to see, goes unnoticed—cervical chancre more common in pregnancy
                iii. Painless firm ulcer with raised edges
                iv. Heals after 2–6 weeks; may have nontender enlarged inguinal lymph nodes
            (c) Clinical manifestations—secondary syphilis
                i. Variable skin rash appears 4–10 weeks after chancre heals
                ii. Not noticed in 25%—may be limited to genitalia
                iii. Condylomata lata—elevated areas that may cause vulvar ulcerations
                iv. Alopecia sometimes occurs
            (d) Etiology
                i. Chronic infection—spirochetes cause lesions in major organs
                ii. Recent infection more likely to affect fetus
                iii. Placental changes—large, pale
            (e) Diagnosis
                i. VDRL or RPR—first prenatal visit
                ii. Fluorescent treponemal antibody absorption test (FTA-ABS) or microhemagglutination assay for antibodies to *Treponema pallidum* (MHA-TP) confirms nonspecific VDRL/RPR

        iii. Repeat, or do a nontreponemal screening at time of delivery
            (f) Treatment—98% effective
                i. Penicillin—dual purpose in pregnancy; eradicate maternal infection and prevent infection in the newborn
                ii. Early syphilis—benzathine penicillin G 2.4 million units IM; some recommend a second dose in 1 week particularly for secondary stage or in third trimester
                iii. Syphilis of more than 1 year duration—benzathine penicillin G 2.4 million units IM weekly $\times$ 3 doses
            (g) Penicillin allergy
                i. Skin test to confirm allergy
                ii. Desensitize, then treat as above
            (h) Congenital syphilis or stillbirth—may be only sign of maternal infection
                i. Incidence—historically accounted for 30% of all stillbirths
                ii. US 1998—30 per 100,000 births
            (i) Jarisch-Herxheimer reaction
                i. Acute febrile reaction often with headache and myalgia occurring within first 24 hours of treatment initiation; not an allergic reaction; most common in early syphilis treatment
                ii. Might induce early labor or cause fetal distress; should not prevent or delay therapy
                iii. Advise pregnant women of this possible reaction
                iv. May use antipyretics for symptoms; resolves in 24 hours
        (2) Herpes Simplex virus (HSV)
            (a) Incidence—at least 50 million in US have been infected with HSV-2 (CDC, 2006)
            (b) Signs and symptoms—primary infection
                i. Incubation—3–6 days
                ii. Pruritic papular eruption that becomes painful and vesicular, multiple lesions
                iii. Inguinal adenopathy

        iv. Transient flu-like symptoms

        v.   By 2–6 weeks all signs and symptoms are gone

    (c) Signs and symptoms—recurrent infection

        i.   Reactivation results in virus shedding

        ii. Signs and symptoms are less intense but occur at same site

    (d) Diagnosis

        i.   Viral culture or PCR detection

        ii. Type-specific serologic tests

    (e) Treatment

        i.   Antivirals—acyclovir, valacyclovir—primary or first episode infection, symptomatic recurrent episode; daily suppression from 36 weeks' gestation until delivery

        ii. Analgesics and topical anesthetics

    (f) Management of birth—Cesarean delivery indicated only if woman has active genital lesions or prodromal symptoms

  (3) Human papillomavirus (HPV)

    (a) Incidence—symptomatic or asymptomatic is common

    (b) HPV type and associated conditions

        i.   HPV-16—cervical, vaginal and vulvar neoplasia

        ii. HPV-6, 11, also 16, 18, 30s, 40s, 50s, 60s—condylomata acuminata

        iii. HPV-16, 18, 45, 56, 31, 33, 35, 39, 51, 52, 58, 66—cervical intraepithelial neoplasia and cancer

    (c) Treatment

        i.   Imiquimod, podophyllin, podofilox are contraindicated in pregnancy

        ii. Cryotherapy, trichloracetic acid (TCA), surgical removal if indicated

    (d) Management of birth—Cesarean delivery should not be used solely to prevent transmission to newborn; Cesarean delivery may be indicated if genital warts obstruct pelvic outlet or if vaginal delivery would result in excessive bleeding

  d. Diseases characterized by urethritis/cervicitis

    (1) Gonorrhea

        (a) Incidence—119 cases per 100,000 population (CDC, 2007); highest in 15–19 year age group

        (b) Prevalence in pregnancy—varies with high at 7%

        (c) Risk factors—single, adolescence, poverty, drug abuse, prostitution, concomitant STD, lack of antepartal care

        (d) GC is marker for chlamydia

        (e) Diagnosis—screen at first visit; repeat at 28 weeks in high-risk groups

        (f) Clinical significance in pregnancy—associated with septic spontaneous or induced abortion

        (g) Treatment

           i.   Single dose ceftriaxone 125 mg IM, or cefixime 400 mg orally or spectinomycin 2 g IM

          ii. Concomitant treatment for chlamydia if infection is not ruled out

    (2) *Chlamydia trachomatis* (CT)

        (a) Incidence—370 cases per 100,000 population (CDC, 2007); most common reportable STD

        (b) Risk factors—age younger than 25, presence or history of STD, multiple partners, new sexual partner in last 3 months

        (c) Signs and symptoms—urethritis, mucopurulent cervicitis, acute salpingitis

        (d) Differential diagnosis—normal pregnancy, cervical mucus

        (e) Diagnosis—NAAT is most specific and sensitive test available

        (f) Treatment

           i.   Tetracyclines and quinolones are contraindicated in pregnancy

          ii. Azithromycin 1 g orally, single dose or amoxicillin 500 mg orally tid for 7 days recommended

          iii. Alternative regimens—various dosing regimens of erythromycin base or ethylsuccinate

          iv. Repeat testing 3 weeks after completion of treatment

  e. Diseases characterized by vaginal discharge

    (1) Bacterial vaginosis (BV)

        (a) Associated with premature rupture of membranes,

chorioamnionitis, preterm labor and birth, intra-amniotic infection, postpartum endometritis, postCesarean wound infection

    (b) Treatment in pregnancy

        i. Treat all symptomatic pregnant women and asymptomatic pregnant women at high risk for preterm delivery

        ii. Metronidazole 250 mg orally tid or 500 mg bid for 7 days

        iii. Clindamycin 300 mg orally bid for 7 days

  (2) Trichomoniasis

    (a) Associated with premature rupture of membranes, preterm delivery, low birth weight

    (b) Treatment in pregnancy

        i. No data to support treatment reduces perinatal morbidity

        ii. Metronidazole 2 g orally single dose or 500 mg bid for 7 days

  (3) Vulvovaginal candidiasis (VVC)

    (a) Treatment of uncomplicated VVC in pregnancy—topical treatment with azoles for 7 days—butoconazole, clotrimazole, miconazole, terconazole, nystatin

    (b) Treatment of recurrent or severe VVC in pregnancy—may require longer duration of therapy with topical azoles

4. Small for gestational age (SGA) and intrauterine growth restriction (IUGR)

  a. Definitions—small for gestational age (SGA), intrauterine growth restriction (IUGR) or fetal growth restriction are terms used interchangeably to describe a fetus or newborn whose size is smaller than the norm. IUGR is used to describe impaired or restricted intrauterine growth and is considered a pathologic process. SGA is a neonatal diagnosis and describes an infant who falls below the 10th percentile. The majority of SGA babies are IUGR.

  b. Differentiation

    (1) The genetic design of a constitutionally small infant (parents are also small)

    (2) Low birth weight secondary to poor nutrition

  c. Incidence—3–8%; leads to 18% mortality rate

  d. Symmetric growth restriction

    (1) Appears around 18–20 weeks

    (2) Caused by

      (a) Congenital infections

      (b) Chromosomal abnormalities

      (c) Maternal drug use—tobacco, alcohol, dilantin, cocaine, heroin

    (3) Increased risk of adverse long-term sequelae

  e. Asymmetric growth restriction

    (1) Appears later in the pregnancy

    (2) Asymmetry is caused by a reduction in cell size, not number of cells resulting in "head-sparing"

    (3) Due to abnormalities in uteroplacental perfusion

    (4) Caused by

      (a) Maternal factors

        i. Hypertension

        ii. Anemia

        iii. Collagen disease

        iv. IDDM

      (b) Placental factors

        i. Previa

        ii. Abruption

        iii. Malformations

        iv. Infarctions

      (c) Fetal factors

        i. Multiple gestation

        ii. Anomalies

    (5) Diagnosis

      (a) Review history

      (b) Physical examination

        i. Fundal height

        ii. EFW

      (c) Ultrasound to confirm diagnosis

        i. Anomalies

        ii. Serial studies for growth

        iii. AFI

        iv. Doppler flow studies

        v. Placenta grading and assessment

    (6) Fetal effects

      (a) Fetus adjusts to conditions by conserving energy and decreasing metabolic requirements

      (b) Fetus stops growing

      (c) Risk of intrauterine fetal demise

    (7) Management

      (a) Consult

      (b) If you are able to identify a cause, counsel and make adjustments

        i. Decrease smoking

        ii. Nutrition evaluation

        iii. Maternal positions that facilitate uteroplacental blood flow, left lateral or sitting

        iv. Emotional support and anticipatory guidance

      (c) Serial ultrasounds for growth

(d) Serial NSTs and AFI or BPPs (weekly or biweekly)

(e) TORCH titer

(f) Amniocentesis, chromosome evaluation of parents

(g) If lungs are mature, consider delivery

5. Large for gestational age (LGA)/macrosomia
   a. Definition—in US babies weighing more than 4000 g at birth (macrosomia) or over the 90th percentile in weight for gestational age
   b. Risk factors
      (1) Ethnic/racial origins
      (2) Obesity
      (3) Previous LGA/macrosomic neonate
      (4) Previous shoulder dystocia
      (5) Size of the father
      (6) Birth weight of both the mother and the father
      (7) Diabetes or history of gestational diabetes
      (8) Previous uterine myomata
      (9) Multiparity
   c. Physical examination
      (1) Fundal height
      (2) EFW and palpation of fetal parts
      (3) Maternal body habitus
   d. Differential diagnosis
      (1) Inaccurate dating
      (2) Polyhydramnios
      (3) Multiple gestation
      (4) Diabetes
      (5) Uterine fibroids
   e. Management
      (1) Discuss risks/challenges
      (2) Diet counseling
      (3) Ultrasound for EFW
      (4) Carefully assess clinical pelvimetry
      (5) Consult
      (6) Monitor for shoulder dystocia

6. Preterm birth
   a. Definition—a combination of prematurity, expressed as a birth at 37 weeks' gestation or earlier and low birth weight, indicated by infant weight of 2500 g or less; with improved neonatal care, the greatest contribution to mortality and serious morbidity comes from infants of less than 34 weeks' gestation
   b. Incidence of preterm birth by gestational age—11.6% of births are 37 weeks or less of which 1.93% are less than 32 weeks (US NCHS, 2000)
   c. Factors associated with preterm birth
      (1) Largely unknown
      (2) Abruptio placenta
      (3) Uterine overdistention—multiple gestation, polyhydramnios
      (4) Cervical incompetence
      (5) Hormonal changes perhaps mediated by fetal or maternal stress
      (6) Acute inflammatory response
      (7) Bacterial infections—urinary tract or genital tract
      (8) Poor nutritional status
      (9) Prepregnancy underweight and inadequate gain during pregnancy
      (10) Previous history of preterm labor and birth
      (11) Short interval between pregnancies
      (12) Substance abuse—cocaine, alcohol, cigarettes
      (13) Chorioamnionitis
      (14) Placenta previa
      (15) Fetal death
      (16) Preterm premature rupture of membranes
      (17) Preeclampsia
   d. Risk scoring systems to identify women at risk for preterm birth have not been successful
   e. Signs and symptoms
      (1) Painful or painless uterine contractions
      (2) Pelvic pressure
      (3) Menstrual-like cramps
      (4) Watery or bloody vaginal discharge
      (5) Low back pain
   f. Markers for predicting preterm birth
      (1) Fetal fibronectin (fFN) screening
         (a) Use only in women at high risk for preterm birth
         (b) fFN normally present in cervical secretions until 16–20 weeks' gestation and then again late in pregnancy
         (c) Negative test results useful in ruling out imminent (within 14 days) preterm birth before 37 weeks' gestation (predictive value up to 94%)
         (d) Positive test at 24–34 weeks may predict imminent preterm birth (predictive value 46%)
      (2) Home uterine activity monitoring—data insufficient to support use in preventing preterm birth
      (3) Endocervical length
         (a) Cervical shortening determined with ultrasound associated with preterm birth

      (b) Usefulness limited by lack of proven treatments to affect outcomes

  g. Diagnosis—ACOG and AAP criteria for 20–37 weeks' gestation

     (1) Contractions—4 in 20 minutes or 8 in 60 minutes plus progressive change in the cervix

     (2) Cervical dilatation greater than 2 cm

     (3) Cervical effacement of 80% or more

  h. Management—goal is to delay preterm birth (prior to 34 weeks) and enhance infant's resources to cope with life outside the uterus

     (1) Premature rupture of membranes—two approaches

       (a) Expectant management/nonintervention until spontaneous labor begins

       (b) Intervention with corticosteroids in conjunction with or without tocolytics to advance fetal maturation

       (c) Birth is inevitable but delaying the birth seems to decrease infant mortality

       (d) Hospitalize

       (e) Corticosteroids

       (f) Antimicrobials

     (2) With intact membranes

       (a) Corticosteroids—clear benefits for birth at 24–34 weeks, but unclear for 34 weeks or longer; treatment is most effective when time interval from rupture to birth is a minimum of 24 hours and a maximum of 7 days

       (b) Bed rest—ineffective to stop labor; associated with increased risk of thromboembolic problems

       (c) Hydration and sedation—ineffective

       (d) Tocolytic drugs

         i. Beta-adrenergic receptor agonists—ritodrine and terbutaline—relatively little effect with serious maternal side-effects, i.e., pulmonary edema, cardiac insufficiency, hyperglycemia, death

         ii. Magnesium sulfate—evidence shows no effect for stopping labor and hypermagnesemia may have toxic effect on mother and fetus

         iii. Prostaglandin inhibitors—indomethacin; adversely affects fetus, i.e., necrotizing enterocolitis, intracranial hemorrhage

         iv. Calcium-channel blockers-nifedipine; shows promise but not adequately researched yet

         v. Oxytocin analog—atosiban; research to date shows it did not improve infant outcomes

7. Multiple gestation—identify as early as possible

  a. Incidence

     (1) Monozygotic—4/1000 worldwide

     (2) Dizygotic—8/1000 worldwide

     (3) Accounts for less than 1% of births but more than 10% of perinatal mortality

     (4) Incidence varies with race and increases with age, parity, and heredity

  b. Dizygotic (DZ) (fraternal)—fertilization of two separate ova by two separate sperm

     (1) Use of fertility drugs increases chance

     (2) Clomid—1/10 risk

     (3) Gonadotropins—1/5 risk

     (4) IVF increases risk

  c. Monozygotic (MZ) (identical)—division of a single egg fertilized by a single sperm

     (1) Risk factors are unknown

     (2) Time of ovum division determines membrane development

       (a) Day 0–3—dichorionic, diamniotic (30%)

       (b) Day 4–8—monochorionic, diamniotic (68%)

       (c) After day 8—monochorionic, monoamniotic (2%)

       (d) After day 13 conjoined twins (< 1%)

  d. Family history increases risk

  e. Clinical skills are important to identify multiple pregnancies

  f. Signs and symptoms

     (1) Fundal height greater than dates

     (2) Earlier or exaggerated discomforts of pregnancy

     (3) Two distinct heart beats

     (4) Outline of more than one fetus

     (5) Palpation of multiple small parts

     (6) Ultrasound of two or more fetuses

  g. Differential diagnosis

     (1) Macrosomia

     (2) Uterine, ovarian, or pelvic mass

     (3) Distended bladder

     (4) Polyhydramnios

     (5) Hydatidiform mole

     (6) Inaccurate dates

  h. Potential complications

(1) Hyperemesis
(2) Preterm labor, PROM, preterm birth
    (a) 36% deliver before 36 weeks' gestation
    (b) 50% deliver before 37 weeks' gestation
(3) Low birth weight—55% are less than 5 lb
(4) Twin-to-twin transfusion
(5) Oligohydramnios
(6) Perinatal asphyxia
(7) Preeclampsia
(8) Postpartum hemorrhage
(9) Pyelonephritis
(10) Maternal anemia
(11) Placental problems
    (a) Previa
    (b) Abruption
(12) Fetal anomalies

  i. Antepartum management
    (1) Consult
    (2) Discuss risks and benefits of management, serial ultrasounds, and regular fetal surveillance
    (3) Counsel about maternal nutrition, rest, exercise, and stress
        (a) Increased nutritional needs
        (b) Increased iron
        (c) Small frequent meals
        (d) Exercise limitations and bed rest are both controversial
    (4) Provide emotional support
    (5) Evaluate weekly for weight, fetal growth, signs/symptoms of preterm labor, and elevated BP
    (6) Preterm labor monitoring
        (a) Possible administration of glucocorticoids for lung maturity
        (b) Tocolytic therapy
        (c) Birth plan should include availability of physician consultant for birth

8. Malpresentations of significance during the prenatal period—breech and shoulder (transverse lie)
  a. Concept—the presentation determines the presenting part
  b. Breech—longitudinal lie with buttocks in the lower pole
    (1) Incidence
        (a) 14% between 29 and 32 weeks
        (b) 3.5% at term
    (2) Variations
        (a) Frank—legs are extended up over the fetal abdomen and chest
        (b) Complete—legs are flexed at the hips and knees

        (c) Footling or incomplete—one or both feet or knees are lowermost
    (3) Etiology—some situation that distorts the shape of the fetus or the uterus
        (a) Uterine septum
        (b) Fetal anomaly, e.g., hydrocephaly
        (c) Fetal attitude, e.g., extention of spinal column or neck
        (d) Placenta previa
        (e) Conditions resulting in abnormal fetal movement or muscle tone
    (4) Diagnosis
        (a) Abdominal examination—Leopold's maneuvers findings (four maneuvers)
          i. Fetal part in the fundus is round, hard, freely moveable and ballotable
          ii. Find back and small parts
          iii. Part in lower pole is large, nodular body
          iv. Determine degree of engagement and reaffirm previous findings by confirming lack of cephalic prominence in lower pole
        (b) Vaginal findings compared to vertex findings
          i. No fetal skull sutures nor fontanels
          ii. Round indentation (anus)
          iii. Tissue texture is softer than head, if complete breech; toes, feet, or knees may be palpated if footling
    (5) Treatment
        (a) External cephalic version
        (b) Moxibustion
        (c) Anticipatory guidance regarding plan for version as well as plans for persistent breech

  c. Shoulder—transverse lie in which the shoulder or arm is found in the lower pole
    (1) Incidence—0.4%
    (2) Etiology
        (a) Multiparity
        (b) Placenta previa
        (c) Polyhydramnios
        (d) Uterine anomalies
9. Hypertensive disorders of pregnancy
  a. Definitions
    (1) Chronic hypertension—BP 140/90 mm Hg or higher diagnosed before pregnancy, before 20 weeks' gestation, or after 12 weeks postpartum
    (2) Chronic hypertension with superimposed preeclampsia—chronic

hypertension with new-onset proteinuria at greater than 300 mg in 24 hours, but no proteinuria before 20 weeks' gestation; or sudden increase in proteinuria or blood pressure or platelet count of less than 100,000/mm³ in women with HTN and proteinuria before 20 weeks' gestation

   (3) Preeclampsia—the development of hypertension with proteinuria after the 20th week of pregnancy; varies in degree (mild vs severe); only exception is if the woman has a hydatidiform mole

   (4) HELLP syndrome—*H*emolytic anemia, *E*levated *L*iver enzymes, and *Low Pl*atelet count

   (5) Eclampsia—seizures that cannot be attributed to other causes in a woman with preeclampsia

  b. Management of chronic hypertension

   (1) Consult—will need to comanage and/or transfer care

   (2) Prepregnancy antihypertensive regimen to be continued (precluding contraindicated medications)

   (3) Diuretics should not be used in pregnancy

   (4) First choice of antihypertensives include labetalol or hydralazine

   (5) Fetal surveillance

     (a) Monitor for IUGR

     (b) NSTs

     (c) AFI/BPP

  c. Classifications of preeclampsia—a range of signs exist

   (1) Minimum criteria

     (a) BP ≥ 140/90 mm Hg

     (b) Proteinuria 300 mg in 24 hours or 1+ dipstick or greater

   (2) Increased likelihood of preeclampsia

     (a) BP 160/110 mm Hg or higher

     (b) Proteinuria 2.0 g/24 hour period or 2+ dipstick or greater

     (c) Serum creatinine at greater than1.2 mg/dL

     (d) Platelets less than 100,000 mm³

     (e) Elevated ALT/AST

     (f) Persistent headache, visual disturbance

     (g) Persistent epigastric pain

   (3) Other signs and symptoms

     (a) Severe headache

     (b) Cerebral or visual disturbances

     (c) Right upper gastric or epigastric pain

     (d) Edema

     (e) Hemoconcentration

     (f) Thrombocytopenia

     (g) Hepatic dysfunction

     (h) Elevated uric acid

  d. Risk factors

   (1) Nulliparity

   (2) Adolescent or advanced maternal age (> 35 years)

   (3) Multiple gestation

   (4) Family history of preeclampsia or eclampsia

   (5) Obesity and insulin resistance

   (6) Chronic hypertension

   (7) Limited exposure to father of baby's sperm—new partner, donor insemination

   (8) Antiphospholipid antibody syndrome and thrombophilia

  e. Theory of causes

   (1) Abnormal trophoblast invasion

   (2) Coagulation abnormalities

   (3) Vascular endothelial damage

   (4) Cardiovascular maladaptation

   (5) Immunologic phenomena

   (6) Genetic predisposition

   (7) Dietary deficiencies or excesses

  f. Antepartum management of preeclampsia

   (1) Consult diet assessment

   (2) Adequate fluids

   (3) Restricted activities (some experts advise)

   (4) Monitor BP, proteinuria, edema, weight, intake and output, DTRs, subjective symptoms

  g. Laboratory tests

   (1) Creatinine

   (2) Hgb/hct

   (3) Platelets

   (4) LFTs

   (5) 24-hour urine for protein

   (6) Creatinine clearance

  h. Assessment of fetus

   (1) Daily fetal movement assessment

   (2) NST

   (3) AFI/BPP

   (4) USG for growth

  i. Intrapartum management

   (1) Goal to prevent seizures

   (2) Magnesium sulfate

     (a) Given IV

     (b) Used as an anticonvulsant

     (c) Side-effects—flushing, somnolence

     (d) Overdosage signs and symptoms

       i. Loss of patellar reflex

       ii. Muscular paralysis

       iii. Respiratory arrest

        iv. Aggravated by decreased urine output (MgSO$_4$ is excreted by kidneys)

    (3) Antidote is calcium gluconate

    (4) Valium as anticonvulsant rarely used

    (5) Antihypertensives

        (a) Hydralazine IV is antihypertensive of choice in severe preeclampsia

        (b) Others—labetalol (beta blocker), nifedipine

    (6) Diuretics are *not* recommended—woman is already volume depleted

  i. HELLP syndrome—affects 10% of patients with severe preeclampsia

    (1) Diagnosis

        (a) Hemolysis

        (b) Abnormal peripheral blood smear

        (c) Increased bilirubin at 1.2 mg/dL or greater

        (d) Elevated liver enzymes—AST, ALT, LDH

        (e) Platelet count at less than 100,000

    (2) Treatment

        (a) Plasma volume expansion

        (b) Bedrest

        (c) Crystalloids

        (d) Albumin 5–25%

        (e) Delivery as indicated

        (f) Magnesium sulfate

  j. Eclampsia

    (1) Signs and symptoms—same as preeclampsia with seizures

    (2) Management—medical management

        (a) Magnesium sulfate

        (b) Administer oxygen

        (c) Safety—prevent injuries and minimize aspiration during seizures

        (d) Stabilize and deliver

  k. Prevention of pregnancy-induced hypertension

    (1) Calcium and vitamin D supplementation if at risk and have low dietary intake

    (2) Low-dose aspirin—consider in high-risk pregnancies

10. Postterm pregnancy

  a. Definition—pregnancy continuing beyond 42 completed weeks' gestation

  b. Incidence

    (1) 6–12% of pregnancies go beyond 42 weeks

    (2) 25% of postterm pregnancies result with babies who have postmaturity syndrome

    (3) Associated with increased morbidity and mortality

  c. Diagnosis

    (1) Based on careful gestational age assessment

        (a) Certain LNMP

        (b) Early examination

        (c) Sizing by bimanual examination

        (d) Fundal height

        (e) Fetal heart tones by doppler and fetoscope

    (2) Report of sexual history

    (3) Report of quickening

    (4) Early USG gestational dating

        (a) CRL best (between 6–14 weeks)

        (b) Or dating using FL, AC, HC, and BPD before 26 weeks

  d. Potential complications

    (1) Shoulder dystocia—if fetus macrosomic

    (2) Problems related to oligohydramnios

    (3) Problems related to utero-placental insufficiency

    (4) Neonatal meconium aspiration

    (5) Stillbirth

  e. Management

    (1) Fetal movement counts between 40 and 41 weeks

        (a) At 41 weeks begin biweekly NST/AFI or BPP

        (b) BPP if abnormal NST (CST used less frequently)

        (c) Doppler velocimetry

        (d) Consult

        (e) Expectant management and delivery

            i. Consider induction when cervix is ripe

           ii. Prostaglandins may be used to promote cervical ripening

          iii. Methods of labor induction—oxytocin, membrane stripping, amniotomy, nipple stimulation

          iv. Deliver if any indication of fetal compromise or oligohydramnios

           v. Be prepared for possible meconium staining of fluid

◻ MEDICAL COMPLICATIONS

- Urinary tract infection (UTI)
  1. Risk factors
     a. History of UTI
     b. Sickle cell trait
     c. Diabetes
     d. Pregnancy

(1) The increased progesterone of pregnancy causes relaxation of the smooth muscles of the GU tract

(2) Decreased ureteral peristalsis and ureteral dilation present

(3) Physical pressure on bladder

(4) Urinary stasis

(5) Incidence

  (a) Occurs in 2–7% of all pregnancies

  (b) 25–30% will progress on to pyelonephritis if left untreated

2. Cystitis; infection of the bladder

  a. May be asymptomatic (asymptomatic bacteriuria)

  b. Usual signs of UTI (although acute cystitis is relatively rare in pregnancy)

  c. Uterine contractions

  d. Suprapubic discomfort

  e. Urgency and frequency

3. Pyelonephritis—infection of the kidneys

  a. Fever and chills

  b. Nausea and vomiting

  c. CVA tenderness

  d. Dysuria

  e. Flu-like symptoms

4. Bacterial causes of UTIs

  a. *E. Coli* (most common)

  b. Klebsiella

  c. Proteus

  d. *Neisseria gonorrhoeae*

  e. Pseudomonas

5. Diagnosis

  a. Symptoms

  b. Urinalysis

  c. Culture and sensitivity

  d. If protein and WBC are present on urine dipstick, consider culture

  e. Screen every 4 weeks in sickle cell trait, diabetes, and previous pyelonephritis in this pregnancy

6. Management

  a. Asymptomatic bacteriuria and UTI

    (1) Treat with antibiotic even if no symptoms

    (2) Adequate fluids

    (3) Cranberry juice

    (4) Antimicrobial therapy

      (a) Ampicillin or amoxicillin

      (b) Cephalosporins

      (c) Nitrofurantoin (contraindicated in late third trimester and in women with G-6-PD)

      (d) Trimethoprim/sulfamethoxazole (contraindicated in third trimester or if have G-6-PD)

    (5) Follow up 2 weeks later with a test of cure

    (6) If recurrent infection, consider suppressive therapy for the remainder of the pregnancy

      (a) Nitrofurantoin 100 mg, orally at night

      (b) Cephalexin 250 mg orally at night

    (7) Patient education

  b. Pyelonephritis

    (1) Hospitalization

    (2) IV antibiotics

    (3) Hydration

    (4) Antipyretics

    (5) Monitor for preterm labor

- Human immunodeficiency virus (HIV) (AIDS)

  1. Etiology—DNA retroviruses termed human immunodeficiency viruses, HIV-1 and HIV-2; most cases worldwide are HIV-1; retroviruses have genomes that encode reverse transcriptase allowing the virus to make DNA copies of itself in the host cells

  2. Incidence—approximately 25% of HIV-positive adults in US are women; HIV/AIDS is number one cause of death for black women 25 to 34 years of age; 40% of HIV-infected infants born to women unaware of HIV status until after delivery

  3. Transmission

    a. Sexual intercourse (80%)

    b. IV drug use (19%)

    c. Other (1%)

    d. Mother to infant

      (1) 15–25% if woman does not receive antiretroviral (ARV) therapy during pregnancy

      (2) Less than 1% if woman receives multi-agent ARV and if has undetectable viral load at delivery

  4. Diagnosis

    a. Risk assessment—drug use/sexual histories

    b. Universal screening of pregnant women for HIV as part of routine prenatal tests with option to decline (opt-out screening) recommended

    c. Repeat screening in third trimester if high risk, high incidence of HIV in reproductive age women in geographic area, signs or symptoms of acute HIV infection

    d. Rapid HIV testing at labor and delivery if status unknown (CDC, 2006)

    e. HIV testing

      (1) Antibody testing

        (a) Screening tests—enzyme immunoassay (EIA) or rapid test

      (b) Confirmatory tests if screening test is positive—Western blot or immunofluorescence assay (IFA)

    (2) Direct viral screens

      (a) Nucleic acid testing if suspect acute retroviral syndrome or recent infection

      (b) Confirm with subsequent antibody testing to document seroconversion

5. Signs and symptoms of initial HIV infection
   a. Incubation period from exposure to clinical disease—days to weeks
   b. Acute viral illness syndrome—lasts 10 days or less
   c. Fever
   d. Night sweats
   e. Fatigue
   f. Rash
   g. Headache
   h. Lymphadenopathy
   i. Pharyngitis
   j. Myalgias
   k. Arthralgias
   l. Nausea
   m. Vomiting
   n. Diarrhea
   o. Becomes asymptomatic and chronic viremia begins
   p. Time to immunodeficiency syndrome is 10 years

6. Signs and symptoms of AIDS
   a. Generalized lymphadenopathy
   b. Oral hairy leukoplakia
   c. Aphthous ulcers
   d. Thrombocytopenia
   e. Opportunistic infections
   f. Esophageal or pulmonary candidiasis
   g. Persistent herpes
   h. Cytomegalovirus
   i. Molluscum contagiosum
   j. Pneumocystis
   k. Toxoplamosis
   l. Neurologic disease—50%
   m. $CD4^+$ count of less than 200 is definitive diagnosis

7. Management of HIV-positive women
   a. Infection control
   b. Initial evaluation
   c. Complete review of systems (ROS)
   d. Physical examination
   e. Initial labs—HIV antibody, $CD4^+$ count, viral load
   f. Follow-up by team of experts; interdisciplinary approach is most effective
   g. Prevention of vertical transmission

    (1) Viral load is strongest predictor for vertical transmission

    (2) Multi-agent ARV therapy during pregnancy—start after first trimester if mother does not need treatment

    (3) Intravenous zidovudine therapy during labor and delivery

    (4) Avoid artificial rupture of membranes if delivery is not imminent

    (5) Consider C-section at 38 weeks if viral load is greater than 1000 copies/ml

    (6) Treat infant with ARV therapy—usual regimen is 6 weeks

  h. Prevention of opportunistic infections

  i. Standard precautions for all blood and body fluid-borne pathogens to include blood, all body fluid secretions and excretions, nonintact skin and mucous membranes

8. Treatment—antepartum
   a. Goals are treatment of maternal infection and reduction of risk for perinatal transmission
   b. Highly active antiretroviral therapy (HAART) that includes:

    (1) Two nucleoside analogues—zidovudine, didanosine, zalcitabine, lamivudine and

    (2) Protease inhibitor—indinavir, ritonavir, saquinavir or non-nucleoside analogue—nevirapine, delavirdine, efavirenz

    (3) Start after first trimester unless mother needs treatment

9. Treatment—intrapartum
   a. Zidovudine IV throughout labor and delivery for vaginal birth
   b. Zidovudine IV starting 3 hours before C-section and through delivery

10. Counseling
    a. Pretest counseling is important
    b. Informed consent
    c. Posttest counseling is also important

11. Legal issues
    a. Confidentiality
    b. Reporting
    c. Partner notification
    d. Discrimination

12. Concurrent disease concerns for HIV-infected women
    a. Syphilis
    b. TB
    c. HPV
    d. Hepatitis B
    e. Pneumococcal infection

13. Possible effects on pregnancy outcome

a. PROM
b. Preterm labor and birth
c. Low birth weight
d. Fetal demise
e. HIV transmission to fetus

14. Fetal assessment as clinically indicated
    a. US
    b. FMC
    c. Serial US as needed
    d. NST with AFI, BPP

15. Intrapartum care
    a. Avoid invasive procedures
    b. Maintain universal body fluid precautions for all births
    c. Cleanse maternal secretions from baby as soon as possible
    d. Drain umbilical cord for cord blood/avoid needles
    e. Breastfeeding is *not* recommended—16% probability of transmission of HIV infection to infant
    f. Give emotional support

- Toxoplasmosis
  1. Incidence—15–40% of pregnant women have antibodies to toxoplasmosis
     a. Primary infection in pregnancy is 1/1000
     b. Most infections are asymptomatic
     c. Of those infected
        (1) 10% will have damage resulting in lower IQ and deafness
        (2) Severe congenital infection occurs 1/10,000
        (3) Infection can also cause abortion, prematurity, and IUGR
  2. Diagnosis
     a. Laboratory data
     b. Testing does not allow diagnosis between primary and secondary infection
     c. Testing for antitoxoplasma IgG antibody is difficult to interpret so not a practical test to perform
  3. Prevention
     a. Fully cook meat
     b. Do not drink unpasteurized milk or cheese
     c. Avoid kitty litter
     d. Good hand washing following gardening or wear gloves

- Rubella
  1. Incidence (CDC, 2006)
     a. Rare in US
     b. Only 11 new cases of rubella (2006)
     c. One half of new cases have occurred in persons born outside US
     d. 10–20% of reproductive women are susceptible to rubella
     e. Four cases of congenital rubella 2001–2004; three of these cases in women born outside US
     f. No reported cases of congenital rubella syndrome (CRS) since 2004
     g. Risk of long-term complications from CRS highest if mother infected in first trimester
     h. Most common complications are deafness, IUGR, cataracts, retinopathy, patent ductus arteriosus
  2. Pathophysiology
     a. Rubella is a single-stranded RNA virus
     b. Acquired respiratory disease
     c. Occurs 2–3 weeks following exposure
     d. Infectious virus is present in respiratory tract 1 week prior to symptom development
  3. Symptoms—rash
     a. Discrete pink-red maculopapular rash
     b. Appears first on face then trunk and extremities
     c. May also have lymphadenopathy, fever, arthralgias
     d. Symptoms last 3 days
     e. Up to 50% of all infections are subclinical
  4. Laboratory testing
     a. Demonstrate serologic conversion
     b. Recent rubella infection will result in specific IgM in the fetal blood
     c. Can use CVS to recover virus
  5. Treatment—prevention
     a. No available antiviral therapy
     b. Vaccination of susceptible reproductive age women preconception or postpartum
     c. No documented cases of CRS from vaccine but recommend giving at least 4 weeks prior to attempting a pregnancy or postpartum; may give while breastfeeding

- Varicella-zoster (VZV)
  1. Herpes virus causing two common infections
     a. Varicella—chicken pox
        (1) Primary infection is rare in pregnancy
        (2) Greatest risk for congenital varicella syndrome is when mother is infected in first 20 weeks
        (3) Maternal infection occurring from 6 days before to 2 days after delivery can be passed to newborn causing serious infection—5% mortality
        (4) Varicella infection causes varicella pneumonia in 10–30% of adults
     b. Herpes zoster—shingles
        (1) Secondary infection
        (2) Poses little risk to mother or baby

2. Incidence
   a. Among pregnant women, 5/1000
   b. VZV is highly contagious and peaks in winter and spring
3. Pathophysiology
   a. Respiratory inhalation of virus particles
   b. Results in a viremia
   c. Incubation period is 10–21 days, usually 14 days
   d. Virus may be transmitted up to 2 days prior to rash
4. Diagnosis
   a. Prior to rash, adults experience fever, malaise, myalgias, and headache
   b. Rash—maculopapular rash that becomes vesicles
   c. New vesicles continue for 3–4 days
   d. Crusted by 1 week
5. Complications
   a. Pneumonia
   b. Increased risk of preterm labor and birth
6. Treatment
   a. Antiviral agent—IV acyclovir for severe infection in woman
   b. Infection in mother 6 days before delivery—give VZIG, prepare for tocolysis to delay delivery, give VZIG to infant
   c. Infection in mother within 3 days postpartum—give infant VZIG
7. Prevention
   a. Varicella vaccination for all susceptible reproductive age women preconception (at least 4 weeks before attempting pregnancy) or postpartum
   b. Varicella-zoster immunoglobulin (VZIG) as early as possible if pregnant woman exposed and susceptible

- Tuberculosis (TB)
  1. Definition—infection, mostly in the lung, by *Mycobacterium tuberculosis;* clinical disease occurs in 10% of those infected
  2. Populations at risk for tuberculosis
     a. HIV-infected women
     b. Foreign-born women from countries with high TB prevalence
     c. Medically underserved low-income populations
     d. Close contacts of persons with active infection
     e. Alcoholics and IV drug users
  3. Incidence (CDC, 2008)
     a. 13,299 new cases in US (2007); 4.4 per 100,000 persons
     b. Foreign-born persons accounted for 58% of new cases

4. Screening tests for tuberculosis
   a. Purified protein derivative (PPD) intradermally
      (1) If negative, i.e., no induration, no further assessment is needed
      (2) Positive test interpreted by risk factors
         (a) 5 mm is positive for very high risk—HIV positive, with abnormal chest radiograph, recent contact with active case
         (b) 10 mm is positive for high risk, i.e., foreign born, HIV negative IV drug user, low-income populations, associated medical problems
         (c) 15 mm is positive for those with none of these risks
      (3) Vaccination with bacillus Calmette-Guerin (BCG) requires special guidance for interpretation
5. Signs and symptoms
   a. Cough with minimal sputum production
   b. Low-grade fever
   c. Hemoptysis
   d. Weight loss
6. Diagnosis
   a. Chest radiograph
   b. Sputum for acid fast bacillus
   c. Extrapulmonary disease occurs in any organ; disseminated disease exists in 40% of HIV-positive patients
7. Treatment (CDC, 2008)
   a. Initiate treatment of pregnant women when probability of TB is moderate to high
      (1) Recent PPD converters—incidence of active infection is 3% the first year
      (2) PPD positive through exposure to active disease because infection is 0.5% per year
      (3) HIV-positive women have annual active disease risk of 8%
   b. Latent TB infection
      (1) Isoniazid daily or twice weekly for 9 months
      (2) Vitamin B_6 (pyridoxine) 50 mg daily during treatment
   c. Active tuberculosis in pregnancy
      (1) Isoniazid, rifampin, and ethambutol daily for 2 months
      (2) After initial 2 months of treatment, Isoniazid and rifampin daily or twice weekly for 7 months
      (3) Pyridoxine 50 mg daily throughout treatment
   d. HIV-infected pregnant woman with suspected TB—consult with infectious disease specialist

e. Breastfeeding is not contraindicated with TB treatment
f. Precautions
   (1) Liver toxicity
   (2) Drug resistance

- Diabetes
  1. Definition—endocrine disorder of abnormal carbohydrate metabolism resulting in inadequate production and/or utilization of insulin
  2. Gestational diabetes
     a. Occurs in 2–12% of pregnancies.
     b. Results from the diabetogenic effect of pregnancy
     c. hPL (human placental lactogen) acts as an insulin antagonist
     d. Estrogen and progesterone may also act as insulin antagonists
  3. Diagnosis
     a. Risk assessment at initial prenatal visit
     b. High risk (American Diabetes Association, 2009)
        (1) Obesity
        (2) Prior history of GDM or large for gestational age infant
        (3) Presence of glycosuria
        (4) Diagnosis of PCOS
        (5) Strong family history of type 2 diabetes
     c. Low risk (American Diabetes Association, 2009)
        (1) Age of younger than 25 years
        (2) Normal weight before pregnancy
        (3) Member of ethnic group with low prevalence of diabetes
        (4) No known diabetes in first-degree relatives
        (5) No history of abnormal glucose tolerance
        (6) No history of poor obstetrical outcome
  4. Screening (American Diabetes Association, 2009)
     a. High risk—screen as soon as possible using standard diagnostic testing
     b. All women not considered low risk—screen at 24–28 weeks
        (1) Two-step approach
           (a) One-hour 50 g glucose challenge test (GCT)
           (b) If 130 mg/dl (90% sensitivity) or more, or greater than 140 mg/dl (80% sensitivity), perform diagnostic 100 g OGTT on another day
        (2) One-step approach
           (a) May prefer if high prevalence of GDM in patient population
           (b) 100 g OGTT
  5. Diagnostic criteria for GDM—presence of at least two of the following plasma glucose values
     a. Fasting 95 mg/dl or greater
     b. 1 hour 180 mg/dl or greater
     c. 2 hour 155 mg/dl or greater
     d. 3 hour 140 mg/dl or greater
  6. Presence of three or more of the following risk factors increases the chance of perinatal mortality:
     a. Uncontrolled hyperglycemia
     b. Ketonuria, nausea, vomiting
     c. PIH, edema, proteinuria
     d. Pyelonephritis
     e. Lack of compliance with care
     f. Maternal age older than 35 years
  7. Management—objective is to maintain strict levels of maternal glucose for optimum perinatal outcomes
     a. Comanage or transfer to perinatal center
     b. Diet
        (1) 30 kcal/kg of actual or ideal body weight
        (2) 25% at breakfast
        (3) 30% at lunch
        (4) 30% at dinner
        (5) 15% at snack
     c. Distribution of calories
        (1) Protein 20% of calories
        (2) Fat 30–35% of calories
        (3) Carbohydrates 45–50% of calories
     d. Medications
        (1) Oral hypoglycemics—glyburide and acarbose are pregnancy category B; others are category C
        (2) Insulin
     e. Maternal monitoring
        (1) PIH
        (2) Changing insulin requirements
        (3) Decreased need in first trimester due to low hPL levels
        (4) Increases in second trimester due to increasing hPL levels
        (5) HgbA$_{1C}$/fasting plasma
     f. Fetal monitoring
        (1) Increased risk of neural tube defects and cardiac anomalies in nongestational diabetics
        (2) Ultrasound for IUGR, macrosomia, polyhydramnios
        (3) FMCs beginning at 28 weeks
        (4) NSTs with AFI or CST beginning at 36 weeks

(5) May consider amniocentesis for L/S ratio (maturity is 3:1 with positive pg)

g. Immediate postpartum—monitor insulin requirements (usually decrease 24–48 hours after delivery of the placenta)

h. 6–12 weeks postpartum—screen for diabetes and then follow with subsequent screening for diabetes or prediabetes

- Thyroid disease
  1. Definition—most common thyroid diseases in pregnancy are nontoxic goiter, hyperthyroidism, hypothyroidism, and thyroiditis
  2. Impact of pregnancy on maternal thyroid physiology is great; structural and functional changes related to pregnancy can cause confusion in defining abnormalities
  3. Thyroid enlarges somewhat due to hyperplasia and increased vascularity but does not cause serious thyromegaly
  4. Thyroid hormones in pregnancy— total serum thyroxine (TT_4) and triiodothyronine (TT_3) concentrations increase; TSH and free thyroxine (FT_4) levels are not affected
  5. Thyrotoxicosis or hyperthyroidism
     a. Incidence—1/2000 pregnancies
     b. Signs and symptoms
        (1) Tachycardia, more than normal in pregnancy
        (2) Elevated sleeping pulse rate
        (3) Thyromegaly
        (4) Exophthalmos
        (5) Failure to gain weight with normal or increased food consumption
     c. Diagnosis
        (1) Elevated serum free thyroxine (FT_4) or free thyroxine index (FTI) levels
        (2) Suppressed TSH levels
     d. Treatment
        (1) Control with thioamide drugs; propylthiouracil or methimazole
        (2) Thyroidectomy if medical approach unsuccessful but easier done outside of pregnancy due to increased vascularity
     e. Maternal and fetal outcomes
        (1) Good if treatment successful
        (2) If not, higher incidence of preeclampsia and heart failure as well as preterm birth, IUGR and stillbirth

- Blood incompatibilities—D(Rh) isoimmunization
  1. Incidence (Rh−)
     a. Highest incidence found in Basques of France and Spain (25–40%)
     b. White Americans approximately 15%

c. African Americans approximately 5–8%
d. American Hispanics approximately 5–10%

2. Types
   a. ABO incompatibility
      (1) 20–25% of pregnancies are ABO incompatible
      (2) Isoimmunization causes 60% of fetal hemolytic disease
   b. Maternal serum contains anti-A or anti-B
      (1) Rarely causes more than fetal anemia with mild to moderate hyperbilirubinemia in the first 24 hours of life
      (2) Due to the fact that the IgM anti-B or IgM anti-A cross the placenta poorly
   c. Sensitization caused by minor antigens
      (1) Some cause hemolytic disease, some do not
      (2) Believed to be the result of incompatible transfusion although may be seen in multiparas
   d. Kell—may have mild to severe with hydrops (K-kills)
   e. Duffy—Fy^a may have mild to severe with hydrops; Fy^b—not associated with problems

3. Pathogenesis for Rh isoimmunization
   a. Three requirements
      (1) Fetus must be D+ and mother D−
      (2) Mother must be able to be sensitized
      (3) Fetal cells must gain access into the mother's blood stream in sufficient quantities
   b. Occurs when
      (1) There is a transfusion of incompatible blood to the mother, usually before pregnancy
      (2) A feto-maternal exchange of blood during
          (a) Delivery
          (b) Spontaneous or induced abortion (woman may not realize she's pregnant)
          (c) Amniocentesis
          (d) Ectopic
          (e) Placental separation
          (f) Unknown cause

4. Implications
   a. Maternal
      (1) No significant maternal complications
      (2) Fetal loss
   b. Fetal
      (1) Mother produces anti-D antibodies (IgG), which cross the placenta
      (2) Hemolysis of fetal RBC then occurs
      (3) Fetal anemia results with hematopoiesis in liver and spleen

(4) Fetal liver and spleen enlarge

(5) Liver and spleen show degenerative changes.

(6) Erythroblastosis fetalis results (ascites, cardiac failure, hydrothorax)

(7) Hydrops fetalis with generalized edema

   c. Newborn

(1) Maternal IgG is still present and attacking RBC

(2) Further RBC breakdown occurs

(3) Fetal liver is immature and unable to clear RBC

(4) Hyperbilirubinemia results

(5) Bilirubin causes kernicterus with CNS damage and possible death

  5. Management

   a. Unsensitized pregnancy—mother Rh negative with negative antibody titer

(1) ABO/D group and antibody titer at first visit

(2) Repeat antibody screen at 28 weeks and give RhoGAM if remains unsensitized

(3) RhoGAM is protective for 12 weeks

(4) If infant is Rh positive, give mother RhoGAM again after delivery

   b. Sensitized pregnancy—mother Rh negative with positive antibody titer (> 1:4)

(1) Consult—comanage or transfer care

(2) Follow fetus with serial ultrasounds to assess for signs of ascites

(3) Follow titers to assess need for amniocentesis

- Acquired anemias

  1. Iron deficiency anemia

   a. Definition—hemoglobin less than 11.0 g/dL first trimester, 10.5 g/dL second trimester, 11.0 mg/dL third trimester and postpartum

   b. Etiology—related to poor nutrition resulting in inadequate iron stores; consequence of expansion of blood volume with inadequate expansion of maternal hemoglobin mass

   c. Signs and symptoms—not apparent unless severely anemic

   d. Differential diagnosis

(1) Anemia associated with chronic disease

(2) Blood loss effect

   e. Diagnostic tests

(1) Serum ferritin levels lower than normal

(2) Microcytic, hypochromic erythrocytes

(3) Serum iron-binding capacity elevated (but not a significant finding since it is elevated in pregnancy in absence of iron deficiency)

   f. Associated with low birth weight, premature delivery, perinatal mortality

   g. Management and treatment—correct the hemoglobin mass deficit and rebuild iron stores

(1) Iron replacement therapy

(2) Ferrous sulfate, ferrous gluconate, ferrous fumarate

(3) Include vitamin C and folic acid

(4) Intramuscular therapy if unable to take orally or if severely anemic

(5) Iron therapy for 3 months after anemia corrected

  2. Anemia from acute blood loss

   a. Definition—drop in hemoglobin due to moderate-to-severe blood loss, which can occur at any time in pregnancy

   b. Etiology—abortion, ectopic pregnancy, hydatidiform mole, placenta previa, abruptio placenta, placenta implantation anomalies, etc.

   c. Management and treatment

(1) Massive hemorrhage requires restoration of volume and cells to maintain perfusion of vital organs

(2) Treat residual iron depletion (Hb 7 g/dL or greater) with oral iron for 3 months as long as woman is afebrile and able to ambulate

  3. Megaloblastic anemia

   a. Definition—group of hematologic disorders characterized by blood and bone marrow abnormalities caused by impaired DNA synthesis

   b. Prevalence—rare in the US

   c. Etiology—in the US, during pregnancy, most always results from folic acid deficiency due to lack of consumption of green leafy vegetables, legumes, and animal protein

   d. Signs and symptoms—nausea, vomiting, and anorexia, which worsen as deficiency increases

   e. Diagnosis—laboratory tests showing hypersegmentation of neutrophils, macrocytic erythrocytes, bone marrow megaloblastic erythropoiesis

   f. Risks to fetus—neural tube defects

   g. Prevention—folic acid (0.4 mg daily for childbearing-aged women; 4 mg daily prior to and during pregnancy for women with history of previous neural tube defect infant), nutritious diet, and iron

- Inherited anemias—hemoglobinopathies
  1. Sickle cell hemoglobinopathies
     a. Sickle cell anemia (SS disease)
     b. Sickle cell–hemoglobin C disease (SC disease)
     c. Sickle cell–β-thalassemia disease (S–β-thalassemia disease)
  2. Etiology—individual inherits a gene for S hemoglobin from each parent, or an S and a C gene from each, or an S and β-thalassemia gene from each
  3. Incidence
     a. SS disease—1 in 12 African Americans has sickle cell trait—SA hemoglobin; incidence is 1 in 576 theoretically but is, in fact, less common
     b. SC disease—1 in 40 African Americans has hemoglobin C gene; incidence of SC disease in African-American pregnant women is 1 in 2000
     c. Sickle cell-β-thalassemia disease—1 in 2000 African-American women
  4. Signs and symptoms—SS is worst of hemoglobinopathies in pregnancy
     a. Sickle cell crisis occurs more frequently in pregnancy
     b. Infections and pulmonary complications more common
     c. Contributes to maternal mortality
  5. Differential diagnosis
     a. Thalassemia
     b. G-6-PD deficiency
  6. Physical findings
     a. Hb 7 g/dL or less
     b. Intense pain of crisis particularly in third trimester, in labor, and in puerperium
     c. Fever due to dehydration or infection
     d. Acute chest syndrome—pleuritic pain, cough, fever, lung infiltrate, and hypoxia
  7. Management and treatment
     a. Consult and comanage
     b. Weekly fetal surveillance after 32–34 weeks
     c. Pain medication
     d. Follow-up (including possible need for paternal blood screening and genetic counseling)
     e. Counseling for current and future pregnancies

- Appendicitis
  1. Incidence—suspected in 1/1000; found in 1/1500 pregnant woman; most common reason for surgical exploration during pregnancy
  2. Pregnancy confounds signs and symptoms of appendicitis
     a. Nausea, vomiting, and anorexia of pregnancy vs appendicitis
     b. Displacement of the appendix by the growing uterus moves the point of pain and tenderness associated with appendicitis
     c. Leukocytosis, to some extent, occurs in pregnancy
     d. Confounding diagnosis, especially in pregnancy; pyelonephritis, renal colic, placental abruption, and degeneration of a myoma
     e. In late pregnancy, symptoms may be very atypical
  3. Diagnosis and management
     a. Persistent abdominal pain and tenderness is most critical symptom
     b. Immediate surgical exploration indicated if suspected
     c. Diagnosis correct in 50–65% of cases; verify to prevent peritonitis

- Neoplastic disease
  1. Incidence of cancer in pregnancy—uncommon; second leading cause of death in women ages 15–44 in US
  2. Most frequent types of cancers in pregnancy—genital tract, breast, and malignant melanoma
  3. Principle of treatment—the woman should not be penalized for being pregnant
  4. Approach to the pregnant woman with cancer
     a. Surgical intervention for diagnosis, staging or therapeutic purposes is well tolerated; oophorectomy may be done after 8 weeks of gestation since placental hormone production is sufficient
     b. Radiation of 15–20 rads may cause microcephaly and mental retardation in the fetus
     c. Chemotherapy risk for the fetus depends on GA, but avoid at 5–10 weeks if possible
  5. Breast cancer
     a. Incidence—most common malignancy at all ages; estimated at 10–30/100,000 pregnancies
     b. Effects of pregnancy on breast cancer; none of note; stage of the disease at time of diagnosis and treatment more important to survival
     c. Diagnosis—same as for nonpregnant women; any suspicious breast mass should be diagnosed immediately using one or more of the following methods:
        (1) Needle aspiration can differentiate a cyst or galactocele from solid tumor
        (2) Tissue biopsy if needle biopsy results are not diagnostic
        (3) Mammography—but more difficult due to denser tissue; requires

adequate shielding; radiation is less than 100 mrad

    (4) Once cancer diagnosis made, limited metastatic search and chest radiogram done; computerized tomography (CAT) bone and liver scans are contraindicated due to ionizing radiation

  d. Treatment

    (1) Surgery as soon as the diagnosis is confirmed

    (2) Radiotherapy not recommended

    (3) Chemotherapy can be given in pregnancy

  e. Recommendations for future pregnancies—little evidence exists to say that survival is adversely affected by pregnancy after mastectomy for breast cancer

6. Malignant melanoma

  a. Incidence—estimated at 0.14 to 2.8 per 1000 live births

  b. Skin changes to watch and report—pigmented lesion that changes

    (1) Contour

    (2) Surface elevation

    (3) Discoloration

    (4) Itching

    (5) Bleeding

    (6) Ulceration

  c. Clinical stages

    (1) Stage I—no positive lymph nodes (85%); tumor thickness is single most important factor in predicting survival at this stage

    (2) Stage II—nodes are positive

    (3) Stage III—distant metastases

  d. Effect of pregnancy—usually have thicker tumors when diagnosed in pregnancy

  e. Treatment—surgery and chemotherapy if indicated

7. Cervical cancer

  a. Incidence—most common form of cancer in pregnancy—carcinoma in situ 1.3/1000; invasive carcinoma 1/2200 pregnancies

  b. Abnormal Pap tests equal 3% during pregnancy

  c. Colposcopy to confirm and identify lesions

  d. Treatment—varies with stage of cancer and duration of pregnancy

    (1) Microinvasive disease follows same guidelines as for nonpregnant intraepithelial disease; continuation of pregnancy and vaginal delivery with postpartum therapy

    (2) Invasive cancer is treated immediately in first half of pregnancy; if detected in latter half, can wait for fetal viability and maturation

- Heart disease

1. Incidence—rheumatic heart disease almost nonexistent in US due to better management and resources; congenital heart disease accounts for half of pregnancy heart problems

2. Heart disease accounts for 5–15% of maternal deaths

3. Etiology—cardiac output increases in pregnancy by 30–50%, half of which occurs by the eighth week; reaches maximum level by midpregnancy

4. Symptoms

  a. Progressive dyspnea

  b. Nocturnal cough

  c. Hemoptysis

  d. Syncope

  e. Chest pain

5. Clinical findings

  a. Cyanosis

  b. Clubbing of fingers

  c. Neck vein distension

  d. Systolic murmur grade 3/6 or greater

  e. Diastolic murmur

  f. Cardiomegaly

  g. Persistent arrhythmia

  h. Persistent split-second sound

6. Diagnosis—normal changes of pregnancy make diagnosis difficult

  a. EKG

  b. Echocardiography

  c. Chest radiograph

7. Functional classification of cardiac disease—based on past and present disability, uninfluenced by physical signs

  a. Class I—uncompromised; no limit on activity; no symptoms of cardiac insufficiency, no anginal pain

  b. Class II—slightly compromised; ordinary activity results in excessive fatigue, palpitation, dyspnea, or anginal pain

  c. Class III—markedly compromised; marked limitation of activity; less than normal activity causes symptoms manifested in Class II

  d. Class IV—severely compromised; symptoms manifested in Class II and III develop at rest and become more intense with activity

8. Antepartum management of the patient with Class I and Class II cardiac disease with regard to the following:

  a. Preventative measures—avoid URI contact; provide pneumococcal and flu vaccines

b. No smoking
c. No illicit drugs, especially cocaine and amphetamines
d. Instruct client regarding signs and symptoms of developing congestive heart failure:
   (1) Nocturnal cough
   (2) Basilar rales

I want to give special thanks to Annie Gibeau, CNM, MS, a faculty colleague of the NYU Midwifery Program, for all that she contributed to the development of this chapter.

◘ QUESTIONS

Select the best answer.

1. M. S. comes to the office indicating her period is 1 month overdue. Her level of pregnancy diagnosis is?
   a. Positive
   b. Presumptive
   c. Possible
   d. Probable

2. R. L. states she is trying to get pregnant and had unprotected intercourse on day 14 of her usual 28-day menstrual cycle. However, the pregnancy test was negative 3 days later. Appropriate management would be to:
   a. Order an ultrasound
   b. Prescribe progesterone
   c. Repeat the test in a week
   d. Order a serum pregnancy test

3. Pregnancy tests detect:
   a. Estrogen
   b. Human chorionic gonadotropin
   c. Human placental lactogen
   d. Progesterone

4. During the first few weeks of pregnancy, progesterone is secreted by the:
   a. Placenta
   b. Corpus luteum
   c. Endometrium
   d. Trophoblasts

5. Blood in the chorionic villi pertains to whose circulation?
   a. Mother
   b. Mother and fetus
   c. Placenta
   d. Fetus

6. The vessels of the umbilical cord are:
   a. One vein with oxygenated blood and two arteries with deoxygenated blood
   b. One vein with deoxygenated blood and two arteries with oxygenated blood
   c. Two veins with oxygenated blood and one artery with deoxygenated blood
   d. Two veins with deoxygenated blood and one artery with oxygenated blood

7. The uterus is palpable at the symphysis pubis at:
   a. 6 weeks
   b. 8 weeks
   c. 12 weeks
   d. 16 weeks

8. Implantation occurs _____ after fertilization.
   a. 24–48 hours
   b. 3–4 days
   c. 6–7 days
   d. 9–10 days

9. Placental transport of substances occurs by:
   a. Simple perfusion
   b. Facilitated diffusion
   c. Active osmosis
   d. Active perfusion

10. The human zygote consists of:
    a. 46 chromosomes from each parent
    b. 2 pairs of sex chromosomes
    c. 23 chromosomes
    d. 23 pairs of chromosomes

11. The trophoblast will ultimately become the:
    a. Placenta
    b. Embryo
    c. Blastocyst
    d. Umbilical cord

12. M. R. presents for an antepartal visit at 26 weeks and wants to know how big the fetus is. Your response would be that the fetus is approximately:
    a. 0.5 lb
    b. 1 lb
    c. 2 lb
    d. 4 lb

13. At her initial visit, M. R. was a healthy primigravida, but you heard a Grade I systolic murmur. Your management would be:
    a. A cardiology consult
    b. Chest radiograph
    c. Immediate referral
    d. No intervention

14. The drop in diastolic blood pressure during normal pregnancy is partly the result of:

    a. Plasma volume expansion
    b. Progesterone's effect on vessel walls
    c. Increased cardiac output
    d. Pooling of plasma in tissues

15. Changes in the respiratory system due to pregnancy may cause:

    a. Tachypnea
    b. Cough
    c. Increased chest diameter
    d. Pale nasal mucosa

16. C. D., a primigravida, came in for a visit at 34 weeks stating she has "a lot of vaginal discharge," but no other problems. On exam you see a white, odorless discharge of moderate quantity. Your next step would be:

    a. Treat for candida
    b. Check for trichomoniasis
    c. Reassure that this is normal
    d. Send a vaginal culture

17. R. P. comes for a 24-week visit and mentions that her interest in sex has increased greatly. You respond to her concern because you know that increased libido is:

    a. A normal variation of response in pregnancy
    b. An abnormal response of changing image
    c. Reflective of repressed desire to disrupt the pregnancy
    d. The early sign of a parenting disorder

18. R. Q., at her 36-week visit, tells you that she is having nightmares that include labor as well as fears of having an abnormal baby. Your best response is:

    a. Tell her there is nothing to worry about, as most babies are fine
    b. Encourage her to tell you more about the nightmares and her fears
    c. Make her an appointment with a mental health nurse practitioner
    d. Reassure her that there are dangers about which we all have to worry

19. Initial management of constipation in pregnancy should include suggestions for:

    a. Increased protein intake
    b. Limitation of calcium rich foods
    c. Use of a laxative
    d. Increased intake of fiber and fluids

20. P. J. has had three spontaneous abortions and is now pregnant for the fourth time. The term that defines her status is:

    a. Multipara
    b. Nullipara
    c. Primigravida
    d. Primipara

21. The calculation of estimated date of birth (EDB) by Naegele's rule is based on:

    a. A 28-day menstrual cycle
    b. Average length of pregnancy of 290 days
    c. 32-day cycle
    d. Length of pregnancy of 270 days

22. A. B. is pregnant for the third time. Her obstetrical history indicates she has had two miscarriages and one twin birth at 36 weeks. One twin died but the other is alive and well. The four-digit descriptor of this history is:

    a. 0121
    b. 0221
    c. 2021
    d. 2201

23. D. M. comes for her first antepartal visit. When asked the date of her last menstrual period, she indicates she has not had one since she has been nursing her 6-month-old daughter. You diagnose that she is pregnant. How would you determine estimated date of birth (EDB)?

    a. Determine when she expected to get her period and calculate from there
    b. Document quickening and extrapolate from there
    c. Send her to fetal assessment unit for an ultrasound
    d. Get good sexual history and use last coitus as the basis for calculation

24. R. P., G1 P0, comes for her 20-week visit. Her abdominal exam shows the uterine fundus to be half way between the symphysis and the umbilicus. This finding leads you to consider:

    a. Intrauterine growth restriction (IUGR)
    b. Nothing, since it is normal
    c. Oligohydramnios
    d. She is not eating and gaining enough weight

25. In your abdominal exam using Leopold's maneuvers, the first step is to determine fetal:

    a. Attitude
    b. Position
    c. Engagement
    d. Lie

26. D. P. presents for her first antepartal visit. She is 9 weeks pregnant and requests that you listen for the FHT. Your response would be:

    a. "No, there's no reason to since it can't be heard yet anyway."
    b. "Sure, I'll listen but we may not hear it yet."
    c. "Sure we can listen since it'll be there now."
    d. "We don't usually do that at this visit."

27. Normal findings on speculum and pelvic examination of a pregnant woman include:

    a. Eversion of the squamocolumnar junction
    b. Pale vaginal mucosa
    c. Open cervical os
    d. Firm, slightly enlarged cervix

28. Clinical pelvimetry of a woman with an adequate pelvis would provide which of the following findings?

    a. Ischial tuberosities of 10 cm and a flat sacrum
    b. Convergent sidewalls
    c. Pubic arch of 90 degrees with diagonal conjugate of greater than 11.5 cm
    d. Protuberant ischial spines

29. The value of clinical pelvimetry rests in its ability to:

    a. Predict successful vaginal birth
    b. Identify the characteristics of the woman's pelvis
    c. Determine if she will have a breech presentation
    d. Predict an occiput posterior position

30. F. R., a primigravida at 16 weeks, states that she is concerned because she has not felt the baby move yet. Your response should be:

    a. "Most women with a first pregnancy don't feel movement until around 20 weeks."
    b. "You're worrying too much, just relax."
    c. "I'll order an ultrasound, just to be sure everything is fine."
    d. "I'd like you to return in a week so we can recheck it."

31. Maternal serum alphafetoprotein screening is performed in what time frame?

    a. 8–12 weeks
    b. 12–15 weeks
    c. 15–19 weeks
    d. 20–24 weeks

32. CDC recommends screening for group B streptococcus (GBS) at what point?

    a. At the first visit
    b. When labor starts
    c. At 20 weeks
    d. At 35–37 weeks

33. The triple screen tests for:

    a. AFP, progesterone, hCG
    b. AFP, estriol, hCG
    c. Estriol, progesterone, hPL
    d. Estradiol, progesterone, AFP

34. A nonstress test containing 2 fetal heart accelerations lasting 15 seconds that are 15 beats per minute above the baseline is:

    a. Negative
    b. Positive
    c. Nonreactive
    d. Reactive

35. The recommended folic acid supplement for a woman with a past history of a baby with a neural tube defect is:

    a. 4 mg per day starting before conception
    b. 0.4 mg per day starting with a missed period
    c. 2 mg per day prior to conception
    d. 0.4 mg per day throughout pregnancy

36. B. D. comes for her first antepartal visit. She is 5 ft 4 in and weighs 190 lb (BMI 33). Weight goal for the pregnancy should be:

    a. Maintain current weight
    b. Gain 11–20 lb
    c. Gain 25–35 lb
    d. Lose 10–15 lb

37. Exercise guidelines for healthy pregnant women include suggestions to:

    a. Discontinue exercise at 20 weeks
    b. Begin intense program of exercise, especially if prepregnant weight was high
    c. Modify the existing program if symptoms occur
    d. Limit fluids before exercising

38. Anticipatory guidance concerning sexual activity during pregnancy includes:

    a. Sexual intercourse may continue until early third trimester in an uncomplicated pregnancy.
    b. Sexual intercourse is contraindicated throughout pregnancy if there is a past history of preterm labor.
    c. The pregnant woman's sexual desire may change throughout pregnancy.
    d. Most pregnant women do not desire sex after the first trimester.

39. Breastfeeding should be encouraged for:

    a. All women whose families strongly support the idea
    b. All pregnant women who are not HIV positive
    c. Those with adequate breast tissue
    d. Women who desire to do so

40. M. D. comes for her first antepartal visit at 8 weeks and tells you she has nausea every morning, but is able to eat and drink in the afternoon. Your management at this point would include:

    a. Prescription for antinausea medicine
    b. Vitamin B_6 50 mg bid
    c. Small frequent meals
    d. Carbonated beverage on rising

41. The fatigue of early pregnancy is best managed by:

    a. Ruling out a thyroid problem
    b. Encouraging increased exercise
    c. Increased amounts of caffeinated drinks
    d. Reassurance and rest

42. Leg cramps may be relieved by:

    a. Pointing the toes
    b. Hot compresses
    c. Flexion of the foot
    d. Hot tub baths

43. R. T. comes for her 36-week visit, during which she mentions that her hands and feet are somewhat swollen. She has gained 2 lb since her visit 2 weeks ago; her BP is 128/76 and she has no protein in her urine. What is your plan?

    a. Refer to perinatologist for impending preeclampsia
    b. Explain the edema at this stage is normal and see her in a week
    c. Order bed rest with return visit in a week
    d. Restrict salt and fluid intake

44. T. G. asks about the value of childbirth preparation classes during a second trimester visit. You tell her that the evidence indicates that they are associated with:

    a. Reduced use of analgesics/anesthesia during labor
    b. Improved parenting skills
    c. Decreased Cesarean rates
    d. Less use of IVs in labor

45. Diabetes screening recommendations during pregnancy for the woman who is obese include:

    a. Fasting blood glucose each trimester
    b. Testing Hemoglobin A_{1c} in the first trimester

    c. Routine screening early in pregnancy and at 24–28 weeks
    d. The same as for the normal weight woman

46. G. H. comes for her 34-week visit, at which time the fundus measures 39 cm. Abdominal palpation reveals a large uterus and difficulty feeling fetal parts. The most likely diagnosis is:

    a. Multiple gestation
    b. Macrosomic fetus
    c. Uterine fibroid
    d. Polyhydramnios

47. W. T., during her initial prenatal visit, mentions that she had a rubella immunization 3 weeks before conceiving this baby. Your plan is to:

    a. Advise her to consider termination of the pregnancy
    b. Continue regular care
    c. Consult with an infectious disease specialist
    d. Referral to perinatologist

48. On physical examination at an initial prenatal visit of a 25-year-old woman who is at 14 weeks' gestation, you feel a 1 cm mobile, nontender mass in the upper, outer quadrant of her right breast. Your plan is:

    a. Explain this is normal with hormonal changes of pregnancy
    b. Advise her you will watch at each visit to assess for any change
    c. Schedule a mammogram to be done in the third trimester
    d. Refer for further evaluation with biopsy

49. A pregnant woman who is 5 ft 3 in in height has a prepregnancy weight of 115 lb. Which of the following represents the most appropriate weight for her by the end of her pregnancy?

    a. 125 lb
    b. 135 lb
    c. 145 lb
    d. 155 lb

50. The biophysical profile (BPP) assesses fetal well-being with:

    a. A combination of nonstress test and ultrasound evaluation to assess five variables
    b. Both a contraction stress test and ultrasound evaluation of amniotic fluid volume
    c. Serial ultrasounds to evaluate amniotic fluid volume as well as fetal breathing and body movement and tone
    d. Evaluation of fetal movement with kick counts after administration of oxytocin or nipple stimulation

51. An appropriate plan of care for a 40-week gestation woman with a BPP score of 8 that includes a 2 score for amniotic fluid volume includes:

    a. Order a contraction stress test
    b. Repeat the BPP in 48 hours
    c. Schedule a return visit after 1 week
    d. Admit for induction of labor and delivery

52. Evaluation of fetal lung maturity is a required procedure for a:

    a. Scheduled delivery before 39 weeks' gestational age
    b. Scheduled delivery before 37 weeks' gestational age
    c. Laboring woman at 37 weeks' gestational age
    d. Laboring woman at 35 weeks' gestational age

53. W. M., who is 11 weeks pregnant, calls you from the ER to say she sustained a laceration, and they want to give her a tetanus booster. You would tell her:

    a. All vaccinations are contraindicated in pregnancy
    b. It is not a problem because she doesn't need it
    c. It can be given in pregnancy if needed
    d. She should wait until the third trimester

54. Drugs from which one of the following categories may be given to a pregnant woman when the potential benefit justifies the potential fetal risk:

    a. Category A
    b. Category B
    c. Category C
    d. Category X

55. A woman who is pregnant for the second time, and her first pregnancy ended with a spontaneous abortion at 10 weeks is a:

    a. Multigravida
    b. Multipara
    c. Primigravida
    d. Primipara

56. A pregnant woman presents for her 24-week visit, at which time she relates that she doesn't feel very interested in sex anymore. Your response is to:

    a. Tell her this is common and she should not be concerned
    b. Assure her the interest will return in the third trimester

    c. Tell her to get more rest and her interest will increase
    d. Get her to talk about what she's feeling and thinking about sex

57. The screening test for group B streptococcus requires that the specimen be obtained from the:

    a. Ectocervix and vaginal side walls
    b. Ectocervix and endocervical os
    c. Endocervical os and rectum
    d. Vaginal introitus and rectum

58. Pregnancy loss and the woman's need for appropriate grieving occur across the reproductive spectrum. Maladaptive grief reactions are best addressed by:

    a. Telling her to put the baby's things away
    b. Listening to whatever the woman has to say
    c. Encouraging her to be strong so she'll get past it
    d. Making her an appointment with a therapist

59. Recommended routine screening tests at an initial antenatal visit during the first trimester include:

    a. Group B streptococcus culture
    b. Syphilis serology
    c. Triple marker screen
    d. Ultrasound

60. Which of the following statements concerning influenza vaccination for pregnant women is correct?

    a. Vaccination is recommended for all women who will be pregnant during the influenza season.
    b. Pregnant women with HIV infection should not receive this vaccination.
    c. The pregnant woman should be offered the option of either the injection or nasal administration of the vaccine.
    d. Vaccination should be given only in the second or third trimester.

61. RDA of calories and protein during pregnancy is:

    a. 3,000 kcal and 50 g/day
    b. 3,500 kcal and 60 g/day
    c. 3,800 kcal and 60 g/day
    d. 2,500 kcal and 60 g/day

62. R. H. presents for her 36-week visit. Abdominal exam reveals a likelihood of polyhydramnios.

In response to her question of where does the fluid come from, you answer:

a. From the mother's blood volume
b. Through a combination of maternal serum and fetal urination
c. Produced by amniotic epithelium and fetal functions
d. From fluid ingested by mother

63. D. B., a 24-year-old primigravida, during her initial visit asks how the fetus has genes from both her husband and herself. Your response is based on what fact?

a. Mitosis occurs producing half the number of chromosomes.
b. Meiosis occurs producing half the number of chromosomes.
c. The egg is a somatic cell.
d. Sperm is a somatic cell.

64. Which of the following are parts of the placenta?

a. Trophoblast, chorion, amnion
b. Trophoblast, chorion, endometrium
c. Chorion, amnion, umbilical cord
d. Intervillous spaces, endometrium, trophoblast

65. The term *conceptus* means:

a. The embryo and placenta
b. The embryo and membranes
c. The embryo, membranes, and placenta
d. The embryo, membranes, placenta, and endometrium

66. What structure in human reproduction produces the most diverse and greatest quantity of steroid and protein hormones?

a. Trophoblast
b. Blastocyst
c. Chorion laeve
d. Deciduas basalis

67. At her 32-week visit, B. R. asks you to tell her what you are looking for or feeling when doing her abdominal exam with Leopold's maneuvers. You respond that you are:

a. Determining the placement of the placenta
b. Finding what direction the fetus is lying
c. Evaluating the size of the uterus
d. Evaluating adequacy of fetal growth

68. T. D. comes for an 18-week visit. Appropriate routine screening tests at this visit include:

a. Gestational diabetes testing
b. Chlamydia and gonorrhea tests

c. CBC or hematocrit
d. Multiple marker screen

69. R. D. at 37 weeks calls to say she feels like the fetus is moving less. After further inquiry you decide to send her for an NST. She asks what this is. You explain that it is an assessment of fetal well-being based on:

a. Evaluation of body movements
b. Breathing movements
c. Fetal heart-rate response to fetal movement
d. Fetal body tone

70. P. R. comes for a first visit at 11 weeks' gestation. Her history reveals her concern about sore gums that sometimes bleed. Your thinking is:

a. She most likely needs to see a periodontist.
b. Gingivitis is common in pregnancy with increased vascularity of connective tissue.
c. She should be started on antibiotics to prevent systemic infection.
d. She should be placed on a soft diet until the problem is resolved.

71. A woman presents at 32 weeks' gestation with vaginal bleeding for the past 6 hours, back pain, and irregular abdominal cramping pain. Exam reveals diffuse abdominal tenderness and increased uterine tone. You suspect:

a. Marginal placenta previa
b. Placental abruption
c. Preterm labor
d. Pyelonephritis

72. A postterm pregnancy is best diagnosed by:

a. Certain LMP
b. Third trimester ultrasound
c. Fundal growth
d. Quickening

73. Serial beta hCG levels are done after uterine evacuation for hydatidiform mole to:

a. Assure that the woman is not pregnant in the first year after treatment
b. Monitor for persistent trophoblastic proliferation
c. Identify a pregnancy early so appropriate care can be provided
d. Assess for a possible undetected ectopic pregnancy

74. P. R. indicates she is afraid of pitocin because her sister had a uterine rupture when she was induced. Your response would be:

a. Reassurance since she won't need induction anyway
b. Discuss how pitocin is given with assurance that nothing will go wrong
c. Discuss alternate methods to promote uterine readiness and contractions
d. Say it is the best way to get through labor and not a problem

75. L. M. is a G2 P1001 whose initial visit reveals a healthy pregnant woman. Her urinalysis and culture and sensitivity (C&S) report indicates a colony count of greater than 100,000 organisms/mL. You would:

a. Refer her to a urologist to evaluate for underlying renal disease
b. Encourage fluids and repeat C&S in 2 weeks
c. Initiate treatment with antibiotics
d. Advise her to contact you if she has any UTI symptoms

76. Antepartal care for the woman who is HIV positive should focus mainly on:

a. Assuring fetal well-being at all cost
b. Frequent drug testing to assure she is not using IV street drugs
c. Getting her partner tested and treated if necessary
d. Maintaining her health and preventing neonatal transmission

77. On reviewing the record of a currently pregnant woman, you see that she is P1112. What obstetrical history can you derive from this information?

a. Two previous pregnancies of which one infant was term and one was a premature stillbirth
b. You are unable to determine an obstetric history from this information
c. Three pregnancies with one term birth and premature twins
d. Three pregnancies of which one was term, one premature and one abortion

78. Polyhydramnios is defined as:

a. AFI greater than 10 cm
b. Single pocket greater than 5 cm
c. AFI greater than 15 cm
d. Single pocket greater than 8 cm

79. Etiology of polyhydramnios is associated with:

a. Maternal over-hydration
b. Fetal anomalies of GI tract
c. Fetal anomalies of cardiovascular system
d. Maternal preeclampsia with edema

80. The fetal system most associated with oligohydramnios is the:

a. GI system
b. Central nervous system
c. Renal system
d. Cardiovascular system

81. When speaking with a primigravida about the way a baby develops, you would describe the embryonic stage as the:

a. Period between the second and eighth weeks
b. Time from implantation to 12 weeks into pregnancy
c. Period when drugs are least likely to affect development
d. Period from fertilization to 4 weeks

82. During the embryonic stage all major organ systems are formed *except*:

a. Heart
b. Reproductive organs
c. Liver
d. Lungs

83. Determining an accurate estimated date of birth (EDB) is critical because:

a. It is the basis for making decisions toward the end of the pregnancy.
b. Mothers want to know the exact date the baby will be born.
c. It is all that is needed to plan a 37-week elective C-section.
d. Families want to make plans around the baby's birth.

84. Which of the following would *not* be a normal physical examination finding during pregnancy?

a. Blue color of vaginal mucosa and cervix
b. Hypertrophy of nasal mucosa and gums
c. Mildly enlarged, nodular thyroid
d. Increased redness on palms of hands

85. During the last 8 weeks of pregnancy, the fetus:

a. Finishes the final formation of the renal system
b. Completes the development of reproductive organs
c. Experiences the closure of the foramen ovale
d. Increases weight through fat accumulation

86. The determination of an accurate EDB is best accomplished by using:

a. The first day of the last menstrual period
b. A complete menstrual history
c. The use of Naegele's rule
d. Date when symptoms of pregnancy began

87. Dating of pregnancy by USG is most accurate in the first trimester using:

    a. Crown rump length (CRL)
    b. Head circumference
    c. Abdominal circumference
    d. Femur length

88. Which of the following statements most accurately reflects the growth of the pregnant uterus?

    a. At 14 weeks it begins to rise out of the pelvis, and at 24 weeks is at the umbilicus.
    b. At 14 weeks it is halfway to the umbilicus, and at 20 weeks is at the umbilicus.
    c. At 12 weeks it begins to rise out of pelvis, and at 20 weeks is at the umbilicus.
    d. At 10 weeks it begins to rise out of the pelvis, and at 16 weeks is at the umbilicus.

89. Which of the following is a presumptive sign of pregnancy seen in the vagina?

    a. Hegar's
    b. Piskacek's
    c. Goodell's
    d. Chadwick's

90. The pregnancy is maintained through hormones produced by:

    a. Egg sac and placenta
    b. Corpus luteum and chorion
    c. Corpus luteum and placenta
    d. Ovary and placenta

91. Of the four pelvic types, which is more likely to lead to a posterior position with higher possibility of dystocia?

    a. Android
    b. Platypelloid
    c. Anthropoid
    d. Gynecoid

92. The characteristic gait of pregnancy results from:

    a. Shift in the center of gravity as uterus enlarges
    b. Effects of relaxin and estrogen
    c. Effects of relaxin and progesterone
    d. Effects of increasing amounts of estrogen and progesterone

93. The effect of pregnancy on the cardiovascular system is most clearly seen in:

    a. Lower diastolic blood pressure in third trimester
    b. 10% cardiac volume increase that peaks in midpregnancy
    c. Resting pulse increase of 10–15 beats in first trimester
    d. Slight decrease in cardiac output in second trimester

94. The usual 1 g drop in hemoglobin during pregnancy is due to:

    a. Blood volume increase of 30–50%
    b. Decrease in iron absorption
    c. Decrease in production of RBC
    d. Increasing iron needs of the fetus

95. Which of the following is considered a risk factor for psychological well-being in pregnancy?

    a. Limited support network
    b. Introversion at any point
    c. Ambivalence anytime
    d. Concern about the danger signs

96. The maternal mortality ratio is defined as the number of maternal deaths that result from the reproductive process per:

    a. 1000 live births
    b. 100,000 live births
    c. 100,000 pregnant women
    d. 100,000 reproductive age women

97. G. R. comes for her first pregnancy visit. Her obstetrical history includes one spontaneous abortion, one termination of pregnancy, one infant born at 36 weeks and one born at 41 weeks. Both infants are living. Her parity is:

    a. 2022
    b. 2122
    c. 1212
    d. 1122

98. The pelvic planes of obstetrical significance are the:

    a. Inlet, midplane, and outlet
    b. Inlet, posterior outlet, and anterior outlet
    c. Inlet, posterior midplane, and anterior midplane
    d. Linea terminalis, posterior outlet, and anterior outlet

99. Which of the elements of clinical pelvimetry defines the midplane?

    a. Diagonal conjugate
    b. Intertuberous diameter
    c. Ischial spines distance and sacrum
    d. Pubic arch

100. Amniocentesis is used in early pregnancy to:

    a. Screen for fetal anomalies
    b. Diagnose fetal genetic well-being
    c. Evaluate maternal genetic problems
    d. Determine AFI and muscle tone

101. Chorionic villous sampling (CVS) has an advantage over amniocentesis because it:

    a. Can be done 3–4 weeks earlier
    b. There is less risk for infection
    c. There is less risk for limb deformities
    d. There is greater specificity in test results

102. When considering the use of fetal movement counting for a particular woman, it is important to know that:

    a. Fetuses move constantly so it can be done at any time.
    b. Fetal movement is strongest at 29–38 weeks.
    c. Most women don't feel the fetus move before 24 weeks.
    d. There is only one way to perform fetal movement counts.

103. The basis for the nonstress test (NST) to assess fetal well-being is that:

    a. Fetal movement will increase the mother's heart rate.
    b. The fetus responds to an increase in heart rate by accelerating movement.
    c. Fetal movement should cause no significant change in FHR.
    d. Fetal heart rate accelerates in association with fetal movement.

104. Contraindications to contraction stress testing (CST) include:

    a. Gestational age greater than 37 weeks
    b. History of ectopic pregnancy
    c. Nonreactive nonstress test (NST)
    d. Placenta previa

105. Cordocentesis may be used:

    a. As an adjunct to chorionic villi sampling (CVS)
    b. To obtain blood samples for fetal fibronectin test
    c. To provide fetal blood transfusion
    d. To relieve pressure on a prolapsed cord

106. Substances classified as addictive:

    a. Are only illegal drugs
    b. Include only those inhaled or injected
    c. Include both legal and illegal drugs
    d. Do not include alcohol

107. Which of the following is most common during pregnancy?

    a. Binge drinking
    b. Cigarette smoking
    c. Marijuana smoking
    d. Occasional alcohol use

108. When faced with a woman who manifests clear evidence of being a victim of violence, your first goal is:

    a. Evaluate her safety
    b. Get her to a shelter
    c. Tell her to press charges
    d. Get photos of all injuries

109. Correct information concerning pregnancies with first trimester bleeding includes:

    a. Approximately 10% of women have some bleeding in the first trimester.
    b. Bleeding that occurs between 10 and 12 weeks is often caused by implantation.
    c. Cervical incompetence is a common cause of first trimester bleeding.
    d. 90% of pregnancies in which FHT are heard will continue to term after early bleeding.

110. A patient presents with an LMP of 8 weeks ago and a positive urine pregnancy test. She is having a small amount of bleeding for the past 12 hours, along with some mild abdominal cramping. A pelvic exam reveals a closed cervix and a slightly enlarged uterus. Differential diagnosis for this woman includes:

    a. Complete abortion and threatened abortion
    b. Ectopic pregnancy and inevitable abortion
    c. Ectopic pregnancy and threatened abortion
    d. Incomplete abortion and inevitable abortion

111. An example of an autosomal recessive disease is:

    a. BRCA 2 breast cancer
    b. Cystic fibrosis
    c. Hemophilia
    d. Trisomy 21

112. A 34-week pregnant woman presents stating she noticed a small amount of blood on her underwear this morning about an hour after having sexual intercourse. She is not having any pain or contractions. Your initial differential diagnosis for this woman would include:

    a. Cervicitis
    b. Incompetent cervix

c. Placental abruption

d. Premature rupture of membranes

113. Risks to the fetus in a postterm pregnancy are related to all of the following *except*:

a. Fetal macrosomia

b. Meconium aspiration

c. Polyhydramnios

d. Uteroplacental insufficiency

114. Symmetric growth restriction is more likely than asymmetric growth restriction to:

a. Be related to multiple gestation

b. First become apparent in late pregnancy

c. Occur as a result of maternal medical illness

d. Result from maternal cigarette smoking

115. Loss of a fetus in the second trimester is most frequently related to:

a. Hydatidiform mole

b. Inevitable abortion

c. Ectopic pregnancy

d. Incompetent cervix

116. As a result of an early USG, a low-lying placenta is verified for B. T. What do you tell her regarding this?

a. Approximately 30% of women with low-lying placenta in early pregnancy will have placenta previa in the third trimester.

b. Approximately 30% of women have a low-lying placenta in the first trimester.

c. Regular vaginal examinations will be done in the third trimester to monitor any obstruction of the cervix.

d. Vaginal delivery is contraindicated if there is a marginal placenta previa.

117. A pregnant woman has the following history: vaginal delivery at 38 wks; spontaneous abortion at 8 wks; elective abortion at 13 wks; vaginal delivery at 34 wks; 2 living children; is now 28 wks pregnant. Her gravity and parity are:

a. G5 P1122

b. G5 P0222

c. G3 P2002

d. G3 P2112

118. Which of the following tests is diagnostic rather than screening?

a. MSAFP

b. Nuchal translucency US

c. Amniocentesis

d. USG at 10 weeks

119. An elevated maternal AFP result is associated with which of the following?

a. Down syndrome

b. Neural tube defect

c. Autosomal recessive gene

d. X-linked recessive inheritance

120. Which of the following factors would predispose a pregnant woman to having a baby with GBS disease?

a. History of previous GBS-positive infant

b. Bacterial vaginosis in current pregnancy

c. Frequent urinary tract infections prior to pregnancy

d. Streptococcal pharyngitis in the third trimester

121. V. R. comes for her 38-week visit, during which she reports that her friend gave birth last week and had a placental abruption. She is now concerned that she might have the same. What information would you share with her about this?

a. In the event of bleeding near term, 50% are related to placental abruption.

b. In the third trimester, she has a 30% chance of having a placental abruption.

c. The likelihood of her having this occur is basically zero at this time.

d. It is associated with risk factors such as hypertension, smoking, and trauma.

122. Genotype refers to:

a. The expression of genes present in an individual

b. The dominant genes that will be inherited by a fetus

c. The pair of genes for each characteristic inherent in an individual

d. The recessive genes that will be passed on to a fetus

123. Which of the following women should receive RhoGAM postpartum?

a. Nonsensitized Rh negative mother with an Rh negative baby

b. Nonsensitized Rh negative mother with an Rh positive baby

c. Sensitized Rh negative mother with an Rh negative baby

d. Sensitized Rh negative mother with an RH positive baby

124. Aneuploidy describes which of the following situations?

a. Down syndrome
b. BRCA 1 and 2 inheritance
c. Cystic fibrosis genes
d. Sickle cell anemia

125. B. T., G2 P0010, comes for her first antepartal visit. Her history indicates she had a pregnancy loss at 18 weeks. She is gravely concerned that it will happen again in this pregnancy. You discuss cervical cerclage, mentioning the following facts:

a. Will be done after 12–14 weeks and is 80–90% successful
b. Will be done after 16–20 weeks and is 80–90% successful
c. Will be done after 16–20 weeks and is 50–60% successful
d. Will be done after 12–14 weeks and is 50–60% successful

126. The CDC's recommended treatment for primary syphilis in a 10-week pregnant woman is:

a. Benzathine penicillin G 2.4 units IM x 1 dose after the first trimester
b. Benzathine penicillin G 2.4 units IM x 1 dose at the time of diagnosis
c. Benzathine penicillin G 2.4 units IM weekly x 3 doses
d. Benzathine penicillin G 2.4 units IM at the time of diagnosis and repeat in 4 weeks if no decline in RPR titer

127. At an initial prenatal visit, a woman is diagnosed with bacterial vaginosis. She is not having any symptoms of vaginal infection. You will advise her that:

a. All pregnant women should be treated if they have asymptomatic bacterial vaginosis.
b. Pregnant women who are at risk for preterm delivery should be treated if they have asymptomatic bacterial vaginosis.
c. Only pregnant women at risk for preterm delivery should be treated for symptomatic bacterial vaginosis.
d. Pregnant women who are at risk for preterm delivery should be tested for asymptomatic bacterial vaginosis in early third trimester.

128. CDC's recommended treatment for trichomoniasis during pregnancy is:

a. Metronidazole 2 g orally
b. Clindamycin 300 mg orally bid x 7 days
c. Azithromycin 1 g orally
d. Ceftriaxone 125 mg IM

129. Symmetric intrauterine growth restriction:

a. Generally becomes evident in midpregnancy
b. Is usually associated with placental abnormalities
c. Is caused by conditions that result in a reduction in cell size
d. Is a neonatal diagnosis made when the infant falls below the 10th percentile

130. M. K. is a 34-year-old G5 P4004. Her 1-hour 50 g glucose challenge test at 28 weeks was 154 mg/dL. Follow-up 100 g glucose tolerance test produced the following results: 100, 192, 185, and 160 mg/dL. Your plan for M. K. includes:

a. Obtaining fasting glucose tests at 32 and 36 weeks to assure that levels stay at or below 100 mg/dL
b. Referring her to a nutritionist to help her limit further weight gain to no more than 10 lb.
c. Referring her to a perinatologist for peri-umbilical blood sampling to determine fetal blood glucose levels
d. Screening for diabetes at 6–12 weeks postpartum

131. At 20 weeks' gestation a pregnant woman was seen and fundal height was 1 cm below the umbilicus. At today's 24-week visit, fundal height is at the umbilicus. She is feeling regular fetal movement and fetal heart rate is 140 bpm. The most appropriate management for this patient is:

a. Ordering a biophysical profile
b. Ordering an ultrasound
c. Performing a nonstress test at this visit
d. Scheduling her next visit for 4 weeks from today

132. Ectopic pregnancy is consistent with no intra-uterine sac on transvaginal ultrasound and an hCG titer of less than:

a. 100 IU/L
b. 1500 IU/L
c. 6500 IU/L
d. 10,000 IU/L

133. L. H. is an 18-year-old female who is 16 weeks pregnant. She has a positive chlamydia test. Appropriate management includes:

a. Erythromycin base 500 mg orally qid for 7 days and ceftrixone 125 mg IM
b. Azithromycin 1 g orally in a single dose and perform test of cure in 3–4 weeks

c. Ofloxacin 300 mg orally bid for 7 days and rescreen in the third trimester

d. Spectinomycin 2 g IM now and repeat in 1 week

134. M. I. is a 29-year-old G4 P2012 at 41 weeks today. She complains of occasional cramping, denies leaking/bleeding, but states she passed her "mucus plug" yesterday. She asks how she'll know if she's in labor since both her previous births were induced. You respond that:

a. True labor occurs when contractions are 7–8 minutes apart and last for 45 seconds.

b. Real labor is when contractions are 2–3 minutes apart and are very painful.

c. Labor contractions usually become more regular and more intense over time.

d. Contractions begin slowly; once they are 4–5 minutes apart, it is real labor.

135. Hyperthyroidism in pregnancy is diagnosed by:

a. Elevated free thyroxine (T_4) levels

b. Low free T_3 levels

c. Elevated TSH

d. Elevated total thyroxine (TT_4) levels

136. ABO incompatibility occurs in what percentage of pregnancies?

a. 15%

b. 20–25%

c. 25–40%

d. 5–8%

137. T. W., a 32-year-old G2 P1001, is Rh negative. Her first pregnancy was uneventful, and she received RhoGAM after the birth. She read on the Internet that problems were much more likely with the second pregnancy. You respond that:

a. Since she reports she has had no transfusions since the previous birth, there is no problem.

b. The RhoGAM she received in the last pregnancy will prevent any problems in this pregnancy.

c. She was not sensitized in the first pregnancy, and you will provide monitoring and treatment to prevent it in this pregnancy.

d. It is likely that her fetus is Rh– so there is no real concern that she will have any problems related to this.

138. At 28 weeks' gestation, a patient's Hgb is 11.2 g/dL. At her initial first trimester visit, her Hgb was 12.8 g/dL. Management will include:

a. Obtaining a CBC and ferritin level

b. Asking if she is having difficulty tolerating her iron supplement and change to a different type if needed

c. Rechecking her history to see if she may be at risk for an inherited anemia

d. Encouraging her to continue getting dietary iron and taking her iron supplement

139. Folic acid deficiency anemia is characterized by:

a. Hemoglobin at 9 g/dL or less

b. Low ferritin levels

c. Elevated serum iron binding capacity

d. Macrocytic erythrocytes

140. Which of the following statements is true concerning sickle cell hemoglobinopathies:

a. Trait indicates that one parent has sickle cell disease.

b. Disease is present when the person inherits a sickle cell gene from each parent.

c. G-6-PD deficiency is a potential complication of sickle cell disease.

d. 1 in 100 African Americans has sickle cell trait.

141. Normal changes of pregnancy may confound a diagnosis of appendicitis. With this in mind, you should note the following as a critical sign or symptom pointing to possible appendicitis in pregnancy:

a. Persistent abdominal pain and tenderness

b. Intermittent lower abdominal cramping

c. Elevated WBC level

d. Nausea and vomiting

142. M. D., a 32-year-old P1, during a discussion of infant care and breastfeeding, says, "My first baby didn't like the breast, then I didn't have enough milk, so I stopped breastfeeding after two weeks." What is your response to her statement?

a. Tell her she probably misinterpreted what was going on and shouldn't have stopped nursing.

b. Delve further into what occurred and how she came to the conclusions that led her to stop breastfeeding.

c. Let her know she probably wasn't drinking enough fluids so didn't have enough milk to feed the baby.

d. Reassure her that she was listening to her body and had done the right thing for herself and her infant.

143. M. B., G1 P0, comes for her 36-week visit with a piece of paper in her hand. "I'm really confused about this birth plan business. What am I supposed to do about my birth? Don't I just show up when I'm in labor?" How will you counsel her today?

    a. "It really doesn't matter what you write because the hospital has its own plan."
    b. "You will need to be very detailed about each element of the birth experience so you get what you want."
    c. "The plan provides the opportunity for you to make choices about events associated with the birth."
    d. "The healthcare provider who is there when you are in labor will tell you what is best for you and how to do it."

144. Y. L., G2 P1001, comes for her first visit. She is concerned about the possibility of a UTI since her sister was recently hospitalized for pyelonephritis. What facts would you give her to enhance her understanding?

    a. UTIs do occur in about 10% of pregnancies.
    b. 25% of women with UTI in pregnancy will develop pyelonephritis.
    c. If she has a history of UTIs before pregnancy, she will be screened with a urine culture each trimester.
    d. Pregnant women are typically screened for asymptomatic bacteruria in early pregnancy.

145. Who is at greatest risk for developing a UTI in pregnancy?

    a. Adolescents
    b. Woman pregnant with twins
    c. Women older than 35 years
    d. Woman with diabetes

146. L. T. returns for the reading of the PPD that was placed during her first prenatal visit. You read the result as 10 mm of induration. L. T. is American-born, healthy, and has no known history of contact with the disease. How do you interpret this result to her?

    a. It is positive and she needs referral to an infectious disease specialist.
    b. It is unclear and she should have a chest radiograph to be certain.
    c. It is positive and you should give her a prescription for INH.
    d. It is negative since she has no high-risk characteristics for the disease.

147. Which of the following statements concerning HIV in women is correct?

    a. The main route of acquiring the infection in women is IV drug use.
    b. Viral load is the strongest predictor for transmission of infection to infant during birth process.
    c. C-section is the recommended route of delivery for all HIV-infected women to reduce the risk of transmission of infection to infant.
    d. Breastfeeding should only be recommended if the mother's viral load is less than 200 copies/ml.

148. S. R. has reached her 39th week of pregnancy. On abdominal exam you measure a fundal height of 42 cm. Leopold's maneuvers provides you with an EFW of 4200 g. What factors would help to ease your mind about the fetal size?

    a. She has wide hips and will have no problem with a big baby.
    b. She is 5 ft 10 in with an anthropoid pelvis and her husband is 6 ft 4 in.
    c. She is totally unconcerned and knows this baby will fit.
    d. The fetus is not yet engaged so the height is greater than expected.

149. Many conditions are associated with preterm birth. Of the 28% of births that occur preterm, what is the condition that contributes most to these births?

    a. IUGR
    b. Preeclampsia
    c. Fetal demise
    d. Abruptio placenta

150. A patient who is 32 weeks pregnant has had symptoms of preterm labor and has a history of preterm delivery at 34 weeks. A fetal fibronectin test is negative. You advise her that:

    a. She has a 60% chance of going into labor within the next week.
    b. It is really too early in her pregnancy for this test to be of much value.
    c. The result offers some reassurance that she will not go into labor in the next 2 weeks.
    d. It is really too late in her pregnancy for this test to be of much value.

151. A decision is made to start tocolytic therapy for a 30-week gestation woman in preterm labor. Betamethasone IM has also been ordered. This is done because the administration of corticosteroids:

a. Decreases the respiratory side-effects of tocolytic drugs
b. Decreases the incidence of premature rupture of membranes
c. Enhances the effects of tocolytic drugs
d. Reduces the incidence of newborn respiratory distress syndrome

152. G. F. comes for her 32-week visit, and you determine she has a breech presentation. Your plan for her is to:

a. Send her to Maternal Fetal Medicine for external cephalic version
b. Refer her to perinatologist for care decision and treatment
c. Send her for ultrasound to confirm breech presentation
d. Wait until 36 weeks to see if spontaneous version has occurred

153. A pregnant woman presents for her 32-week visit with no complaints. All findings from previous visits have been normal. Today she has blood pressure of 145/95. Expected additional findings if she has mild preeclampsia include:

a. Lower extremity edema
b. 1 to 2+ proteinuria on dipstick urine
c. Right upper epigastric pain
d. Elevated liver function tests

❏ ANSWERS

1. b	25. d	49. c	102. b
2. c	26. b	50. a	103. d
3. b	27. a	51. c	104. d
4. b	28. c	52. a	105. c
5. d	29. b	53. c	106. c
6. a	30. a	54. c	107. b
7. c	31. c	55. a	108. a
8. c	32. d	56. d	109. d
9. b	33. b	57. d	110. c
10. d	34. d	58. b	111. b
11. a	35. a	59. b	112. a
12. c	36. b	60. a	113. c
13. d	37. c	61. d	114. d
14. b	38. c	62. c	115. d
15. c	39. b	63. b	116. b
16. c	40. c	64. a	117. a
17. a	41. d	65. c	118. c
18. b	42. c	66. a	119. b
19. d	43. b	67. b	120. a
20. b	44. a	68. d	121. d
21. a	45. c	69. c	122. c
22. b	46. d	70. b	123. b
23. c	47. b	71. b	124. a
24. a	48. b	72. a	125. a
		73. b	126. b
		74. c	127. b
		75. c	128. a
		76. d	129. a
		77. d	130. d
		78. d	131. b
		79. b	132. c
		80. c	133. b
		81. a	134. c
		82. d	135. a
		83. a	136. b
		84. c	137. c
		85. d	138. d
		86. b	139. d
		87. a	140. b
		88. c	141. a
		89. d	142. b
		90. c	143. c
		91. a	144. d
		92. c	145. d
		93. b	146. d
		94. a	147. b
		95. a	148. b
		96. b	149. b
		97. d	150. c
		98. a	151. d
		99. c	152. d
		100. b	153. b
		101. a	

◘ BIBLIOGRAPHY

Advisory Committee on Immunization Practices (ACIP). (2009). *Recommended adult immunization schedule United States.* Atlanta, GA: Department of Health and Human Services—Centers for Disease Control and Prevention.

American College of Obstetricians and Gynecologists (ACOG). (2008). Anemia in pregnancy. *Practice Bulletin No. 95.* Washington, DC: Author.

American College of Obstetricians and Gynecologists (ACOG). (2007). Management of herpes in pregnancy. *Practice Bulletin No. 82.* Washington, DC: Author.

American College of Obstetricians and Gynecologists (ACOG). (2004). Management of postterm pregnancy. *Practice Bulletin No. 55.* Washington, DC: Author.

American College of Obstetricians and Gynecologists (ACOG). (2000). Intrauterine growth restriction. *Practice Bulletin No. 10.* Washington, DC: Author.

American College of Obstetricians and Gynecologists (ACOG). (2001). Management of recurrent early pregnancy loss. *Practice Bulletin No. 24.* Washington, DC: Author.

American College of Obstetricians and Gynecologists (ACOG). (2001). Chronic hypertension in pregnancy. *Practice Bulletin No. 29.* Washington, DC: Author.

American College of Obstetricians and Gynecologists (ACOG). (2001). Gestational diabetes. *Practice Bulletin No. 30.* Washington, DC: Author.

American College of Obstetricians and Gynecologists (ACOG). (2002). Diagnosis and management of preeclampsia/eclampsia. *Practice Bulletin No. 33.* Washington, DC: Author.

American College of Obstetricians and Gynecologists (ACOG). (2004). Nausea and vomiting of pregnancy. *Practice Bulletin No. 52.* Washington, DC: Author.

American College of Obstetricians and Gynecologists (ACOG). (2001). Assessment of risk factors for preterm birth. *Practice Bulletin No. 31.* Washington, DC: Author.

American Diabetes Association. (2009). Standards of medical care in diabetes—2009. *Diabetes Care, 32* (Suppl 1), S13–S61.

Branson, B., Handsfield, H., Lampe, M. et al. (2006). Revised recommendations for HIV testing of adults, adolescents, and pregnant women in healthcare settings. *MMWR, 55*(RR14), 1–17.

Centers for Disease Control and Prevention (CDC). (2005). Achievements in public health: Elimination of rubella and congenital rubella syndrome—United States, 1969–2004. *MMWR, 54*(RR11), 279–282.

Centers for Disease Control and Prevention (CDC). (2008). *STD surveillance 2007.* Atlanta, GA: Author. Retrieved on May 2, 2010 from http://www.cdc.gov/std/stats07/main.htm.

Centers for Disease Control and Prevention (CDC). (2008). *Reported tuberculosis in the United States, 2007.* Atlanta, GA: Author.

Centers for Disease Control and Prevention (CDC). (2008). *TB elimination: Tuberculosis and pregnancy.* Atlanta, GA: Author. Retrieved on May 2, 2010 from http://www.cdc.gov/tb/publications/factsheets/specpop/pregnancy.htm.

Chernecky, C., & Berger, B. (2008). *Laboratory tests and diagnostic procedures* (5th ed.). St. Louis: Saunders Elsevier.

Coad, J., & Dunstall, M. (2005). *Anatomy and physiology for midwives* (2nd ed.). St. Louis: Mosby, Inc.

Coustan, D. (2007). Pharmacologic management of gestational diabetes. *Diabetes Care, 30* (Suppl 2), 206–208.

Cunningham, F., Leveno, K., Bloom, S., Hauth, I., Rouse, D., & Spong, C. (2009). *Williams obstetrics* (23rd ed.). New York: McGraw-Hill.

Enkin, M., Kreiree, M., Nelison, J., & Crowther, C. (2000). *A guide to effective care in pregnancy and childbirth* (3rd ed.). Oxford, UK: Oxford University Press.

Gibbs, R., Karlan, B., Haney, A., & Nygaard, I. (2008). *Danforth's obstetrics and gynecology* (10th ed.). Philadelphia, PA: Lippincott, Williams, and Wilkins.

HIV/AIDS Bureau. (2005). *A guide to the clinical care of women with HIV/AIDS, 2005 edition.* Washington, DC: US Department of Health and Human Services.

Hunter, L., Sullivan, C., Young, R., & Weber, C. (2007). Nausea and vomiting of pregnancy: Clinical management. *The American Journal of Nurse Practitioners, 11*(8), 57–67.

Institute of Medicine. (2009). *Weight gain during pregnancy: Reexamining the guidelines.* Washington, DC: Institute of Medicine.

King, T., & Murphy, P. (2009). Evidence-based approaches to managing nausea and vomiting in early pregnancy. *Journal of Midwifery and Women's Health, 54*(6), 430–444.

Naegele, M. A., & D'Avanza, C. E. (2001). *Addictions and substance abuse.* Upper Saddle River, NJ: Prentice Hall.

Sibai, B. (2005). Preeclampsia. *Lancet, 365*(9461), 785–799.

Substance Abuse and Mental Health Services Administration (SAMHSA) (2009). Results from the 2008 national survey on drug use and health: National findings. *NSDUH Series H-36, HHS Publication No. SMA 09-4434.*

Tharpe, N., & Farley, C. (2009). *Clinical practice guidelines for midwifery and women's health* (3rd ed.). Sudbury, MA: Jones and Bartlett.

Varney, H., Kriebs, J., & Gegor, C. (2004). *Varney's midwifery* (4th ed.). Sudbury, MA: Jones and Bartlett.

Wynne, A., Woo, T., & Olyaei, A. (2007). *Pharmacotherapeutics for nurse practitioner prescribers* (2nd ed.). Philadelphia, PA: F. A. Davis.

5

Midwifery Care of the Newborn

Anthony A. Lathrop

☐ PHYSIOLOGIC TRANSITION TO EXTRAUTERINE LIFE

- Immediate extrauterine transition—immediate transition from intrauterine to extrauterine life depends on changes in four major areas: respiration, circulation, thermoregulation, and glucose regulation

- Respiratory changes
  1. Must immediately begin respiration upon delivery
  2. Factors in initiation of respiration
     a. Biochemical—relative hypoxia at the end of labor
     b. Physical stimuli—cold, gravity, pain, light, noise
     c. Recoil from pressure on thorax while passing through vagina
  3. Sustained respiration depends on coordinated response of the following:
     a. Central nervous system (CNS) respiratory center
     b. Aortic and carotid chemoreceptors
     c. Thoracic mechanoreceptors
     d. Diaphragm and respiratory muscles
  4. Initial breathing serves the following purposes:
     a. Assist in conversion from fetal to extrauterine circulation
     b. Clear lungs of fluid
     c. Establish lung volume and expand alveoli
  5. Characteristics of normal newborn respiration
     a. Respiratory rate 30 to 60 breaths per minute
     b. Irregular/fluctuating pattern
     c. Diaphragmatic and abdominal breathing
     d. Obligate nose breathing
     e. Absence of nasal flaring, grunting, and retractions

- Circulatory changes
  1. Transition from fetal to adult circulation begins with clamping of the umbilical cord and continues throughout the first weeks of life
  2. Characteristics of fetal circulation
     a. Low-pressure system, including placenta (low-resistance circuit)
     b. Minimal circulation to lungs; bypassed via foramen ovale
     c. Ductus arteriosus favors circulation to the brain
  3. Transition from fetal to neonatal circulation
     a. Increased systemic resistance due to loss of placental circuit
     b. Increased pressure in left atrium causes functional closure of foramen ovale
     c. Initial respiration opens pulmonary vasculature, favoring circulation to lungs
     d. Increased oxygenation of circulating blood causes constriction and functional closure of ductus arteriosus
     e. Absence of placental circulation closes ductus venosus

- Thermoregulation
  1. Mechanisms of neonatal heat loss
     a. Convection
     b. Conduction

c. Radiation

d. Evaporation

2. Neonate creates heat in three ways:

a. Shivering (inefficient)

b. Muscle activity (limited benefit)

c. Thermogenesis by metabolism of brown adipose tissue (BAT)

(1) BAT stores are decreased in preterm and growth-restricted fetuses

(2) BAT stores are nonrenewable

(3) Hypoglycemia decreases efficiency of BAT metabolism

3. Consequences of cold stress

a. Increased oxygen consumption, leading to relative hypoxia and acidosis

b. Metabolism of BAT and release of fatty acids decreases pH

c. Increased use of glucose, depletion of glycogen stores, and hypoglycemia

d. Worsening hypoglycemia and acidosis may result in respiratory distress

4. Management

a. Skin-to-skin on mother's chest or abdomen with blanket over both

b. Pre-warm blankets and resuscitation area

c. Dry the newborn immediately and replace wet blankets

d. Regulate room temperature and minimize exposure to air convection

e. Postpone newborn bath at least 2 hours

f. Keep newborn warm and wrapped

- Glucose regulation

1. Glycogen stores

a. Predominantly in liver

b. Accumulated in third trimester

2. Risk factors for neonatal hypoglycemia

a. Infants of diabetic mothers

b. Intrauterine growth restriction

c. Preterm or postterm

d. Intrapartum—fetal distress, beta-agonist tocolysis, IV glucose administration

e. Maternal substance abuse

3. Glucose regulation in the healthy neonate

a. Normal physiologic decrease in blood glucose

(1) Lowest at 1 to 1.5 to 5 hours after birth

(2) Stabilizes at 3 to 4 hours after birth

(3) Should not drop below 40 mg/dL (some place cutoff at 60 mg/dL)

b. Mean glucose levels from 4 to 72 hours are 60 to 70 mg/dL

c. Sources and mechanisms of glucose maintenance

(1) Intake of human milk or formula

(2) Glycogenolysis (use of glycogen stores)

(3) Gluconeogenesis (use of lipid stores)

4. Signs and symptoms of hypoglycemia

a. Weak cry

b. Jitteriness

c. Cyanosis

d. Apnea

e. Lethargy

f. Poor feeding

5. Management

a. Encourage feeding as soon as possible

b. Observe for signs/symptoms of hypoglycemia

c. Assess glucose levels if signs/symptoms or risk factors are present

(1) Profound severity at less than 20–25 mg/dL

(2) Moderate severity at 25–34 mg/dL

(3) Minimal severity at 35–45 mg/dL

d. Indications for treatment with intravenous dextrose

(1) Symptomatic infants, or those with initial serum glucose less than 25 mg/dL

(2) Asymptomatic infants with persistent serum glucose less than 40 mg/dL

◘ ONGOING EXTRAUTERINE TRANSITION

- Changes in the blood

1. Red blood cells (RBC)

a. Hemoglobin F

(1) Predominates in fetal circulation

(2) High affinity for oxygen

(3) Gradually eliminated in first month of life

b. Short RBC life span leads to increased bilirubin and physiologic jaundice

c. Infant position at cord clamping

(1) Below introitus—may cause placental transfusion and polycythemia

(2) Neutral position on maternal abdomen is preferable

d. Normal values

(1) Hemoglobin

(a) Newborn 13.7–20.0 g/dL

(b) Slight rise in first few days of life due to decreased plasma volume

(c) Mean value at 2 months of age 12.0 g/dL

(2) Hematocrit 43–63%

(3) RBC count 4.2–5.8 million/mm³

(4) Reticulocytes 3–7%

2. White blood cells (WBC) normal value—10–30,000/mm³

3. Platelets

a. Normal value—150–350,000/mm³

b. Relatively low levels of vitamin-K–dependent clotting factors

4. Obtaining blood samples
   a. Venous stasis in extremities may lead to false values from heel-stick samples
   b. Maximize blood flow by using heel warmer before obtaining sample
   c. Confirm abnormal results with venipuncture sample

- Changes in the gastrointestinal (GI) system
  1. Relatively mature aspects of the neonatal GI system
     a. Suckling/swallowing
     b. Gag and cough reflexes
  2. Relatively immature aspects of the neonatal GI system
     a. Limited ability to digest fats and proteins
     b. Better absorption of monosaccharides than polysaccharides
     c. Frequent regurgitation due to
        (1) Incomplete development of cardiac sphincter
        (2) Limited stomach capacity (less than 30 cc)
     d. "Gut closure"
        (1) Maturation process of intestinal lining and its enzymes and antibodies
        (2) Vulnerability to bacteria, viruses, and allergens until process is complete
        (3) Promoted by breastfeeding
     e. Large intestine
        (1) Less efficient water conservation than adult
        (2) Predisposes infant to dehydration

- Changes in the immune system
  1. Natural immunity
     a. Physical and chemical barriers (skin, mucosa, gastric acid)
     b. Phagocytes (neutrophils, monocytes, macrophages)
        (1) Immature phagocytic response
        (2) Relative inability to localize infection
  2. Acquired immunity
     a. Maternal IgG crosses placenta, conferring passive immunity to viruses the mother has encountered
     b. Breast milk provides maternal antibodies
     c. Active production of IgG develops slowly throughout childhood as passive immunity diminishes
  3. Immaturity of natural and acquired immune systems predisposes the newborn to infection and sepsis

- Changes in the renal system
  1. Limited renal circulation
  2. Decreased glomerular filtration rate

3. Immature tubular function
   a. Relative inability to concentrate urine
   b. Predisposition to fluid and electrolyte imbalances

▢ IMMEDIATE CARE AND ASSESSMENT OF THE HEALTHY NEWBORN

- Assessment prior to birth of pertinent maternal history
  1. Genetic history
     a. Family history of structural or metabolic defects
     b. History of genetic syndromes
  2. Maternal elements
     a. Demographic factors
        (1) Maternal age of younger than 16 or older than 35 years
        (2) Overweight or underweight prior to pregnancy
        (3) Maternal education less than 11 years
        (4) Family history of inherited disorders
     b. Medical factors
        (1) Cardiac disease
        (2) Pulmonary disease
        (3) Renal disease
        (4) Gastrointestinal disease
        (5) Endocrine disorders, particularly diabetes or thyroid disease
        (6) Chronic hypertension
        (7) Hemoglobinopathies
        (8) Seizure or other neurologic disorders
     c. History of present pregnancy
        (1) Late or no prenatal care
        (2) Rh sensitization
        (3) Fetus large or small for gestational age
        (4) Premature labor or delivery
        (5) Pregnancy-induced hypertension
        (6) Multiple gestation
        (7) Polyhydramnios
        (8) Premature or prolonged rupture of membranes
        (9) Antepartum bleeding
        (10) Abnormal presentation
        (11) Postmaturity
        (12) Abnormal results in fetal testing
        (13) Anemia
     d. Psychosocial history
        (1) Inadequate financial, housing, or social resources
        (2) Minority status
        (3) Malnutrition
        (4) Parental occupation
        (5) Significant relationships, marriage status
        (6) Violence or abuse

(7) Smoking during pregnancy

(8) Alcohol use during pregnancy

(9) Drug use/abuse

- Assessment at birth
  1. During and immediately following birth
     a. Assess tone and skin color
     b. Gross inspection of anatomy
     c. Place infant on maternal abdomen or radiant warmer
     d. Palpate cord to assess heart rate
  2. Apgar scoring
     a. Scale—0 to 10
        (1) Heart rate—0 = absent, 1 = <100, 2 = >100
        (2) Respiratory effort—0 = absent, 1 = slow/irregular, 2 = strong cry
        (3) Tone—0 = flaccid, 1 = flexion of extremities, 2 = active motion
        (4) Reflex irritability—0 = no response, 1 = grimace, 2 = strong cry
        (5) Color—0 = general cyanosis, 1 = acrocyanosis, 2 = completely pink
     b. Assigned at 1 and 5 minutes; may be assigned at additional 5-minute intervals when prolonged resuscitation efforts are required
     c. Primary purpose of Apgar score—objective method of quantifying the newborn's condition and response to resuscitation
     d. Poor predictor of long-term outcome
     e. Poor predictor of acidemia
     f. Apgar score is not used to determine the need for resuscitation, what resuscitation steps are necessary, or when to use them (Neonatal Resuscitation Steering Committee, 2000)

- Review of neonatal resuscitation (American Academy of Pediatrics, 2006)
  1. Midwives and nurse practitioners who care for women in the intrapartum setting should be trained and certified in neonatal resuscitation; the information presented here is a review, not a substitute for training and certification
  2. Approximately 10% of newborns require some assistance to begin breathing at birth; about 1% require extensive resuscitation
  3. Evaluation is based upon three signs
     a. Respirations
     b. Heart rate
     c. Color
  4. ABCs of resuscitation
     a. Establish an open *A*irway
        (1) Position the infant on back or side with the neck slightly extended
        (2) Suction mouth and nose, and trachea as indicated
        (3) Insert endotracheal (ET) tube to ensure open airway if necessary
     b. Initiate *B*reathing
        (1) Use tactile stimulation to initiate respirations
        (2) Use positive pressure ventilation (PPV) with 100% oxygen when necessary
     c. Maintain *C*irculation—stimulate and maintain circulation with chest compressions and/or medications when necessary
  5. Overview of resuscitation in the delivery room
     a. Initial steps
        (1) Place infant under radiant heater
        (2) Suction trachea if meconium aspiration is suspected
        (3) Dry infant; remove wet linen
        (4) Suction mouth and nose
        (5) Provide tactile stimulation
     b. Evaluate respirations, heart rate, and color
        (1) If no respirations, or heart rate less than 100 beats per minute (bpm), provide positive-pressure ventilation (PPV) with oxygen
           (a) If heart rate is below 60 bpm, continue PPV and initiate chest compressions
           (b) If heart rate is above 60 bpm, continue PPV without chest compressions
     c. Medications
        (1) Medications are initiated when the heart rate remains below 60 bpm after 30 seconds of coordinated chest compressions and PPV
        (2) Dosage based on infant weight
        (3) Medications include
           (a) Epinephrine—increases strength and rate of cardiac contractions and causes peripheral vasoconstriction
           (b) Volume expanders—recommended solution is normal saline
           (c) Sodium bicarbonate—may be beneficial in correcting acidosis during prolonged resuscitation
           (d) Naloxone—narcotic antagonist used when there is severe respiratory depression and a history of maternal narcotic administration within the last 4 hours
  6. Newborns with meconium-stained amniotic fluid

a. Suction mouth, nose, and posterior pharynx after delivery of head but before delivery of shoulders

b. If the baby has a normal respiratory effort, normal tone, and heart rate greater than 100 bpm, use bulb syringe or suction catheter to clear secretions and meconium from mouth and nose—endotracheal suctioning is not indicated

c. If the baby has depressed respirations, depressed tone, or heart rate less than 100 bpm, endotracheal suctioning of meconium is indicated

◘ CARE DURING THE FIRST HOURS AFTER BIRTH

- Transitional period
  1. Time when the infant stabilizes and adjusts to extrauterine life
  2. Three stages
     a. First period of reactivity
     b. Period of unresponsive sleep
     c. Second period of reactivity
  3. May be altered when the infant is significantly stressed in labor and delivery
  4. Preferred management for first hour of life; some say during hospital stay
     a. Maintain contact with the mother
     b. Limit or defer examinations and procedures, or perform them unobtrusively

- First period of reactivity
  1. Begins immediately after birth
  2. Lasts approximately 30 minutes
  3. Assessment findings
     a. Rapid heart rate and respirations—near upper limits of normal
     b. Respiratory rales present, disappearing by 20 minutes of age
     c. Behavior—alert, eyes open, may exhibit startle, cry, and/or rooting
     d. Bowel sounds usually present by 30 minutes after birth; may pass stool
  4. Encourage breastfeeding during first period of reactivity
     a. Facilitated by infant's alert, active state
     b. Ameliorates physiologic drop in blood glucose at 1 to 1.5 hours after birth

- Period of unresponsive sleep
  1. Lasts from 30 minutes to 2 hours after birth
  2. Assessment findings
     a. Heart rate decreases—usually to less than 140 bpm
     b. Murmur due to incomplete closure of ductus arteriosus

c. Slower, more regular respirations

d. Bowel sounds present but diminished

- Second period of reactivity
  1. Lasts from 2 to 6 hours after birth
  2. Assessment findings
     a. Labile heart rate
     b. Rapid changes in color
     c. Respiration—rate less than 60/min without rales or rhonchi
  3. Early feeding
     a. Infant may be interested in feeding during the second period of reactivity
     b. Prevention of hypoglycemia
     c. Stimulation of stool passage
     d. Prevention of jaundice

- Bonding and parent–newborn attachment
  1. Definitions vary; generally referring to the process occurring in the time after birth whereby the mother (and/or other family members) form a unique, lasting relationship with the newborn
  2. Factors that may influence bonding
     a. Parental background
        (1) Care that parents received from their parents
        (2) Social/cultural factors
        (3) Couple and family relationships
        (4) Experiences in previous pregnancies
     b. Care practices
        (1) Interventions and assessments before and after birth
        (2) Behavior of healthcare providers
        (3) Care and support received in labor and delivery
        (4) Institutional rules and policies
     c. Facilitating factors
        (1) Skin-to-skin contact
        (2) Breastfeeding
        (3) Visual contact
        (4) Holding, touching, "getting acquainted"
  3. Limitations of bonding and attachment theories
     a. Formation of relationships probably evolves out of many experiences rather than a single critical event
     b. Little evidence that early separation has permanent effects on mother–infant or parent–child relationships
     c. May lead to judgmental responses among healthcare providers, or guilt among parents, when bonding expectations are not met

◘ PLAN OF CARE FOR THE FIRST FEW DAYS OF LIFE

- Feeding
  1. Demand feeding
     a. Indicated for both breast- and bottle-fed infants
     b. Most infants will stop sucking and may fall asleep when full and satisfied
  2. Breastfeeding
     a. Breast-fed infants average 8 to 10 feedings per day
     b. Intake is adequate if the infant seems satisfied and wets 4 to 6 diapers per day
     c. Frequent assessment, reassurance, and anticipatory guidance are essential for breastfeeding mothers and infants in the first few days of life
     d. Discourage supplementary bottle feedings to promote development of maternal and infant breastfeeding skills and to ensure adequate milk supply
  3. Formula feeding
     a. Formula-fed infants average 6 to 8 feedings per day
     b. Limited stomach capacity
        (1) Infant may take only 20 to 30 mL of formula at initial feedings
        (2) Most infants should take 60 to 120 mL formula per feeding by the third day of life
     c. Demonstrate positioning and burping techniques

- Voiding/Stooling
  1. Record time and characteristics of first passage of urine and stool
  2. Stool will progress from meconium to yellow-green
  3. Absence of voiding for 24 hours is an indication for pediatric evaluation

- Skin
  1. Full baths and use of antibacterial soap are discouraged
  2. "Dry care"—skin is dried and skin folds are wiped clean with gauze
  3. Warm sponge bath late in first day of life to clear blood and meconium
  4. Discourage use of skin lotions, powders, creams, oils

- Medications
  1. Gonorrhea/chlamydia prophylaxis
     a. 0.5% erythromycin ointment
     b. Should be deferred until after the first period of reactivity
  2. Vitamin K
     a. Prevention of hemorrhagic disease
     b. May be administered intramuscularly or orally
  3. Hepatitis B vaccination
     a. First dose prior to discharge
     b. Second dose at 1 to 2 months of age
     c. Third dose no earlier than 24 weeks of age

- Health promotion and safety
  1. All caregivers should wash hands thoroughly before handling infant
  2. Follow policies/procedures for infant identification
  3. Follow policies/procedures for infant security
  4. Teaching—safety and signs of illness (see Discharge teaching section in this chapter)

◘ DISCHARGE PLANNING

- Discharge teaching
  1. Formula feeding
     a. Use iron-fortified formula
     b. Clean nipples and bottles thoroughly prior to use
     c. 1.5 oz every 3 to 4 hours, increasing gradually
     d. Supplementary water or juice not recommended
  2. Breastfeeding
     a. On demand, at least every 2 to 5 hours
     b. Average 8 to 10 feeds every 24 hours
     c. 10 to 15 minutes suckling on each side, each feeding
     d. Adequate maternal rest and fluid intake
     e. Sore nipples indicate incorrect positioning or latch-on
  3. Voiding/Stooling
     a. Bottle-fed infant stools—yellow-green, firm to pasty, straining is normal and not necessarily indicative of constipation
     b. Breast-fed infant stools—yellow-gold, loose or liquid, frequency varies, stooling with each feed or every other day
     c. 4 to 6 wet diapers per day is usually indicative of adequate intake
  4. Jaundice
     a. Occurs in more than 50% of newborns; more often in breast-fed infants
     b. Temporary condition, rarely indicative of disease
     c. Usually peaks at 3 to 4 days of life
     d. Yellowing of sclera should be evaluated by pediatric provider
  5. Skin
     a. Sponge bath every day or every other day
     b. Tub baths after cord stump falls off

    c. Mild, unscented soap

    d. Lotions, oils, and powders are unnecessary

    e. Dry/peeling skin is normal and resolves spontaneously

    f. Diaper rash may be treated with petroleum jelly and air exposure, but notify pediatric provider if persistent

6. Cord care

    a. Apply rubbing alcohol to cord stump several times per day

    b. Diaper should be fastened below cord

    c. Avoid immersion of cord stump in water

    d. Cord will usually drop off at approximately 2 weeks

    e. Redness around the cord base, foul odor, or drainage from cord should be reported to pediatric provider

7. Safety

    a. Infant car seats for every car ride

    b. Hand-held carrier vs body carrier—pros and cons

    c. Bottle propping is dangerous due to choking risk

    d. Avoid handling hot liquids while handling newborn

    e. Avoid exposure to direct sunshine; sunscreens are not necessarily safe for newborns

    f. Install smoke detectors

    g. Avoid exposure to cigarette smoke

    h. Infant should sleep in supine or side-lying position

8. Expected infant behavior

    a. Hiccups are common and do not require treatment

    b. Sneezing is normal and does not necessarily indicate illness

9. Signs of illness

    a. Poor feeding, irritability, lethargy, skin rash, cord problems, vomiting, diarrhea, decreased urine output, rectal temperature greater than 100°F, or change in infant's behavior

    b. Emphasize that neonatal infection is not always accompanied by fever

- Psychosocial barriers/considerations to discharge

1. Current maternal substance abuse
2. Present or historical maternal psychiatric illness
3. Severe illness or physical disability of the mother
4. History of abuse or neglect of a previous child
5. Inappropriate maternal behavior
6. Homelessness or inadequate living arrangements

- Physical barriers to discharge

1. Feedings—newborn must demonstrate adequate intake of human milk or formula prior to discharge
2. Prematurity

    a. Any newborn less than 37 weeks' gestation or less than 2500 g should be observed for minimum of 3 days or in accord with Pediatric Department policy

    b. Premature infants must demonstrate ability to maintain normal body temperature outside incubator for 24 hours prior to discharge

3. Neonatal drug withdrawal

    a. Newborn should be held for observation

    b. Social work evaluation and referral to drug treatment are indicated

    c. Referral to child protective services is indicated if withdrawal symptoms occur or if newborn's urine toxicology is positive

    d. If medication is required to treat withdrawal, newborn must be held until medication is no longer necessary

    e. Newborn should be asymptomatic for 48 to 72 hours

4. Congenital abnormalities

    a. Heart murmurs suspected to be pathologic should be evaluated prior to discharge

    b. Dislocated hips should be evaluated by orthopedic specialist and treatment begun prior to discharge

    c. Abnormal renal findings on prenatal ultrasound should be evaluated prior to discharge

5. Infections

    a. Sepsis—infant at risk for sepsis should be treated with antibiotics until blood cultures negative for 72 hours

    b. Syphilis—infants with congenital syphilis or infants of mothers with untreated syphilis should receive spinal tap and be treated within 10 days with intramuscular or intravenous penicillin

    c. Pneumonia—infants with pneumonia should be held in hospital for 7 to 14 days for antibiotic treatment

6. Hyperbilirubinemia

    a. Physiologic jaundice

      (1) Not visible in first 24 hours

      (2) Rises slowly and peaks at day 3 or 4 of life

      (3) Total bilirubin peaks at less than 13 mg/dL

      (4) Lab tests reveal predominance of unconjugated (indirect) bilirubin

      (5) Not visible after 10 days

b. Possible pathologic jaundice
   (1) Visible during first 24 hours
   (2) May rise quickly to greater than 5 mg/dL/24 hours
   (3) Total bilirubin is greater than 13 mg/dL
   (4) Greater amounts of conjugated (direct) bilirubin
   (5) Visible jaundice persists after 1 week
c. Labs—serum total bilirubin (STB), blood type, Rh, Coombs
d. Phototherapy, if indicated, may be arranged through home healthcare agency
e. Infants with elevated bilirubin but without hemolytic disease may be discharged if outpatient pediatric follow-up can be arranged

- Criteria for early discharge
  1. General criteria
     a. Following uncomplicated birth, most infants may be discharged at 12–24 hours after birth depending on hospital policy
     b. Joint decision by midwife, pediatric provider, and family
     c. Uncomplicated antepartum, intrapartum, and postpartum course
     d. Early discharge increases importance of patient and family education to assess newborn
     e. Adequate support for mother at home, including home healthcare referral
  2. Neonatal criteria
     a. Uncomplicated vaginal delivery
     b. Full-term infant with adequate growth (2500 to 4500 g)
     c. Normal findings on neonatal examination
     d. May be minimum 6-hour hospitalization but at least sufficient time under provider care to demonstrate:
        (1) Thermal homeostasis
        (2) Ability to feed
     e. Normal laboratory results confirmed
  3. Maternal criteria
     a. Demonstrated ability with chosen feeding method
     b. Demonstrated ability with cord care
     c. Demonstrated ability to assess newborn's temperature with thermometer
     d. Verbalizes understanding of signs of newborn well-being and illness

- Discharge evaluation
  1. Complete physical examination with emphasis on the following:

a. Frequency and duration of breast feedings, or frequency and amount of bottle feedings
b. Number of voids/stools
c. Present weight and birth weight
2. Discharge evaluation should be performed in the presence of parents for teaching, answering questions, and providing anticipatory guidance

- Follow-up care
  1. Pediatric follow-up should be arranged prior to discharge
  2. Factors influencing time of first pediatric visit
     a. Medical condition of newborn
     b. Length of hospital stay
     c. Experience of mother and family in caring for newborns
     d. Size of newborn
     e. Mother/family psychosocial factors
     f. Adequacy of newborn feeding

◻ NEWBORN ASSESSMENT

- History—see Immediate Care and Assessment of the Healthy Newborn section

- Physical examination
  1. General
     a. Whole
        (1) Proportions
        (2) Symmetry
        (3) Facies
        (4) Gestational age (approximate)
     b. Skin
        (1) Color
        (2) Subcutaneous tissue
        (3) Imperfections (bands and birthmarks)
        (4) Vernix and lanugo
        (5) Cysts and masses
     c. Neuromuscular
        (1) Movements
        (2) Responses
        (3) Tone (flexor)
  2. Head and neck
     a. Head
        (1) Shape
        (2) Circumference
        (3) Molding
        (4) Swellings
        (5) Depressions
        (6) Occipital overhang
     b. Fontanelles, sutures
        (1) Size
        (2) Tension
     c. Eyes
        (1) Size

      (2) Separation
      (3) Cataracts
  d. Ears
      (1) Placement
      (2) Complexity
      (3) Preauricular tags
  e. Mouth
      (1) Symmetry
      (2) Size
      (3) Clefts
  f. Neck
      (1) Swellings
      (2) Fistulas

3. Chest
  a. Inspect for deformities (nipples, clavicles, sternum)
  b. Observe respiratory function with abdomen
  c. Palpate—breast bud size; clavicle for crepitus and/or swelling

4. Lungs and respiration
  a. Retraction
  b. Grunt
  c. Quality of breath sounds

5. Heart and circulation
  a. Rate
  b. Rhythm
  c. Murmurs—usually present for 1–2 days after birth until ductus arteriosus closes
  d. Sounds

6. Abdomen
  a. Musculature
  b. Bowel sounds
  c. Cord vessels—number and type
  d. Distension
  e. Scaphoid shape
  f. Masses
  g. Liver edge may be palpable at 2–3 cm below right costal margin
  h. Normal spleen and kidneys are not easily felt
  i. Femoral pulses are felt when the infant is quiet

7. Genitalia and anus
  a. Placement
  b. Identify ambiguous genitalia
  c. Scrotum—size, skin is wrinkled; determine if testes are descended
  d. Phallus—size, placement of urethra
  e. Labia—palpate for masses; identify all structures and determine patency of vaginal orifice
  f. Anus—determine patency and relative position to other genital structures

8. Musculoskeletal
  a. Posture

  b. Hands—digits; polydactyly, syndactyly, webbing, overlapping, shape and texture; "fisting"
  c. Feet—degree of flexion, shape, position
  d. Neck—rotation
  e. Joints—normal range of motion
  f. Long bone fractures—distortion, swelling, crepitus

9. Spine
  a. Symmetry
  b. Scoliosis
  c. Sinuses

- Gestational age assessment
1. Dubowitz (detailed assessment of gestational age) and Ballard (abbreviated version of Dubowitz) scales
  a. Estimation of gestational age and maturity based on observation and examination—score for 40-week infant total equals 40
  b. Elements include posture and tone, and characteristics of skin, lanugo, plantar surface, breast tissue, eyes/ears, and genitals

2. Posture and tone—premature infant generally demonstrates extended posture, less tone, and less resistance to flexion of extremities

3. Skin—premature infant has redder/pinker, translucent skin; postmature infant has cracked, wrinkled skin

4. Lanugo is sparse to absent in the postmature or very premature infant and is most abundant in midterm infant (28 to 30 weeks)

5. Plantar surface
  a. Assessed by length of foot from heel to tip of great toe in the premature infant
  b. Creases appear by 28 to 30 weeks of gestation and cover the entire surface at term

6. Breast tissue and areola—progressive development throughout gestation
  a. Preterm—flat areola with no palpable breast bud
  b. Term infant—raised areola with 3 to 4 mm palpable breast bud

7. Eye/ear
  a. Eyelids are fused in very premature neonate
  b. More mature infants will exhibit more cartilaginous ear tissue that exhibits greater firmness and recoil when flexed

8. Male genitalia—increasing rugation of scrotum and descent of testes with advancing gestational age

9. Female genitalia—increasing development of labia majora and decreasing prominence of clitoris and labia minora with advancing gestational age

10. Anterior vascular capsule of ocular lens—more prominent vasculature at early gestational ages

- Measurements
  1. Weight
     a. Normal weight for a term newborn is 2501 to 4000 g
     b. Less-than-normal birth weight—definitions
        (1) Extremely low birth weight—less than 1000 g
        (2) Very low birth weight—1000–1500 g
        (3) Low birth weight—1501–2500 g
     c. Usual growth patterns
        (1) Infants typically lose 10 to 15% of birth weight in first 3 days of life
        (2) Should regain birth weight by 10 to 14 days of age
        (3) Double birth weight by 4 to 6 months of age
        (4) Triple birth weight by 12 months of age
  2. Length
     a. Most accurately measured by placing head against a firm surface, extending legs, then marking the surface
     b. Normal length for a term newborn is 48 to 53 cm
  3. Head circumference
     a. Measured from the occiput around head and above eyebrows
     b. Normal head circumference for a term newborn is 33 to 35 cm
  4. Chest circumference
     a. Measured under armpits across nipple line
     b. Normal chest circumference is 30 to 33 cm and 2 to 3 cm less than head circumference
  5. Be aware of genetic pool of parents, i.e., one or both of small stature

- Assessment for birth defects
  1. Minor malformations are relatively common, but three or more minor malformations on physical examination is suggestive of a major underlying condition
  2. Minor malformations
     a. Large fontanelles
     b. Epicanthic eye fold
     c. Hair whorls
     d. Widow's peak
     e. Low posterior hair line
     f. Preauricular skin tags or pits
     g. Minor ear anomalies—low-set, rotated, protruding
     h. Darwinian tubercule—small nodule on upper helix of ear
     i. Digital anomalies—curved, webbed, or bent fingers
     j. Transverse palmar crease
     k. Shawl scrotum
     l. Redundant umbilicus
     m. Widespread or supernumerary nipples

- Neurologic examination
  1. Level of alertness
     a. Most sensitive of all neurologic functions
     b. Varies depending on gestational age, time of last feeding, sleep patterns, recent stimuli, and recent experiences
     c. Findings associated with level of alertness
        (1) Response to arousal attempts (e.g., gentle shaking, sound, light)
        (2) Level and character of motility
  2. Neuromotor findings
     a. Tone and posture
     b. Motility and power
     c. Tendon reflexes—pectoralis major, brachioradialis, patellar, achilles
     d. Plantar response—flexion or extension of toes
     e. Eyes—red reflex, pupillary reflex, doll's eye reflex, blink reflex
  3. Assess for normal, absent, diminished or exaggerated reflexes—abnormal reflexes suggest nervous system depression, spinal lesion, or central nervous system disorder or lesion
  4. Primary neonatal reflexes (Volpe, 2008)
     a. Palmar grasp
        (1) Newborn grasps object or finger placed on his/her palm
        (2) Typically disappears by 2 months of age
     b. Tonic neck response
        (1) Elicited by rotation of the head to one side
        (2) Newborn extends arm on the side to which the head is rotated and flexes the contralateral arm ("fencing posture")
        (3) Typically disappears by 7 months of age
     c. Moro reflex
        (1) "Startle" response, evidenced by abduction and extension of arms with hands open and thumb and index finger semiflexed to form a C
        (2) Elicited by jarring examination table, allowing the infant to fall backward onto the examiner's hand, or making a loud noise

(3) Typically disappears by 6 months of age

d. Placing and stepping ("walking")

(1) Elicited by holding the infant upright and placing soles of feet in contact with flat surface or table edge

(2) Typically disappears by 4 weeks of age

- Metabolic screening
  1. No federal guidelines; requirements vary state to state
  2. Metabolic screening tests mandated in most states, e.g.:
     a. Phenylketonuria
     b. Biotinidase deficiency
     c. Congenital adrenal hyperplasia
     d. Congenital hypothyroidism
     e. Cystic fibrosis
     f. Galactosemia
     g. Homocystinuria
     h. Branched-chain ketoaciduria
     i. Sickle cell disease
     j. Tyrosinemia
  3. Timing of metabolic screening
     a. Generally, after 24 hours of age—allowing time for feeding to be established and accumulation of toxic metabolites if disease is present
     b. Preferably 48 to 72 hours of age
     c. Recommended repeat screening at 2 to 4-week pediatric visit
     d. Law may mandate screening before discharge—for early discharge, repeat screening must be done

◨ PRIMARY CARE OF THE NEWBORN FOR THE FIRST 6 WEEKS

- Well child surveillance
  1. All newborns should have at least two physical examinations before discharge
  2. Well child visit
     a. Within 3 to 5 days for early-discharged newborns
     b. Within 10 to 14 days for newborns held 48 hours
     c. Purpose—reexamine newborn, review teaching, perform metabolic screening
     d. Assessment includes
        (1) Review of maternal, perinatal, and newborn history
        (2) Observation of parents and assessment of family adjustment
        (3) Newborn interval history, including feeding, behavior, voiding/stooling
        (4) Physical examination
     e. Schedule follow-up visits

- Newborn behavior
  1. Sleep-wake states as classified by Brazelton
     a. Quiet sleep
     b. Active sleep
     c. Drowsy
     d. Quiet alert
     e. Active alert
     f. Crying
  2. Alert state
     a. Determine infant's ability to feed and interact with environment
     b. Comprises approximately 15% of daytime hours
  3. Crying
     a. May express need for feeding, holding, stimulation, or sleep
     b. May be indicative of pain
     c. Parental responsiveness to crying does not promote "spoiling" of infant—responsiveness is essential to newborn's development
  4. Sleeping
     a. Infant may exhibit varying respiratory patterns while sleeping e.g., decreased depth and rate or periodic breathing (intermittent cessation of breathing for up to 10 seconds)
     b. Normal infants sleep up to 60% of the time

- Sensory capabilities
  1. Sensory threshold—level of tolerance for stimuli within which the infant can respond appropriately
     a. Infant may become fatigued or stressed when overstimulated; signs of stress and fatigue include:
        (1) Color changes
        (2) Irregular respiration
        (3) Irritability or lethargy
        (4) Vomiting
     b. Varies significantly among individuals; markedly low in premature or neurologically impaired newborns
  2. Visual capabilities
     a. Normal term infant can visually fix and track objects
     b. Sharp focus limited to distance of 10 to 12 inches
     c. Preference for striped patterns and strong contrasts
     d. Limited color perception
     e. Ability to recognize mother visually and respond to facial expressions within the first few weeks of life
  3. Newborns can detect and discriminate odors
  4. Taste capabilities

a. Newborns react strongly to variations in taste

b. Preference for sweet

5. Hearing is acute, with ability to localize sounds and preference for mother's voice

6. Touch—sensitive to light touch, as demonstrated by reflex responses

- Regulation of behavior
  1. Ability to respond appropriately to stimuli and maintain behavioral states
  2. Full-term infants should demonstrate smooth transition between states from sleep to active alertness; consistently abrupt or unpredictable changes are a cause for concern
  3. Ability to maintain active alert state varies among individuals—some have difficulty becoming or remaining alert, while irritable infants progress rapidly from alertness to crying
  4. Overstimulated infants may require "time-out"; relative isolation from stimuli and time to recover
  5. Organization—ability to integrate physiologic and behavioral systems in response to the environment without disruption in state or physiologic functions
     a. Maintenance of stable vital signs
     b. Smooth state transitions
     c. Coordination of movements and responses in interacting with environment
     d. Consolable with ability for self-consolation (frequently characterized by hand-to-mouth movements)
     e. Habituation—ability to block out noxious stimuli

- Developmental milestones in first 6 weeks as measured by Denver II
  1. Personal/social skills—spontaneous and responsive smiling, attentiveness to a face
  2. Visual tracking—follows dangling object from midline through 45°
  3. Spontaneous vocalization
  4. Response to sound of bell
  5. Gross motor—lifting head momentarily and symmetrical body movements

- Psychological tasks of early infancy as defined by Erikson
  1. Development of basic trust
     a. Birth through 12 to 18 months
     b. Definition—belief that world is a place where people and things can be relied upon and needs and wishes will be met
     c. Essential for formation of human attachments throughout life

  2. Development of differentiation—ability to discriminate between self and other
  3. Ability to elicit care giving is essential to early development
  4. Secure attachment depends on caregivers':
     a. Emotional availability
     b. Sensitivity and stimulation
     c. Appropriate response to infant cues
     d. Consistency
  5. In the first year of life, securely attached infants will venture out and return to mother
  6. Results of insecure attachment
     a. Anxious or unable to cope with changes or distance from mother
     b. More negative infant behavior
     c. Avoidance/detachment
     d. Research suggests long-term impairment, including school problems and delinquency
  7. Counseling or parenting classes may be helpful when mothers/caregivers are experiencing problems in forming secure attachment

- Circumcision
  1. Increased prevalence in United States during 1950s
  2. Significant role of cultural, religious, and family traditions
  3. Medical complications are rare but serious; include bleeding, infection, and inappropriate operative result
  4. Controversial impact on sexual and psychological functioning; no clear evidence
  5. Unclear evidence as to risks/benefits; routine circumcision for medical reasons is no longer recommended
  6. Provide pain control if family chooses circumcision
  7. Care of circumcised infant
     a. Apply petroleum jelly gauze strip to prevent adhesion of tissue to diaper
     b. Continue to use petroleum jelly on affected tissue until healed
     c. Notify care provider if bleeding, exudate, swelling, or inability to void occur
  8. Uncircumcised infant
     a. Foreskin should separate and become freely mobile by 4 to 7 years of age
     b. Never forcefully retract the foreskin
     c. Infant hygiene—"only clean what can be seen"
     d. As the child matures, he should be taught to retract the foreskin and clean

- Nonnutritive sucking
  1. Thumb sucking and use of pacifiers subject to mother/family preferences and attitudes

2. Common behavior in utero
3. Infant may use nonnutritive sucking to regulate behavior state or self-console
4. Avoid
   a. Use of empty bottle for nonnutritive sucking (promotes ingestion of air, dental caries, and may contribute to otitis)
   b. Placing pacifier on string around baby's neck
   c. Prolonged use of and serious dependence on pacifiers

◘ COMMON VARIATIONS FROM NORMAL NEWBORN FINDINGS

- Jaundice
  1. Incidence—up to 50% of newborns
  2. Physiologic vs pathologic jaundice
     a. Physiologic jaundice does not occur within first 24 hours of life
     b. Total serum bilirubin concentrations increasing by more than 5 mg/dL per day indicate pathologic jaundice
     c. Physiologic jaundice rarely results in total serum bilirubin concentrations greater than 15 mg/dL
     d. Direct serum bilirubin levels greater than 1.5 mg/dL indicate pathologic jaundice
  3. More common and slower to resolve in breast-fed infants
  4. Can be detected by blanching skin of nose, palms, or soles of feet—if jaundiced, skin will blanch yellow
  5. Treatment
     a. Supplementation of breast-fed infants with oral glucose water is not helpful and may be harmful
     b. Frequent feeding to stimulate GI elimination
     c. Management algorithm (values reflect total serum bilirubin concentrations)
        (1) Consider phototherapy for values of 12 to 17 mg/dL
        (2) Phototherapy indicated for values of 15 to 20 mg/dL
        (3) Exchange transfusion indicated for values of 20 to 25 mg/dL
        (4) Treatment thresholds are lower at earlier ages (24 to 48 hours after birth)
     d. Phototherapy may be indicated; some sources recommend exposing newborn to indirect sunlight for short periods several times per day

- Obstructed lacrimal ducts
  1. Incidence—50% of newborns will exhibit excessive tearing and mucoid discharge from eyes

  2. Treatment
     a. Massage—apply gentle, firm pressure in a circular motion on the lateral aspect of the nose adjacent to inner canthus of eye
     b. Clear drainage with cotton ball moistened with warm water, proceeding from inner to outer canthus
     c. Repeat treatment 3 to 4 times per day

- Dacryocystitis
  1. Definition—acute infection of lacrimal ducts
  2. Presentation—purulent discharge, swelling, tenderness adjacent to inner canthus of eye
  3. Treatment
     a. Same hygiene routine as described for obstructed lacrimal ducts
     b. Aseptic technique to prevent cross-contamination
     c. Topical or systemic antibiotics are indicated

- Skin problems
  1. Cradle cap
     a. Definition—dermatitis resulting from accumulation of sebum on scalp
     b. Presentation—characteristic yellow, crusting patches on anterior scalp, often in area of anterior fontanelle
     c. Treatment
        (1) Vigorous cleansing with mild shampoo and washcloth
        (2) Apply baby oil to area 30 minutes prior to shampooing
        (3) Rub affected area with dry washcloth gently but firmly to remove crusting
        (4) If severe, antiseborrheic shampoo may be indicated
  2. Diaper dermatitis
     a. Definition—general term for a variety of skin conditions that can occur in the diaper area
     b. Primary—caused by exposure to moisture and friction
     c. Secondary
        (1) Caused by colonization of affected area by pathogen; most commonly *Candida albicans*
        (2) Presentation—"fire-engine red" erythema, circumscribed pustulovesicular lesions, often with satellite lesions
     d. Treatment
        (1) Change diapers frequently
        (2) Avoid use of baby wipes
        (3) Rinse area with tepid water after every voiding; use tepid water and mild soap after stooling
        (4) Clean and dry skin thoroughly

(5) Allow exposure of skin to air, especially before reapplying diaper

(6) Some infants are sensitive to irritants in disposable diapers; change brands or use cloth diapers

(7) For infants with diarrhea, apply zinc oxide ointment to clean, dry skin to provide a barrier

(8) Severe irritation may be treated with 1% topical hydrocortisone

(9) Nystatin topical cream, applied at each diaper change, for *Candida albicans* dermatitis

- Thrush
  1. Definition—oral fungal infection usually caused by *Candida albicans*
  2. Peak incidence around second week of life
  3. Often occurs after antibiotic therapy
  4. Presentation—characteristic white patches on the buccal mucosa, gums, tongue, and/or palate; lesions may be friable
  5. May cause feeding difficulty if extensive
  6. Treatment
     a. Nystatin suspension orally 4 times a day for 1 week
     b. Instill one dropper-full into each buccal pocket
     c. "Paint" lesions with cotton-tipped applicator
     d. Bottle-fed infants—boil nipples after use
     e. Breast-fed infants—treat mother's nipples simultaneously with topical antifungal agents (nystatin, miconazole, clotrimazole)

- Regurgitation
  1. Definition—effortless "spitting up" of small amount of formula or breast milk
  2. Exacerbated by excessive swallowing of air, resulting from underfeeding or delayed feeding and prolonged crying, improper positioning, sucking on empty formula bottle
  3. Treatment
     a. Normal self-limiting condition, no treatment necessary
     b. May be reduced if infant is positioned sitting upright at 50 to 60-degree angle for 30 to 60 minutes after feeding

- Colic
  1. Definition—sudden, loud, and/or continuous unexplained crying often accompanied by flushed facies, mild abdominal distension, adduction of legs, or clenched fists
  2. Affects 10% of infants

3. No proven organic basis; suggested but unproved causative factors include:
   a. Overfeeding, especially in bottle-fed infants
   b. Allergy to constituents of formula or breastfeeding mother's diet (milk products often suggested)
   c. Anxiety in primary caregiver or tension in household; possibly symptomatic rather than etiologic
   d. Immaturity of digestive system
4. Treatment
   a. Attempt to identify factors associated with colic episodes for the individual infant
   b. Correct overfeeding
   c. Trial elimination of milk products from breastfeeding mother's diet
      (1) Efficacy is unknown; anecdotally effective in many cases
      (2) If bovine allergens are implicated, a trial longer than 1 week is necessary to clear mother's system
      (3) Maternal calcium supplementation is suggested with this approach
   d. Some infants respond to warmth, wrapping in a blanket, limitation of stimuli, rhythmic soothing motion, gentle repetitive massage, or soft monotonous music
   e. Probably most important factor is supportive care for parents, including reassurance and respite opportunities
   f. As a last resort for exhausted parents, infant may be positioned safely and left to cry for limited periods of time

◘ DEVIATIONS FROM NORMAL

- Danger signs of neonatal morbidity
  1. Central nervous system signs
     a. Lethargy
     b. High-pitched cry
     c. Jitteriness
     d. Abnormal eye movement
     e. Seizure activity
     f. Abnormal fontanelle size or bulging fontanelles
  2. Respiratory signs
     a. Apnea of more than 15 seconds accompanied by bradycardia or cyanosis
     b. Tachypnea
     c. Nasal flaring, expiratory grunting, and/or chest retractions
     d. Persistent rales and/or rhonchi
     e. Asynchronous breathing movements
  3. Cardiovascular signs
     a. Abnormal rate and rhythm
     b. Murmurs

c. Changes in blood pressure

d. Marked differential between upper and lower extremity blood pressure

e. Alterations and/or differentials in pulses

f. Changes in perfusion and skin color

4. Gastrointestinal signs

   a. Refusal to feed

   b. Absent or uncoordinated feeding reflexes

   c. Vomiting

   d. Abdominal distension

   e. Changes in stool patterns

5. Genitourinary signs

   a. Hematuria

   b. Absence of urine or failure to pass urine

6. Metabolic alterations

   a. Hypoglycemia

   b. Hypocalcemia

   c. Hyperbilirubinemia and jaundice, especially jaundice occurring within the first 24 hours of life

7. Fluid balance alterations

   a. Decreased urine output

   b. 5–15% weight loss in one day

   c. Dry mucous membranes

   d. Sunken fontanelles

   e. Poor skin turgor

   f. Increased hematocrit

8. Temperature instability

- Preterm infants

  1. Definition—infants born before 37 completed weeks of gestation

  2. Associated complications

     a. Respiratory complications

     b. Necrotizing enterocolitis

     c. Intraventricular hemorrhage

     d. Hypothermia

     e. Hypoglycemia

     f. Infection

     g. Hyperbilirubinemia

  3. Maternal factors associated with prematurity

     a. Obstetric—uterine malformation, multiple gestation, incompetent cervix, premature rupture of membranes, pregnancy-induced hypertension, placenta previa, history of previous preterm birth, isoimmunization

     b. Medical—diabetes, hypertension, urinary tract infection, other acute illness

     c. Psychosocial—poor prenatal care, low socioeconomic status, malnutrition, adolescent pregnancy, substance abuse

- Small for gestational age infants

  1. Definition—birth weight below 10th percentile or two standard deviations below mean for gestational age

2. Symmetric growth restriction

   a. Results from early and prolonged insult(s)

   b. Associated with decreased brain size and mental retardation

   c. Growth restriction continues after birth

3. Asymmetric growth restriction

   a. Results from insult(s) late in pregnancy

   b. Head circumference is near normal for gestational age

   c. Rapid postnatal growth and development with normal cognitive development

4. Maternal factors associated with growth restriction

   a. Obstetric—history of infertility, history of abortions, grand multiparity, pregnancy-induced hypertension

   b. Medical—heart disease, renal disease, hypertension, sickle cell disease, phenylketonuria, diabetes

   c. Psychosocial—malnutrition, low socioeconomic status, extremes of maternal age, poor prenatal care, substance abuse

- Postterm infants

  1. Definition—born after 42 completed weeks' gestation

  2. Associated complications

     a. Meconium aspiration

        (1) Physical barrier to gas exchange

        (2) Causes chemical irritation and thickening of the alveolar walls

        (3) Vasoconstriction/vasospasm may cause pulmonary hypertension and persistent fetal circulation

     b. Hypoglycemia

     c. Polycythemia

     d. Hypothermia

  3. Associated maternal and fetal factors

     a. Maternal—primigravid, grand multiparity, previous postterm delivery

     b. Fetal—anencephaly, trisomies

- Large for gestational age infants

  1. Definition—birth weight above 90th percentile or two standard deviations above the mean; sometimes defined as birth weight above 4000 or 4500 g

  2. Associated complications

     a. Birth injuries, including fractures and intracranial hemorrhage

     b. Hypoglycemia (resulting from increased activity and hypertrophy of pancreatic islet cells)

     c. Polycythemia

     d. Perinatal asphyxia

  3. Maternal factors associated with excessive fetal growth

a. Gestational diabetes

b. Genetic predisposition

c. Excessive maternal weight gain during pregnancy

4. Infants of diabetic mothers (IDM)

a. Chronic or severe maternal diabetes with vascular changes more likely to result in growth restriction

b. Gestational diabetes and hyperglycemia more likely to result in excessive fetal growth

c. Associated with congenital anomalies, including central nervous system anomalies, congenital heart defects, and tracheo-esophageal fistula

- Neonatal infection

1. Signs of infection in the newborn

a. Often subtle and nonspecific

b. Early signs—lethargy, refusal to feed, vomiting, temperature instability

c. May show subtle changes in color—cyanosis, pallor, mottling

d. May be related to involved organ system(s)

(1) CNS infections—jitteriness, seizures

(2) Pulmonary infections—respiratory distress, apnea

(3) Intestinal infections—diarrhea

2. Signs of chronic intrauterine infection

a. Growth retardation

b. Microcephaly

c. Hepatosplenomegaly

3. Sepsis

a. Increased susceptibility due to immature immune function

b. Evaluation includes blood and CSF cultures, CBC with differential, IgM titer, chest radiograph, and toxoplasmosis, rubella, cytomegalovirus, and herpes screening

4. Bacterial infections

a. Group B β-hemolytic streptococcus (GBS)

(1) Most common pathogen in neonatal infections

(2) Etiology—maternal colonization, transmitted to neonate during labor and delivery

(3) Preterm newborns at highest risk

(4) Early-onset GBS disease—develops within first 24 hours of life, characterized by respiratory involvement, may be fatal

(5) Late-onset GBS disease—onset usually after second week of life, characterized by CNS involvement, rarely fatal, but may result in permanent neurologic damage

b. Listeria

(1) Presentation—diffuse papular rash on trunk and pharynx, respiratory distress, cyanosis, sepsis

(2) Etiology—maternal colonization, transmitted to neonate during labor and delivery

c. *Escherichia coli*

(1) Major cause of neonatal meningitis and sepsis

(2) Etiology—maternal colonization, transmitted to neonate during labor and delivery

d. *Neissieria gonorrhoeae*

(1) Pathogenic for ophthalmia neonatorium

(2) May cause blindness if untreated

(3) Prophylaxis—administration of silver nitrate or erythromycin ointment to eyes after birth

(4) Rarely, may invade joint capsules causing septic arthritis

e. Tuberculosis

(1) Congenital disease is rare unless mother has untreated, advanced disease

(2) Primarily affects newborn liver when acquired before birth

(3) Separation of newborn from mother is unnecessary if mother has negative chest radiograph, negative sputum culture, and is receiving treatment

5. Viral and protozoan infections

a. Toxoplasmosis

(1) Associated with raw meat and infected feces, especially cat

(2) Mother is often asymptomatic

(3) Signs of infection in the newborn include microcephaly, cerebral calcifications, chorioretinitis, hepatosplenomegaly, and jaundice

(4) Treatment limits further disease but does not correct damage to the central nervous system

b. Syphilis

(1) Signs of infection in the newborn include intrauterine growth restriction (IUGR), ascites, rhinitis, jaundice, anemia

(2) Spontaneous abortion, stillbirth, or newborn demise occur in 40% of cases when mother is untreated; another 40% will result in congenital syphilis

(3) Congenital syphilis may result in multisystem organ damage and/or death

c. Rubella
   (1) Infection in utero may result in IUGR, cardiac anomalies, deafness, blindness, and/or mental retardation
   (2) Effects depend on gestational age at transmission and duration of infection
d. Cytomegalovirus (CMV)
   (1) No effective means of treatment or prevention
   (2) Effects of congenital CMV infection—30% incidence of death in infancy, 90% of survivors will have CNS, visual, and/or auditory damage
e. Herpes
   (1) Transmission typically occurs during intrapartum period; prenatal infection is rare
   (2) Newborns are susceptible to systemic disease, which may involve hepatitis, pneumonia, encephalitis, and/or disseminated intravascular coagulopathy
   (3) Primary maternal infection is associated with 50% newborn mortality rate and high rates of permanent neurologic damage
   (4) Recurrent maternal infection rarely results in severe systemic disease
f. Hepatitis B
   (1) Often results in prematurity and low birth weight
   (2) Onset of disease occurs 4 to 6 weeks after birth and is marked by poor feeding, jaundice, and hepatomegaly
   (3) Most infants infected perinatally demonstrate carrier state without acute disease
g. Chlamydia
   (1) Most common cause of blindness worldwide
   (2) Intrapartum transmission may result in conjunctivitis, pneumonia, and/or otitis media
   (3) Chlamydial conjunctivitis is not prevented by ocular administration of silver nitrate; erythromycin ophthalmic ointment is preferred
h. Human immunodeficiency virus (HIV) and acquired immune deficiency syndrome (AIDS)
   (1) Maternal antiretroviral therapy significantly reduces vertical transmission; elective cesarean section may also reduce vertical transmission
   (2) Can be transmitted via breast milk
   (3) May result in prematurity, growth restriction, and/or microcephaly
   (4) Opportunistic infection usually manifests within the first months of life

- Plexus injuries—prognosis is good; 88–92% of affected infants recover fully within first year of life
  1. Thought to result from lateral traction on shoulder or head during delivery; some evidence of intrauterine effect also exists
  2. Erb's palsy
     a. Accounts for 90% of all plexus injuries
     b. Involves upper part of the plexus (C5 through C7 and occasionally C4)
     c. Shoulder and upper arm are affected
     d. Decreased biceps reflex is present
     e. When C4 is involved, diaphragmatic dysfunction is present
  3. Total palsy
     a. Accounts for 8–9% of all plexus injuries
     b. Diffuse plexus involvement (C5 to T1)
     c. Upper arm, lower arm, and hand are affected
     d. Biceps and triceps reflexes are decreased
  4. Klumpke's paralysis
     a. Accounts for less than 2% of all plexus injuries
     b. Involves C8 to T1
     c. Lower arm and hand are affected
  5. Associated injuries—clavicle fracture, humerus fracture, shoulder dislocation, facial nerve injury
  6. Management usually consists initially of limiting movement of the affected extremity, then gradual introduction of gentle range-of-motion exercises

- Neonatal fractures
  1. Fracture of the clavicle—not a significant newborn fracture
     a. Most common neonatal fracture
     b. Signs—hematoma, crepitus, asymmetric tone/movement of upper extremities
     c. Sometimes associated with plexus injuries
  2. Fracture of humerus or femur—significant fractures, may be nosocomial
     a. Rare; usually associated with breech deliveries
     b. Ecchymosis, hematoma, or hemorrhage may occur at fracture site
  3. Skull fracture
     a. Rare; may be associated with forceps delivery
     b. Linear fracture—usually benign, resolves without treatment

    c. Depressed fracture—may be associated with seizures and/or permanent neurologic injury

    d. Signs—cephalohematoma, palpable depression in bone

- Infants with hemolytic disease
  1. Definition—destruction of red blood cells resulting in hyperbilirubinemia and jaundice
  2. Causes—maternal antibodies, enzymatic disorders, infections
  3. Rh incompatibility
     a. Occurs when mother is Rh negative and fetus is Rh positive
     b. Positive result on direct Coombs' test indicates presence of maternal antibodies
     c. May necessitate exchange transfusion
  4. ABO incompatibility
     a. Occurs when mother is serologic type O and fetus is type A or B; infrequently when mother is type A and fetus is type B
     b. Very rare incidence of hydrops or stillbirth
     c. May result in neonatal jaundice; rarely causes severe hemolysis or anemia

- Hyperbilirubinemia and severe jaundice
  1. Associated with many neonatal complications, including hemolytic disease, prematurity, impaired hepatic function, sepsis, metabolic disorders, hematomas, impaired intestinal function, and others
  2. Kernicterus
     a. Encephalopathy caused by deposition of bilirubin in brain cells
     b. Classic signs—lethargy, diminished reflexes, hypotonia, and seizures
     c. Contributing factors—prematurity, hypothermia, asphyxia, acidosis, sepsis
     d. Complications include hearing impairment, cerebral palsy, and mental retardation
  3. Phototherapy
     a. Oxidizes unconjugated bilirubin in the skin, rendering it water soluble and facilitating elimination
     b. Precautions
        (1) Protect infant's eyes from high-intensity light
        (2) Monitor fluid status and temperature

- Infants affected by maternal substance abuse
  1. Fetal alcohol syndrome
     a. Fetal/neonatal effects—microcephaly, facial abnormalities, cardiac defects, malformation of joints, failure to thrive, mental retardation

    b. May result in withdrawal syndrome in the neonate characterized by irritability, tremors, tachypnea, tachycardia, poor feeding

  2. Cocaine abuse
     a. Fetal/neonatal effects—prematurity, low birth weight, IUGR, genitourinary abnormalities, seizures, congenital heart disease, irritability, frantic or poor feeding
     b. May result in long-term behavioral impairment
  3. Opiate abuse
     a. Minimal long-term effects compared to cocaine and alcohol; primarily affects immediate neonatal period
     b. Abstinence syndrome (opiate withdrawal)
        (1) Onset shortly after birth
        (2) CNS signs—irritability, tremors, high-pitched cry, hyperstimulability, possible seizure activity
        (3) Other signs—tachypnea, tachycardia, poor or disorganized feeding, hyperthermia, vasomotor instability
        (4) Care is primarily supportive
  4. Marijuana abuse
     a. Little or no evidence for teratogenic effects
     b. Possible newborn behavioral effects—fine tremor, prolonged startle response, irritability, poor habituation to visual stimuli
     c. No behavioral effects demonstrated to persist beyond infancy
  5. Prescription drugs of abuse potential
     a. Amphetamines
        (1) Fetal/neonatal effects—genitourinary, cardiac, and/or central nervous system abnormalities, behavioral state disorganization
        (2) May result in long-term learning disabilities
     b. Benzodiazepines—fetal/neonatal effects include hypotonia, hypothermia, low Apgar scores, respiratory depression, poor feeding, possible association with midline cleft defects

- Congenital anomalies
  1. Central nervous system anomalies
     a. Spina bifida occulta
        (1) Absent or incomplete closure of one or more vertebral arches
        (2) Dimple or hair tuft may be present over site
        (3) Often asymptomatic without requiring treatment
     b. Meningocele/myelomeningocele
        (1) Meningocele—extrusion of meninges and cerebrospinal fluid (CSF) through defect in vertebral column

      (2) Myelomeningocele—meningocele with extrusion of spinal cord

      (3) Surgical repair is necessary to prevent rupture and infection

      (4) Myelomeningocele results in loss of sensory and motor function below the level of the defect

  c. Anencephaly

      (1) Congenital absence of cranial vault and underlying brain tissue

      (2) Newborn may manifest heart rate and respiration but will die within a few hours after birth

  d. Hydrocephalus

      (1) Abnormal accumulation of cerebrospinal fluid in ventricles of the brain

      (2) Signs—increased head circumference, separation of cranial sutures, bulging tense fontanelles, high pitched cry, and downward deviation of eyes ("setting sun sign")

      (3) Surgical treatment involves placement of a shunt to drain excess fluid

2. Respiratory anomalies

  a. Choanal atresia

      (1) Definition—congenital blockage of posterior nasal passages

      (2) Respiratory distress will be evident at birth if both nares are blocked

      (3) Treatment includes respiratory support and surgical repair

  b. Diaphragmatic hernia

      (1) Definition—defect of diaphragm, allowing herniation of abdominal contents into thoracic cavity and displacement of heart and lung tissue

      (2) Presentation—respiratory distress and scaphoid abdomen apparent at birth

      (3) Treatment is surgical repair

  c. Pulmonary hypoplasia/agenesis

      (1) Definition—underdevelopment or absence of one or both lungs

      (2) Strong association with other anomalies

      (3) Rare condition with high mortality rate

      (4) Presentation—acute respiratory distress with thoracic asymmetry

3. Cardiovascular anomalies

  a. Anomalies resulting in acyanotic heart disease

      (1) Atrial septal defect, ventricular septal defect, patent ductus arteriosus, and coarctation of the aorta

      (2) Surgical repair required

      (3) Prognosis is usually good for isolated defects

  b. Anomalies resulting in cyanotic heart disease

      (1) Tetralogy of Fallot—pulmonary stenosis, ventricular septal defect, overriding aorta, and right ventricular hypertrophy

      (2) Transposition of the great vessels—aorta arises from right ventricle and pulmonary artery arises from left ventricle, resulting in circulatory bypass of lungs and circulation of unoxygenated blood to the body

      (3) Tricuspid atresia—results in no direct communication between right atrium and right ventricle; further resulting in hypoplastic right ventricle and enlarged left ventricle

      (4) Truncus arteriosus—failure of embryonic structure to divide into aorta and pulmonary artery

      (5) Surgery is more complicated, with generally poorer outcomes (except Tetralogy of Fallot)

4. Gastrointestinal anomalies

  a. Cleft lip and palate

      (1) Definition—incomplete fusion of lip and palate during prenatal development

      (2) May interfere with feeding and weight gain

      (3) Surgical repair usually results in good cosmetic and functional results

  b. Esophageal atresia and tracheoesophageal fistula

      (1) Definition—abnormal development of trachea and esophagus, resulting in "blind pouch" esophagus and/or communication between the two structures

      (2) Presentation—copious drooling, poor feeding with reflux, acute respiratory distress and cyanosis with feeding

      (3) Repaired surgically, with good prognosis

  c. Pyloric stenosis

      (1) Definition—obstruction of pylorus (distal opening of stomach)

      (2) Affects males three to four times more often than females

      (3) Presentation—vomiting, visible gastric peristalsis, constipation

      (4) Repaired surgically, with good prognosis

  d. Omphalocele

      (1) Definition—defect of abdominal wall with herniation of abdominal viscera through umbilical ring

(2) Protruding abdominal viscera usually covered by membrane

(3) Frequently associated with other anomalies

(4) Repaired surgically; prognosis depends on extent of lesion and nature and extent of associated anomalies

e. Gastroschisis

(1) Definition—defect of abdominal wall and evisceration of abdominal organs

(2) Rarely associated with other anomalies

(3) Management at birth—cover eviscerated organs with sterile gauze moistened with sterile saline solution

(4) No oral intake until after repair; IV therapy for fluid and electrolyte maintenance

(5) Repair may require several surgeries; prognosis depends on extent of lesion

5. Genitourinary anomalies

a. Hypospadias

(1) Definition—in males, urethral opening is located on ventral aspect of penis

(2) Circumcision contraindicated—foreskin tissue is often used in surgical repair

(3) Rare in females, with urethral opening located in the vagina

b. Epispadias

(1) Definition—congenital absence of anterior urethral wall

(2) Often associated with other genitourinary anomalies

(3) Repaired surgically

c. Ambiguous genitalia

(1) Definition—anomalies of the external genitalia precluding identification of the newborn's sex

(2) May be associated with anomalies of the internal genitalia

(3) Chromosome studies can determine genotypic sex

(4) Gender identity problems are frequent; reconstructive surgery is controversial

d. Exstrophy of the bladder

(1) Definition—exposure of bladder outside the abdominal wall

(2) Repaired surgically; often complicated by associated genitourinary anomalies

e. Patent urachus

(1) Definition—persistence of fetal opening between bladder and umbilical cord

(2) Repaired surgically

6. Musculoskeletal anomalies

a. Congenital hip dysplasia

(1) Definition—abnormal development of the acetabulum, resulting in dislocation of femoral head

(2) Presentation—asymmetry of gluteal folds, positive Ortolani sign

(3) Treatment—reduction and stabilization of femoral head into acetabulum to allow development of stable hip capsule

(4) Stabilization is accomplished by use of Frejka splint or Pavlik harness

b. Talipes equinovarus

(1) Definition—congenital deformity of ankle and foot

(2) Orthopedic treatment involves application of splints or successive plaster casts to correct position of foot and allow normal development

(3) Success of treatment depends on early treatment; with early treatment prognosis is good

7. Chromosomal abnormalities

a. Down syndrome

(1) Results from extra chromosome at pair 21 or 22 or translocation of pairs 15 and 21

(2) Signs include close-set slanting eyes, narrow palpebral fissures, flattened nose, large protuberant tongue, short thick fingers with incurving of fifth digit, simian palmar crease, nuchal thickening

(3) Involves varying degrees of mental impairment

(4) Associated with multiple congenital anomalies, including cardiac and GI tract defects

b. Trisomies 13 and 18

(1) Clinically similar to but more severe than Down syndrome

(2) High mortality rates; poor life expectancy

8. Inborn errors of metabolism

a. Phenylketonuria

(1) Definition—deficiency of phenylalanine hydroxylase, resulting in inability to metabolize phenylalanine

(2) Results in toxic accumulation of abnormal metabolites of phenylalanine, eventually leading to CNS damage

(3) Treatment—dietary restriction of foods high in phenylalanine

(4) Should be identified and treated before 3 weeks of age

b. Galactosemia
(1) Definition—inability to convert galactose to glucose
(2) Results in toxic accumulation of galactose in the bloodstream
(3) Treatment—dietary restriction of foods containing galactose

- Sudden infant death syndrome (SIDS)
  1. Definition—sudden unexplained death of infant between birth and 1 year of age
  2. Prevalence—2 out of 1000 infants
     a. Most prevalent between 2 and 4 months of age
     b. Rarely occurs before 3 weeks or after 9 months
  3. Unknown cause
     a. "Apnea hypothesis"—theory that sleep-associated apnea is the primary mechanism of SIDS
     b. Apnea hypothesis has led to increased use of home cardiorespiratory monitors
     c. No evidence that home cardiorespiratory monitoring saves lives
     d. Subsequent research has not shown a strong association between apnea and SIDS
  4. Risk factors
     a. Gender—SIDS occurs more often in male than female infants
     b. Premature birth
     c. IUGR
     d. Low socioeconomic status
     e. Young maternal age
     f. Short interpregnancy interval
     g. Maternal smoking or use of cocaine or opiates
     h. More common in cold weather months
     i. More common after midnight and before 8:00 a.m.
     j. Higher incidence in African-American or Native-American infants
  5. Recommendations
     a. "Back to sleep"—infants should be positioned in supine or side-lying position to sleep
     b. Avoidance or reduction of modifiable risk factors
     c. Infants should sleep on a firm surface
     d. Avoid loose bedclothing

❏ QUESTIONS

Select the best answer.

1. Which of the following infants is *least* at risk for neonatal hypoglycemia?
   a. The infant of a mother with diabetes mellitus
   b. The infant of a mother with gestational diabetes
   c. An infant who had intrapartum fetal monitoring findings suggestive of fetal distress
   d. The infant of an opioid-abusing mother

2. Which of the following best describes the appearance and behavior of an overstimulated infant?
   a. Tremors, tachycardia, nonnutritive sucking, nasal flaring, and grunting
   b. Color changes, irregular respiration, irritability or lethargy, and vomiting
   c. Lethargy, flaccid tone, pallor, and inability to maintain alert active state
   d. Habituation to noxious stimuli and attempts to self-console

3. The midwife performs a physical examination on a newborn 2 hours after birth. Which of the following findings indicate a need for pediatric consultation?
   a. Respiratory rate of 50 breaths per minute
   b. Intermittent episodes of apnea, lasting less than 10 seconds each
   c. Yellow blanching of skin when pressure is applied to the infant's nose
   d. Preauricular skin tag

4. Ms. G. has just given birth, and the midwife's initial impression is that resuscitation may be necessary. According to American Academy of Pediatrics (AAP) and American Heart Association (AHA) guidelines, the midwife's initial steps are, in sequential order:
   a. Place the infant under a radiant heater, dry the infant and remove wet linen, suction the mouth and nose, and provide tactile stimulation while assessing for the presence or absence of spontaneous respirations
   b. Place the infant under a radiant heater, suction the mouth and nose, and evaluate heart rate by palpating the base of the umbilical cord or femoral pulse
   c. Place the infant under a radiant heater, evaluate heart rate by palpating the base of the umbilical cord or femoral pulse, dry the infant and remove wet linen, suction the mouth and nose, and continue to provide tactile stimulation
   d. Place the infant under a radiant heater, suction the mouth and nose, evaluate for the presence or absence of spontaneous respirations, and dry the infant and remove wet linen

5. Following the steps listed in question 4, the midwife notes that spontaneous respiration and tone are normal and the heart rate is 120 beats per minute. Continuing to follow AAP/AHA guidelines, the midwife then:

   a. Initiates positive pressure ventilation with 100% oxygen
   b. Returns the infant to the mother to facilitate bonding and initiate breastfeeding
   c. Evaluates the infant's color and provides oxygen if acrocyanosis or general cyanosis are present
   d. Evaluates the infant's color and provides oxygen only if general cyanosis is present

6. With respect to question 5, how would the midwife proceed differently if meconium staining of the amniotic fluid had been noted on rupture of membranes?

   a. Suction the trachea after drying the infant and removing wet linen
   b. Suction the trachea on the perineum before delivery of the thorax
   c. Suction the mouth, nose, and pharynx only—endotracheal suctioning is not indicated
   d. Suction the trachea after drying the infant and providing tactile stimulation

7. Which of the following statements about the newborn transitional period is *not* true?

   a. Rapid changes in the infant's color during the period from 2 to 6 hours after birth are an ominous sign and require further evaluation.
   b. The three stages, in order, are: (1) the first period of reactivity, (2) the period of unresponsive sleep, and (3) the second period of reactivity
   c. Respiratory rales are normally present during the first 20 minutes of life
   d. A period of unresponsive sleep typically begins within 30 minutes after birth and continues until about 2 hours after birth

8. Ms. F., a primipara, is discussing infant feeding with her midwife. Which statement would indicate to the midwife that further teaching is necessary to correct a misunderstanding?

   a. "As long as my baby is suckling well and wetting diapers, I don't have to worry about whether he's getting enough milk."
   b. "Because I'm bottle feeding, I'm going to stick to a regular 2-hour feeding schedule."

   c. "My baby is 5 days old, but according to the scale on the side of the bottle, she's only taking about 20 or 30 mL of formula at each feeding. I'm worried: shouldn't she be eating more than that by now?"
   d. "I'm letting my baby feed for 10 or 15 minutes on each breast, at every feeding."

9. Which of the following statements about prophylaxis for newborn eye infections is *untrue*?

   a. Due to the rapid onset of ophthalmia neonatorum, administration of silver nitrate or erythromycin should take priority over family bonding and initiation of breastfeeding.
   b. Erythromycin is preferred over silver nitrate, because it provides coverage against the two most common pathogens.
   c. Chlamydial conjunctivitis is the most common cause of blindness worldwide.
   d. The two major pathogens for newborn eye infections are *Nessieria gonorrhoeae* and *Chlamydia trachomatis.*

10. Ms. H., who has a 1-month-old infant, contacts the midwife on call. Ms. H. sounds distraught, and tells the midwife that her baby "just cries and cries, all the time, and cries so hard that he gets red in the face. He's starting to drive me crazy!" The midwife asks questions about the baby's temperature, feeding habits, and voiding and stooling, all of which appear to be normal despite the baby's behavior. The midwife correctly tells Ms. H. that:

    a. She should take the baby to the emergency room immediately.
    b. The baby's behavior is normal and getting used to the demands of an infant is a normal part of adjusting to motherhood.
    c. Some babies are prone to this behavior, and one of the biggest problems is the effect on the baby's parents—when it gets to be too much, position the baby safely in his crib and go outside for a "sanity break."
    d. The baby's problem results from lack of stimulation—put on some upbeat music, turn on all the lights, make sure he can move freely, and engage him in active play.

11. At her 6-month well child checkup, Ms. J.'s baby weighs 12 lb, compared to a birthweight of 6 lb. Ms. J. says that she seems to breastfeed well, but frequently spits up afterward. The midwife:

    a. Obtains a consultation with the pediatrician
    b. Recommends supplementation of formula in addition to continuing breastfeeding

c. Orders metabolic screening, including screening for phenylketonuria

d. Reassures Ms. J. that the baby's weight gain is normal and reinforces her breastfeeding technique

12. Which of the following is *not* characteristic of normal newborn behavior states?

a. Abrupt, unpredictable changes between Brazelton's sleep-wake states

b. Difficulty becoming and remaining alert

c. Irritability and rapid progression from alertness to crying

d. Overstimulation, requiring "time out" with limitation of stimuli

13. The midwife wishes to estimate a newborn's gestational age. Which standard instrument is appropriate?

a. Denver II

b. Ballard

c. Erikson

d. Erb-Duchene

14. Which of the following statements about the major psychological tasks of early infancy is *untrue*?

a. Secure attachment is facilitated by caregivers who demonstrate predictable responses and emotional availability.

b. The development of basic trust is essential for formation of relationships later in life.

c. Research has not been able to demonstrate any long-term effects of insecure attachment in early infancy.

d. A major issue is the infant's ability to elicit caregiving responses from his or her mother.

15. The midwife's discussion about circumcision with the infant's parents should acknowledge that:

a. The medical benefits of circumcision are well-established and outweigh the risks, which are rare.

b. The risks of circumcision, while rare, are potentially serious and outweigh any possible medical benefit.

c. Research has proven that circumcision has a negative impact on long-term psychological and sexual functioning.

d. Decisions about circumcision are largely based on personal, cultural, and religious considerations.

16. Which of the following statements about hemolytic disease is true?

a. ABO incompatibility is most common when the maternal blood type is A and the fetus' blood type is B.

b. Rh incompatibility may result in neonatal jaundice, but rarely causes severe hemolysis or anemia.

c. A positive result on the direct Coombs' test indicates the presence of fetal blood cells in maternal circulation.

d. Hemolytic disease in the infant can be caused by maternal antibodies, enzymatic disorders, and some infections.

17. The midwife suspects maternal opiate abuse due to which of the following clusters of newborn signs and conditions?

a. Prematurity, low birth weight, genitourinary abnormalities, congenital heart disease, irritability, and frantic ineffective sucking

b. Irritability, tremors, high-pitched cry, hyperstimulability, tachypnea, tachycardia, disorganized feeding, hyperthermia, and vasomotor instability

c. Microcephaly, facial abnormalities, cardiac defects, and malformation of joints

d. Lethargy, diminished reflexes, and hypotonia

18. Which of the following assessment findings are most consistent with prematurity?

a. Translucent skin, sparse lanugo, flat areolae, prominent clitoris and labia minora, and highly flexible, nonrecoiling ear tissue

b. Scant rugation of scrotum, undescended testes, and wrinkled, cracked, peeling skin

c. Extended posture, flaccid tone, little resistance to flexion of extremities, and increased recoil of ear tissue

d. Abundant lanugo, flexed posture, skin creases covering entire plantar surface, and relatively low-set position of ears

19. Prominent vasculature of the anterior lens capsule is most suggestive of which condition?

a. Herpes virus exposure in the intrapartum period

b. Relatively immature gestational age

c. Gonococcal or chlamydial conjunctivitis

d. Elevated total serum bilirubin concentration

20. Compared to fetal circulation, which of the following is *not* characteristic of circulation after birth?

a. Increased pressure in the left atrium facilitating closure of the foramen ovale
b. Relatively low pulmonary vascular resistance resulting in increased circulation to the lungs
c. Decreased systemic vascular resistance due to loss of high-resistance placental circuit
d. Increased oxygenation of circulating blood causing constriction of the ductus arteriosus

21. Mr. N. is concerned about Ms. N.'s positive tuberculosis screening result. While awaiting results from Ms. N.'s chest radiograph and sputum culture, the midwife tells Mr. N. that:

a. Even if the chest radiograph is negative, Ms. N.'s exposure will necessitate a period of isolation from the newborn which may interfere with the initiation of breastfeeding.
b. Congenital tuberculosis is unlikely to be a problem for the newborn, since Ms. N. shows no signs of active disease.
c. If the newborn acquires tuberculosis in utero, the most serious risk is for respiratory problems in the neonatal period.
d. Subclinical maternal tuberculosis infection is associated with a number of congenital malformations.

22. Which of the following newborn assessment findings is/are *least* likely to be related to maternal gestational diabetes?

a. High-pitched cry, plethora, tachypnea, and inconsolability
b. Weak cry, jitteriness, cyanosis, apnea, poor feeding, and lethargy
c. Serum glucose level below 40 mg/dL
d. Absent Moro reflex on right side, and palpable crepitus between the right shoulder and neck

23. A defect in the vertebral column resulting in extrusion of meninges and cerebrospinal fluid is best described as:

a. Spina bifida occulta
b. Hydrocephaly
c. Myelomeningocele
d. Meningocele

24. Which of the following conditions is most likely to result in loss of sensory and motor function below the level of the defect?

a. Spina bifida occulta
b. Hydrocephaly
c. Myelomeningocele
d. Meningocele

25. Within the first day of life, the midwife notices that Ms. O.'s baby drools copiously, feeds poorly with excessive reflux, and turns bluish-grey while feeding. Which condition does the midwife suspect?

a. Tracheoesophageal malformation
b. Pyloric stenosis
c. Gastroschisis
d. Oomphalocele

26. Increased oxygen consumption, hypoglycemia, hypoxia, acidosis, and respiratory distress can be caused in the immediate newborn period by:

a. Congenital bacterial infections
b. Maternal opioid abuse
c. Patent ductus arteriosus
d. Cold stress in the birthing room

27. Relatively mature capabilities of the newborn's gastrointestinal system include:

a. Suckling, swallowing, and gag reflex
b. Ability to digest fats and proteins
c. Absorption of complex sugars
d. Cardiac sphincter tone

28. At 1 minute of age, Baby P exhibits a strong cry, some flexion of the arms and legs, heart rate of 136 beats per minute, and acrocyanosis. Baby P's 1-minute Apgar score is:

a. 6
b. 7
c. 8
d. 9

29. At 5 minutes of age, Baby Q exhibits slow irregular respirations, some flexion of extremities, heart rate of 96 beats per minute, grimace in response to suction, and generalized cyanosis. Baby Q's 5-minute Apgar score is:

a. 4
b. 5
c. 6
d. 7

30. Which of the following statements about Apgar scores is true?

a. The infant's Apgar score indicates whether or not resuscitation is needed and which steps of resuscitation procedure should be initiated.
b. The 1-minute Apgar score is more predictive of cord pH and long-term outcome than is the 5-minute Apgar score.

c. The 1-minute Apgar score is more predictive of cord pH, while the 5-minute Apgar score is more predictive of long-term outcome.

d. The Apgar score is only useful as a systematic way to assess the newborn's immediate adaptation to extrauterine life.

31. In the initial examination of a male infant, the midwife notes drainage of urine from the stump of the umbilical cord. The newborn's condition is most likely:

a. Patent urachus
b. Epispadias
c. Hypospadias
d. Exstrophy of the bladder

32. Which of the following is *not* a true statement about the newborn's first breaths?

a. The first inhalation requires less ventilatory pressure than later breaths.
b. The first breaths trigger the conversion from fetal to extrauterine circulation.
c. Initial breathing serves to clear the lungs of fluid.
d. The first breaths establish lung volume and expand the alveoli.

33. Which of the following is a true statement about thermoregulation in the transitional period?

a. Shivering and muscular activity are the newborn's most effective means of thermogenesis.
b. Convection, conduction, radiation, and evaporation are important thermoregulatory mechanisms in the newborn period.
c. Metabolism of BAT is limited as a means of thermoregulation, because BAT stores cannot be renewed once they are used.
d. Alkalosis is a potentially serious consequence of ineffective thermoregulation in the newborn.

34. Patient education about newborn skin care includes:

a. "Cradle cap," a crusty yellowish-white accumulation on the anterior scalp, is caused by *Candida albicans* and must be treated with a topical antifungal agent.
b. Dry or peeling skin can be treated with baby oil, but if the condition does not resolve quickly the healthcare provider should be notified.

c. Primary diaper dermatitis, characterized by circumscribed areas of bright red erythema and smaller outlying lesions, can be treated with thorough cleaning, baby powder, and air exposure.
d. Tub baths should be avoided for the first 2 weeks of life or so until the cord stump has fallen off.

35. Which of the following newborns is *not* a candidate for early discharge?

a. Metabolic screening tests have not been completed; the baby has an appointment with the pediatric provider in 2 days.
b. Congenital hip dislocation is suspected; the baby has an orthopedic appointment in 2 weeks for evaluation and treatment.
c. The infant's birth weight was 2625 g; gestational age assessment indicates term infant.
d. The infant requires phototherapy; a home health agency referral has been made.

36. The midwife is examining Baby S prior to discharge. She notes that the head circumference is 34 cm, while the chest circumference is 31 cm. The midwife should:

a. Assess for further signs of hydrocephalus, including separation of cranial sutures, bulging fontanelles, high-pitched cry, and downward deviation of the eyes
b. Repeat the measurements—these findings are extremely unlikely
c. Suspect diaphragmatic hernia—measurement of abdominal circumference and location of heart, lung, and bowel sounds may give some indication
d. Proceed to the next component of the examination without further investigation of these findings

37. Evaluation of the newborn begins:

a. Before the infant is born
b. When the presenting part is crowning
c. At the moment of birth
d. After initial stabilization and resuscitation, if necessary

38. Which of the following statements is true of small for gestational age infants?

a. Symmetric growth restriction results from chronic conditions, and is typically associated with "catch-up growth" and good long-term outcome.
b. An infant is considered small for gestational age if he/she weighs less than 1500 grams at birth.

c. An infant with head circumference above the 45th percentile and birth weight below the 10th percentile for gestational age would be described as asymmetrically growth restricted.

d. Asymmetric growth restriction is associated with acute insults in late pregnancy, and is associated with poor long-term outcome.

39. Baby U has the most abundant lanugo the midwife has ever seen. Baby U's gestational age is probably:

a. 24 to 26 weeks
b. 26 to 28 weeks
c. 32 to 34 weeks
d. 36 to 38 weeks

40. Which of the following is *not* associated with microcephaly?

a. Prenatally acquired toxoplasmosis
b. Prenatally acquired hepatitis B
c. Fetal alcohol syndrome
d. Prenatally acquired HIV

41. Ms. V. asks her midwife about sudden infant death syndrome (SIDS) during her 6-week postpartum visit. In discussing SIDS with Ms. V., the midwife states that:

a. SIDS almost never occurs after 6 weeks of age, so her baby is "in the clear."
b. SIDS is extremely rare, affecting less than 2 in 100,000 infants.
c. The exact cause of SIDS is unknown.
d. Infants should be put to sleep in a prone or side-lying position.

42. The normal newborn's sensory capacities are most limited in:

a. Color perception
b. Hearing
c. Taste sensation
d. Near vision focus

43. The organized infant is able to:

a. Form significant relationships with others throughout life
b. Hear high-pitched sounds
c. Self-console and return to a stable behavioral state
d. Sleep for 20–25% of daytime hours

44. Which of the following is a true statement about newborn metabolic disorders?

a. Federal law mandates testing for phenylketonuria, galactosemia, and cystic fibrosis
b. For early-discharge neonates, screening at 8 hours of life is acceptably reliable

c. Most are characterized by enzyme deficiency, resulting in toxic accumulation of metabolites
d. Breastfeeding is strongly recommended for infants with galactosemia.

45. Which of the following is *not* an associated combination of intrapartum factor and neonatal finding?

a. Forceps delivery—cephalohematoma
b. Vertex presentation—asymmetry of gluteal folds
c. Shoulder dystocia—asymmetric Moro reflex
d. Breech presentation—positive Ortolani sign

46. Visible gastric peristalsis on observation of the abdomen is most suggestive of:

a. Pyloric stenosis
b. Esophageal fistula
c. Colic
d. Normal finding

47. Normal newborn respiratory findings include:

a. Nasal flaring, expiratory grunting, and retractions
b. Diaphragmatic and abdominal breathing
c. Respiratory rate 40 to 80 breaths per minute
d. Ventilation primarily through the mouth

48. Nonnutritive sucking

a. Is *not* known to occur before birth
b. Should be discouraged to prevent dental and facial malformations
c. Is an example of behavioral self-regulation
d. Can be promoted by placing a pacifier on a string around the baby's neck

◻ ANSWERS

1.	**d**	14.	**c**
2.	**b**	15.	**d**
3.	**c**	16.	**d**
4.	**a**	17.	**b**
5.	**d**	18.	**a**
6.	**c**	19.	**b**
7.	**a**	20.	**c**
8.	**b**	21.	**b**
9.	**a**	22.	**a**
10.	**c**	23.	**d**
11.	**d**	24.	**c**
12.	**a**	25.	**a**
13.	**b**	26.	**d**

27. **a**	38. **c**
28. **c**	39. **b**
29. **a**	40. **b**
30. **d**	41. **c**
31. **a**	42. **a**
32. **a**	43. **c**
33. **c**	44. **c**
34. **d**	45. **b**
35. **b**	46. **a**
36. **d**	47. **b**
37. **a**	48. **c**

◘ BIBLIOGRAPHY

American Academy of Pediatrics. (2006). *Textbook of neonatal resuscitation* (5th ed.). Elk Grove, IL: American Academy of Pediatrics.

Centers for Disease Control and Prevention (CDC). (2010). *Recommended immunization schedule for persons age 0 through 6 years—United States.* Atlanta, GA: Author. Retrieved on May 5, 2010 from www.cdc.gov/vaccines/recs/schedules.

Kenner, C. (2004). *Neonatal nursing* (1st ed.). Philadelphia, PA: W. B. Saunders.

Lowdermilk, D., & Perry, S. (2007). *Maternity and women's health* (9th ed.). St. Louis: Mosby, Inc.

Papalia, D. E., Olds, S. W., & Feldman, R. (2009). *Human development* (11th ed.). New York: McGraw-Hill.

Polin, R. A., Fox, W. W., & Abman, S. (2004). *Fetal and neonatal physiology* (3rd ed.). Philadelphia, PA: W. B. Saunders.

Riordan, J., & Auerbach, K. G. (2010). *Breastfeeding and human lactation* (4th ed.). Sudbury, MA: Jones and Bartlett.

Rudolph, C. D., & Abraham, M. R. (Eds.). (2010). *Rudolph's pediatrics* (22nd ed.). Chicago: McGraw-Hill.

Seidel, H. M., Rosenstein, B. J., & Pathak, A. (2006). *Primary care of the newborn* (4th ed.). St. Louis: Mosby, Inc.

Tappero, E. P., & Honeyfield, M. E. (2009). *Physical assessment of the newborn* (4th ed.). Petaluma, CA: NICU Ink.

Varney, H., Kriebs, J. M., & Gegor, C. L. (2004). *Varney's midwifery* (4th ed.). Sudbury, MA: Jones and Bartlett.

Volpe, J. J. (2008). *Neurology of the newborn* (5th ed.). Philadelphia, PA: W. B. Saunders.

6

Intrapartum and Postpartum

Susan P. Shannon

☐ INITIAL ASSESSMENT

- Sociodemographics
  1. Age—opposite ends of the age spectrum create risks
     a. Adolescents
        (1) Prone to late entry to care and poor compliance with prenatal care schedule
        (2) At risk for low birth weight and prematurity
        (3) Increased risk of
            (a) Pregnancy-induced hypertension
            (b) Premature labor
            (c) Preterm birth
            (d) Intrauterine growth restriction (IUGR)
            (e) Infant mortality
        (4) Risk probably multifactorial with associated socioeconomic factors
            (a) Parity
            (b) Race
            (c) Marital status
            (d) Educational level
     b. Advanced maternal age for pregnancy is older than age 35
        (1) Higher incidence of infertility and first trimester spontaneous abortion and ectopic pregnancy
        (2) Proportional increase in rates of genetic abnormalities with advancing age
        (3) Increased rates of complications including:
            (a) Pregnancy-induced hypertension
            (b) Preterm delivery
            (c) Gestational diabetes
            (d) Dysfunctional labor leading to Cesarean section
            (e) Relationship to underlying disease processes
            (f) Placenta previa and abruption
  2. Race/Ethnicity
     a. Increased rate of low birth weight babies born to African-American and Hispanic women
     b. Certain genetic disorders are increased within specific ethnic groups
  3. Socioeconomic status
     a. Lower socioeconomic status directly proportional to poor obstetrical outcome including premature labor and delivery
     b. Can be related to limited access to prenatal care and necessary resources such as appropriate food sources

- Gravidity and parity
  1. Length of labor
     a. Nullipara average longer labors
     b. Multipara average shorter labors
     c. Grand multiparous women (parity > 5) can have prolonged dysfunctional labors
  2. Obstetrical complications
     a. Increased parity associated with increased rates of
        (1) Abruptio placenta
        (2) Placenta previa
        (3) Multifetal pregnancy

(4) Postpartum hemorrhage
    b. Grand multiparity can contribute to abnormal presentation including transverse lie

- Estimated gestational age—determination of estimated date of confinement (EDC)
    1. Menstrual dating (using Naegele's rule)—add 7 days to the first day of the last menstrual period and subtract 3 months
    2. Ultrasound dating—most accurate if performed in the first trimester
    3. Anatomical dating by fundal height measurement

- Review of the antepartum course—preferably using prenatal chart
    1. History of prenatal visits
        a. Timing of first visit
        b. Compliance with visit schedule
        c. Unscheduled visits/consults
    2. Weight gain
        a. Prepregnancy weight
        b. Appropriateness of interval weight gain
        c. Total weight gain
    3. Blood pressure
        a. Initial blood pressure
        b. Changes in blood pressure values throughout pregnancy
    4. Fundal height growth
    5. Ultrasound results
    6. Current medications
    7. Obstetrical complications/unscheduled visits

- Laboratory data
    1. Blood type and Rh factor
    2. Hemoglobin/hematocrit
    3. Hepatitis B antigen status
    4. Rubella status
    5. Pap test result
    6. STD screening results
    7. Glucose screening
    8. Group B streptococcus culture
    9. Genetic testing results
        a. Chorionic villus sampling
        b. Amniocentesis
        c. Triple screen

- Family history
    1. Obstetrical complications
    2. Genetic diseases including chromosomal abnormalities and ethnicity-based disorders
    3. Congenital defects or syndromes
    4. Medical disorders
        a. Hypertension (HTN)
        b. Diabetes
        c. Cardiac disease

- Obstetrical history
    1. Gravidity—total number of pregnancies
    2. Parity—outcome of previous pregnancies
        a. Expressed as a four-digit number (TPAL)
        b. First digit is full-term infant (T); second digit is preterm infant (P); third digit is abortions/terminations (A); fourth digit is living children (L)
    3. Description of previous pregnancies
        a. Duration of gestation
        b. Birth weight
        c. Duration of labor
        d. Type of delivery
        e. Analgesia/anesthesia
        f. Complications of the prenatal, intrapartum, or postpartum period
        g. Place of delivery
        h. Provider

- Past medical history
    1. Allergies
    2. Medical conditions
    3. Previous surgeries
    4. Medication and herb use

- Review of systems
    1. Genitourinary
    2. Respiratory
    3. Cardiovascular
    4. Gastrointestinal
    5. Neurologic
    6. Musculoskeletal

- Labor status
    1. Onset of contractions
    2. Description of contractions
        a. Frequency
        b. Duration
        c. Intensity
    3. Status of membranes
        a. Time of rupture
        b. Amount
        c. Color
    4. Frequency of fetal movements
    5. Presence or absence of bloody show
    6. Other subjective symptoms
        a. Nausea and vomiting
        b. Rectal pressure

◻ PHYSICAL EXAMINATION

- Vital signs

- Abdominal examination
    1. Leopold's maneuver for fetal presentation and position during labor

a. Determination of attitude is more difficult secondary to fetal descent
b. Location of fetal back provides best determination of fetal position without pelvic examination
2. Palpation of contraction intensity
3. Presence of fetal movement
4. Location of fetal heart tones

- Pelvic examination
  1. External perineal inspection
     a. Presence of bloody show
     b. Presence of amniotic fluid
     c. Presence of lesions
  2. Internal examination
     a. Sterile speculum examination—*before digital examination* if ruptured membranes are suspected, frank bleeding is present, or inspection for herpetic lesions is necessary
     b. Digital examination
        (1) Dilation
        (2) Effacement
        (3) Station—relationship of the fetal presenting part to the ischial spines (in centimeters)
            (a) 0 station—the presenting part is at the level of the spines
            (b) –3, –2, –1 station—presenting part above the level of the ischial spines
            (c) +1, +2, +3 station—presenting part below the level of the ischial spines
        (4) Presenting part—the anatomical part of the fetus that first descends into the pelvis
        (5) Position—relationship between the denominator of the presenting part and the maternal pelvis
            (a) Cephalic presentation—the denominator is the occiput
            (b) Breech presentation—the denominator is the sacrum
            (c) Shoulder presentation—the denominator is the scapula
            (d) Face presentation—the denominator is the mentum
        (6) Status of membranes
        (7) Clinical pelvimetry—determination of adequacy of bony pelvis
            (a) The pelvis is composed of four bones
                i. Two innominate
                ii. Sacrum
                iii. Coccyx

(b) Symphysis pubis joins the two innominate (pubic) bones anteriorly
(c) True pelvis defines the birth canal
    i. Inlet is at the level of the sacral promontory, linea terminalis, and the upper margins of the pubic bones
    ii. Midplane of the pelvis is the inferior margins of the ischial tuberosities and the tip of the coccyx
    iii. Outlet is the anterior surfaces of the sacrum and coccyx
(d) Classification of pelvic types
    i. Gynecoid
        a) Round shaped pelvis
        b) Transverse diameter only slightly longer than anteroposterior
        c) Incidence—50% of white women
        d) Excellent prognosis for vaginal birth
    ii. Android
        a) Heart shaped or triangular shaped pelvis
        b) Posterior pelvis wider than anterior
        c) Poor prognosis for vaginal birth requiring operative delivery or C-section
    iii. Anthropoid
        a) Oval shaped pelvis
        b) Anteroposterior diameter is longer than transverse diameter
        c) Incidence—50% of nonwhite
        d) Good prognosis of vaginal birth—higher incidence of occiput posterior position
    iv. Platypelloid
        a) Flattened gynecoid shape pelvis
        b) Wide transverse diameter with very short anteroposterior diameter
        c) Incidence—3%
        d) Very poor prognosis for vaginal birth

- Fetal heart rate assessment
  1. Continuous—by external electronic fetal monitor
     a. Determination of the fetal heart rate

b. Assessment of long-term variability

c. Determine presence or absence of periodic changes including decelerations, tachycardia, or bradycardia

2. Continuous—by internal monitoring via fetal scalp electrode

a. Measures the actual R-to-R interval of the fetal QRS complex; more accurate surveillance

b. Can determine short-term variability

3. Intermittent by Doppler

a. Auscultation of fetal heart rate at prescribed intervals based upon stage of labor to assess fetal tolerance of labor

b. Unable to determine variability or isolated decelerations

- Head-to-toe examination
  1. General affect and coping abilities
  2. Head, eyes, ears, nose, and throat
     a. Absence of facial edema
     b. Absence of URI signs
  3. Heart and lungs
     a. Heart sounds without murmurs, rubs, or gallops—may have split S1, I/VI systolic murmur, audible S3
     b. Lungs clear to auscultation
  4. Abdomen
     a. Fundal height and appropriateness to gestational age
     b. Leopold's maneuver if not performed previously
     c. Presence of scars or lesions
     d. Intensity of contractions by palpation
     e. Location of fetal heart tones
  5. Pelvic examination—described in detail in this chapter
  6. Extremities
     a. Presence or absence of edema
     b. Presence or absence of varicosities
     c. Reflexes

◘ DIAGNOSTIC STUDIES

- Type of studies—dependent upon policies of birthing facility
  1. Complete blood count
  2. Blood type and Rh—may need to type and screen or cross-match depending on maternal risk status
  3. Repeat testing for HIV, syphilis, or hepatitis if indicated by history or examination findings

- Urine testing
  1. Protein
  2. Glucose
  3. Ketones

- Cervical/Vaginal/Perineal cultures performed during sterile speculum examination, if indicated
  1. Cervical culture if suspect active infection or has prolonged rupture of membranes (PROM)
  2. Culture of any suspicious lesions
  3. Vaginal and rectal cultures for group B streptococcus (GBS) if rupture of membranes before 37 weeks and not yet laboring

◘ MANAGEMENT AND TEACHING

- Based upon birth facility's policies, client desire, and risk status for discussion, consultation and management options

- Admission vs outpatient management
  1. Generally admit during active labor; client may desire outpatient management
  2. Factors to consider in decision making
     a. Stage of labor
     b. Nullipara vs multipara
     c. Functional vs prodromal labor
     d. Labor support at home
     e. Need for increased fetal surveillance

- Intravenous access
  1. If intravenous access is necessary via saline lock or IV catheter, most-common IV fluids are:
     a. 5% Dextrose solution
     b. 5% Dextrose with Lactated Ringer's
     c. Lactated Ringer's
  2. Factors to consider in decision making
     a. Hydration status, including presence of ketonuria
     b. Need for oxytocin induction or augmentation
     c. Need for antibiotics
     d. Predisposing factors for postpartum hemorrhage such as an overdistended uterus
     e. Abnormal placentation
     f. Grand multiparity
     g. Need for pain medication or regional anesthesia

- Limitations of activity level
  1. Clients can be encouraged to ambulate to help labor progress and coping abilities
  2. Factors to consider in decision making
     a. Unstable lie or malpresentation
     b. Need for increased fetal surveillance and monitoring
     c. Membrane status and station of the presenting part
     d. Pregnancy induced hypertension
     e. Maternal exhaustion level

- Nutrition and fluid status
  1. Energy levels can be positively influenced by oral intake
  2. Factors to consider in decision making
     a. Gastrointestinal motility/absorption
     b. Potential need for anesthesia during labor
     c. Birthing facility policy
  3. Can consider gastrointestinal protective agents such as magnesium/aluminum hydroxide, calcium carbonate/magnesium hydroxide, and sodium citrate/citric acid combinations

- Monitoring of vital signs
  1. Dependent upon stage of labor and risk status
  2. Patients with ruptured membranes require more frequent vital signs, especially temperature

- Pain management during labor and delivery
  1. Nonpharmacologic methods
     a. Have no effect on fetus or progress of labor, can allow the woman to feel more in control of the birth process
     b. Can be used in the latent phase of labor without detrimental effect—especially helpful in latent labor
        (1) Ambulation and movement
        (2) Hydrotherapy
        (3) Breathing and relaxation/hypnotherapy
        (4) Music
        (5) Position changes
  2. Analgesia
     a. Used to ameliorate the pain sensation; may change and alter consciousness; some medications have amnesiac effect
     b. Can be used in latent and active phase
     c. Avoid within 1 hour of birth due to the potential respiratory depressant effect on the fetus
        (1) Hypnotic
        (2) Sedatives
        (3) Narcotics
  3. Anesthesia
     a. Provides complete neurologic block
     b. Can interfere with muscular action
     c. Possible effect on the labor progress; may cause an increase in need for obstetrical intervention due to interference with uterine contractility
     d. Can have systemic effects, including fever and hypotension
     e. Can cause spinal headache
        (1) Spinal/intrathecal
        (2) Epidural
  4. Local blocks—provide pain blockade at site of pain for brief periods of time
     a. Paracervical
     b. Pudendal
     c. Local infiltration

- Fetal well-being monitoring—method used dependent upon risk status of mother, policy of the birth facility, and provider preferences in combination with mother's desires
  1. Intermittent auscultation
     a. Facilitates increased mobility
     b. Increased patient comfort
     c. Equivalent to continuous fetal monitoring when performed at appropriate intervals
     d. Requires one-to-one labor attendance
     e. Associated with decreased rates of intervention
  2. Continuous fetal monitoring
     a. May be indicated for antepartum or intrapartum risk factors
     b. Reactive fetal monitor tracing is predictive of a well-oxygenated fetus
     c. Interpretation of fetal well-being can be equivocal in the presence of nonreassuring fetal heart rate tracing

- Support people and their roles
  1. Labor support can improve a woman's perception of her labor
  2. One-to-one labor support can assist the woman to cope better with labor
  3. Dedicated labor support has been found to decrease use of obstetrical intervention

- Management of membranes
  1. Intact membranes provide a barrier to bacterial introduction to the uterus
  2. Intact membranes can facilitate rotation of the head during pelvic descent
  3. Early rupture of membranes with unengaged vertex can increase risk of cord prolapse
  4. The prostaglandin content in the amniotic fluid can assist in the augmentation of labor if dysfunctional or arrested

- Physician role
  1. Clarify with the client the CNM role in relation to the consulting physician
  2. Indications for physician involvement should be reviewed

- Birth preferences
  1. Birth plan should be reviewed with client upon admission and discussed in relation to status at that time
  2. Discussion with client regarding inability to control labor process

◻ MECHANISMS OF LABOR

- The 4 Ps of labor
  1. Power of contractile efforts
     a. Adequacy of strength
     b. Need for augmentation of labor
  2. Passenger
     a. Lie
     b. Presentation
     c. Position
     d. Size
     e. Synclitism vs asynclitism
        (1) The relationship of the sagittal suture line to the maternal sacrum and symphysis pubis
        (2) Synclitism denotes the sagittal suture is midway between these two bones; biparietal diameter is parallel to the planes of the pelvis
        (3) Asynclitism denotes that the sagittal suture is oriented towards the pubis or the sacrum
            (a) Posterior asynclitism—the sagittal suture is closer to the symphysis pubis
            (b) Anterior asynclitism—the sagittal suture is closer to the sacrum
            (c) Can be the cause of labor dystocia
            (d) Lax abdominal musculature contributes to asynclitism
  3. Passage
     a. Clinical pelvimetry
     b. Classification of the pelvic structure
  4. Psyche
     a. Woman's view of labor/birth and her ability to handle it
     b. Appropriateness of emotional support
     c. Education or preparation of labor
     d. Meaning of the pregnancy
     e. Ability to achieve birth plan
     f. History of sexual abuse

- Labor assessment and progress
  1. Stages of labor—Friedman's concepts
     a. First stage—from onset of regular contractions through full dilatation (10 cm)
        (1) Latent labor—from onset of labor until 4 cm
            (a) Contraction pattern
                i. Every 10–20 minutes lasting 15–20 seconds to every 5–7 minutes lasting 30–40 seconds
                ii. Mild to moderate intensity
            (b) Length
                i. Nullipara should be 20 hours or less
                ii. Multipara should be 14 hours or less
        (2) Active labor—from 4 to 10 cm, begins with the acceleration phase and ends with the deceleration phase just prior to complete dilatation
            (a) Contraction pattern
                i. Become more frequent, regular, and intense
                ii. In active labor, every 2 to 3 minutes lasting at least 60 seconds
                iii. Moderate to strong by palpation
            (b) Length
                i. Nullipara at least 1.2 cm/hour; average is 3 cm/hour during maximum slope
                ii. Multipara at least 1.5 cm/hour; average is 5.7 cm/hour
            (c) Strength of contractions
                i. Externally measured by palpation
                ii. Internally
                    a) By intrauterine pressure catheter (IUPC)
                    b) Adequacy is considered 200 Montevideo (mVu) in a 10-minute period
            (d) Descent
                i. Nullipara at 1 cm/hr or greater, average 1.6 cm/hr
                ii. Multipara at 2.1 cm/hr or greater, average 5.4 cm/hr
     b. Second stage of labor—from full dilatation until the birth of the baby; pushing or expulsive phase
  2. Abnormal labor progress—according to Friedman
     a. Abnormal latent phase
        (1) Nullipara, more than 20 hours
        (2) Multipara, more than 14 hours
     b. Abnormal active phase
        (1) Nullipara progress, less than 1.2 cm/hr
        (2) Multipara progress, less than 1.5 cm/hr
        (3) Less than 200 mVu in 10 minutes by IUPC
     c. Descent
        (1) Nullipara, less than 1 cm/hr
        (2) Multipara, less than 2.1 cm/hr
  3. Evidence growing that challenges Friedman's parameters

☐ MANAGEMENT OF THE FIRST STAGE OF LABOR

- Assessment of maternal status
    1. Psychological status of client
        a. Perception of pain
        b. Coping ability and coping strategies
        c. Presence and support of people
        d. Client's perception of need for admission to the birthing facility
    2. Physical status of the client
        a. Vital signs
            (1) Temperature
                (a) Slightly elevated (< 100°F) during labor, highest in the time preceding and immediately following the birth
                (b) Epidural anesthesia can artificially elevate temperature
            (2) Blood pressure
                (a) Systolic blood pressure increases 10–20 mm Hg during contractions
                (b) Diastolic blood pressure increases 5–10 mm Hg during contractions
                (c) Blood pressure returns to prelabor levels between contractions
                (d) Pain and fear can contribute to elevations in blood pressure
            (3) Pulse
                (a) Due to the increased metabolic rate during labor, pulse rate is slightly elevated
                (b) Inversely proportional to action of the contraction, increases during increment and decreases at acme
            (4) Respiration
                (a) Slightly increased rate during labor
                (b) Hyperventilation is common and related to pain response and can lead to alkalosis

- Assessment of labor progress
    1. Vaginal examinations
        a. Allows assessment of labor progress related to cervical dilatation and/or fetal descent
        b. Frequency of vaginal examinations dependent upon phase of labor, provider choice, client's wishes, and status of membranes
    2. Partographs—graph of labor curve
        a. Designed by Dr. Emmanuel Friedman to chart labor progress to assure adequacy
        b. Expectation of standard progress of labor by Friedman's formula not universally accepted

- Pain management
    1. Basis of labor pain
        a. Physiologic
            (1) Intensity of contractions
            (2) Degree of cervical dilatation
            (3) Descent of fetus causing pressure on pelvic structures
            (4) Fetal size
            (5) Fetal position
            (6) Hypoxia of uterine muscle cells during action of contractions
        b. Psychological
            (1) Fear
            (2) Anxiety
            (3) Lack of knowledge regarding labor process
            (4) Lack of support
            (5) Cultural influences
    2. Negative physiologic responses related to labor pain
        a. Hyperventilation causing decreased oxygenation
        b. Stress responses—related psychological effect causes increased cortisol and decreased placental perfusion
        c. Increased cardiac output and blood pressure
    3. Factors influencing pain management decisions
        a. Patient choice or birth plan
        b. Stage of labor
        c. Fetal status
        d. Other factors contributing to pain response
        e. Possible routes of medication administration
        f. Availability of pain medication modalities
        g. Nursing staff availability
    4. Pain management methods
        a. Nonpharmacologic pain relief
            (1) Relaxation and breathing techniques
            (2) Hydrotherapy—tub, shower, Jacuzzi
            (3) Position changes; ambulation
            (4) Massage
            (5) Environmental measures, i.e., quiet surroundings, aromatherapy, music
            (6) Acupuncture
            (7) Hypnosis
        b. Pharmacologic pain relief
            (1) Sedatives used for false labor or prodromal labor, facilitate rest/relaxation
                (a) Diphenhydramine 25–50 mg
                (b) Zolpidem 5–10 mg
                (c) Pentobarbital 100 mg
            (2) Ataractics—do not affect contraction pattern, have a calming effect

(a) Promethazine 25–50 mg IM or 25 mg IV

(b) Hydroxine 25–50 mg IM

(3) Narcotic analgesics given in active labor but should be avoided within 1 hour of birth

(a) Meperidine 50 mg IM or 25–50 mg IV

(b) Morphine sulfate for prodromal labor 10–15 mg IM or active labors 3–5 mg IV

(4) Nonnarcotic analgesics—cause less neonatal respiratory depression than narcotics

(a) Butorphanol 1–2 mg IV or 1–4 mg IM

(b) Nalbuphine 10–20 mg IM or 5 mg IV

c. Anesthesia

(1) Spinal/intrathecal

(2) Epidural

(3) Pudendal

- Assessment and evaluation of fetal well-being
  1. Physiology of fetal heart rate (FHR) regulation
     a. Parasympathetic nervous system—responsible for the beat-to-beat variability of the FHR
     b. Baroreceptors
        (1) Increased pressures can cause vagal response in the fetus
        (2) Located in the carotid arteries
     c. Chemoreceptors
        (1) Located in the aortic arch and carotid sinus
        (2) Sensitive to changes in the fetal pH, O_2 and CO_2 levels, and respond by increasing fetal blood pressure and heart rate
     d. Sympathetic nervous system—controls the baseline fetal heart rate
  2. Evaluation of the FHR in labor
     a. Baseline
        (1) Normal range for a fetus at term 120–160 beats per minute (bpm)
        (2) FHR between 110–120 bpm can be normal at term with appropriate variability
        (3) Judged over approximately 10–20 minutes, the mean FHR in the absence of periodic changes
        (4) Should be documented as a 5 bpm range
     b. Bradycardia
        (1) FHR at less than 120 bpm for 10 or more minutes

(2) Marked bradycardia is less than 100 bpm for 10 or more minutes

(a) Causes
  i. Cord compression
  ii. Rapid descent
  iii. Vagal stimulation
  iv. Medications
  v. Anesthesia or medications
  vi. Placental insufficiency
  vii. Fetal cardiac anomalies
  viii. Terminal condition of the fetus

c. Tachycardia
   (1) FHR of more than 160 bpm for more than 10 minutes
      (a) Causes
         i. Maternal fever
         ii. Infection
         iii. Medications, especially beta sympathomimetics
         iv. Chronic fetal hypoxia
         v. Can be compensatory after temporary fetal hypoxia event
         vi. Undiagnosed prematurity
         vii. Excessive fetal movement

d. Variability
   (1) Combination of influences between the sympathetic and parasympathetic nervous systems
      (a) Long-term variability (LTV)—fluctuations of the fetal heart rate over the course of 1 minute
         i. Absent, less than 2 bpm from baseline
         ii. Decreased, 2–6 bpm from baseline
         iii. Average, 6–10 bpm from baseline
         iv. Increased, 15–25 bpm from baseline
         v. Marked, more than 25 bpm from baseline
      (b) Short-term variability (STV)—changes in fetal heart rate between individual beats of the fetal heart
         i. Beat-to-beat variability
         ii. Cannot be assessed by external fetal monitoring; must have fetal scalp electrode (FSE)

e. Periodic changes
   (1) Variable decelerations
      (a) Periodic or nonperiodic decrease in the FHR that differs in shape from one deceleration to another

(b) FHR deceleration does not reflect the shape of the contraction

(c) Can occur at any time in relation to the contractions

(d) Nonconsistent shape; can look like a U, V, or W

(e) Generally with an abrupt drop below the FHR baseline and a rapid return to baseline

(f) Generally caused by cord compression

(g) Implications

  i. With rapid recovery to baseline and good STV, generally considered an uncompromised fetus

  ii. Suspect fetal compromise with slow recovery to baseline, increasing length or depth of deceleration, absent STV or compensatory "overshoot" of baseline, or increasing frequency of deceleration

(h) Management

  i. Position change

  ii. IV fluid bolus

  iii. O_2 at 10 liters per minute (LPM) via face mask

  iv. Pelvic examination, to rule out cord prolapse and provide scalp stimulation

  v. Contact consulting physician if warranted

  vi. Consider amnioinfusion

(2) Early decelerations

(a) Uniformly shaped slowing of the FHR that mirrors the contractions

(b) Gradual descent to the nadir with gradual return

(c) FHR usually remains within the normal range and deceleration usually less than 90 seconds

(d) Deceleration begins, peaks, and ends with the contraction

(e) Generally caused by head compression, vagal stimulation

(f) Generally not considered an ominous pattern

(g) Management

  i. Position change

  ii. Surveillance

(3) Late decelerations

(a) Uniformly shaped slowing of the FHR which begins with the peak of the contraction and does not return to baseline until after the completion of the contraction

(b) FHR may or may not remain within the normal fetal heart range

(c) Can occur in an isolated fashion but more ominous when occurs repetitively

(d) Possible causes

  i. Uteroplacental insufficiency

  ii. Fetal hypoxia

  iii. Uterine hyperstimulation

  iv. Decreased placental blood flow

  v. Maternal hypotension

  vi. Abruptio placenta

  vii. Medication effect

(e) Management

  i. Left lateral position

  ii. IV fluid bolus

  iii. O_2 at 10 LPM

  iv. Attempt to correct underlying cause

  v. Consult with physician

3. Fetal monitoring techniques

a. All women require some method of fetal monitoring in labor

b. Modality is based upon maternal/fetal risk status, birth site, and client desire

c. For low-risk women, intermittent auscultation is equivalent to continuous fetal monitoring to detect fetal compromise

d. FHR monitoring techniques

(1) Intermittent FHR auscultation by fetoscope or Doppler

(a) Should be considered for low-risk pregnancies

(b) Frequency of auscultation—dependent also on facility protocol

  i. Auscultate for 60 seconds after a contraction every 30 minutes in the first stage of labor, if low risk; every 15 minutes if high risk

  ii. Every 15 minutes during the second stage of labor if low risk, every 5 minutes if high risk

(2) Continuous fetal monitoring

(a) Recommended for high-risk pregnancies or when intermittent monitoring is not indicated

(b) Frequency of FHR tracing review

  i. Every 15 minutes in the first stage

  ii. Every 5 minutes in the second stage

(c) Modalities for continuous fetal monitoring

i.   External FHR—ultrasound detection and tracing of the FHR through the abdominal wall

ii. Internal FHR
  a) Via FSE
  b) Directly measures fetal heartbeat by measuring the R-to-R interval during heartbeats
  c) Indications include inability to externally monitor, fetal distress, meconium stained fluid

e. Direct fetal testing
  (1) Fetal scalp sampling
    (a) Small amount of fetal blood is obtained from the fetal scalp for pH testing to rule out acidosis
    (b) Limiting factors
      i.   Inadequate cervical dilation
      ii.   Fetal head too high
      iii. Intact membranes
      iv.   Sampling errors due to developing caput or hematoma
    (c) Results
      i.   Normal, more than 7.25
      ii.   Prepathologic, 7.20–7.25
      iii. Pathologic, less than 7.20
    (d) Results are time limited and must be repeated every 20–30 minutes if indications of distress persist
    (e) Validity and reliability are questionable
  (2) Fetal scalp stimulation
    (a) During vaginal examination, fetal head is stimulated
    (b) Expected result should be FHR acceleration of more than 15 beats off baseline for more than 15 seconds
    (c) Expected result correlates to fetal pH of more than 7.20
    (d) Cannot be reliably performed during deceleration or bradycardia; must wait for FHR recovery
    (e) Validity and reliability not well established
  (3) Fetal pulse oximetry
    (a) Provides ongoing measure of fetal oxygenation
    (b) Research indicates no change in rate of Cesarean section with knowledge of fetal oxygen saturation

4. External uterine monitoring
  a. Tocodynameter—senses the changes in pressures against the strain gauge resulting from the change in abdominal wall contour
    (1) Records contraction interval and duration
    (2) Cannot determine intensity of contractions
  b. Palpation
  c. IUPC

- Fetal positions during birthing process
  1. Mechanisms of labor and cardinal movements based on occiput anterior (OA) position
    a. Left occiput anterior (LOA) is the most common position of birth
    b. Position and appropriate cardinal movements are facilitated in the gynecoid pelvis
    c. Cardinal movements of labor
      (1) Descent—usually in the ROA position, if engagement occurs during labor
      (2) Flexion—vertex begins partially flexed, is completely flexed when reaches pelvic floor, changing presenting diameter to suboccipitobregmatic of 9.5 cm
      (3) Internal rotation—rotation of 45° to OA allows the head to maximize the anterior posterior diameter of the gynecoid pelvis
      (4) Extension—fulcrum of the neck under the symphysis pubis allows birth of the head
      (5) Restitution—vertex reassumes the orientation of a 90° angle with the shoulders as the shoulders begin entering the AP diameter
      (6) External rotation—as head rotates, shoulders complete the remainder of the rotation to allow delivery in direct anterior posterior position
  2. Mechanisms of labor and cardinal movements based upon occiput posterior (OP) position
    a. Incidence of OP presentation is 15–30%
    b. Right occiput posterior (ROP) is five times more common than left occiput posterior
    c. More common in android and anthropoid pelvis
    d. 90% of OP presentations rotate to OA via long arc rotation of 135° (ROP to ROT to ROA to OA)
    e. Short arc rotation of 45° results in direct OP or deep transverse pelvic arrest
    f. Cardinal movements
      (1) Descent—head enters pelvis in an oblique angle

(2) Flexion does not occur until the head meets the pelvic floor, unflexed head can cause cephalopelvic disproportion (CPD)

(3) Internal rotation—head must rotate 135°

(4) Extension—once rotation is complete, head can be born by normal extension

(5) Restitution—may be delayed due to the slower rotation of the fetal shoulders

(6) External rotation—as rotation occurs, fetus rotates shoulders to the anterior–posterior diameter of the outlet to facilitate birth

- Emotional support
  1. Psychological
     a. Calm environment
     b. Perception of safety and support for mother and baby
     c. Maintenance of privacy and modesty
     d. Participation in the plan of care
  2. Role of the labor support person
     a. Reinforcement of and positive encouragement for the laboring woman
     b. Participation in the birth process
        (1) Providing oral fluids and/or ice chips
        (2) Encouraging position changes
        (3) Relaxation techniques
        (4) Massage
        (5) Coaching with breathing techniques

◻ MANAGEMENT OF THE SECOND STAGE OF LABOR

- Begins with complete dilatation and ends with the birth of the infant

- Maternal status
  1. Vital signs
     a. BP every 15 minutes in low-risk women, every 5 minutes in high-risk women
        (1) BP must be taken between contractions
        (2) BP can be elevated 10 mm Hg in the second stage of labor due to pushing effort
     b. Pulse and respiratory rate every hour
     c. Temperature every 2 hours
  2. Hydration and fluid status
     a. IV or oral fluids should be encouraged due to
        (1) Increased metabolism
        (2) Increased respiratory efforts/hyperventilation of transition
        (3) Diaphoresis
        (4) Nausea and vomiting
     b. Bladder status
        (1) Bladder distention can compromise pelvic capacity
        (2) Inability to void may require catheterization
        (3) Prevent problem by having client void when full dilatation approaches
  3. Behaviors and coping ability
     a. Assessment of maternal fatigue
     b. Coping ability
     c. Response to pain and pressure
  4. Pain control
     a. Evaluate level of sensation in epiduralized client to determine if anesthetic level is hindering pushing efforts
     b. Pudendal anesthesia may be necessary as fetal descent occurs causing perineal distention and pain
  5. Expulsive effort
     a. Client should be coached to achieve effective pushing effort
     b. Assessment of which type of pushing is most effective for the client
        (1) Open glottis physiologic pushing
        (2) Closed glottis "Valsalva" pushing
     c. Client should be instructed to pant at the time of crowning; "control the mother, not the head"
  6. Integrity of the perineum
     a. Maternal preference is generally avoidance of episiotomy
     b. Contributing factors to need for episiotomy
        (1) Fetal malposition
        (2) Anticipation of large baby
        (3) Anticipation of shoulder dystocia
        (4) Poor distensibility of the perineal tissues
        (5) Difficulty in maintaining adequate control of client's expulsive efforts

- Fetal status
  1. Vaginal examination
     a. Evaluation of descent with pushing effort
     b. Normalcy of fetal position and adaptation to the maternal pelvis
        (1) Molding/caput succedaneum
        (2) Synclitism vs asynclitism
        (3) Appropriate rotation to facilitate delivery
  2. FHR monitoring
     a. Need for increased frequency of FHR evaluation
        (1) Evaluation at least every 15 minutes

(2) More commonly every 5 minutes or after each contraction

b. Periodic changes (early and variable decelerations) in FHR common

(1) Decelerations secondary to head compressions

(2) Not indicative of acute fetal distress

- Pain relief
  1. Breathing techniques
     a. Controlled breathing as contraction begins and ends assists in focusing efforts
     b. Promote relaxation between pushing efforts
  2. Narcotic analgesia
     a. Should *not* be given within 1 hour of birth
     b. Can cause respiratory depression in the neonate
  3. Regional anesthesia
     a. Effectively lessens the pain and pressure sensations of the second stage
     b. Can lengthen second stage secondary to pelvic musculature relaxation and decreased pressure sensations
     c. Pudendal—lidocaine 1–2% up to 10 cc on each side
        (1) Provides dense nerve block to the perineum
        (2) Does not inhibit pushing efforts
        (3) Needs to be timed well for best anesthetic effect
           (a) Primiparas when vertex is at +2
           (b) Multiparas shortly before complete dilation
  4. Local anesthesia
     a. Perineal infiltration—lidocaine 1–2% up to 10 cc in divided dosing
        (1) Used prior to cutting of an episiotomy
        (2) For repair of episiotomy or laceration(s)

- Emotional support
  1. Encouragement
  2. Participation of labor support persons
  3. Adherence to birth plan

- Cardinal movements of labor
  1. Eight basic movements that take place to allow birth in vertex presentation
     a. Engagement—biparietal diameter of fetal head passes through pelvic inlet
     b. Descent—occurs secondary to forces of uterine contractions, change in the tone of pelvic musculature and maternal pushing

c. Flexion—occurs when the fetal head meets the resistance of the pelvic floor during descent and forces the smaller sub-occipitobregmatic diameter to enter the pelvis first

d. Internal rotation—causes the anteroposterior diameters of the fetal head and the maternal pelvis to align, most commonly causing the occiput to rotate to the anterior portion of the pelvis

e. Extension—mechanism by which the birth of the fetal head occurs; the fetal head follows the curve of Carus; the suboccipital region of the fetal head pivots under the maternal pubic symphysis

f. Restitution—rotation of the head 45° and realignment 90° to the shoulders

g. External rotation—occurs as the shoulders rotate 45° bringing the shoulders into the anteroposterior diameter of the pelvis; the head also rotates another 45°

h. Birth of the body occurs by lateral flexion of the shoulders via the curve of Carus

◻ DELIVERY MANAGEMENT

- Maintenance of pelvic integrity
  1. Anatomy
     a. Pelvic floor musculature
        (1) Function to support pelvic organs
        (2) Aids in the anterior rotation of the fetus during pelvic descent and birth
        (3) Consists of two muscle groups
           (a) The levator ani, made up of:
              i. Pubococcygeus, made up of:
                 a) Pubovaginalis
                 b) Puborectalis
                 c) Pubococcygeus proper
              ii. Illiococcygeus
           (b) Coccygeus
     b. Perineal musculature
        (1) Perineum is divided into two triangles and is more superficial than the pelvic floor musculature
           (a) Anteriorly as the urogenital triangle
              i. Superficial transverse perineal muscle
              ii. Ischiocavernosus muscle
              iii. Bulbocavernosus
              iv. Deep transverse perineal muscle
           (b) Posteriorly as the anal triangle
              i. Sphincter ani externus
              ii. Anococcygeal body

(2) Separation is the transverse perineal muscles and the base of the pelvic floor musculature

2. Factors interfering with perineal integrity
   a. Size of fetus
   b. Distensibility of perineum
   c. Control of expulsive efforts
   d. Operative delivery modalities, i.e., forceps or vacuum extraction
   e. Occiput posterior position
   f. Use of lubricants
   g. Maternal position for birth
   h. Episiotomy (median or mediolateral)
3. Strategies to minimize perineal trauma
   a. Antepartum perineal massage
      (1) Begin at 36–37 weeks
      (2) Increases elasticity and maternal tolerance to perineal stretching
   b. External perineal massage from the time of perineal distension
   c. Warm compresses during second stage
      (1) Increases circulation to perineum
      (2) Promotes elasticity
      (3) Assists in the relaxation of the musculature
   d. Lateral positioning for birth
   e. Counter pressure to maintain flexion of the fetal head during birth
   f. Education of the mother regarding the importance of controlled delivery of the head
   g. Support of the perineum at the time of birth (this is controversial, some providers adopt a "hands-off" approach to birth)

- Episiotomy—surgical incision performed to enlarge the vaginal opening to allow delivery of the fetal head
  1. Anatomy
     a. Muscles cut during median episiotomy
        (1) Bulbocavernosus (sphincter vaginalis)
        (2) Ischiocavernosus
        (3) Superficial and deep transverse perineal muscles
  2. Technique
     a. Median episiotomy
        (1) Place index and middle fingers, slightly separated and palm side down, in vagina
        (2) Insert scissors into the introitus in an up and down position with one blade placed externally and one blade placed internally
        (3) Depth of insertion should correspond to the length of intended episiotomy
        (4) Cut tissue in one motion deliberately and purposefully

(5) Evaluate adequacy of incision; repeat if indicated
   b. Mediolateral episiotomy—generally used if patient has a short perineum to avoid a laceration into the anal sphincter
      (1) Used much less frequently in US—less than 10%
      (2) Same procedure except that the direction of the scissors is a 45° angle from the base of the introitus directed either right or left
      (3) The angle of the incision should be aimed toward the corresponding ischial tuberosity
      (4) Much more difficult to repair
3. Lacerations
   a. First degree—involves the vaginal mucosa, posterior fourchette, and perineal skin
   b. Second degree—involves same structures as above plus perineal muscles
   c. Third degree—involves same structures as a second degree plus tearing through the entire thickness of the rectal sphincter
   d. Fourth degree—involves all the structures as above plus tearing of the anterior rectal wall
4. Repair
   a. Fundamentals of repair
      (1) Use of aseptic technique
      (2) Adequate anesthesia
      (3) Visibility through good hemostasis
      (4) Appropriate suture material including needle size
      (5) Minimize local tissue trauma through gentle and limited blotting
      (6) Minimize the amount of suture used
      (7) Good approximation of tissues decreasing dead space
   b. Suture material
      (1) Chromic catgut is the most common suture material
      (2) Vicryl is alternately used for repair
      (3) Suture gauge
         (a) 3-0 chromic catgut
            i. Vaginal mucosa
            ii. Subcutaneous tissue
            iii. Subcuticular tissue
         (b) 4-0 chromic catgut for finer repairs
            i. Periurethral
            ii. Periclitoral
            iii. Anterior wall of the rectum
         (c) 2-0 chromic catgut for areas requiring more tensile strength
            i. Vaginal wall lacerations
            ii. Cervical lacerations

    iii. Deep interrupted sutures for repair of pelvic musculature
  (4) Needle selection
    (a) Atraumatic general closure needles are preferable
    (b) Small, fine GI needles should be used for fine stitching
    (b) Cutting needles should not be used
  c. Mechanisms of repair of median episiotomy or second-degree laceration
    (1) Inspection of tissues to assess depth and extent of laceration
    (2) Identify all appropriate anatomical structures
    (3) Begin repair approximately 1 cm beyond the apex of the laceration to the vaginal mucosa
    (4) Close the mucosa using continuous locked stitches to the level of the hymenal ring
    (5) Pass needle under hymenal ring and continue using blanket stitches (nonlocked) to the level of the bulbocavernosus muscle
    (6) Repair bulbocavernosus muscle with a crown stitch using a separate 2-0 chromic, if desired
    (7) If laceration is deep, consider several deep interrupted stitches using 2-0 chromic
    (8) Using the 3-0 chromic suture again, repair the perineal fascia with continuous stitching to the perineal apex
    (9) Using mattress stitches, perform subcuticular closure
    (10) At the level of the hymenal ring, bury the suture and tie off

- Management decisions for birth
  1. Timing for the preparation of the birth related to location, i. e., moving to a delivery room
  2. Delivery position for birth
    a. Semi-sitting
    b. Squatting
    c. Lateral
    d. Hands and knees
    e. Supine or lithotomy (least appropriate, but commonly used)
  3. Determine need for an episiotomy
  4. Need for/type of additional anesthesia/analgesia
  5. Use of perineal support during birth
  6. Use of the Ritgen maneuver—assistance, if needed, in delivering fetal head by applying upward pressure to the fetal chin through the perineum during extension

  7. Need for additional personnel, i. e., nurse, second midwife, consulting physician, pediatric provider
  8. Placement of newborn upon delivery
  9. Timing of umbilical cord cutting

- Hand maneuvers for birth in the OA position
  1. Apply counter pressure to the fetal head during crowning to maintain flexion and control extension using nondominant hand
  2. If using perineal support, place thumb and index finger laterally on the distended perineum with palmar surface supporting perineal body
  3. Control birth of head during extension
  4. After birth of head, slide fingers of dominant hand around fetal head to posterior neck to feel for umbilical cord
  5. If nuchal cord is present:
    a. Gently slip over baby's head if loose
    b. If not easily reduced over the head, slip cord over baby's shoulders as the baby is born
    c. If tight, doubly clamp and cut and unwind cord before delivery of the shoulders
  6. Suction baby's mouth and nose with bulb syringe, if needed
  7. After restitution and external rotation, place the palmar surface of each hand laterally on the baby's head
  8. With gentle downward traction, and maternal pushing effort, deliver anterior shoulder. Some recommend waiting for the next contraction
  9. With upward traction, lift the baby's head toward ceiling to deliver the posterior shoulder while observing the perineum
  10. Glide posterior hand along head and posterior shoulder to control the posterior arm as it delivers
  11. As the baby delivers, maintain posterior hand under the baby's neck with the baby's head supported by the wrist and forearm
  12. The anterior hand follows the body of the baby during birth and grasps the lower leg of the baby
  13. Rotate the baby into the football hold with the head in the palm, and the legs between what was the posterior arm and attendant's body
  14. Keep the baby's head below its hips, and slightly to the side, to facilitate drainage and suctioning

- Suctioning—ensuring a clear airway
  1. Routine suctioning of nasal and oral passages has not been assessed in clinical trials so its value is uncertain
  2. Most healthy babies can clear their airways with no additional help

3. Bulb syringe
   a. Generally sufficient to clear oral and nasal passages of fluid and mucus after birth
   b. Minimize pharyngeal stimulation and tissue trauma
   c. After birth of baby, sometimes additional suctioning is necessary
4. DeLee mucous trap suctioning
   a. Indicated for meconium stained amniotic fluid
   b. Occurs after birth of head to clear oro- and nasopharynx
   c. Mucous trap allows amount and color of fluid to be assessed
   d. Mother should be instructed to pant and not push during this suctioning

◻ MANAGEMENT OF THE THIRD STAGE

- Begins with delivery of the infant and ends with the delivery of the placenta

- Delivery of the placenta
   1. Timing—generally 5–30 minutes after the birth
   2. Method of placental separation
      a. Placenta separates from the uterine wall due to change in uterine size
      b. Hematoma forms behind the placenta along the uterine wall
      c. Separation of the placenta completes
      d. Descent of the placenta to the lower uterine segment or vagina
      e. Expulsion
   3. Signs and symptoms of placental separation
      a. Sudden increase in vaginal bleeding
      b. Lengthening of the umbilical cord
      c. Uterine shape from discoid to globular
      d. Uterus rises in the abdomen
   4. Mechanisms of placental delivery
      a. Schultz
         (1) Presents at the introitus with fetal side showing
         (2) More common than Duncan
         (3) Separation is thought to occur centrally first
         (4) Majority of bleeding is contained
      b. Duncan
         (1) Presents at the introitus with maternal side showing
         (2) Less common
         (3) Separation occurs initially at placental margin
         (4) Bleeding is more visible
         (5) Higher incidence of hemorrhage due to incomplete separation of placenta

5. Management of placenta delivery
   a. Obtain cord bloods after clamping of the cord
   b. Inspect cord for number of vessels
   c. Guard the uterus while waiting for placenta separation
      (1) No fundal massage before separation
      (2) No traction on umbilical cord until separation
   d. Use modified Brandt-Andrews to assess for separation
   e. When separation has occurred, use Brandt-Andrews maneuver to stabilize the uterus and control cord traction to deliver the placenta
   f. May have mother push to assist expulsion
   g. Deliver placenta via the curve of Carus
   h. If membranes are trailing behind the placenta, carefully deliver membranes by:
      (1) Using a Kelly clamp or sponge stick clamp onto membranes, gently apply lateral and outward traction
      (2) Holding the bulk of the placenta and twisting the placenta over and over until the membranes are delivered
      (3) Inspecting placenta and membranes for completeness

- Appropriate diagnostic tests
   1. Cord blood
      a. Fetal blood type and Rh
      b. Direct Coombs testing
   2. Maternal blood
      a. Kleihauer-Betke stain, if mother is Rh negative
      b. CBC, if hemorrhage suspected

- Use of oxytocics
   1. Oxytocin
      a. Used prophylactically against postpartum hemorrhage
      b. Causes intermittent uterine contractions to decrease uterine size and the placental bed exposure
      c. Administration
         (1) Intravenous
            (a) 20 units in 1000 cc of IV fluid with first liter running as rapidly as possible, second liter at 150 cc/hr
            (b) Can use up to 30 units per liter
            (c) Total no more than 100 units
         (2) Intramuscular—10 units intramuscularly if no IV access
   2. Methylergonovine
      a. Causes a sustained, tetanic uterine contraction

b. Can be used emergently as one-time dosing or as a series of doses for sustained effect

c. Contraindicated in hypertensive patients because it causes peripheral vasoconstriction

d. Administration
   (1) Intramuscular—0.2 mg IM, can be repeated once
   (2) Oral
      (a) Generally given as a series of 6 doses over the first 24 hours postpartum
      (b) 0.2 mg orally every 6 hours

3. Carboprost
   a. Used only in severe hemorrhage situations
   b. Administration
      (1) 250 mcg
      (2) Can be given IM or intramyometrially

- Placental abnormalities and variations
  1. Battledore placenta—peripheral cord insertion, at placental margin
  2. Succenturiate lobe
     a. Most common abnormality—occurrence 3%
     b. Accessory placental lobe within the fetal sac that had continuous vascular connections with main placenta
     c. Can cause retained placenta or hemorrhage
  3. Velamentous cord insertion
     a. Cord insertion into fetal sac, not directly into placental bed, generally 5–10 cm away from placenta
     b. Can cause shearing of blood vessels during labor or delivery of placenta, causing hemorrhage
     c. More common in multiple gestation
  4. Circumvallate placenta
     a. Opaque ring of fibrous-appearing tissue on fetal side of the placenta, caused by a double layer of chorion and amnion
     b. Can be seen in IUGR pregnancies but usually of no clinical significance

◻ MANAGEMENT OF IMMEDIATE NEWBORN TRANSITION—SEE ALSO CHAPTER 5

- Apgar scoring
  1. Devised in 1952 by Dr. Virginia Apgar to identify infants requiring assistance adapting to the extrauterine environment
  2. Comparable to the biophysical profile scoring in utero

3. Significance of scoring
   a. One-minute Apgar scoring used to determine level of resuscitation required
   b. Five-minute Apgar scoring has a relationship to neonatal morbidity and mortality
      (1) Apgars of less than 7 at 5 minutes indicate need for pediatric involvement
      (2) Apgars of less than 4 at 5 minutes correlate with neonatal mortality
      (3) Low Apgar scores by themselves are not predictive of later neurologic dysfunction
   c. Not as valid an assessment for preterm infants

- Indications for pediatric involvement
  1. Any condition or circumstance that may compromise the adaptation of the neonate to extrauterine life
     a. Obstetrical conditions
        (1) Known IUGR
        (2) Birth prior to 37 weeks
        (3) Oligohydramnios
        (4) Maternal systemic disease
        (5) Congenital abnormalities
     b. Intrapartum conditions
        (1) Narcotic analgesia at less than 1 hour prior to birth
        (2) Chorioamnionitis
        (3) Operative delivery including Cesarean section
        (4) Nonreassuring fetal heart rate

◻ SPECIAL CONSIDERATIONS AND DEVIATIONS FROM NORMAL

- Premature labor
  1. Definitions
     a. Premature labor—onset of regular uterine contractions between 20 and 37 weeks' gestation with spontaneous rupture of membranes or progressive cervical changes (ACOG, 2003).
     b. Premature birth—delivery prior to 37 weeks' gestation
     c. Term birth—delivery between 37 and 42 weeks' gestation
     d. Small for gestational age (SGA)—birth weight at less than 10th percentile for gestational age; corresponds to IUGR
  2. Incidence—approximately 10% of all births in the United States
  3. Etiology
     a. Idiopathic and multifactorial; in most cases the cause of premature labor is unknown
     b. Maternal factors

(1) Systemic diseases
   (a) Pregnancy-induced hypertension
   (b) Renal disease
   (c) Autoimmune disease
   (d) Infection
(2) Structural uterine abnormalities
   (a) Müllerian defects
   (b) Fibroids
(3) Overdistended uterus
   (a) Multiple gestation
   (b) Polyhydramnios
(4) Cervical incompetence
(5) History of premature labor
(6) Low socioeconomic factors
c. Fetal factors
   (1) Premature rupture of membranes—implicated in 30% of all premature labor
   (2) Fetal anomalies
   (3) Placental insufficiency

4. Signs and symptoms
   a. Menstrual-like cramping with increasing frequency and intensity
   b. Pelvic pressure, especially suprapubic
   c. Backache
   d. Passage of amniotic fluid
   e. Change in the character of vaginal secretions
   f. Bloody show/spotting
   g. Progressive cervical dilatation

5. Physical findings
   a. Uterine contractions documented by EFM or palpation
   b. Cervical dilation on digital examination
   c. Documented ruptured membranes

6. Differential diagnosis
   a. Urinary tract infection/pyelonephritis
   b. Round ligament pain
   c. Braxton Hicks contractions
   d. Renal colic
   e. Appendicitis

7. Diagnostic tests to consider
   a. Fern and/or nitrazine test if suspect rupture of membranes
   b. Urinalysis with culture and sensitivity
   c. Other tests for suspected infections—Chlamydia, GC, wet prep
   d. Fetal fibronectin—collect before digital examination; recent sexual activity or blood may affect results
   e. Ultrasound—cervical length and funneling, placental location and status, biophysical profile, and amniotic fluid index
   f. Amniocentesis—fetal surfactant and lecithin/sphingomyelin (L/S) ratio
   g. CBC with differential

8. Management—consultation with physician regarding need for transfer of care versus comanagement
   a. Nonpharmacologic
      (1) Hydration
      (2) Left-lateral bed rest
   b. Tocolysis—generally used to delay birth more than 48 hours in order to give steroids to hasten lung maturity
      (1) Contraindications to tocolysis—any conditions causing a hostile uterine environment
         (a) Placental abruption
         (b) Chorioamnionitis
         (c) Severe preeclampsia
         (d) Placenta previa
         (e) Fetal distress
         (f) Lethal fetal anomalies
         (g) IUGR without interval growth
      (2) Beta agonists (terbutaline, ritodrine)
         (a) Drug action—interferes with smooth muscle contractility
         (b) Side-effects
            i. Palpitations/tachycardia
            ii. Tremors
            iii. Anxiety
            iv. Hyperglycemia
            v. Hypokalemia
            vi. Pulmonary edema
            vii. Fetal tachycardia
         (c) Drug interactions
            i. MAO inhibitors
            ii. Diuretics
            iii. Beta blockers
         (d) Contraindications
            i. Use of drugs causing untoward interactions
            ii. Underlying cardiac disease, especially conduction disorders
         (e) Administration and dosing
            i. Routes—PO, SQ, SQ infusion pump, IV
            ii. Terbutaline PO 2.5–5 mg, SQ 0.25
            iii. Ritodrine PO 5–10 mg, IV rarely used any longer
      (3) Magnesium sulfate (MgSO$_4$)
         (a) Drug action—acts on vascular smooth muscle causing vasodilatation
         (b) Side-effects
            i. Flushing
            ii. Palpitations
            iii. Feeling of warmth
            iv. Lethargy
            v. Muscle weakness

vi.   Dizziness
vii. Nausea/vomiting
viii. Respiratory depression
ix.   Pulmonary edema

(c) Drug interactions—calcium channel blockers

(d) Contraindications
   i.   Use of calcium channel blockers
   ii. Toxic effects at serum level of more than 7 mg/dL
   iii. Antidote is calcium gluconate

(e) Administration and dosing
   i.   Generally IV, can be given IM
   ii. Loading dose 4–6 g in 100 cc IVF over 20–30 minutes
   iii. Initial maintenance dose 2 g/hr
   iv. If contractions continue, increase by 0.5 g/hr every 30 minutes to a max dose of 4 g/hr
   v.   Maintain at effective level for 12 to 24 hours after contractions stop
   vi. No benefit for weaning when discontinued

(4) Calcium channel blockers (nifedipine)

(a) Drug action—nonspecific smooth muscle relaxant; prevents influx of extracellular calcium ions into myometrial cells; effect not specific to uterus

(b) Side-effects
   i.   Maternal hypotension
   ii. Flushing
   iii. Nausea/vomiting

(c) Drug interactions
   i.   Beta-agonists
   ii. Magnesium sulfate

(d) Contraindications
   i.   Do not use in presence of intrauterine infection, maternal hypertension, or cardiac disease
   ii. Do not use in combination with beta-agonists or magnesium sulfate

(e) Administration and dosing
   i.   Route—PO
   ii. Initial dose of 10 mg
   iii. If contractions continue, repeat doses every 20 minutes for total of 30 mg in 1 hour
   iv. Once contractions decrease, may give 10 mg every 6 hours or 30–60 mg sustained release dose per day

c. Other management decisions
   (1) Group B streptococcal prophylaxis
     (a) Penicillin 5 million units IV followed by 2.5 million units every 4 hours until delivery or negative culture
     (b) Clindamycin as alternative therapy if allergic to penicillin
   (2) Corticosteroid administration
     (a) Stimulates fetal lung maturity and possibly protection from intraventricular hemorrhage
     (b) Dexamethasone 6 mg IM every 12 hours for 4 doses
     (c) Betamethasone 12 mg IM × 2 doses 24 hours apart
     (d) Should attempt to delay birth until 24 hours post administration

- Umbilical cord prolapse
  1. Definition—umbilical cord lies below or beside the presenting part; danger is compression of the umbilical cord, thus compromising the blood supply to the fetus
  2. Etiology/incidence
     a. Presenting part does not fill the pelvic inlet; can occur with the rupturing of membranes
     b. Incidence—1 in 400 pregnancies
  3. Signs and symptoms/physical findings
     a. Umbilical cord visible at or outside introitus
     b. Palpation of cord during vaginal examination
     c. Presumptive diagnosis of occult prolapse if fetal distress occurs immediately following rupture of membranes
  4. Management
     a. Elevate presenting part off cord by continuous vaginal examination
     b. Assist mother into knee–chest position or steep left-lateral Trendelenburg
     c. Do not attempt to manipulate the cord as this may cause cord spasm; if protruding, wrap loosely with warm normal saline-soaked gauze
     d. Do not rely on cord pulsations as indicator of fetal status—obtain ultrasound if unable to detect fetal heart tones
     e. Immediately alert consulting physician and other staff of emergency
     f. O_2 at 10 L/min
     g. Intravenous fluid bolus
     h. Monitor FHR
     i. Consider terbutaline for tocolysis
     j. Prepare for Cesarean section

- Placenta previa
  1. Definition—placenta is located over or very near the internal os
     a. Complete placenta previa—placenta completely covers the cervical os
     b. Partial placenta previa—cervical os partially covered by placenta
     c. Marginal placenta previa—edge of placenta within 1 cm of cervical os
  2. Etiology/predisposing factors
     a. Increased parity
     b. Advanced maternal age
     c. Previous Cesarean section
     d. Multiple gestation
  3. Signs and symptoms
     a. *Painless* vaginal bleeding during the third trimester 70–80% of the time
     b. Bleeding with contractions 10–20%
     c. Can be diagnosed before hallmark bleed with ultrasound
  4. Physical findings—no digital vaginal exam until placenta location is known; contraindicated with placenta previa
  5. Differential diagnosis—placental abruption
  6. Diagnostic testing—ultrasound confirmation
  7. Management
     a. Acute bleeding requires emergency Cesarean section
     b. Otherwise dependent on severity of symptoms and gestational age
     c. Bedrest and/or hospitalization usually indicated
     d. Rhogam for unsensitized Rh negative mother
     e. Generally delivered by C-section

- Placental abruption
  1. Definition—premature separation of the placenta from the uterine wall prior to delivery of the fetus
  2. Etiology
     a. Maternal hypertension
     b. Severe abdominal trauma
     c. Sudden decrease in uterine volume such as rupture of membranes with polyhydramnios or multiple gestation
     d. Cocaine use
     e. Previous abruption
  3. Incidence
     a. 1 in 80 deliveries
     b. Can be marginal abruption and not catastrophic
  4. Signs and symptoms/physical findings
     a. With complete abruption, *painful* vaginal bleeding, uterine rigidity, shock
     b. Less than complete abruptions have less severe presentations
     c. Bleeding can be concealed

  5. Differential diagnosis—placenta previa
  6. Diagnostic testing—ultrasound confirmation of condition of placenta
  7. Management
     a. Complete abruption
        (1) Notify consulting physician
        (2) Insert two large-bore IV catheters
        (3) Prepare for STAT C-section
        (4) Obtain blood type and cross-match for blood products including clotting factors
        (5) Trendelenberg position
        (6) O_2 at 10 L/min
        (7) Monitor fetal status
     b. Partial abruption
        (1) IV access
        (2) Monitor fetal status
        (3) Preparation in the event immediate surgical intervention is required

- Shoulder dystocia
  1. Definition—difficulty in delivery of shoulders secondary to anterior shoulder becoming impacted on the pelvic rim
  2. Etiology/risk factors
     a. Gestational diabetes
     b. History of macrosomic babies
     c. Maternal obesity
     d. Increased weight gain during pregnancy
     e. Small/abnormal/contracted pelvis
     f. Prior history of shoulder dystocia
     g. Estimated weight of fetus 1 pound larger than previous infants if a multiparous woman
  3. Incidence—less than 1% of all births
  4. Morbidity and mortality
     a. Maternal—extensive vaginal and perineal lacerations
     b. Fetal
        (1) Fractured clavicle
        (2) Brachial plexus injury
        (3) Hypoxia/anoxia
        (4) Fetal death
  5. Signs and symptoms
     a. "Turtle sign"—the immediate retraction of the fetal head against the perineum after extension
     b. Delayed restitution or need for facilitated restitution without descent
     c. Inability to deliver anterior shoulder with usual traction effort
  6. Management
     a. Anticipation of shoulder dystocia should be an indication or signal of need for emergency preparedness
     b. Immediately have any physician paged STAT

c. Notify other staff including anesthesia and the pediatrics team

d. Perform McRobert's maneuver—place mother in exaggerated lithotomy position (knees to shoulders)

e. Have suprapubic pressure (*not* fundal pressure) applied while exerting downward traction on baby's head while mother is pushing

f. Cut or extend episiotomy—controversial; catheterize woman to empty bladder

g. Attempt to rotate shoulders to oblique and repeat McRobert's maneuver and suprapubic pressure—insert a hand on either side of the fetal chest and attempt to rotate shoulders out of the anteroposterior diameter

h. Attempt Wood's screw maneuver
   (1) Using the same techniques
   (2) Rotate fetus 180° (keeping the back anterior)
   (3) If still impacted, continue rotation another 180°

i. Knee–chest position

j. Deliver posterior arm
   (1) Insert hand behind posterior shoulder
   (2) Splint arm and sweep across abdomen and chest until the hand can be grasped externally

k. Break the anterior clavicle—place thumbs along clavicle and force clavicle outward; controversial as have possibility of puncturing lung or injuring subclavian vessels

l. Zavanelli maneuver—rotate and flex head while replacing fetus into pelvic cavity followed by immediate C-section; controversial as associated with significant risk of infant morbidity and mortality

- Breech delivery—the elective vaginal delivery of infants in the breech presentation is no longer recommended by the American College of Obstetricians and Gynecologists. Vaginal delivery of breech presentation should be reserved only for breeches that present emergently and when birth is essentially inevitable.
  1. Definition—delivery of infant presenting with buttocks, feet, or knees
     a. Complete breech—legs and thighs are flexed with buttocks presenting
     b. Frank breech—legs extended on abdomen with flexed thighs and buttocks presenting; most common type of breech presentation
     c. Footling breech—one or both feet presenting
     d. Knee presentation—single or double knee(s) are presenting (most rare)
     e. Spontaneous vaginal breech delivery—birth without additional external assistance
     f. Assisted vaginal delivery (partial breech extraction)—spontaneous delivery to the umbilicus, remainder of the body delivered with assistance
     g. Total breech extraction—entire body extracted by birth attendant
  2. Incidence
     a. 3–4% at term
     b. At 28 weeks, 25% of all fetuses are breech
     c. Most convert to cephalic by 34 weeks' gestation
  3. Etiology/risk factors
     a. Presentation possibly related to the fetus accommodating to the shape of the uterus
        (1) Preterm fetuses position the head in the upper portion of the uterus being the larger portion of the body
        (2) At term, the largest part of the fetus is the head, thus causing it to descend into the pelvis
     b. Maternal indications
        (1) Gestational age
        (2) Fibroids
        (3) Uterine anomalies
        (4) Abnormal placentation
           (a) Placenta previa
           (b) Cornual fundal implantation
        (5) Oligohydramnios/polyhydramnios
     c. Fetal factors
        (1) Congenital anomalies—three-fold increase in anomalies with breech presentation
        (2) Short umbilical cord
  4. Morbidity/mortality
     a. Cord prolapse (1.5% of frank breech and 10% in other breech presentations)
     b. Traumatic vaginal delivery
        (1) Largest part of the fetus is delivered last
        (2) Head entrapment causing injury to organs, brain, and skull
     c. Increased perinatal morbidity and mortality
  5. Management and treatment
     a. Vaginal breech birth is a comanagement situation
     b. Criteria for candidates of vaginal breech birth
        (1) Frank breech presentation
        (2) EFW 2500–3800 g
        (3) Flexion of the fetal head
     c. Management decisions
        (1) Continuous fetal monitoring
        (2) IV access

(3) Use of oxytocin for protraction disorders very controversial; generally Cesarean section is indicated

(4) Generous episiotomy

(5) Empty bladder before second stage

(6) Should deliver as a double set-up in operating room

6. Delivery sequence for partial breech extraction

   a. "Hands off the breech" until the body is born to the umbilicus

   b. Second provider should be maintaining head flexion through the abdominal wall during entire descent

   c. Wrap the body with a warm dry towel for remainder of birth

   d. Pull down loop of cord

   e. From this point on, the mother is instructed to push continuously

   f. If the legs have not delivered spontaneously, they should be gently guided out of the vagina

   g. Downward traction then applied with the hands to baby's hips with thumbs in the sacroiliac region to encourage delivery of the anterior scapula

   h. If necessary, provider can encourage rotation to LSA

   i. Attendant delivers anterior arm by moving hand up the infant's back and over the top of the anterior shoulder sweeping the arm down across the chest and under the pubis with attendant's finger

   j. The infant is raised so the posterior arm can be delivered in the same manner

   k. The back should spontaneously rotate anteriorly

   l. Employ the Mauriceau-Smellie-Veit maneuver to maintain flexion of the head

     (1) With dominant hand palmar side up, place extended index finger in baby's mouth with chest and body resting on palm and legs straddling forearm

     (2) The other hand is placed on top of the baby with the index finger on one side and middle finger on the other side of the neck extending over the shoulder for traction

   m. Again apply downward traction until the suboccipital region (the hairline is seen coming under the pubic symphysis)

   n. Now apply upward traction while elevating body to deliver the head via the curve of Carus

- Face presentation

1. Definition—cephalic presentation with attitude of head in complete extension with occiput proximal to the spine; usually begins labor as a brow presentation

2. Incidence 1 in 250 births, higher in multiparas

3. Etiology

   a. Can be an indicator of CPD

   b. Multiple loops of nuchal cord

   c. Tumors of the neck

   d. Anencephalic fetus

4. Risk factors

   a. Can cause CPD because of the longer presenting diameter being obstructed in the pelvis

   b. If mentum is not anterior, fetus is unable to pass under the pubic symphysis

5. Diagnosis

   a. During Leopold's maneuver, occipital bone is easily palpated and prominent; head feels larger than expected

   b. During vaginal examination, facial landmarks can be palpated

6. Management

   a. Review clinical pelvimetry to assure pelvic adequacy

   b. Confirm position is mentum anterior as mentum posterior is contraindicated for vaginal birth

   c. Collaborate with consulting physician if protraction disorder occurs

   d. Pediatric attendance at the birth

- Twin gestation—intrapartum twins are always a collaborative management situation

1. Definitions—multiple gestation with two fetuses in the uterus

   a. Monozygotic twins—zygotic division between 4 and 8 days

     (1) Identical twins

     (2) One placenta

     (3) Generally one chorion, two amnions

   b. Dizygotic twins

     (1) Fraternal twins

     (2) Two placentas

     (3) Two chorions, two amnions

2. Incidence

   a. Monozygotic twinning rate stable at 1 per 250 births

   b. Dizygotic twinning rates increasing due to assisted reproductive technologies

3. Predisposing factors

   a. Family history

   b. Ovulation induction/in vitro fertilization

   c. Sub-Saharan African descent

4. Diagnosis

   a. Size larger than dates

   b. Auscultation of more than one fetal heart beat

   c. Abnormal Leopold's maneuver findings

   d. Ultimate diagnosis by ultrasound

5. Morbidity
   a. Premature labor and birth
   b. Premature rupture of membranes
   c. Malpresentation of second twin
   d. Cord prolapse
   e. Operative delivery for second twin
   f. SGA and IUGR babies
   g. Twin-to-twin transfusion
6. Management decisions
   a. Physician should be collaborating for all intrapartum decisions and present for the birth
   b. Ultrasound confirmation of presentation
   c. Intravenous catheter insertion
   d. Type and screen blood upon admission; some facilities require type and cross-match
   e. Continuous fetal monitoring
   f. Anesthesia presence for birth
   g. Pediatric attendance for birth
   h. Ultrasound machine in delivery room
   i. Bladder should be emptied prior to pushing
7. Management
   a. Birth of the first twin in usual fashion—if nuchal cord is present, DO NOT cut cord, attempt birth with cord intact
   b. Upon delivery, clamp cord and transfer baby to pediatric team
   c. Via fundal pressure, assistant can guide second twin into the pelvis depending upon presentation
   d. Confirm presentation of second twin based on ultrasound
   e. Timing of delivery is dependent upon fetal status
   f. Oxytocin augmentation can be used if contractions do not resume
   g. Birth of second twin
   h. Observe for postpartum hemorrhage

- Retained placenta
  1. Definition—placenta that has not separated from uterine wall after 60 minutes
  2. Predisposing factors
     a. Premature delivery
     b. Chorioamnionitis
     c. Prior Cesarean section
     d. Placenta previa
     e. Grand multiparity
  3. Etiology
     a. Structurally abnormal uterus
     b. Abnormal placentation—incidence has increased with increasing Cesarean rates
        (1) Placenta accreta—adherence to myometrium due to partial or total absence of decidua
        (2) Placenta increta—further extension into the myometrium with penetration into the uterine wall
        (3) Placenta percreta—further extension through the uterine wall to the serosa layer
  4. Management
     a. Facilitate usual methods of placental separation
        (1) Allow baby to nurse/nipple stimulation
        (2) Assist mother into squatting position
        (3) Empty maternal bladder
        (4) Injection of oxytocin solution (10 units in 20 cc normal saline) into the umbilical vein
     b. If third stage is more than 30 minutes, consider that placenta is retained; notify consulting physician
     c. Management in preparation for consulting physician
        (1) Monitor for bleeding or shock
        (2) Insert IV if none in place
        (3) Prepare mother for manual placenta removal
        (4) Notify anesthesia

- Postpartum hemorrhage
  1. Definition—blood loss of more than 500 cc
     a. Immediate—within first 24 hours
     b. Delayed—after the first 24 hours but within the first 6 weeks
  2. Etiology
     a. Predisposing factors
        (1) History of postpartum hemorrhage
        (2) Grand multiparity
        (3) Overdistended uterus
           (a) Multiple gestation
           (b) Polyhydramnios
           (c) Macrosomia
     b. Intrapartum factors
        (1) Induced or augmented labor
        (2) Prolonged labor
        (3) Precipitous labor
        (4) Uterine atony
  3. Management
     a. Notify consulting physician
     b. Uterine massage, if related to atony
     c. Medications
        (1) Oxytocin
        (2) Methylergonovine
        (3) Carboprost
     d. IV fluid bolus
     e. Bimanual compression if other measures unsuccessful
     f. Consider manual removal of placenta, if not delivered

g. Consider vaginal, sulcus, cervical lacerations as cause of bleeding

◘ THE NORMAL POSTPARTUM

- Data base
  1. Pregnancy highlights
     a. Gravidity/parity
     b. Obstetrical history
     c. Pertinent medical history
     d. Pertinent pregnancy diagnostic tests
        (1) Blood type and Rh
        (2) Rubella titer status
        (3) Hepatitis B status
        (4) HIV status
  2. Birth information
     a. Type of birth
        (1) Type of episiotomy/laceration
        (2) Type of operative birth
        (3) Reason for interventions
     b. Type of anesthesia/analgesia
     c. Sex of baby
     d. Weight of baby
     e. Apgar scores
     f. Method of feeding

- Physiologic and anatomical changes
  1. Uterus
     a. Immediately contracts to 1–2 fingerbreadths below the umbilicus but by 12 hours postdelivery, is at the level of the umbilicus
     b. By 2 weeks, no longer palpated abdominally
     c. By 6 weeks, returns to slightly larger than prepregnant size
     d. Involution—process of the uterus returning to the prepregnant state
        (1) Involves three steps
           (a) Contraction of the uterus
           (b) Autolysis of myometrial cells
           (c) Regeneration of the epithelium
        (2) Results from cell size reduction not cell number reduction
  2. Lochia
     a. Consists of the breakdown of myometrial placental bed eschar and decidual cells
     b. Three stages of discharge
        (1) Rubra—first 24–72 hours, superficial layer of decidua sloughs with debris and necrotic remains of the placenta
        (2) Serosa—from day 3 to day 10, serous to serosanguinous secretion
        (3) Alba—until cessation of flow, yellowish or white discharge

     c. Flow increases with additional activity initially but decreases progressively over the puerperium
     d. Total amount 150 to 400 cc
  3. Cervix, vagina, and perineum
     a. Cervix
        (1) Initially appears edematous, dilated 3–4 cm and bruised
        (2) At 7 days, 1 cm dilated and by day 10–12, fingertip dilated
        (3) Nonpregnant appearance and texture 1 month postdelivery
        (4) Multiparous—at completion of involution, external os does not return to its prepregnant appearance; remains somewhat wider with a transverse opening resembling a "fish-mouth"
     b. Vagina
        (1) Initially edematous, relaxed, sometimes bruised with decreased tone
        (2) Rugae return by 3 weeks postpartum
     c. Perineum
        (1) Edematous with decreased tone immediately after birth
        (2) Laceration and episiotomy repair should be well approximated
        (3) Skin should appear healed at 7 days with only linear scarring at 6 weeks
  4. Breasts
     a. Colostrum is produced upon birth of baby
     b. Engorgement occurs approximately 72 hours after birth
        (1) Human milk production begins in the upper-outer milk glands
        (2) Filling then occurs medially and inferiorly
        (3) Distention and stasis of vascular and lymphatic circulation causes engorgement as the ducts, lobules, and alveoli fill with milk
     c. "Let-down" reflex develops within the first 1 to 2 weeks
  5. Hematologic
     a. Within the first hours post delivery, cardiac output increases 60–80%
     b. Over first 48 hours, as diuresis occurs plasma volume decreases and cardiac output normalizes by 2 weeks
     c. Transient bradycardia occurs in first 1–2 days postpartum
     d. Can have transient leukocytosis in initial 48 hours
  6. Renal system changes
     a. Diuresis occurs within first 5 days due to extravascular fluid shifts

b. Bladder can be hypotonic and edematous immediately after the birth; resolves within 24 hours

7. Weight loss
   a. Weight loss of up to 15 pounds initially, may return to prepregnant weight by 6 weeks postpartum
   b. Weight loss facilitated by breastfeeding secondary to increased caloric requirements (350 calories more per day)

8. Gastrointestinal changes
   a. Peristalsis decreased in first 24 hours; increases risk of ileus after Cesarean section
   b. Liver enzymes including AST and ALT return to prepregnant values within 2 weeks

9. Abdominal changes
   a. Diastasis recti found in 75–80% of postpartum women—if diastasis after the postpartum period, future pregnancies will lack sufficient abdominal support leading to back pain
   b. Striae common in most postpartum women

10. Endocrine
    a. Breastfeeding women
       (1) Lactation is stimulated and prolactin secreted
       (2) By negative feedback mechanism, ovulation and menstruation are inhibited by increased prolactin and resulting estrogen suppression
       (3) Resumption of menses is variable with supplementation or food introduction
           (a) Generally ovulation occurs 14–30 days after weaning
           (b) First menses 14 days later
           (c) Mean time to ovulation is 190 days
    b. Nonbreastfeeding women
       (1) Prolactin levels fall after initial engorgement
       (2) Hormonal shifts to stimulate ovulation begin approximately 3–4 weeks postpartum
       (3) First menses at 6–8 weeks postpartum, 70% by 12 weeks

11. Vital signs
    a. Temperature
       (1) Stabilizes during the first 24 hours postpartum
       (2) Should not be over 100.4°F
    b. Pulse
       (1) Should remain within normal limits
       (2) More than 100 bpm could be significant for infection or posthemorrhage anemia
    c. Respiratory rate—remains normal

d. Blood pressure
   (1) Remains normal
   (2) Blood pressure of greater than 140/90, evaluate for postpartum preeclampsia
   (3) Blood pressure of less than 90/60, evaluate causes of hypotension
       (a) Blood loss
       (b) Medication reaction

◘ ASSESSMENT OF MATERNAL RESPONSE TO BABY

- Early attachment and bonding
  1. First hour after birth—maternal sensitive period
     a. Initial bonding occurs during this time
     b. Mother and baby should *not* be separated
     c. Signs of attachment
        (1) Initial touching with fingertips progressing to entire hand with stroking and massaging baby
        (2) "En face" posturing between mother and baby
        (3) Using high-pitched speaking voice
        (4) Bonding is facilitated during the first hour of life, the quiet alert phase for the baby
  2. Attachment
     a. Privacy should be arranged for parents as soon as possible after the birth
     b. Attachment is a progressive process during the initial postpartum period

- Psychological response to childbearing
  1. Positive reactions
     a. Sense of achievement in giving birth
     b. Sense of empowerment and strength
     c. Thrill of new baby
  2. Negative reactions
     a. Sense of loss if birth was not as anticipated
     b. Feeling of mistrust of body if unable to complete the birth process or if birth was premature

- Postpartum blues and depression
  1. Postpartum blues
     a. 80% of all women
     b. Begins within 3–5 days of birth, concurrent with profound hormonal shifts
     c. Very labile emotions (giddiness thru sadness and crying), usually defy explanation
     d. Generally time limited over 1–2 weeks
     e. Supportive, sensitive care is usually all that is required
  3. Postpartum depression/psychosis
     a. Approximately 10% incidence of depression, true postpartum psychosis in less than 1% of women

   b. Onset of symptoms around 4–6 weeks, generally worsen over time
   c. Symptoms are the same as for major depression in nonpostpartum woman
   d. Symptoms can incapacitate women
      (1) Unable to perform activities of daily living
      (2) Can have suicidal or homicidal ideation
      (3) Apathy towards themselves and their babies
   e. Symptoms do not improve over time; more likely they worsen
   f. Diagnosis—screen all postpartum women for depression with Edinburgh Postnatal Depression Scale; rule out postpartum thyroiditis, anemia, infection, sleep deprivation
   g. Require psychiatric evaluation and treatment usually including medication
   h. Women previously treated for clinical depression have increased risk of postpartum depression
   i. Psychosis—disorganized thinking, behavior, speech; auditory or visual perceptual disturbances; delusions—medical emergency

- Grief
  1. Can be related to losing a pregnancy, having a viable baby but not meeting expectations, i.e., congenital anomalies or organic cause such as postpartum depression
  2. Stages of grief
     a. Shock
     b. Suffering
     c. Resolution

◘ MANAGEMENT PLAN FOR THE POSTPARTUM PERIOD

- Evaluation of maternal well-being

- Chart review

- History
  1. Family history
  2. Past medical, surgical, and obstetrical history
  3. Review of prenatal care
  4. Review of intrapartum period
  5. Infant data

- Physical examination
  1. Vital signs
  2. General appearance and affect
  3. Breasts
     a. Condition of breasts and nipples
     b. Status of milk production
  4. Abdominal examination
     a. Uterine fundal examination
     b. Abdominal musculature
     c. Bladder status
  5. Perineum
     a. REEDA (redness, ecchymosis, erythema, drainage, and approximation)
     b. Lochia
     c. Status of lacerations/episiotomy
     d. Hemorrhoids
  6. Extremities
     a. Calf tenderness and warmth
     b. Edema
     c. Varicosities
  7. Pain assessment
  8. Emotional status

- Diet—after normal birth, regular diet immediately postpartum

- Activity
  1. Out of bed as desired
  2. Should be escorted out of bed for the first time, secondary to risk of syncope

- Hygiene
  1. Should receive instructions in perineal care
  2. Topical anesthetics, if indicated

- Contraception
  1. Nonbreastfeeding women generally have menses prior to the 6-week visit; therefore, birth control should be initiated prior to discharge
  2. Hormonal methods (combination hormonal methods—pills, patch, vaginal ring; progestin-only methods—progestin-only pills, depo medroxyprogesterone DMPA, subdermal implant)
     a. Combination hormonal methods not indicated for breastfeeding women initially postpartum
     b. DMPA, progestin-only pills, and subdermal implant good choices for breastfeeding women
  3. Barrier methods
     a. Cervical cap/diaphragm—cannot be fit until involution is complete
     b. Male and female condoms—can be used immediately
  4. Spermicides
     a. Foam, cream, vaginal contraceptive film, sponge
     b. Should delay use until lochia ceases
  5. Intrauterine contraception (IUC)—levonorgestrel or copper-containing
     a. Can be placed immediately postdelivery but has a 30% expulsion rate
     b. If not placed within 48 hours postpartum, need to wait until 6 weeks postpartum

6. Lactational amenorrhea method
   a. Full or nearly full breastfeeding
   b. Infant less than 6 months old
   c. No menses
   d. Choose alternative method if woman and infant do not fit all three criteria
7. Tubal ligation
   a. Permanent method of contraception
   b. Most easily accomplished during hospital stay
   c. Generally need to obtain consent prior to birth

- Diagnostic tests
  1. Complete blood count
     a. Commonly performed first morning after birth
     b. Only profound anemia will change management
  2. Cord blood testing for blood type, Rh, and Coombs
  3. Kleihauer-Betke screen if Rh negative

- Immunizations
  1. Rubella vaccine may be given prior to discharge if not immune to rubella
  2. RhoGAM prior to discharge if indicated

▫ POSTPARTAL DISCOMFORTS

- Involutional pain
  1. Uncommon in primigravidas, increases in intensity with each subsequent birth
  2. Increases with nursing
  3. Nonpharmacologic relief
     a. Maintain empty bladder and bowels
     b. Prone position may relieve pain
  4. Pharmacologic relief
     a. Acetaminophen, ibuprofen, codeine
     b. Ketorolac

- Diuresis—maintain fluids to prevent dehydration

- Breast engorgement
  1. Initiate breastfeeding early and often
  2. Supportive brassiere
  3. Warm compresses
  4. If bottle feeding, tight brassiere, ice packs, analgesics, reassurance about time limitation, iced cabbage leaves for comfort

- Perineal pain
  1. Evaluate by REEDA
  2. Topical medications
     a. Witch hazel pads
     b. Dibucaine, benzocaine

- Constipation
  1. Increase fluids and fiber; stool softener
  2. Encourage ambulation
  3. Laxatives

- Hemorrhoids
  1. Ice packs
  2. Topical anesthetics
  3. Referral if thrombosed

▫ QUESTIONS

Select the best answer.

1. At 38 weeks' gestation, Ms. Jones presents to your birth center complaining of a small amount of watery, clear-to-whitish vaginal discharge for the past 8 hours. She has been having Braxton Hicks contractions for a couple of days; the baby is moving on a regular basis, but now she just "doesn't feel right." What would you do in your initial assessment related to her presenting symptoms?

   a. Obtain 20-minute fetal monitor strip to assure reactivity.
   b. Perform sterile speculum exam to R/O rupture of membranes versus vaginal infection.
   c. Contact consulting physician regarding premature rupture of membranes protocol.
   d. Send Ms. Jones home with reassurance and instructions to rest until better labor pattern is established.

2. Mrs. Hogan, a 37-year-old G4 P0 at 35 weeks, presents saying she is having bright red bleeding and clots for 2 hours since intercourse with her husband. She has saturated 2 pads in 2 hours. She is *not* having any pain. The most probable diagnosis is:

   a. Placenta previa
   b. Cervical irritation from intercourse
   c. Placental abruption
   d. Normal bloody show

3. Tocolysis of premature labor contractions is most effectively achieved by:

   a. NSAIDS
   b. Beta sympathomimetics such as terbutaline
   c. Intravenous fluids
   d. Oxytocics

4. Which client is most at risk for placental abruption?

   a. 19-year-old G2 P0010 in preterm labor at 35 weeks

b. 28-year-old G1 pregnant with twins with spontaneous rupture of membranes at 37 weeks

c. 28-year-old G3 P2002 with induced labor at 41 weeks

d. 41-year-old G1 pregnant who had low-lying placenta in first trimester

5. What is the major risk of multifetal gestation?

a. Eclampsia
b. Gestational diabetes
c. Cephalopelvic disproportion
d. Preterm birth

6. The cardinal movements of labor and birth are which of the following?

a. Flexion, descent, internal rotation, extension, restitution, external rotation
b. Descent, flexion, extension, internal rotation, external rotation, restitution
c. Descent, flexion, internal rotation, extension, restitution, external rotation
d. Descent, flexion, internal rotation, extension, external rotation, restitution

7. The cardinal movement responsible for the birth of the fetal head in the vertex presentation is:

a. Flexion
b. Restitution
c. Extension
d. External rotation

8. The definition of postpartum hemorrhage is:

a. Blood loss in excess of 500 cc or more after the third stage of labor
b. Blood loss in excess of 750 cc during the entire labor
c. Blood loss of more than 500 cc before a C-section
d. Blood loss of 750 cc or more after the third stage of labor

9. Which of the following statements concerning Apgar scores is correct?

a. Scoring is especially useful in assessment of the preterm infant.
b. Scoring is less useful when the infant is postterm.
c. A score of less than 7 at 1 minute correlates with increased neonatal morbidity.
d. Five-minute scoring has a relationship to neonatal morbidity and mortality.

10. Infants born to mothers with gestational diabetes are at increased risk for:

a. Hyperbilirubinema
b. IUGR
c. Hyperglycemia
d. Shoulder dystocia

A client who is a G3 P2002 at 38 weeks presents with regular uterine contractions every 4–6 minutes for 60 seconds for the past 6 hours. Her vaginal exam is 1–2 cm/30%/–2, vertex with intact membranes.

11. At this time, the patient is in:

a. Prodromal labor
b. Latent labor
c. Active labor
d. Not in labor

12. Your management plan at this time is:

a. Discharge home with instructions
b. Ambulate for 2 hours and then reassess
c. Contact consulting physician for augmentation of labor
d. Need additional information prior to formulating plan

Three hours later, you re-assess this client. Contractions are now every 4 minutes for 60 seconds. Her exam is 2 cm/50%/–2, vertex with intact membranes. The fetal heart rate is 150 with audible accelerations by Doppler.

13. At this time your client is in:

a. Prolonged latent phase
b. Latent phase of labor
c. Active phase of labor
d. Cannot make a determination based on this information

Six hours later the client has the same contraction pattern every 4 minutes for 60 seconds. Her exam is now 2–3 cm/100%/0, vertex with intact membranes. The fetal heart rate remains in the 140s to 150s with audible accelerations. The client is exhausted and is no longer coping well with the contractions and "just wants it over."

14. Your diagnosis at this time is:

a. Latent phase of labor
b. Prolonged latent phase of labor
c. Arrested labor
d. Protracted active phase of labor

15. Your management plan at this time is:

a. Discharge home with encouragement and instructions to return when the contractions become closer

b.   Contact consulting physician regarding your plan for oxytocin augmentation

c.   Encourage her to continue with her original plan for an unmedicated childbirth

d.   Offer medication of morphine 10 mg IM so she can get some sleep and potentially correct this dysfunctional labor pattern

16. C. S. presents to your office stating she is pregnant and wants to know her due date. The first day of her last period was February 4. Her due date by menstrual dating (Naegele's rule) would be:

a.   November 11
b.   October 28
c.   May 11
d.   November 4

17. The denominator of breech presentation is the:

a.   Symphysis pubis
b.   Sacrum
c.   Feet
d.   Shoulders

18. Your client is in active labor making appropriate progress thus far. Currently her exam is 6 cm/100%/−2, vertex with intact membranes. During your exam, you notice the position of the vertex is LOT and sagittal suture of the fetus is closer to the maternal sacrum. Your diagnosis at this time is:

a.   Deep transverse pelvic arrest
b.   Anterior asynclitism
c.   Failure to descend
d.   Posterior asynclitism

19. Your management plan for this patient would be:

a.   Artificial rupture of membranes
b.   Epidural anesthesia
c.   Pitocin augmentation
d.   Encourage movement and position change

20. On the monitor strip of the same client, you notice the fetal heart rate has intermittently been 100–110 bpm for 20–30 seconds at a time for 10–15 minutes with good return to baseline. You would document this as:

a.   Variable decelerations
b.   Late decelerations
c.   Fetal bradycardia
d.   Cannot determine from this information

21. The largest diameter of the fetal head is the:

a.   Verticomental
b.   Submentobregmatic
c.   Occipitofrontal
d.   Suboccipitobregmatic

22. Intermittent auscultation of the fetal heart rate during labor is:

a.   Inferior to continuous electronic fetal monitoring
b.   Acceptable only for out-of-hospital birth
c.   Acceptable for the fetal monitoring of certain patients
d.   Correlated to lower Apgar scores than babies born after continuous fetal monitoring

23. Your patient states that she does *not* want an episiotomy no matter what happens. Your management of this situation would be:

a.   Discuss the indications for episiotomy and reinforce that you would obtain consent prior to performing the procedure, if necessary
b.   Teach her perineal massage antenatally and hope that she will not need an episiotomy
c.   Explain to her that skilled midwives never perform episiotomies
d.   Explain that since this is her first baby, that she will probably need an episiotomy to prevent serious laceration

24. A client presents while you are covering Labor and Delivery. She is a 33-year-old G3 P2002 at term in labor with ruptured membranes. Your exam reveals 5 cm/90% effaced/0 station but you are unable to palpate fontanels or sutures. You suspect that you feel the orbital ridge in the anteroposterior diameter and the chin at 3 o'clock. If this is the case, what is the presentation?

a.   ROT
b.   LMT
c.   RMT
d.   ROA

25. Three hours later, the same client is completely dilated/100% effaced/0 station. Your exam now reveals that the presentation is MA. What would your next step be?

a.   Prepare client for urgent C-section
b.   Manually attempt to flex the fetal head
c.   Encourage patient to push as effectively as possible
d.   Allow patient to only push in the hands and knees position to allow the fetal head to rotate

26. During an assisted breech birth, if a nuchal arm is encountered, what should you do?

a.   Exert steady downward traction on the entire fetus
b.   Slowly rotate the infant 180° to attempt to dislodge the arm

c. Raise the baby in a warm towel above the plane of the vagina

d. Sweep the arm down by hooking the elbow and pulling the arm down

27. The most common cause of postpartum hemorrhage is:

a. Sulcus tears
b. Episiotomy extensions to third- and fourth-degree lacerations
c. Uterine atony
d. Cervical lacerations

28. The process of involution takes place over which of the following time frames?

a. The first 6 weeks postpartum
b. The first 24 hours postpartum
c. The first 2 weeks postpartum
d. The first year postpartum

The following is the clinical picture of your client. She is a G1 P0 at 39 weeks with an uncomplicated pregnancy. Her labor started at 4:00 a.m. with regular contractions. She was admitted at 8:00 a.m. when her exam was 2–3 cm/100%/–2 station, vertex, membranes intact.

At 12:00 p.m. her exam was 3–4 cm/100%/–2, intact.

At 4:00 p.m., her exam was 4 cm/100%/–2, intact.

At 7:30 p.m. her exam was 5–6 cm/100%/–1, intact.

At 8:15 p.m., she ruptured membranes for light meconium stained fluid.

At 10:00 p.m., her exam was 8 cm/100%/0 station.

29. Based on the information provided above, at 12:00 p.m. what was the most appropriate diagnosis related to your client's labor progress?

a. Latent phase
b. Protracted latent phase
c. Unable to make determination with this information
d. Active labor

30. At 7:30 p.m., what was the most appropriate diagnosis?

a. Unable to make determination based on the information provided
b. Protracted active phase of labor
c. Arrest of labor in the active phase
d. Active phase of labor

31. At 10:00 p.m., she requests something for pain because she states the pain is intolerable now and she is feeling increased pelvic pressure. What would *not* be indicated for pain relief at this time?

a. Epidural anesthesia
b. Intravenous narcotics
c. Pudendal anesthesia
d. Paracervical block

32. At 10:50 p.m., you notice on the fetal monitor strip early decelerations that occur with every contraction. The baseline heart rate is in the 140s with average variability. What do you suspect the cause of these decelerations is?

a. Maternal hypotension
b. Head compression
c. Uteroplacental insufficiency
d. Fetal distress related to the meconium fluid

33. The benefit of placing an internal scalp electrode on a fetus in labor is:

a. The ability to assess short-term variability
b. The ability to detect decelerations
c. It keeps the client in bed
d. The ability to assess long-term variability

34. If you are performing a fetal scalp sample to assess fetal pH, what level would cause you to immediately prepare the patient for a C-section?

a. 7.41
b. 7.21
c. 7.20
d. 7.16

35. What is the most common position for birth?

a. ROA
b. LOA
c. ROP
d. LOP

36. The long arc rotation is most commonly performed by babies beginning labor in which presentation?

a. LOP
b. LSA
c. ROA
d. LOA

37. In the second stage of labor, how frequently should the BP of low-risk women be checked?

a. Every 30 minutes
b. Every 5 minutes
c. Every 60 minutes
d. Every 15 minutes

38. When is the most appropriate time to administer pudendal anesthesia for perineal pain relief in the multiparous client?

    a. For the repair of any laceration or episiotomy
    b. When the head distends the perineum and client complains of the "ring of fire"
    c. When the vertex is at +2
    d. At approximately 8–9 cm dilated

39. What is the largest group of muscles in the pelvic musculature?

    a. Levator ani
    b. Pubococcygeus
    c. Bulbocavernosus
    d. Sphincter ani

40. In a second-degree laceration, which structure is *not* involved?

    a. Vaginal mucosa
    b. Deep transverse perineal muscles
    c. Rectal sphincter
    d. Hymenal ring

41. The Ritgen maneuver is used to:

    a. Slow down the descent of the fetal head during birth
    b. To control expulsion of the fetal head at the time of birth
    c. To avoid lacerations or the need for an episiotomy
    d. To assist in the delivery of the fetal head during extension

42. What complication may be encountered if a placenta is delivered by the Duncan mechanism?

    a. Increased perineal lacerations
    b. Increased bleeding
    c. Increased hemorrhoids due to extra maternal pushing effort
    d. Uterine inversion

43. Which of the following would *not* be included in the differential diagnosis of premature labor?

    a. Urinary tract infection
    b. Appendicitis
    c. Renal colic
    d. Heartburn

44. The fetal heart rate variability is predominantly controlled by:

    a. The parasympathetic nervous system
    b. The baroreceptors
    c. The chemorectors
    d. The sympathetic nervous system

45. During uterine contractions, intervillous blood flow to the placenta

    a. Increases
    b. Decreases
    c. Remains unchanged
    d. Has not been studied in humans

46. Average long-term variability of the fetal heart rate is a change of how many beats per minute from the baseline?

    a. Less than 2
    b. 2–6
    c. 6–10
    d. 10–15

47. Which of the following would *not* cause an alteration in the LTV of the fetal heart rate?

    a. Medications
    b. Congenital cardiac anomalies of the fetus
    c. Placenta previa
    d. Fetal activity patterns

48. Your client, who you are comanaging with your consulting physician, is 33 weeks and 4 days pregnant admitted with premature labor with a cervical exam of 2–3cm/80%/–1, vertex, intact. She is currently on $MgSO_4$ at 3.0 g/hour with occasional contractions. During rounds, she complains of feeling flushed and hot, lethargic and sort of short of breath, which usually gets better when she changes position. Which response would be best to address her complaints?

    a. "The $MgSO_4$ commonly makes you feel like this, but hopefully they will start weaning the medication today."
    b. "Well, since you are almost 34 weeks, I could ask the doctor if we can discontinue the medication now."
    c. "I don't think that you should be having shortness of breath like you are; I am going to have the physician see you and order a chest radiograph."
    d. "Being a little uncomfortable is so much better than giving birth to a 33-week-old infant."

49. Which of the following conditions would *not* necessitate continuous fetal monitoring?

    a. Labor at 41 weeks and 1 day
    b. Thick meconium stained fluid
    c. Nonreactive NST who is now in labor
    d. IV narcotics

50. Mothers in premature labor are given glucocorticosteroids to:

    a. Help stop the uterine contractions
    b. Prevent infections especially chorioamnionitis

c. Speed the maturation of the fetal respiratory system, including the production of surfactant

d. Prevent muscle wasting commonly seen in bedrest patients

51. Kelly Jones, a G3 P2002 at 37 weeks and 1 day, presents to Labor and Delivery with regular contractions every 2–3 minutes for 5 hours. Your vaginal exam reveals 6 cm/100%/–2, LSA with ruptured membranes positive for light meconium. What is your next step:

a. Admit for expectant management

b. Discuss with Kelly her birth plan

c. Await a reactive tracing before making a management plan

d. Notify your consulting physician and prepare for a C-section

52. A complete breech presentation is described as:

a. One or two feet are the presenting part

b. Legs and thighs are flexed with buttocks presenting

c. The baby is flexed at the hips

d. The knees are the presenting part

53. Your client, who is 41 weeks and 5 days pregnant, presents for postdates testing including a nonstress test. When you assess the tracing after 20 minutes, the FHR is 140-145/min, there are no decelerations, the LTV is average but the tracing does not meet criteria for reactivity. What would you do?

a. Admit the client and induce labor

b. Begin a contraction stress test

c. Use the vibroacoustic stimulator

d. Continue nonstress test for another 20 minutes

54. The same client as above is now in labor, at 4 cm/100%/+1, vertex, and she is having contractions every 3–5 minutes for 50–70 sec, which are moderate to palpation. The FHR baseline is still in the 140s, but she is having variable decelerations to the 110s with good return to baseline and average variability. What action would be contraindicated at this time?

a. Allowing the patient to get into the Jacuzzi

b. Beginning oxytocin augmentation

c. Inserting an intravenous catheter

d. Expectant management

55. The definition of engagement is:

a. The fetal head reaches the pelvic floor

b. The head descends to the level of the ischial spines

c. The biparietal diameter is at the level of the pelvic inlet

d. The head is on the perineum

56. When an IUPC is used for the assessment of uterine contractions, the adequacy is quantified in:

a. Millimeters of mercury

b. Mild, moderate, and strong

c. Montevideo units

d. Centimeters

57. By internal monitoring of uterine contractions, which of the following must be achieved in the course of 10 minutes in order to be considered adequate contractile strength to dilate the cervix?

a. 80–100 Montevideo units

b. 80–100 mm Hg

c. 180–200 Montevideo units

d. 180–200 mm Hg

58. Which of the following would represent a contraindication for the use of an IUPC?

a. Maternal birth plan

b. Breech presentation

c. HIV

d. Lack of labor progress

59. In the first stage of labor, for low-risk laboring women, the interval for intermittent fetal heart rate auscultation is:

a. 15 minutes

b. 20 minutes

c. 30 minutes

d. 60 minutes

60. All of the following are risk factors for preterm labor except:

a. Age

b. Smoking

c. Race

d. Sex of fetus

61. Shelley Blank is seen in Labor and Delivery at 33 weeks and 1 day complaining of menstrual-type cramping for the past 3 hours. She denies bleeding or ruptured membranes. The fetus is active. The EFM reveals occasional uterine contractions approximately every 8–12 minutes. The FHR is 135–140/min. Which of the following tests would be most important in formulating your management plan?

a. Complete blood count

b. Cervical culture

c. Urine culture

d. Ultrasound

62. What would be the next step in your management plan?

    a. Expectant management until the lab results are back
    b. Tocolysis
    c. Pain management
    d. Additional information is necessary to formulate the management plan

63. Which of the following represents a risk factor for shoulder dystocia?

    a. Advanced maternal age
    b. Epidural anesthesia
    c. Polyhydramnios
    d. Maternal obesity

64. Which of the following elective vaginal births is no longer recommended?

    a. Brow presentation
    b. Face presentation
    c. Breech presentation
    d. Vertex presentation

65. During the birth of twins, which represents a maneuver that should *not* be performed?

    a. Artificial rupture of membranes
    b. Clamping and cutting of a nuchal cord
    c. McRobert's maneuver
    d. Breech delivery of the second twin

66. Which of the following represents a risk factor for retained placenta?

    a. Preterm delivery
    b. Multiple gestation
    c. Multiparity
    d. Postterm pregnancy

67. While repairing a first-degree laceration, you notice a continual "trickle" of bright red blood from the vagina. As you continue your repair the bleeding becomes more brisk. What would be the next step after fundal massage in your management plan?

    a. Bimanual compression
    b. Adding 20 additional units of oxytocin in the IV
    c. Discussion with the consulting physician regarding management plan
    d. Methylergonovine IM if BP is normotensive

68. Thirty six hours after birth, you find Megan, a 16-year-old, crying quietly with the baby in her room as you perform a.m. rounds. What would be the most helpful response?

    a. Prescribe an SSRI because adolescents are prone to postpartum depression
    b. Encourage her to focus on her baby's needs as her first priority now
    c. Explain that it is normal to have a combination of sadness and euphoria so close to the time of the birth
    d. Conduct a screening test for possible postpartum depression

69. During postpartum rounds, your multiparous client is very pleased with her birth and is clearly bonding with her new baby girl. She is successfully nursing her baby every 3 hours for 5 minutes. She is asking about early discharge and wants to go home as soon as possible. Her only complaint is that her left leg is sore because of her need to deliver in stirrups. What would be the most important piece of your assessment?

    a. Availability of assistance at home with her two other children to assure her rest
    b. Breast exam and assessment to check for milk production to ensure adequacy of feeding prior to discharge
    c. Dietary recall to insure adequate kcal and fluids to produce adequate human milk
    d. Examination of the lower legs to be sure that the muscle strain that she is complaining about is simply related to positioning

70. The same client would like to resume birth control prior to discharge. Which method would be most appropriate for this client?

    a. DMPA
    b. IUD
    c. Combination birth control pills
    d. Diaphragm with spermicidal cream

71. During the second stage of labor, for the low-risk client, the fetal heart rate should be monitored:

    a. Every 5 minutes
    b. Every 15 minutes
    c. Every 30 minutes
    d. Continuously

72. A sudden bradycardia seen in the second stage of labor after an uneventful labor course and previously normal fetal heart tracing is commonly caused by:

    a. A vagal response in the fetus related to descent
    b. Fetal hypoxia related to length of labor
    c. Cord prolapse
    d. Uteroplacental insufficiency

73. Which of the following FHR tracings are indicative of nonreassuring fetal status?

    a. A prolonged deceleration with recovery to baseline with average short-term variability
    b. Variable decelerations that become more pronounced during the second stage but with normal FHR between pushing efforts
    c. A rising baseline and absence of short-term variability
    d. Late decelerations with return to baseline and average long-term variability between decelerations

74. The risk factor that is most predictive of a preterm birth during a current pregnancy is:

    a. Uterine contractions
    b. Prior preterm labor
    c. Prior preterm birth
    d. Preeclampsia

75. The pain of the second stage of labor is caused by:

    a. Uterine muscle hypoxia with lactic acid build-up and distention of the musculature of the pelvic floor
    b. Cervical and lower uterine segment stretching and traction on the ovaries, fallopian tubes, and pelvic ligaments
    c. Pressure on the bony pelvis, urethra, bladder, and rectum
    d. Fundal uterine displacement and extension of the fetal lie

76. Hemodynamic changes during the initial postpartum period include:

    a. Elevated cardiac output for up to 48 hours after the birth
    b. Decreased WBC during the first 72 hours postpartum
    c. Elevated blood pressure for 48 hours after the birth
    d. Decreased urine output for the first 24 hours

77. In the initial newborn period, a 10-minute Apgar score is performed:

    a. Routinely
    b. If the 1-minute Apgar score was less than 7
    c. If the 5-minute Apgar score was less than 7
    d. If the combined Apgar score at 1 and five minutes is less than 16

78. The bluish discoloration of the baby's hands and feet within the first 24–48 hours after birth is:

    a. Acrocyanosis
    b. Circumoral cyanosis
    c. Central cyanosis
    d. Mongolian spots

◻ ANSWERS

1.	b	40.	c
2.	a	41.	d
3.	b	42.	b
4.	b	43.	d
5.	d	44.	a
6.	c	45.	b
7.	c	46.	c
8.	a	47.	c
9.	d	48.	c
10.	d	49.	a
11.	b	50.	c
12.	b	51.	d
13.	b	52.	b
14.	b	53.	d
15.	d	54.	a
16.	a	55.	b
17.	b	56.	c
18.	b	57.	c
19.	d	58.	c
20.	a	59.	c
21.	d	60.	d
22.	c	61.	c
23.	a	62.	d
24.	b	63.	d
25.	c	64.	c
26.	d	65.	b
27.	c	66.	a
28.	a	67.	d
29.	a	68.	c
30.	b	69.	d
31.	b	70.	a
32.	b	71.	b
33.	a	72.	a
34.	d	73.	c
35.	b	74.	c
36.	a	75.	c
37.	d	76.	a
38.	d	77.	c
39.	a	78.	a

◘ BIBLIOGRAPHY

Albers, L. (2007). The evidence for physiologic management of the active phase of the first stage of labor. *Journal of Midwifery and Women's Health, 52*(3), 207–215.

American College of Obstetricians and Gynecologists (ACOG). (2006). The Apgar score. *Committee Opinion No. 333.* Washington, DC: Author.

American College of Obstetricians and Gynecologists (ACOG). (2006). Episiotomy. *Practice Bulletin No. 71.* Washington, DC: Author.

American College of Obstetricians and Gynecologists (ACOG). (2003). Management of preterm labor. *Practice Bulletin No. 43.* Washington, DC: Author.

American College of Obstetricians and Gynecologists (ACOG). (2002). Shoulder dystocia. *Practice Bulletin No 40.* Washington, DC: Author.

Blackburn, S. T. (2002). *Maternal, fetal and neonatal physiology: A clinical perspective* (2nd ed.). Philadelphia, PA: W. B. Saunders.

Butarro, T. M., Trybulski, J., Bailey, P. P., & Sandberg-Cook, J. (2008). *Primary care: A collaborative practice* (3rd ed.). Philadelphia, PA: Mosby Elsevier.

Coad, J. (2001). *Anatomy and physiology for midwives.* Edinburgh, UK: Mosby, Inc.

Creasy, R., & Resnik, R. (2009). *Maternal fetal medicine: Principles and practice* (6th ed.). Philadelphia, PA: W. B. Saunders.

Cunningham, F. G. et al. (Eds.). (2001). *Williams Obstetrics* (21st ed.). New York: McGraw-Hill.

Enkin, M., Krurse, M. J. N. C., Nelison, J., Crowther, C. (2000). *A guide to effective care in pregnancy and childbirth* (3rd ed.). Oxford, UK: Oxford University Press.

Gabbe, S., Simpson, J., Niebyl, J., Galen, H. et al. (2007). *Obstetrics: Normal and problem pregnancies* (5th ed.). Philadelphia, PA: Mosby Elsevier.

Gibbs, R., Karlan, B., Haney, A., & Nygaard, I. (2008). *Danforth's obstetrics and gynecology* (10th ed.). Philadelphia, PA: Lippincott, Williams, and Wilkins.

Hatcher, R. A. et al. (2007). *Contraceptive technology* (19th ed.). New York: Ardent Media.

Lowdermilk, D., & Perry, S. (2007). *Maternity and women's health* (9th ed.). Philadelphia, PA: Mosby Elsevier.

Riordan, J., & Auerbach, K. (2010). *Breastfeeding and human lactation* (4th ed.). Sudbury, MA: Jones and Bartlett.

Seidel, H. M., Rosenstein, B. J., & Pathal, A. (2001). *Primary care of the newborn* (3rd ed.). St. Louis: Mosby, Inc.

Tharpe, N., & Farley, C. (2009). *Clinical practice guidelines for midwifery and women's health* (3rd ed.). Sudbury, MA: Jones and Bartlett.

Varney, H., Kreibs, J., & Gegor, C. (2004). *Varney's midwifery* (4th ed.). Sudbury, MA: Jones and Bartlett.

7

Gynecological Disorders

Penelope Morrison Bosarge

◻ MENSTRUAL AND ENDOCRINE DISORDERS

Premenstrual Syndrome (PMS)

- Definition—the cyclic occurrence, in luteal phase, of a group of distressing physical and psychological symptoms, which begin at or after ovulation and resolve shortly after onset of menses and that disrupt normal activities and interpersonal relationships

- Etiology/Incidence
  1. Unknown etiology; multifactorial and multiorgan disorder; suggested causes include metabolic and endocrine disorders, alterations in estrogen or progesterone levels, withdrawal of endogenous endorphins, fluid imbalance, vitamin and mineral deficiencies, and altered carbohydrate metabolism
  2. Prevalence may be greater than 50% with most women not requiring treatment; severe cases occur in 3–10% of women with PMS

- Signs and symptoms
  1. Symptoms recur cyclically in the luteal phase with symptom-free period in the follicular phase
  2. Range from mild to severe, resulting in interference with normal activities and personal relationships
     a. Physical
        (1) Headache
        (2) Breast changes
        (3) Fluid retention
        (4) Swelling
        (5) Abdominal bloating
        (6) Nausea/vomiting
        (7) Alterations in appetite
        (8) Food cravings
        (9) Lethargy/fatigue
        (10) Exacerbations of preexisting conditions, such as asthma
     b. Psychological
        (1) Irritability
        (2) Depression
        (3) Anxiety
        (4) Sleep alterations
        (5) Inability to concentrate
        (6) Anger
        (7) Violent behavior
        (8) Crying
        (9) Confusion
        (10) Changes in libido

- Physical findings—no specific physical findings

- Differential diagnosis
  1. A diagnosis of exclusion; all others must be ruled out
  2. Depression and/or anxiety
  3. Bipolar affective disorder
  4. Alcohol or substance abuse
  5. Personality disorders
  6. Chronic fatigue syndrome
  7. Fibromyalgia
  8. Diabetes
  9. Brain tumor

10. Thyroid disease
11. Hyperprolactinemia
12. Perimenopause

- Diagnostic tests/findings
  1. Documentation of symptoms in a diary fashion for 2 to 3 months, to evaluate for symptom consistency with ovulation and menses; retrospective recall inaccurate
  2. Individualized testing, based upon symptoms, may include glucose tolerance test and thyroid profile; hormone levels of little value

- Management/Treatment
  1. Nonmedical management
     a. No standard treatment; goal is to isolate symptom groups from history and diary and treat symptomatically
     b. Options for treatment
        (1) Self-help strategies recommended as first line therapy; help client understand the possible causes of symptoms, reassuring her that no serious health threats exist, and there are no quick cures; patience and team effort are key
        (2) Suggested dietary revisions are restriction of salt to 3 g, refined sugar to 5 tsp, and red meat intake to 3 oz or less per day; limit caffeine, alcohol, and fat intake; hypoglycemic diet may be of value
        (3) Vitamin and mineral supplementation as a treatment is poorly documented; magnesium or magnesium-rich foods, pyridoxine (no more than 100 to 300 mg a day), vitamin A and E may relieve some breast symptoms and are often suggested; large doses of supplements may be toxic
        (4) Calcium supplementation marginally superior to placebo in randomized placebo-controlled trial
        (5) Aerobic exercise 20 to 30 minutes at least 4 times a week
        (6) Avoidance of known physical or emotional triggers
        (7) Self-help, support groups, psychological counseling valuable in treatment
  2. Medical management
     a. Selection of medications based on type and intensity of symptoms
     b. Spironolactone during luteal phase to reduce swelling and bloating
     c. Mefenamic acid (antiprostaglandin) menstrually and premenstrually may reduce fluid retention and menstrual pain

        d. Combined oral contraceptives may be helpful in decreasing physical symptoms—especially type containing drospirenone (spironolactone derivative)
        e. Danazol in low doses for luteal phase only may relieve breast pain
        f. Selective serotonin reuptake inhibitors (SSRI) or selective serotonin and norepinephrine reuptake inhibitors (SNRI) antidepressant medications have been shown to alleviate severe PMS; may choose to take only in luteal phase each month
        g. Gonadotropin-releasing hormone agonists (GnRH) to inhibit cyclic gonadotropin release; long-term therapy may predispose to heart disease or osteoporosis—limit use to 4 to 6 months unless combined with combination hormonal therapy

- Premenstrual dysphoric disorder (PMDD)
  1. At least 5 PMS-type symptoms severe enough to markedly disrupt normal functioning in most if not all menstrual cycles
  2. Occurs in luteal phase and resolves within 1 week after menses
  3. Must include at least one of these symptoms—markedly depressed mood, marked anxiety, marked affective lability, persistent and marked anger
  4. Prevalence, 3–10% of reproductive age women
  5. Treatment—SSRI/SNRI, combination oral contraceptives containing drospirenone if also desires contraception, other hormonal interventions

Dysmenorrhea

- Definition
  1. Painful menstruation—a sensation of cramping in lower abdomen during or just before menses; most severe on first day, usually lasts 2 days, may radiate to back and thighs
  2. Primary—dysmenorrhea occurs unassociated with underlying pelvic pathology, rarely begins after age 20, associated with ovulatory cycles, is stimulated by prostaglandin release
  3. Secondary—an underlying pelvic pathologic condition thought to be the cause
  4. May occur at any age in menstruating women

- Etiology/Incidence
  1. Primary—seen in 50–75% of all menstruating women with 10–20% severe; prostaglandins stimulate contractile response on smooth muscles
  2. Secondary—onset may be many years after menarche; most often in women older than age 20; organic disease is related

- Signs and symptoms
  1. Primary
     a. Pain begins shortly before the onset of menses and usually lasts no longer than 2 days
     b. Described as colicky, crampy, and spasmodic pain in the lower abdomen, sometimes radiating to lower back and thighs
     c. May interfere with work or school (15–29%)
  2. Secondary
     a. Pain may begin at any time during the cycle; may notice change in duration and amount of menstrual flow
     b. Unlikely to be relieved by over-the-counter measures
     c. Symptoms often persist longer then primary; related to organic pathology

- Physical findings
  1. Primary—characterized by no abnormalities found on examination
  2. Secondary—has findings consistent with pathologic condition

- Differential diagnosis
  1. Imperforate hymen
  2. Endometriosis
  3. Cervical stenosis
  4. Uterine abnormalities
  5. Pelvic infection
  6. Ovarian cysts
  7. Pelvic congestion
  8. Chronic pelvic pain
  9. Adhesions
  10. Sexually transmitted infections
  11. Urinary tract infections

- Diagnostic tests/findings
  1. Primary—no specific tests are ordered
  2. Secondary
     a. Analyze pain description to help determine etiology
     b. Tests according to history and physical examination findings may include:
        (1) Vaginal ultrasound and hysterosalpingogram to evaluate pelvic structures
        (2) Laparoscopy to evaluate endometrial cavity
        (3) Cultures, smears to evaluate infections
        (4) Lower gastrointestinal (GI) evaluation

- Management/Treatment
  1. Primary
     a. Prostaglandin synthetase inhibitors, nonsteroidal anti-inflammatory drugs (NSAIDs) are treatment of choice; best if begun at onset of menses, continuing for 48 to 72 hours; choices shown to be effective are mefenamic acid, naproxyn sodium, ibuprofen, and indomethacin
     b. Oral contraceptive pills (OCPs) are good choice if contraception is needed; act by reducing prostaglandins and menstrual flow; may consider extended or continuous dosing regimens
     c. NSAIDs and OCPs may be used in combination
     d. Other hormonal contraceptives may also relieve symptoms by decreasing or eliminating menstrual bleeding—depo medroxyprogesterone acetate (DMPA), levonorgestrel-releasing intrauterine system (LNG-IUS)
     e. Self-help measures include exercise, warm heat, relaxation exercises
  2. Secondary treatment consistent with pathology

Amenorrhea

- Definition
  1. Absence of menses during reproductive years
  2. Primary—no menstruation previously; no menstruation by age 14 in absence of development of secondary sex characteristics; no menstruation by age 16 regardless of secondary sex characteristics
  3. Secondary—absence of menses in a previously menstruating woman; no menses for 6 months in a woman who usually has normal periods or for a length of time equivalent to three cycles
  4. A symptom, not a diagnosis

- Etiology/Incidence
  1. Vaginal agenesis
  2. Imperforate hymen
  3. Atrophy
  4. Infection
  5. Irradiation and surgery resulting in destruction of endometrium (Asherman's syndrome)
  6. Stress
  7. Genetic anomalies
  8. Endocrine imbalances
  9. Weight abnormalities
  10. Medications
  11. Chronic illness
  12. Excessive exercise
  13. Incidence is approximately 5% in women who are not pregnant, lactating, or menopausal

- Signs and symptoms—absence of menses at the expected time

- Physical findings
  1. Abnormal vital signs may indicate chronic illness
  2. Abnormal visual fields, enlarged or nodular thyroid, or breast discharge may indicate endocrine disorder
  3. Enlarged uterus may indicate pregnancy
  4. Delay in Tanner stage progression may indicate altered development of secondary sex characteristics, while hirsutism, clitoral enlargement, and acne may mean androgen excess
  5. Normal estrogen production manifested by pink, moist, rugated vaginal mucosa as seen on speculum examination

- Differential diagnosis
  1. Pregnancy
  2. Menopause
  3. Anorexia nervosa
  4. Disorders of ovary, anterior pituitary and/or hypothalamus such as pituitary tumors, gonadotropin deficiency, polycystic ovarian syndrome, ovarian failure, Sheehan's syndrome
  5. Anatomical disorders such as genetic or congenital anomalies (Turner's syndrome, androgen insensitivity syndrome) and destructive changes such as Asherman's syndrome
  6. Chronic illness—hypothyroidism, hyperthyroidism, tuberculosis, alcohol abuse, type 1 diabetes mellitus, disorders of adrenal glands, obesity
  7. Medication effects—hormonal contraceptives, psychotrophic drugs (phenothiazines), reserpine, dilantin

- Diagnostic tests/findings
  1. Pregnancy test
  2. Serum prolactin level
  3. Thyroid stimulating hormone (TSH)
  4. If above tests are normal, may evaluate availability of estrogen with progestin challenge test
     a. Progesterone each day for 5 to 10 days—wait for bleeding, which should occur within 7 days; will indicate adequate estrogen production and stimulation as well as no problem with outflow tract
     b. Should withdrawal bleeding not occur, prime endometrium with estrogen to ensure proliferation; estrogen orally for 21 days, add progesterone orally for last 5 days
     c. Repeat challenge test; if bleeding occurs, order specific test to determine if problem is in pituitary or ovary, or refer

- Management/Treatment
  1. Primary amenorrhea, refer to endocrinologist
  2. Treat thyroid abnormalities or refer
  3. If prolactin and TSH are normal and bleeding occurs after progestin challenge, initiate treatment for anovulation based on age, contraceptive needs, and lifestyle
  4. Treatment may include combination hormonal contraceptives or cyclic progestins
  5. Referral for ovulation induction if desires pregnancy

Oligomenorrhea

- Definition—infrequent uterine bleeding in which interval between bleeding episodes may vary from 35 days to 6 months

- Etiology/Incidence
  1. Occurs frequently in perimenopause
  2. Ovarian-pituitary-hypothalamus abnormalities
  3. Endocrine disorders such as thyroid or adrenal problems
  4. Systemic causes such as chronic illness, weight loss or gain, extreme stress, excessive exercise
  5. Drug use or abuse

- Signs and symptoms
  1. May alternate with episodes of amenorrhea or heavy vaginal bleeding
  2. May present as normal menstrual pattern during first year of menstruation or for several years prior to menopause

- Differential diagnosis
  1. Pregnancy
  2. Menopause
  3. Thyroid disorder
  4. Disturbance with hypothalamic-pituitary-ovarian axis

- Physical findings—consistent with pathology found in Differential diagnosis section

- Diagnostic tests/findings
  1. Pregnancy test (beta hCG) to rule out pregnancy
  2. Tests to evaluate function of thyroid, ovaries, pituitary or hypothalamus, e.g., TSH, prolactin level, gonadotropin levels

- Management/Treatment
  1. If pregnant, discuss options
  2. Treat underlying cause, e.g., stress, weight—possibly refer to an endocrinologist

3. Prevent unopposed estrogen complications by giving progesterone therapy—medroxyprogesterone acetate 10 days of each month or combination hormonal contraceptives

Polycystic Ovarian Syndrome (PCOS)

- Definition—a symptom complex associated with oligo-ovulation or anovulation and clinical or biochemical signs of hyperandrogenism

- Etiology/Incidence
  1. Etiology is unclear
  2. Primary hormonal abnormality is increased luteinizing hormone (LH) with low or normal follicle stimulating hormone (FSH)—ratio is more than 3:1; results in dysregulation of androgen secretion with increased testosterone and androstenedione production
  3. Another cause may be hyperinsulinemia associated with insulin resistance; insulin has effects at both the ovarian stroma and the follicle; can have a significant impact on promoting or disrupting follicles
  4. Approximately 25% of normal women will demonstrate ultrasonographic evidence typical of polycystic ovaries
  5. Prevalence in reproductive women is approximately 6–7% (most common endocrine disorder in this population)
  6. Women are at risk for future development of endometrial cancer, diabetes mellitus, and heart disease; obesity increases risk of metabolic complications

- Signs and symptoms
  1. History of irregular menses (amenorrhea or oligomenorrhea)
  2. Gradual onset of hirsutism around puberty or in early 20s
  3. Signs of androgen excess—acne, hirsutism, deep voice, male pattern baldness
  4. May have acanthosis nigricans
  5. Obesity may be present (40%)
  6. Infertility

- Differential diagnosis
  1. Dysfunctional uterine bleeding
  2. Obesity
  3. Hyperprolactinemia
  4. Thyroid dysfunction
  5. Cushing's disease
  6. Adrenal or ovarian tumors

- Physical findings
  1. Physical findings may be normal
  2. Ovaries may not always be palpable—50% will have enlarged ovaries
  3. Virilization—hirsutism, increased muscle mass, frontal balding, enlargement of clitoris, deepening of voice, and decreased breast size
  4. Abdominal obesity
  5. Acne
  6. Acanthosis nigricans and skin tags usually in neck area

- Diagnostic tests/findings
  1. Serum beta hCG to rule out pregnancy
  2. Progesterone challenge test resulting in bleeding
  3. LH elevated; FSH normal or low (3:1 ratio)
  4. Prolactin mildly elevated or normal
  5. Serum total testosterone and free testosterone—mild to moderate elevation, which may mean androgen excess
  6. Thyroid function tests—high or low TSH
  7. Dehydroepiandrosterone sulfate (DHEAS)—normal to elevated
  8. Endometrial biopsy—to rule out hyperplasia
  9. Basal body temperature reading to indicate evidence of ovulation—use to schedule endometrial biopsy
  10. Assess ovaries with ultrasonography
  11. Laparoscopy to determine and manage fertility
  12. Glucose and lipid levels

- Management/Treatment
  1. Initial goal is to lower androgen levels and decrease risk for long-term effects of hyperandrogenism
  2. May be determined by desire for pregnancy and symptom patterns
  3. If pregnancy desired, refer to reproductive endocrinologist
  4. If pregnancy not desired, direct therapy on prevention of endometrial hyperplasia and pregnancy
     a. Endometrial biopsy may be indicated
     b. Medroxyprogesterone acetate for 10 days of month induces withdrawal bleeding
     c. Low dose combined OCP with low androgenicity is an option for women under 35 and those older than 35 who do not smoke
  5. Be observant for signs of diabetes, heart disease, breast cancer, and endometrial cancer
  6. Weight loss if obese
  7. Insulin sensitizing agents—metformin
  8. Excess hair removal—mechanical or eflornithine HCl topical cream for facial hair

Endometriosis

- Definition—the presence of endometrial stroma and glands outside uterus

- Etiology/Incidence
  1. Etiology is not clearly understood
  2. Possible causes include
     a. Retrograde menstruation (Sampsom's theory)
     b. Immunologic factors
     c. Genetics
     d. Hormonal factors
  3. Found in 5–15% of surgeries performed on reproductive age women and up to 30% of infertile women
  4. Typical patient is 20 to 30 years old, Caucasian, nulliparous (60–70%)
  5. Occurs in all races
  6. 7–10% of premenopausal women are affected; most common cause of chronic pelvic pain
  7. Endometriosis has been found in areas other than pelvis, such as lungs, nose and spinal column; most common sites are cul-de-sac, ovary, posterior uterus and uterosacral ligaments
  8. Majority have a positive family history

- Signs and symptoms
  1. Wide range of clinical symptoms; severity does not correlate with extent of disease
  2. Most common complaints
     a. Dysmenorrhea
     b. Infertility
     c. Premenstrual spotting
     d. Menorrhagia
     e. Pelvic pain
     f. Dyspareunia
  3. Symptoms seen less often include:
     a. Low back pain
     b. Diarrhea
     c. Dysuria
     d. Hematuria
     e. Dyschezia
     f. Rectal bleeding
  4. Symptoms classically occur before or during menses
  5. Pain may be localized to involved area
  6. Infertility

- Physical findings
  1. Fixed, retroverted uterus
  2. Bilateral, fixed, tender adnexal masses
  3. Nodularity and tenderness of uterosacral ligaments and cul-de-sac
  4. Tenderness, thickening, and nodularity of rectal–vaginal septum
  5. Lesions may be visible on laparoscopy or laparotomy
  6. Cervical motion tenderness associated with menses

- Differential diagnosis
  1. Chronic pelvic inflammatory infection
  2. Acute salpingitis
  3. Adenomyosis
  4. Ectopic pregnancy
  5. Benign or malignant ovarian neoplasm

- Diagnostic tests/findings
  1. Direct visualization with laparoscopy or laparotomy may reveal classic implants; classified as Stage I-minimal, Stage II-mild, Stage III-moderate, Stage IV-severe
  2. CT and MRI provide only presumptive evidence
  3. CA-125 levels correlate with degree of disease and response to therapy, cannot be used for diagnosis due to low sensitivity and specificity

- Management/Treatment
  1. No medical management provides universal cure; goal is to relieve pain, restore fertility and prevent progression
  2. Medical management includes
     a. Analgesics (NSAID first choice)
     b. GnRH agonists and danazol induce regression of endometrial implants
     c. Progestins—Sub Q 104 DMPA is FDA approved for treatment; IM DMPA also effective
     d. Continuous use of combined oral contraceptive pills produces atrophy of implants and acyclic hormone environment
     e. Laser surgery may be employed
     f. Hysterectomy, bilateral salpingoophorectomy is curative
     g. May combine surgery and medication
  3. Key points
     a. May need long term emotional support due to pain and infertility
     b. Delayed childbirth may lead to development of endometriosis
     c. Treatment is long term; may become a chronic illness
     d. Counsel regarding the risk of infertility

Adenomyosis

- Definition—benign condition in which ectopic endometrium is found within the myometrium; often is considered a type of endometriosis

- Etiology/Incidence
  1. May be related to breakdown of the endometrium during labor and delivery; the cells of the endometrial basal layer grow downward losing connection with the endometrium
  2. Incidence varies widely from 10–90% of hysterectomies revealing adenomyosis
  3. Diagnosis most common in parous women between ages 40 and 50

- Signs and symptoms
  1. Increasingly severe dysmenorrhea and heavy bleeding during menses are common
  2. Infertility

- Physical findings
  1. Boggy tender uterus
  2. Diffuse, globular enlargement—may be 8 to 10 weeks size
  3. May see evidence of anemia

- Differential diagnosis
  1. Endometriosis
  2. Leiomyomata
  3. Pregnancy
  4. Adhesions

- Diagnostic tests/findings
  1. Ultrasonography or MRI may rule out other pathology
  2. Endometrial biopsy for abnormal bleeding

- Management/Treatment
  1. Symptomatic relief may be only requirement
  2. Hysterectomy may be indicated and is curative
  3. NSAID for pain
  4. Hormone suppression—symptoms usually subside after hormone production ceases

Hyperprolactinemia, Galactorrhea, and Pituitary Adenoma

- Definition
  1. Hyperprolactinemia—elevated levels of prolactin
  2. Galactorrhea—secretion of a nonphysiologic, milky fluid from the breast, unrelated to pregnancy
  3. Pituitary adenoma—benign tumor of pituitary; most common type secretes prolactin

- Etiology/Incidence
  1. Etiology and incidence of pituitary adenoma is unknown; rarely malignant, can grow for years
  2. Prolactin-secreting adenomas account for 50% of all identified at autopsy

  3. Most common age for pituitary adenoma is sixth decade
  4. High prolactin level found in around one-third of women with amenorrhea of unknown origin; about one-third of women with secondary amenorrhea will have pituitary adenoma; one-third of women with high levels of prolactin will have galactorrhea
  5. Galactorrhea should be evaluated in a nulliparous woman or in a parous woman if 12 months has passed since last pregnancy

- Signs and symptoms
  1. Hyperprolactinemia/galactorrhea
     a. Spontaneous clear or milky bilateral or unilateral breast secretions from multiple ducts
     b. Normal or irregular menses; secondary amenorrhea may occur
     c. Disturbances of vision and headaches may be present (if adenoma is cause)
  2. Pituitary adenoma
     a. Breast secretions
     b. Menstrual changes as described
     c. Severe vascular headaches and blurred vision

- Physical findings
  1. Normal funduscopic examination—if no adenoma
  2. Funduscopic examination may show papilledema if adenoma present
  3. Normal physical and gynecological examination

- Differential diagnosis
  1. Pregnancy/breast feeding
  2. Breast cancer
  3. Hypothyroidism, hyperthyroidism
  4. Pituitary adenoma
  5. Excessive breast stimulation
  6. Disorders or injury of chest wall
  7. Medication effect (e.g., endogenous opiates, cannabis, heterocyclic antidepressants)
  8. Disturbances of ovarian function
  9. Benign and malignant brain neoplasm

- Diagnostic tests/findings
  1. Thyroid screening—e.g., TSH, T_4
  2. Serum prolactin—refer if more than 20 ng/mL; if in 100 to 300 ng/mL range—very suspicious for adenoma
  3. Serum hCG to rule out pregnancy
  4. Microscopy of breast secretions—milk indicated by fat globules
  5. CT or MRI of sella turcica to rule out adenoma

- Management/Treatment
  1. Management may best be accomplished by referral to a reproductive endocrinologist
  2. If prolactin level is less than 20 ng/mL, may follow with yearly prolactin levels
  3. Pharmacologic
     a. Dopamine agonist (e.g., bromocriptine, which inhibits prolactin, provides symptomatic relief, decreases or stops galactorrhea); treatment of choice with highest cure
     b. Treat hypo/hyperthyroidism
  4. Surgical
     a. If medical management has failed to relieve symptoms of adenoma, transphenoid neurosurgery may be indicated
     b. Recurrence rate is 10–70%; requires close follow-up
  5. Radiation
     a. Results are less satisfactory than surgery
     b. May take several years for prolactin level to fall
     c. Should be reserved for recurrences or those not responsive to medical management
  6. Patient education
     a. Discontinue breast stimulation
     b. Disclose all drugs and medications being used

Dysfunctional Uterine Bleeding (DUB)

- Definition—a variety of bleeding manifestations secondary to chronic anovulation

- Etiology/Incidence
  1. Disturbances of hypothalamic-pituitary-axis may cause continuous endometrial stimulation
  2. DUB is abnormal bleeding that is unrelated to organic pathology, systemic conditions, medications, genital tract pathology, or pregnancy
  3. Risk factors—postpubertal and perimenopause phase, overweight or underweight, chronic illness, excessive stress
  4. Most common menstrual abnormality in reproductive age women

- Signs and symptoms
  1. Usually occurs at the extremes of reproductive age—adolescence and perimenopause
  2. Patterns of dysfunctional bleeding
     a. Oligomenorrhea—normal bleeding at intervals greater than 35 days
     b. Polymenorrhea—bleeding that is normal, occurring at intervals less than 21 days

     c. Hypomenorrhea—too little bleeding at normal intervals
     d. Menorrhagia—regular, normal intervals, excessive flow and duration
     e. Metrorrhagia—intermenstrual bleeding or bleeding occurring at times other than normal intervals

- Physical findings—none specific

- Differential diagnosis
  1. Diagnosis of exclusion
  2. Pregnancy (ectopic or intrauterine)
  3. Cervical and endometrial cancer, polycystic ovarian syndrome (PCOS), liver disease, thyroid disease, blood dyscrasia, leiomyomata, adenomyosis, trauma, vaginitis, foreign body, medication interaction
  4. Severe stress, drug abuse

- Diagnostic tests/findings
  1. hCG for pregnancy
  2. Pap test for cervical cancer
  3. Complete blood count
  4. FSH and LH to evaluate estrogen stimulation
  5. TSH
  6. Sexually transmitted disease testing as indicated
  7. Endometrial evaluation—biopsy, transvaginal ultrasound, saline infusion sonohysteroscopy
  8. Coagulation studies if indicated

- Management/Treatment
  1. Hormonal
     a. Acute excessive bleeding—parenteral estrogen or high-dose oral estrogen gradually tapered then medroxyprogesterone acetate (MPA) added last 10 days to initiate withdrawal bleeding
     b. Moderate bleeding, not currently bleeding, and maintenance control—OCP cyclic, extended, or continuous regimens; DMPA; cyclic MPA; LNG-IUS
  2. Nonhormonal
     a. Treat anemia
     b. Nonsteroidal anti-inflammatory drugs (NSAIDS)—start at menses onset and continue for 5 days or until cessation of menstruation
  3. Surgical management
     a. Hysterectomy
     b. Endometrial ablation
     c. Dilatation and curettage is diagnostic and therapeutic

◘ BENIGN AND MALIGNANT TUMORS/NEOPLASMS

Cervical Polyps

- Definition—pedunculated growths arising from the mucosal surface of the endocervix

- Etiology/Incidence
  1. Inflammation
  2. Trauma
  3. Pregnancy
  4. Abnormal local response to hypoestrogenic state
  5. Occurs in 4% of all gynecological patients
  6. Most common benign neoplasm of the cervix; and most often seen in perimenopause and multigravida women between ages 30 and 50
  7. Malignant changes are rare

- Signs and symptoms
  1. May be asymptomatic
  2. Leukorrhea
  3. Abnormal vaginal bleeding—intermenstrual, postcoital

- Physical findings
  1. Single or multiple, painless polypoid lesions at cervix
  2. Size ranges from a few millimeters to 2 to 3 cm
  3. Reddish-purple to cherry red in color; smooth and soft; bleeds easily
  4. Otherwise normal pelvic examination

- Differential diagnosis
  1. Adenocarcinoma
  2. Cervical carcinoma
  3. Prolapsed myoma
  4. Squamous papilloma
  5. Retained products of conception
  6. Sarcoma

- Diagnostic tests/findings
  1. Pap test to rule out premalignant cervical lesions or cancer
  2. Biopsy to rule out cancer

- Management/Treatment
  1. Excisional polypoidectomy is usually curative
  2. Recur frequently

Leiomyomata Uteri (Fibroid, Myoma)

- Definition—nodular, discrete tumors varying in size from microscopic to large multiple, nodular masses; classified according to location
  1. Submucosal—protrude into the uterine cavity
  2. Subserosal—bulge through the outer uterine wall
  3. Intraligamentous—within the broad ligament
  4. Interstitial (intramural)—stays within the uterine wall as it grows; most common form of myoma
  5. Pedunculated—on a thin pedicle or stalk attached to the uterus

- Etiology/Incidence
  1. Etiology unknown
  2. May arise from smooth muscle cells in the myometrium
  3. Most common benign gynecological pelvic neoplasm
  4. Affects approximately 20% of women in their reproductive years
  5. Occurs more frequently in African-American women than in Caucasian
  6. Asymptomatic fibroids may be seen in 40–50% of women over age 40
  7. Increased family incidence

- Signs and symptoms
  1. Usually asymptomatic
  2. Menorrhagia—most common sign
  3. Pelvic pain is most often chronic—presents as dysmenorrhea, pelvic pressure, or dyspareunia; if pedunculated, twisted, and infarcted may cause acute pain
  4. Large fibroids may cause constipation; intestinal obstruction may result from compression; venous stasis may occur from pressure; pressure on bladder may result in urinary retention or overflow incontinence

- Physical findings
  1. Abdominal enlargement
  2. Enlarged, irregularly shaped, firm uterus; may be displaced
  3. Pedunculated tumor may protrude from cervix
  4. Tumors usually painless on palpation
  5. Wide variance in size (3 to 4 mm up to 15 lb)
  6. Potential complications
     a. Spontaneous abortion
     b. Premature labor
     c. Anemia
     d. Infertility

- Differential diagnosis
  1. Ovarian mass (benign or malignant)
  2. Pregnancy
  3. Leiomyosarcoma
  4. Uterine malignancy
  5. Adenomyosis
  6. Endometriosis
  7. Colon or rectal tumor (benign or malignant)

- Diagnostic tests/findings
  1. Pap test to rule out cervical cancer
  2. Pregnancy test to rule out pregnancy
  3. CBC if anemia suspected
  4. Occult blood test if rectal or colon symptoms or gastrointestinal problems
  5. Endometrial biopsy or D & C when abnormal bleeding present
  6. Ultrasound, sonohysterogram, CT, MRI confirm diagnosis
  7. Hysteroscopy to provide visualization of uterine cavity

- Management/Treatment
  1. May require no treatment if asymptomatic
  2. Periodic observation and follow-up with bimanual examination may be indicated to insure tumors are not growing or undergoing abnormal changes
  3. Pharmacologic
     a. GnRH agonist results in 40–60% reduction in volume; regrowth occurs about half the time; may be used to reduce volume preoperatively, before attempting pregnancy, when surgery is contraindicated, or in perimenopausal women to avoid surgery
     b. Progestational agents such as medroxyprogesterone acetate (MPA) may decrease fibroid size and bleeding
     c. Treat anemia if indicated
  4. Surgical
     a. Indications for surgery
        (1) Abnormal bleeding
        (2) Rapid growth
        (3) Definitive decision concerning mass if impossible without visualization
        (4) Encroachment of organs
     b. Hysterectomy when symptoms cannot be controlled
     c. Myomectomy through hysteroscopic resection can preserve fertility; up to 30% recurrence with this method

Ovarian Cysts

- Definition:
  1. Functional—cysts of the ovary that occur secondary to hormonal stimulation
     a. Follicular—occur in the follicular phase of the menstrual cycle when continued hormonal stimulation prevents fluid resorption
     b. Corpus luteum—occur in the luteal phase, when corpus luteum fails to degenerate
  2. Dermoid (benign cystic teratoma)—most common ovarian germ cell tumor

- Etiology/Incidence
  1. Follicular cysts
     a. Rare before menarche or after menopause
     b. Account for 20–50% of ovarian cysts; most common adnexal mass in reproductive years
     c. Often found incidentally during routine pelvic examination or ultrasound
     d. Usually resolves in 2 to 3 menstrual cycles, may rupture or undergo torsion causing pain
  2. Corpus luteum cysts
     a. Forms following the failure of the corpus luteum to degenerate after 14 days
     b. May hemorrhage into the cystic cavity
  3. Dermoid cysts (benign cystic teratoma)
     a. One of the most common neoplasms of the ovary (10–20%)
     b. Occurs during the reproductive years
     c. Composed usually of well-differentiated tissue from all three germ layers
     d. Usually measures 5 to 10 cm in diameter; 10–15% are bilateral

- Signs and symptoms
  1. Functional cysts
     a. Usually asymptomatic
     b. May cause irregular menses, pelvic pressure, fullness (if mass is large), increase in abdominal girth/distention
     c. Acute pain if ruptures or if torsion occurs
     d. Large cysts may cause feeling of fullness, heaviness, and dull ache on affected side
  2. Dermoid (benign cystic teratoma)
     a. Usually asymptomatic
     b. Acute pain if twists or ruptures; may experience peritonitis
     c. May cause vague feelings of local pelvic pressure if large
     d. Abnormal uterine bleeding (rare)
  3. Signs of rupture include severe, sudden abdominal pain; mimics ruptured ectopic

- Physical findings
  1. Functional cysts are usually smaller than 8 cm, cystic to firm, mobile, sometimes tender, usually unilateral adnexal mass
  2. Dermoid cysts may measure 5 to 10 cm, usually unilateral, firm to cystic, often anterior to uterus

- Differential diagnosis
  1. Pregnancy; ectopic pregnancy
  2. Ovarian torsion
  3. Uterine fibroid; endometrioma
  4. Tubo-ovarian abscess
  5. Diverticulitis/abscess

6. Distended bladder
7. Congenital anomaly (pelvic kidney)
8. Lymphadenopathy
9. Malignant neoplasm (most often in older women)

- Diagnostic tests/findings
  1. Pregnancy test
  2. Ultrasound to evaluate mass—cystic or solid; septate, irregular, presence of papillations, bilateral or unilateral; rule out ectopic pregnancy
  3. CT scan with contrast or IVP to evaluate kidney

- Management/Treatment
  1. Functional cyst
     a. In reproductive years; cyst less than 6 cm in diameter, examine after next menses
     b. Combination hormonal contraceptives to suppress gonadotropin levels
     c. Mass between 6 and 8 cm, or is fixed or feels solid, pelvic ultrasound to assure is unilocular
     d. If painful, multilocular, or partially solid, surgery indicated
     e. 8 cm, surgery indicated
     f. If 40 years old or older, use more caution and observe
  2. Dermoid cyst—determined by age, desire for pregnancy and potential for malignancy; cystectomy or abdominal hysterectomy and bilateral salpingo-oophrectomy

Cervical Carcinoma

- Definition—slow penetration of the basement membrane and infiltration of malignant cells into the uterine cervix; characterized by histologically defineable stages

- Etiology/Incidence
  1. Approximately 14,500 new cases diagnosed annually with 4000 to 5000 deaths
  2. Highest incidence in Hispanics, then African Americans, then Caucasians
  3. Peak incidence between 45 and 55 years of age; increasing in young women
  4. Time between initial exposure to a carcinogen and subsequent development of carcinoma in-situ considered to be 5 to 10 years
  5. HPV is the primary agent in the development of cervical intraepithelial neoplasia (CIN) and cervical cancer
  6. Risk factors
     a. Smoking

b. Presence of HPV types with malignant potential (types 16, 18, and 31 most common)
     c. First coitus at early age (< 18 years)
     d. Multiple sexual partners or sexual partners with multiple partners
     e. Nonbarrier method of contraception
     f. Immunosuppression
     g. Long-term oral contraceptive use (≥ 5 years)
     h. Never had Pap test or infrequent Pap tests

- Signs and symptoms
  1. May be asymptomatic
  2. Postcoital or irregular, painless bleeding
  3. Odorous bloody or purulent discharge
  4. Late symptoms
     a. Pelvic or epigastric pain
     b. Urinary or rectal symptoms

- Physical findings
  1. Appearance of cervix ranges from normal to severely ulcerated, necrotic or large bulky lesion filling the vagina
  2. Cervix may be firm or "rock like" to soft and spongy
  3. Sanguineous or purulent, odorous vaginal discharge
  4. Anemia if bleeding heavy

- Differential diagnosis
  1. Metastasis from another primary site
  2. Cervicitis/sexually transmitted infections
  3. Cervical polyp
  4. Cervical ectopy
  5. Pre-invasive lesion of cervix
  6. *Condyloma acuminata*

- Diagnostic tests/findings
  1. Pap test is gold standard for cost-effective screening
  2. Biopsy of gross lesions
  3. If malignancy is suspected, but no gross lesion visible, colposcopy is suggested with biopsy
  4. Colposcopic evaluation of vulva and vagina to rule out other lesions
  5. CT, MRI, cystoscopy, sigmoidoscopy, and barium enema may be indicated

- Management/Treatment
  1. Management should be by a gynecological oncologist involving staging, appropriate treatment and follow-up
  2. Treatment may consist of surgery, radiation, chemotherapy, or a combination

Endometrial Carcinoma

- Definition—carcinoma of the body of the uterus; malignant transformation of endometrial glands and/or stroma

- Etiology/Incidence
  1. Most common gynecological malignancy—accounts for 90–95% of malignancies of the uterine corpus
  2. 30,000 new cases annually and 6000 deaths
  3. Median age is 63 years at onset—5% occurring in women younger than age 40
  4. Risk factors are linked to exposure to unopposed estrogen either endogenous or exogenous
     a. Diabetes, obesity, hypertension
     b. Family history
     c. Early menarche; late menopause
     d. Unopposed estrogen therapy
     e. Oligo-ovulation, anovulation
     f. Estrogen secreting tumors (granulosa cell)
  5. Protective factors—multiparity, use of oral contraceptive pills, use of depot medroxyprogesterone acetate (DMPA)

- Signs and symptoms
  1. Painless vaginal bleeding is typically the first symptom
  2. Serous, odorous discharge (watery leukorrhea), soon replaced by bloody discharge, intermittent spotting, spotting-to-steady painless bleeding, then hemorrhage
  3. Lower abdominal pain (10%)

- Physical findings
  1. Blood may be present in the vaginal vault
  2. Advanced disease may have pelvic mass present, ascites
  3. Anemia may be present
  4. Uterus may be enlarged and soft

- Differential diagnosis
  1. Atrophic vaginitis
  2. Cervical or endometrial polyps
  3. Benign endometrial pathology (hyperplasia)
  4. Dysfunctional uterine bleeding
  5. Bleeding from hormone replacement therapy
  6. Leiomyomas
  7. Other genital/gynecological cancers

- Diagnostic tests/findings
  1. Pap test may show glandular abnormalities
  2. Endometrial aspiration biopsy
  3. Ultrasound to measure endometrial stripe; if less than 5 mm thick, likelihood of endometrial cancer is rare
  4. Fractional dilatation and curettage is the gold standard for diagnosis
  5. Hysteroscopy may be useful in identifying lesions/polyps not found on biopsy

- Management/Treatment
  1. Refer to gynecologist for early stage disease or oncologist
  2. Hysterectomy, bilateral salpingo-oophorectomy
  3. Surgical staging to determine treatment
  4. Radiation, chemotherapy, steroids (progesterone), or combination

Ovarian Carcinoma

- Definition—a malignant neoplasm of the ovary

- Etiology/Incidence
  1. Malignancies of the ovary arise from any type of cell found in the ovary; epithelial carcinoma is the most common type (80–85%)
  2. Ovary may be site for metastasis from non-ovarian cancers
  3. Etiology unknown
  4. Risk factors
     a. Family history in one first-degree relative—10% chance
     b. Family history in two first-degree relatives—50% chance
     c. Family susceptibility shown with the BRCA1 gene
     d. Low parity
     e. Early menarche; late menopause
     f. Ovulation induction agents (possibly)
     g. Perineal talc use (suggested)
     h. High socioeconomic class
     i. High dietary fat consumption
     j. History of breast, colon, or endometrial cancer
  5. Use of oral contraceptives reduces risk—protection lasts up to 2 decades after last use
  6. Fifth most common cancer in women
  7. Second most common genital tract cancer
  8. 25,000 new cases annually
  9. Usual age of onset is near the perimenopause or menopause—median age 61 years, peaks at 75 to 79
  10. Mortality rate exceeds all other genital tract malignancies; presents in advanced stage

- Signs and symptoms
  1. Early
     a. Often asymptomatic; may be detected on routine pelvic examination
     b. Symptoms are often mild, vague, and inconsistent

    c.   Abdominal discomfort or pain

    d.   Pressure sensation on the bladder or rectum

    e.   Pelvic fullness or bloating

    f.   Vague gastrointestinal symptoms

  2. Late

    a.   Increasing abdominal girth

    b.   Abdominal pain

    c.   Abnormal vaginal bleeding

    d.   Gastrointestinal symptoms; nausea, loss of appetite, dyspepsia

- Physical findings
  1. Palpation of fixed, irregular, nontender adnexal mass—usually bilateral (usually first diagnostic finding)
  2. Ascites
  3. Pleural effusion and subclavicular lymphadenopathy if advanced
  4. Cachexia

- Differential diagnosis
  1. Primary peritoneal cancer
  2. Benign ovarian tumor
  3. Endometriosis
  4. Functional ovarian cyst
  5. Ovarian torsion
  6. Pelvic kidney
  7. Pedunculated uterine fibroid

- Diagnostic tests/findings
  1. Pelvic ultrasonography/CT/MRI
  2. CA-125—elevated levels not diagnostic for ovarian cancers (elevations can occur with endometriosis, leiomyomata, pelvic inflammatory infection, hepatitis, and other malignancies); helpful to follow response to treatment with chemotherapy and subsequent follow-up
  3. Definitive diagnosis is made with laparotomy

- Management/Treatment
  1. Surgical
     a. Total abdominal hysterectomy, bilateral salpingo-oophorectomy, and omentectomy—establishes histologic staging and grading of tumor
     b. Goal is removal of as much tumor as possible
  2. Chemotherapy and/or radiation
  3. Rule out metastasis with diagnostic evaluation of other organ systems

Vaginal Carcinoma

- Definition—abnormal proliferation of vaginal epithelium with malignant cells extending below the basement membrane

- Etiology/Incidence
  1. Comprises about 2% of malignancies—vaginal cancer is the rarest of gynecological cancers
  2. Mean age of diagnosis 65 years with a range of 30 to 90 years
  3. Etiology is multifactorial; risk factors include presence of HPV infection, other genital cancers, DES exposure, prior radiation
  4. Vaginal intraepithelial neoplasm is thought to be a precurser
  5. Five-year survival ranges from 80% for stage I to 17% for stage V

- Signs and symptoms
  1. May present with vaginal bleeding or odorous blood tinged discharge—may cause vulvitis or pruritus
  2. May have palpable or visible mass or lesion
  3. Urinary problems if bladder involved

- Physical findings
  1. Early lesions are raised, granular and may be white
  2. Late lesions are friable, granular, cauliflower-like and may be palpable; ulceration may be superficial or deep
  3. Most common site is upper one-third of vagina
  4. If lesion darkly pigmented—suspect melanoma

- Differential diagnosis
  1. Malignancy of another site extended or metastatic to the vagina
  2. Vaginitis
  3. Bleeding from uterus
  4. Ulceration from foreign object (pessary, tampon)

- Diagnostic tests/findings
  1. Pap test to evaluate for cervical cancer
  2. Colposcopy and biopsy of lesions
  3. For staging use cystoscopy, proctosigmoidoscopy, IV urography, chest radiography, barium enema
  4. CT scan and MRI are used to evaluate metastasis

- Management/Treatment
  1. Treatment should be by a gynecological oncologist
  2. Accurate diagnosis and stage is to be determined before treatment is planned
  3. If lesion is precancerous (VAIN I, II, III), laser is appropriate
  4. Local excision (partial vaginectomy) may be appropriate for early lesions

5. Radiation is mainstay of treatment
6. Radical surgery may be followed with radiation

Vulvar Carcinoma

- Definition—proliferation of malignant cells of vulva

- Etiology/Incidence
  1. Multifactorial
  2. Increased risk in women with the human papillomavirus (HPV) (30–50%)
  3. Risk factors
     a. History of abnormal Pap test
     b. Multiple sexual partners
     c. Cigarette smoking
     d. Chronic irritation
     e. Vulvar dermatoses
  4. May be associated with other urogenital cancers
  5. Accounts for 1–2% of all gynecological cancer deaths per year
  6. Vulvar malignancies arise from squamous cell carcinoma, melanoma, adenocarcinoma, basal cell carcinoma, and sarcomas
  7. Mean age 65 with a range of 30 to 90 years; incidence in young women is rising

- Signs and symptoms
  1. May be asymptomatic
  2. Lesions may be darkly or irregularly pigmented, white or red; multifocal or singular; flat, wart like, or scaly
  3. Ulceration, erythema, irritation
  4. Pruritus (most common), pain, burning, bleeding
  5. Odorous discharge, may be blood-tinged

- Physical findings
  1. White, red, pigmented or ulcerated lesion
  2. Hyperkeratotic patches (leukoplakia)
  3. Excoriation and erythema
  4. Most common sites are labia majora and minora
  5. Bartholin's gland enlargement
  6. Inguinal lymphadenopathy

- Differential diagnosis
  1. Vulvar dermatoses
  2. Atrophy
  3. *Condyloma acuminata*
  4. Vulvar infection/inflammation
  5. Lymphogranuloma inguinale
  6. Paget's disease

- Diagnostic tests/findings
  1. Pap test, colposcopy to rule out other sites of disease
  2. Biopsy/wide resection to make definitive diagnosis
  3. CT and MRI, chest radiography to evaluate for metastasis

- Management/Treatment
  1. Appropriate evaluation by a gynecological oncologist
  2. Local excision
  3. Simple or radical vulvectomy
  4. Topical treatment—immunologic agents, chemotherapy
  5. Careful follow-up—recurrence is common

Choriocarcinoma

- Definition—a frankly malignant form of gestational trophoblastic disease or may be primary in the ovary

- Etiology/Incidence
  1. Gestational trophoblastic disease
     a. May follow any gestational event—intrauterine or ectopic pregnancy, abortion (50%); hydatidiform mole (50%)
     b. Malignant transformation occurs in the chorion
     c. One of the few metastatic tumors that is curable
  2. Nongestational—mixed germ cell tumor of ovary occurring in childhood or early adolescence; unusual in ages 20 to 30
  3. Disseminates by blood to the lungs, vagina, brain, liver, kidneys, and gastrointestinal tract

- Signs and symptoms—often masquerades as other disease due to metastasis to other organs
  1. Irregular vaginal bleeding—intermittent to hemorrhage; continuing after immediate postpartum period; uterine subinvolution
  2. Amenorrhea (from gonadotropin secretion)
  3. Hemoptysis, cough, dyspnea with lung metastasis
  4. Evidence of central nervous system metastasis—headache, dizziness, fainting
  5. Gastrointestinal—rectal bleeding/tarry stools
  6. Abdominal pain
  7. Hematuria from renal metastasis

- Physical findings
  1. Abdominal mass/ascites
  2. Blood in vaginal vault
  3. Vaginal or vulvar lesion may indicate metastasis

4. Enlarged, soft uterus
5. Abnormalities of multiple organs if metastatic

- Differential diagnosis
  1. May imitate other diseases—suspect strongly if follows a pregnancy event
  2. Intrauterine pregnancy
  3. Invasive mole
  4. Benign ovarian tumor
  5. Other gynecological malignancies

- Diagnostic tests/findings
  1. Quantitative hCG
  2. Abnormal beta hCG regression titers following molar pregnancy
  3. CT scan abdomen, pelvis, and head
  4. Lumbar puncture may be necessary
  5. Chest radiography

- Management/Treatment
  1. Should be managed by a gynecological oncologist
  2. Treatment is usually with surgery and chemotherapy or chemotherapy alone
  3. Appropriate follow-up to monitor side-effects, disease improvement, and recurrence
  4. Nonmetastatic—good prognosis; metastatic—good to poor prognosis

◻ VAGINAL INFECTIONS

Bacterial Vaginosis (BV)

- Definition—an alteration of the normal flora of the vagina with dominance of anaerobic bacteria

- Etiology/Incidence
  1. Loss of lactobacilli (hydrogen producing strains) results in elevated pH and subsequent overgrowth of bacteria—bacteria concentrations are 100- to 1000-fold
  2. No single offending organism—*Gardnerella vaginalis, Mycoplasma nominis, Bacteroides species, Haemophilus, mobiluncus, corynebacterium* are among the anaerobes
  3. BV is not a "vaginitis" and is not sexually transmitted; increased bacteria numbers without inflammation (no increase in white blood cells, WBC); succinic acid produced by organisms alter migration of WBC to bacteria at elevated pH
  4. Risk factors include multiple sexual partners, new sex partner, shared sex toys, and douching
  5. May be associated with intra-amniotic infection, postpartum and postoperative infection, endometritis, pelvic inflammatory disease (PID)

6. Most common vaginal infection in the US, about 10 million patient visits per year

- Signs and symptoms
  1. Most often asymptomatic
  2. Pruritus occasionally
  3. Heavy grayish, yellowish, whitish, odorous, homogenous vaginal discharge; may coat the vulva
  4. Rancid or fishy odor during menses and postcoitally

- Physical findings
  1. Copious amount of homogenous, whitish gray vaginal discharge
  2. Normal appearing vulva and vaginal mucosa
  3. Discharge may coat vulva
  4. Presence of foul odor

- Differential diagnosis
  1. Trichomoniasis
  2. Candidiasis

- Diagnostic tests/findings
  1. Wet mount of vaginal secretions
  2. Presence of three of the following criteria is diagnostic:
     a. Vaginal pH greater than or equal to 4.5
     b. Clue cells on saline wet mount (epithelial cells with borders obscured as a result of stippling with bacteria)
     c. Homogeneous discharge, white, noninflammatory discharge smoothly coating vaginal wall
     d. Positive "whiff test"—fishy odor of vaginal discharge before and after addition of 10% KOH; (caused when anaerobic bacteria combined with potassium hydroxide); may also have positive whiff test in the presence of blood, semen, and trichomonas
  3. Commercially available card tests for detection of elevated pH, presence of amine
  4. Gram stain reveals true clue cells, numerous abnormal bacteria
  5. Cultures for anaerobes are unnecessary

- Management/Treatment
  1. Metronidazole orally for 7 days
  2. Metronidazole gel one full applicator intravaginally at bedtime for 5 days
  3. Clindamycin cream one full applicator intravaginally at bedtime for 7 days
  4. Alternative regimens
     a. Clindamycin orally for 7 days
     b. Clindamycin ovules intravaginally at bedtime for 3 days

5. Treatment of partner will not change course of disease or prevent recurrences
6. Key points concerning metronidazole
   a. May cause a disulfiram effect (flushing, vomiting) if taken when alcohol is consumed
   b. Side-effects; metallic taste, nausea, headache, dry mouth, dark colored urine
   c. May cause disturbance in depth perception
   d. Not to be taken with anticoagulants—may prolong prothrombin time
7. Treatment in pregnancy—see Pregnancy chapter

Trichomoniasis

- Definition—vaginal infection caused by an anaerobic flagellated protozoan parasite

- Etiology/Incidence
  1. Pathogenesis unknown; humans are the only host
  2. Caused by the trichomonas organism; survives best in a pH of 5.6 to 7.5
  3. Sexually transmitted; theoretically possible fomite spread but unlikely
  4. Responsible for 25% of vaginal infections—females symptomatic (25%); men rarely symptomatic
  5. Risk factors include multiple sexual partners, presence of another STD, noncondom use
  6. Use of barrier contraceptive methods may decrease prevalence
  7. May be associated with premature rupture of the membranes and preterm labor

- Signs and symptoms
  1. Symptoms variable; may be asymptomatic
  2. Any combination of the following symptoms may be seen; copious, homogeneous, malodorous, yellowish-green discharge, vulva irritation, pruritus and edema, and occasionally dysuria, urgency, frequency of urination, postcoital and intermenstrual bleeding
  3. Erythema of vulva and vagina with excoriation may be seen
  4. Onset of symptoms often occurs after menses

- Physical findings
  1. Erythema, edema, excoriation of vulva may be seen
  2. Red stipples—"strawberry spots"—on vagina and cervix (punctate lesions called colpitis macularis)

3. Infection may be found in endocervix, vagina, bladder, Bartholin's glands, and periurethral glands
4. Homogeneous, watery, yellowish green, grayish, frothy vaginal discharge
5. pH greater than or equal to 5.0
6. Cervix may bleed easily when touched

- Differential diagnosis
  1. Bacterial vaginosis
  2. Candidiasis
  3. Trauma from foreign body

- Diagnostic tests/findings
  1. Saline wet mount (60–70% sensitive), higher sensitivity with immediate evaluation of wet preparation slide—motile trichomonads; increased WBC
  2. Gram stain—no advantage over wet mount
  3. Definitive test—culture
  4. Urine microscopic examination may reveal live trichomonads
  5. Detection on Pap test 40% positive predictive value
  6. Rapid tests (results in 10–45 minutes) on vaginal secretions (> 82% sensitive, > 97% specific)

- Management/Treatment
  1. Metronidazole orally in a single dose
  2. Tinidazole orally in single dose
  3. Alternative regimen—metronidazole orally twice daily for seven days
  4. For treatment failures—exclude reinfection; retreat with metronidazole orally twice a day for 7 days or tinidazole orally in a single dose
  5. All sexual partners should be treated
  6. Pregnancy—see Pregnancy chapter
  7. Screen for other sexually transmitted infections as indicated
  8. Encourage "safer sex practices" to reduce reinfection and chance of other STD

Vulvovaginal Candidiasis (VVC)

- Definition—inflammatory vulvovaginal process caused by the yeast organism, candida species, which superficially invades the epithelium cells

- Etiology/Incidence
  1. Second most common vulvovaginal infection—caused by candida, a dimorphic fungi
  2. 75% of women will have at least one episode in their reproductive years; 45% will have a second episode; 5% or less will have recurrent intractable episodes; up to 20% of women in their childbearing years will have yeast

isolated; 20–30% will have dual or multiple pathogens

3. *C. albicans* species is responsible 85–90% of the time; *C. glabrata* and *C. tropicalis* are responsible for majority of remaining infections and more resistant to therapy

4. Predisposing factors to candidal overgrowth include pregnancy, reproductive age group, uncontrolled diabetes, immunosuppressive disorders, frequent intercourse, antibiotic use, high-dose corticosteroids

- Signs and symptoms
  1. May have a combination of the following:
     a. Irritation of vulva, pruritus, soreness, external dysuria, excoriation
     b. Edema
     c. Erythema
     d. Discharge may be thick, curdy, thin or watery, with yeast odor
     e. Dyspareunia (upon penetration)

- Physical findings
  1. Discharge is usually adherent to the vaginal wall
  2. Erythema of vulva and vagina
  3. Cervix appears normal on speculum examination

- Differential diagnosis
  1. Trichomoniasis
  2. Bacterial vaginosis
  3. Vulvar dermatoses
  4. Allergic reaction
  5. Urethritis/cystitis

- Diagnostic tests/findings
  1. Wet mount of vaginal secretions with 10% potassium hydroxide (KOH) will reveal mycelia, spores, and pseudohyphae
  2. Vaginal pH usually normal (< 4.5); amine test negative
  3. Increased WBC on wet mount
  4. Fungal culture confirms diagnosis
  5. Gram stain may be positive
  6. Pap test 50% sensitive
  7. Routine cultures may detect asymptomatic colonization; not performed routinely—may be used in recurrences

- Management/Treatment
  1. Treatment indicated if:
     a. Symptomatic
     b. Patient desires
     c. Is immunosuppressed

2. Azole family of antifungals is usual treatment and more effective than nystatin
3. Single dose or 3-day topical azole regimens effective for uncomplicated VVC
4. Fluconazole orally in a single dose
5. Treatment for recurrent VVC—if four or more symptomatic episodes in one year; usually no apparent predisposing factor; culture to determine if nonalbicans candida species; consider longer duration therapy and maintenance regimens (several regimens suggested with both topical azoles and oral fluconazole)
6. Key points
   a. Azole creams and suppositories are oil-based and may weaken latex condoms and diaphragms
   b. Treatment of partner is not recommended unless male has balanitis
   c. Severe VVC (extensive erythema, edema, fissure formation) usually requires 7–14 day topical azole regimen or repeat dose of fluconazole 72 hours after initial dose
   d. Women with uncontrolled diabetes or receiving corticosteroid therapy who have VVC may require 7–14 day treatment regimen
   e. Pregnancy—see Pregnancy chapter

◻ SEXUALLY TRANSMITTED DISEASES (STDs)

Chlamydia

- Definition—infection of epithelial cells of the genital tract of men and women; may cause pneumonia and/or conjunctivitis in neonates

- Etiology/Incidence
  1. Caused by an intracellular organism, *Chlamydia trachomatis,* which replicates in the host causing inclusions in stained cells
  2. Most common STD in the US—approximately 4 million acquired infections annually (reporting not required in all states)
  3. Chlamydia infection may be the etiology of 50% of pelvic infections
  4. May be transmitted vertically to the neonate in up to 70% of untreated women (conjunctival or pneumonic infection)
  5. Sequelae of chlamydia include cervicitis, endometritis, PID, ectopic pregnancy, infertility, acute urethral syndrome, postpartum infections, premature labor and delivery, premature rupture of the membranes, and perinatal morbidity

6. Risk factors
   a. Sexually active women under age 25
   b. Multiple partners or partners with multiple sexual partners
   c. Nonuse of barrier methods of contraception

- Signs and symptoms
  1. May be asymptomatic
  2. Postcoital bleeding; intermenstrual bleeding or spotting
  3. Symptoms of urinary tract infection—dysuria, frequency
  4. Vaginal discharge
  5. Abdominal pain

- Physical findings
  1. Mucopurulent endocervical discharge; edematous, tender cervix with easily induced bleeding
  2. Suprapubic pain or slight tenderness upon palpation

- Differential diagnosis
  1. Gonococcal infection
  2. Urethritis or urinary tract infection
  3. Salpingitis

- Diagnostic tests/findings—presence of organism in various laboratory tests is basis for diagnosis
  1. Culture—expensive
  2. Nonculture methods—nucleic acid amplification test (NAAT) recommended by CDC (2006)
  3. Gonococcal (GC) culture or nonculture test to rule out concomitant gonorrhea
  4. Serologic testing for syphilis, wet mount testing for vaginal infection, consider HIV screen

- Management/Treatment
  1. CDC (2006) recommendations
     a. Azithromycin orally, single dose
     b. Doxycycline orally for 7 days
  2. Alternative regimens
     a. Erythromycin base orally for 7 days
     b. Erythromycin ethylsuccinate orally 7 days
     c. Ofloxacin orally 7 days
     d. Levofloxacin orally for 7 days
  3. Treatment in pregnancy—see Pregnancy chapter
  4. Doxycycline should not be used in pregnancy; may cause discoloration of teeth in children
  5. Erythromycin estolate is contraindicated in pregnancy because of drug-related hepatotoxicity
  6. Quinolones (ofloxacin, levofloxacin) are contraindicated in pregnancy

7. Sex partners should be evaluated, tested, and treated if they had sex contact with patient during the 60 days preceding onset of symptoms in the patient or diagnosis of chlamydia
8. The most recent sex partner should be evaluated and treated even if the time of the last sexual contact was more than 60 days before symptom onset or diagnosis (CDC 2006)
9. Avoid intercourse until all partners have been treated
10. Test of cure
    a. Not recommended if treated with CDC-recommended or alternative regimens and not pregnant
    b. Consider test of cure if suspect noncompliance with treatment or if symptoms persist
    c. Wait at least 3 weeks after treatment to do test of cure—prior to 3 weeks may get false negative
    d. Majority of posttreatment infections are reinfection—retest at 3 months posttreatment or next office visit

Condyloma Acuminata, Venereal Warts

- Definition—a sexually transmitted, viral disease affecting the vulva, vagina, cervix, and perianal area

- Etiology/Incidence
  1. Caused by human papillomavirus (HPV)
  2. Approximately 100 species of HPV; more than 30 types infect anogenital mucosal surfaces; potential for malignancy is variable (low-risk and high-risk HPV types); may be infected with multiple types simultaneously
  3. Sexually transmitted by skin-to-skin contact through viral shedding; fomite spread is possible but rare
  4. Highly contagious—25–65% of partners develop HPV
  5. Incubation period 4 to 6 weeks
  6. The most common viral, sexually transmitted infection in the US
  7. Genital warts most commonly associated with low-risk types of HPV (6, 11)
  8. Persistent infection with high-risk types of HPV is associated with almost all cervical cancers and many vulvar, vaginal, and anal cancers
  9. About 10% of women infected with HPV develop persistent HPV infections
  10. Risk factors
      a. Previous or current other STD
      b. First intercourse at an early age (< 16 years); multiple sexual partners

    c.   Male partner who has (or has had) multiple partners

    d.   Factors that suppress the immune system—diabetes, pregnancy, steroid hormones, folate deficiencies, immunosuppressive diseases

- Signs and symptoms
  1. Wartlike lesions—pedunculated conical or cauliflower appearance; granular, rough texture to skin
  2. Lesions may be singular, multiple, or in clusters on perineum, vulva, vagina, cervix, and peri-anal area
  3. Perianal area may bleed easily, be painful, odorous, and pruritic
  4. Color usually whitish to pinkish gray
  5. May have associated heavy, malodorous discharge (BV)

- Physical findings
  1. Wartlike lesions—conical, cauliflower appearance; may be multiple anywhere on perineum, perianal area, vagina, and cervix
  2. May appear granular, macular, or cobblestone; may be subclinical or microscopic
  3. Color varies pink to gray; darkly pigmented—have high suspicion for malignancy
  4. Many times will have concomitant BV

- Differential diagnosis
  1. Verrucous carcinoma
  2. Normal variants of skin tags
  3. *Molluscum contagiosum*
  4. *Condyloma lata*
  5. Seborrheic keratosis or other benign skin disorders

- Diagnostic tests/findings
  1. Diagnosis is made by visual inspection
  2. Biopsy if diagnosis uncertain; no response to or worsening during standard therapy; patient immunocompromised; warts pigmented, indurated, bleeding, ulcerated
  3. Serologic testing for syphilis; testing for other STDs; wet mount testing for vaginal infections; consider HIV testing

- Management/Treatment
  1. Goal of treatment is to eliminate present visible disease
  2. If untreated may resolve on own, persist, remain unchanged, or increase in size or number
  3. Keep area dry and clean
  4. Advise condom use
  5. Physical agents
     a. Cryotherapy with liquid nitrogen; repeat every 1 to 2 weeks for 6 weeks
     b. Excision with tangential shave excision, curettage, electrocautery, or scissors or excision with laser
  6. Chemical or keratolytic agents
     a. Trichloracetic or bichloracetic acid (80–90% solution); apply small amount carefully to wart, allow to dry; will turn white; apply sodium bicarbonate or talc to neutralize or remove unreacted acid; may reapply weekly; safe in pregnancy
     b. Podophyllin resin (10–25%) in compound tincture of benzoin—CDC recommends application of small amount to each wart, wash off in 1 to 4 hours; repeat weekly up to 6 weeks; pregnancy risk category C; contraindicated when breastfeeding
     c. If lesions are not resolved at the end of 6 weeks of treatment, reevaluate, change treatment, or refer
  7. Patient-applied treatment
     a. Imiquimod 5% cream applied sparingly at bedtime three times a week; area washed with mild soap 6 to 10 hours after application; safety in pregnancy is unknown
     b. Podophilox 0.5% gel or solution; applied sparingly to visible warts; safety in pregnancy is unknown
     c. Use only on external warts
  8. Immunotherapy—interferon
  9. Combination therapy may be useful, especially in single-treatment failures
  10. Refer if treatment fails or if lesions are darkly pigmented, indurated, ulcerated, suspicious, or biopsy positive for HPV type with malignant potential
  11. Rule out high grade squamous intraepithelial lesion (HGSIL) before treating cervical condyloma
  12. Emphasize importance of regular Pap test
  13. HPV vaccination of all young girls and women (recommended for ages 11–26)

Gonorrhea (GC)

- Definition—a sexually transmitted bacterial infection with an affinity for columnar and transitional epithelium

- Etiology/Incidence
  1. *Neisseria gonorrhea*—gram negative, intracellular diplococcus requiring carbon dioxide environment to survive
  2. Sites for uncomplicated GC may be urethra, endocervix (most common), Skene's glands, Bartholin's glands, and/or anus

3. Most commonly sexually transmitted; neonate may become infected during birth
4. Incubation period 3 to 5 days
5. Over 1 million cases reported annually, may be as many as 2 million
6. Occurs in individuals under age 30 approximately 80% of the time
7. Male-to-female transmission estimated at 50–90%; female to male transmission 20–25%
8. Since 1976 penicillinase-producing strains have been present—some are now resistant to tetracycline, spectinomycin, or quinolones
9. Risk factors
   a. Sexually active women under age 25
   b. Multiple sexual partners or partners with multiple partners
   c. History of STD
   d. Inconsistent condom use
   e. Commercial sex work
   f. Illicit drug use

- Signs and symptoms
  1. May be asymptomatic or symptomatic at several sites—anal, vaginal, pharynx, joints
  2. Anal bleeding
  3. Pharyngeal erythema and exudate
  4. Pelvic discomfort; dysuria
  5. Vulvar pain (Skene's, Bartholin's glands)
  6. Joint pain; erythema and inflammation of joints
  7. Potential complications
     a. Septic arthritis and bacteremia
     b. Skin lesions, pharyngitis; proctitis
     c. PID; perihepatitis
     d. Infections of glands (Skene's, Bartholin's)
     e. Gonorrhea ophthalmia neonatorum (in neonates)
     f. Premature rupture of the membranes, chorioamnionitis, and prematurity

- Physical findings
  1. May have purulent discharge, inflamed Skene's or Bartholin's glands
  2. 20% invade uterus after menses with symptoms of endometritis, salpingitis, or pelvic peritonitis

- Differential diagnosis
  1. Nongonococcal mucopurulent cervicitis (MPC)
  2. Chlamydia
  3. Vaginitis

- Diagnostic tests/findings
  1. Gram stain of no value in women (60–70% false negative)

2. Culture on Thayer-Martin medium
3. Nonculture methods—nucleic acid amplification test (NAAT) recommended by CDC (2006)
4. Serologic testing for syphilis; chlamydia testing; consider HIV screen

- Management/Treatment
  1. CDC recommendations for uncomplicated infections of cervix, urethra, and rectum
     a. Cefixime orally in single dose (97.1% cure)
     b. Ceftriaxone IM in a single dose (99.1% cure)
     c. Alternative regimen if can not tolerate cephalosporins—spectinomycin IM in a single dose (98.2% cure)
     d. Patient should also be treated for chlamydia if not ruled out
  2. Treatment in pregnancy—see Pregnancy chapter
  3. Key points
     a. Patients treated for GC routinely also treated with a regimen effective against uncomplicated chlamydia
     b. Avoid sexual intercourse until all partners are treated
     c. Treat all sexual partners presumptively

Herpes Simplex (Genital Herpes Simplex, HSV)

- Definition—a common, incurable, recurrent, viral disease

- Etiology/Incidence
  1. Causative organism—two serotypes of the herpes simplex virus
     a. Type I (HSV-I) commonly found in the mouth, accounts for 15% of genital infections
     b. Type II (HSV-II) causes 85% of genital infections
  2. Approximately 45 million people infected; 1 million new cases each year
  3. 80–90% of people with HSV-II infection report no history of signs/symptoms
  4. Asymptomatic shedding of virus accounts for the majority of transmission
  5. Usually transmitted by skin-to-skin contact; rarely spread by fomite transmission
  6. 80–90% chance a female will develop herpes following sexual contact with an infected male
  7. Risk factors
     a. Previous or present infection with an STD
     b. Trauma to skin (port of entry of virus)
     c. Immunosuppressed individual
     d. Multiple sexual partners

8. Complications
   a. Herpes encephalitis
   b. Herpes meningitis
   c. Diffuse infection in immunocompromised individuals
   d. Perinatal infection
9. Genital herpes and pregnancy
   a. Most women who infect their neonates have no known history of HSV
   b. Infection is transmitted during labor and delivery

- Signs and symptoms—three HSV syndromes (primary infection, nonprimary first episode infection and recurrent infection)
  1. Primary infection
     a. Systemic symptoms—two-thirds will have systemic symptoms; fever, malaise, headache; symptoms usually begin within 1 week of exposure, peak within 4 days and subside over the next week
     b. Localized genital pain
     c. Course of genital lesions
        (1) Local prodrome; pruritus, erythema about 1 to 2 days before appearance of lesions
        (2) Formation of small, painful vesicles over labia majora, minora, mons pubis and occasionally vagina (4 to 10 days)
        (3) Vesicles rupture forming shallow, painful, wet ulcerations lasting 1 to 2 weeks
        (4) Lesions heal without scarring
     d. Tender inguinal lymphadenopathy may be the last symptom to resolve
     e. 75% will have a discharge
     f. 90% will have cervical involvement characterized by vesiculation and tendency to bleed easily
  2. First episode nonprimary—initial clinical episode in patients with previously circulating antibodies to HSV-I or HSV II
     a. Symptoms same as primary
     b. Few constitutional symptoms
     c. Shorter, milder course
  3. Recurrent genital herpes infection
     a. Symptoms same as primary—usually milder (resolve 7 to 10 days)
     b. Usually no constitutional symptoms
     c. Shorter durations of symptoms
        (1) Prodrome—1–2 days
        (2) Vesicles—3–5 days
        (3) Dry-out days—2–3 days

- Physical findings
  1. Small, painful, vesicles, and ulceration at varying stages of progression
  2. Exquisite pain at site of lesion
  3. Inguinal lymphadenopathy

- Diagnostic tests/findings
  1. Gold standard is an HSV culture properly collected from the base of the vesicle or ulcer and properly transported to a high-quality laboratory
  2. Pap test—low sensitivity, high specificity
  3. Nonculture methods—PCR assay for HSV DNA
  4. Type-specific serologic tests (TSST) are available to identify HSV-I and HSV-II antibodies; sensitivity 91–100%, specificity 92–98% at 6–12 weeks after initial infection
  5. Serologic testing for syphilis; tests for other STD; consider HIV testing

- Management/Treatment
  1. HSV-I and II have no cure; systemic antiviral drugs partially control symptoms; do not eradicate the latent virus nor affect the risk, recurrence, frequency, or severity of the symptoms once drug is discontinued; suppressive therapy may reduce viral shedding
  2. Medical management
     a. Acute treatment
        (1) Acyclovir orally for 7 to 10 days
        (2) Famciclovir orally for 7 to 10 days
        (3) Valacyclovir orally for 7 to 10 days
     b. Episodic recurrent treatment
        (1) Acyclovir orally for 5 days
        (2) Famciclovir orally for 5 days
        (3) Valacyclovir orally for 5 days
     c. Daily suppressive therapy
        (1) Acyclovir orally twice a day
        (2) Famciclovir orally twice a day
        (3) Valacyclovir orally once a day
     d. Severe—hospitalize for IV therapy
     e. Sexual partners
        (1) Asymptomatic—counsel, encourage self-examination; condoms
        (2) Symptomatic—use same treatment regimen
     f. Pregnancy—see Pregnancy chapter
     g. Special considerations
        (1) Allergy, intolerance, and adverse reaction; rare—desensitization may be necessary
        (2) HIV infection
            (a) Episodic infection may be prolonged or more severe in persons infected with HIV
            (b) Episodic or suppressive therapy is often beneficial

(c) Acyclovir, famciclovir and vala-cyclovir are safe for use in immunocompromised individuals in recommended doses

3. Nonpharmacologic symptom relief
   a. Cool, topical compresses with Burow's solution as needed; will reduce swelling and inflammation
   b. Local hygiene; topical anesthetics; cool air with fan or hair dryer

Molluscum Contagiosum

- Definition—a mildly contagious viral epithelium proliferation of the skin

- Etiology/Incidence
  1. Caused by the virus *Molluscum contagiosum*, an unassigned pox virus containing double-stranded DNA
  2. Occurs worldwide—more common in tropical and subtropical regions
  3. Most common in children and young adults
  4. Transmitted by skin to skin, fomite, and autoinoculation
  5. Incubation period 2 to 7 weeks

- Signs and symptoms
  1. Reddish to yellow, waxy, smooth, firm, spherical papules; umbilicated apex contains central plug; usually less than 20 lesions ranging from pinhead size to 1 cm in diameter
  2. Presents on trunk and lower extremities in children
  3. Presents on lower abdominal wall, inner thigh, pubic area, genitalia in adults
  4. Usually asymptomatic; may have pain, pruritus, and inflammation

- Physical findings
  1. Lesions are multiple, but usually number less than 20
  2. Characteristic light-colored papules with an umbilicated center
  3. Lesions found on trunk, lower extremities, abdomen, inner thigh, genital area

- Differential diagnosis
  1. Varicella
  2. Lichens planus
  3. Warts/condyloma
  4. Keratoacanthomas
  5. Subepidermal fibrosis
  6. Epidermal cysts

- Diagnostic tests/findings
  1. Biopsy—cytoplasmic inclusions—molluscum bodies
  2. Test for other STD in young adults

- Management/Treatment
  1. Usually resolve spontaneously without scarring
  2. Superficial incision; express contents with comedo extractor
  3. Curettage with cautery
  4. For multiple lesions, cryotherapy with liquid nitrogen, silver nitrate
  5. Treatment may cause scarring

Syphilis

- Definition—a chronic infectious, sexually transmitted process that progresses predictably through distinct stages

- Etiology/Incidence
  1. Caused by *Treponema pallidum*
  2. Organism enters skin through microscopic breaks in the skin during sexual contact
  3. Incubation period 10 to 90 days, average 21 days
  4. Occurs worldwide, primarily involving adults 20 to 35 years of age; has become epidemic in the US; includes syphilis in pregnancy and congenital syphilis
  5. Increased incidence associated with greater use of illicit drugs and high-risk behavior associated with drug use
  6. Racial differences in incidence are associated with social factors; higher incidence in urban areas
  7. Approximately 90,000 cases annually in the US

- Signs and symptoms
  1. Four stages of syphilis
     a. Primary
        (1) May be asymptomatic
        (2) Primary lesion (chancre) arises at the point of entry—evident 10 to 90 days following contact
        (3) Painless, ulcerated with raised border and indurated base, rolled edges—spontaneously disappears in 1 to 6 weeks
        (4) May appear anywhere the organism enters, primary genitals, mouth, or anus
        (5) Painless lymphadenopathy may occur
     b. Secondary
        (1) Follows resolution of the primary stage, symptoms become systemic

(2) Localized or diffuse mucocutaneous lesions (palms, soles [60–80%], mucous patches [21–58] and *condyloma lata*) with generalized lymphadenopathy along with flulike symptoms (low-grade fever, headache, sore throat, malaise, arthralgias)

(3) May begin 4 to 6 weeks after appearance of primary lesion and resolve in 1 week to 2 months

c. Latent

(1) Begins after spontaneous resolution of secondary stage

(2) If no treatment, patient goes into early latent phase for less than 1 year duration (asymptomatic)

(3) Late latent phase (after 1 year duration)

(4) May remain in this stage or progress to tertiary stage

d. Tertiary

(1) Characterized by gummas (nodular lesions) involving skin, mucous membranes, skeletal system, and viscera

(2) Cardiac symptoms, aortitis, aneurysm, or aortic regurgitation

(3) Neurosyphilis may present without symptoms or with tabes dorsalis, meningovascular syphilis, general paralysis, insanity, iritis, chorioretinitis, and leukoplakia

(4) Not infectious

- Physical findings
  1. Chancre on vulva, vagina, cervix, or at site of entry of organism—begins primary stage
  2. Secondary stage manifestations may be generalized maculopapular rash, mucocutaneous lesion, adenopathy
  3. *Condyloma lata*—wartlike lesions on vulva, perianal region, and upper thighs
  4. Tertiary may be manifested by multiple organ involvement
  5. Gummas of vulva—tertiary manifestation; appear as nodules that enlarge, ulcerate and become necrotic

- Differential diagnosis
  1. Other genitoulcerative diseases; herpes, chancroid, lymphogranuloma venereum, granuloma inguinale
  2. Genital carcinoma
  3. Trauma

- Diagnostic tests/findings
  1. Dark field microscopy of fluid from lesions reveals treponema

2. Serologic testing

   a. Nontreponemal—Venereal Disease Research Laboratory (VDRL), rapid plasma reagin (RPR); 80–90% accurate in making a diagnosis

   b. Treponemal—fluorescent treponemal antibody absorption test (FTA-ABS), *T. pallidum* particle agglutination (TP-PA)

   c. A positive RPR or VDRL must be confirmed with a FTA-ABS or TP-PA

   d. Nontreponemal test titers usually correlate with disease activity, and results should be reported quantitatively; a fourfold change in titer is equal to two dilutions (e.g., 1:16 to 1:4 or 1:8 to 1:32)

3. Lumbar puncture—late or tertiary

4. False positives for serologic testing (1%); caused by viral infections, IV drug use, pregnancy

5. Tests for other STDs, consider HIV testing

- Management/Treatment
  1. Who must be treated
     a. Pregnant women
     b. Individuals with positive darkfield examination or positive treponemal antibody test
     c. People treated previously who have a fourfold rise in quantitative nontreponemal test
     d. Patients with uncertain diagnosis
     e. Persons who were exposed within the 90 days preceding the diagnosis of primary, secondary, or early latent syphilis in a sexual partner—treat presumptively even if seronegative
     f. Persons who were exposed more than 90 days before the diagnosis of any stage of syphilis in a sexual partner—treat presumptively if test results not immediately available and opportunity for follow-up is uncertain
  2. Treatment (CDC)
     a. Primary or secondary
        (1) Benzathine penicillin G IM in a single dose
        (2) Doxycycline orally bid for 2 weeks or tetracycline orally qid for 2 weeks, for penicillin allergic
     b. Latent
        (1) Early latent—Benzathine penicillin G IM in a single dose
        (2) Late latent or latent of unknown duration—Benzathine penicillin G given IM as three doses at 1-week intervals
     c. Pregnancy—see Pregnancy chapter
     d. HIV-positive individuals

(1) May have a higher incidence of neurologic involvement and higher rate of treatment failure—careful follow-up is important

(2) Serologic test results may be atypical

(3) When clinical picture is positive and serologic test is negative, biopsy, dark field, or direct fluorescent antibody staining is done

3. Follow-up

   a. Quantitative nontreponemal serologic tests are repeated at 6, 12, and 24 months

   b. Titers should decline at least fourfold within 12 to 24 months

   c. A fourfold increase indicates inadequate treatment or a new infection

   d. Pregnant women without a fourfold drop in titer in a 3-month period, need repeat treatment

   e. Treponemal tests remain positive for lifetime in most individuals regardless of treatment or disease activity

   f. Report all cases to proper agency for follow-up of sexual contacts

Chancroid

- Definition—an acute, contagious, ulcerative, bacterial infection that is sexually transmitted

- Etiology/Incidence
  1. *Haemophilus ducreyi* is a short, nonmotile, gram-negative rod (anaerobe) that grows in chains known as "school of fish" pattern
  2. Incubation period 4 to 5 days
  3. Occurs only in a few areas of the US in discrete outbreaks; endemic in some areas
  4. Most often seen in tropical and subtropical climates
  5. Known cofactor is heterosexual transmission of HIV—strongly associated with increase in incidence of HIV rates in the US and other countries
  6. 10% will be co-infected with syphilis and HSV
  7. Recent increases in the US associated with drug use, urban poverty, prostitution, and those acquiring chancroid outside the US

- Signs and symptoms
  1. May be asymptomatic
  2. Papules or painful ulcerations on labia, anogenital skin, vagina, cervix in women; around the prepuce, frenulum, on coronal sulcus in men
  3. May be foul odor

4. One week after onset, bilateral, tender, suppurant inguinal lymphadenopathy (bubo) develops (30–60%)

5. Lesions resolve in 1 to 2 weeks if treated; 1 to 3 months if untreated

- Physical findings
  1. Deep ulcerations with irregular, scalloped borders
  2. Bilateral, tender, suppurant inguinal lymphadenopathy
  3. Lesions found on labia, vagina, anogenital skin, and cervix
  4. May have foul odor

- Differential diagnosis
  1. Genital herpes
  2. Syphilis
  3. Malignancy of vulva
  4. Trauma
  5. Donovanosis

- Diagnostic tests/findings
  1. Gram's stain reveals gram-negative rods or chains
  2. Definitive test is culture to identify *H. ducreyi*—collect from lesion or bubo; difficult to isolate on culture; use specific medium (sensitivity ≤ 80%)
  3. Clinical signs pathognomonic
     a. Genital ulcers with typical characteristics
     b. Regional lymphadenopathy
     c. Negative test for HSV
     d. Suppurant inguinal adenopathy
  4. Serologic testing for syphilis and HIV

- Management/Treatment
  1. Cured with treatment; may leave scarring in severe cases
  2. CDC recommendations
     a. Azithromycin orally in a single dose
     b. Ceftriaxone IM in a single dose
     c. Ciprofloxacin orally for 3 days
     d. Erythromycin base orally for 7 days
  3. Ciprofloxacin is contraindicated for pregnant and lactating women and for persons younger than 18 years
  4. Follow-up—reexamine in 3 to 7 days; if ulcerations have not improved reevaluate
  5. Management of sexual partners—if sexual contact occurred during 10 days preceding onset of patient's symptoms, evaluate and treat

Lymphogranuloma Venereum (LGV)

- Definition—an ulcerative, bacterial, sexually transmitted disease

- Etiology/Incidence
  1. Caused by serotypes L1, L2, and L3 of *Chlamydia trachomatis*; a bacterium; an obligate, intracellular parasite that infects columnar epithelium
  2. Occurs infrequently in the US
  3. Endemic in tropical areas and travelers to endemic areas
  4. Incubation period 5 to 21 days or longer
  5. Infects men more than women (5:1)

- Signs and symptoms
  1. May be asymptomatic
  2. May report painless ulcerations that may go unnoticed and heal within days (50%)
  3. Tender adenopathy usually occurs 1 to 4 weeks after ulcer; may have fever, malaise, headache, myalgia

- Physical findings
  1. Painless ulceration on vulva at site of inoculation; disappears in a few days
  2. Tender inguinal and/or femoral lymphadenopathy; most commonly unilateral
  3. Rectal exposure in women or men who have sex with men (MSM) may result in proctocolitis or inflammatory involvement of perirectal or perianal lymphatic tissues resulting in fistulas and strictures

- Differential diagnosis
  1. Inguinal or suppurant adenitis
  2. Chancroid
  3. HSV
  4. Syphilis
  5. Vulvar cancer

- Diagnostic tests/findings
  1. Aspiration and culture of material from fluctuant lymph nodes—50% of cases will show chlamydia
  2. Serologic testing—titer of more than 1:64 shows active disease
  3. Complete blood count will show mild leukocytosis or monocytosis
  4. Elevated sedimentation rate
  5. Screening for other STDs
  6. Encourage HIV screen

- Management/Treatment
  1. CDC recommends:
     a. Doxycycline orally for 21 days
     b. Erythromycin base orally for 21 days
  2. Follow-up—follow clinically until signs and symptoms have resolved
  3. Management of sexual partner

    a. Treat those who had sexual contact with the patient during the 30 days prior to onset of symptoms
    b. Evaluate for other STDs

Pelvic Inflammatory Disease (PID)

- Definition—comprises a spectrum of inflammatory disorders of the upper female genital tract, including any combination of salpingitis, endometritis, tubo-ovarian abscess, and pelvic peritonitis

- Etiology/Incidence
  1. Causative organisms include *Chlamydia trachomatis, Neisseria gonorrhea,* polymicrobial infection *(E coli, G. vaginalis, H. Influenzae, M. hominis)*
  2. One million cases are diagnosed annually
  3. 200,000 hospitalizations at a cost of 5 billion dollars
  4. 25% of cases result in infertility, ectopic pregnancy, chronic pelvic pain, and are at risk for major abdominal surgery
  5. One-third of women with gonorrhea or chlamydia cervicitis will progress to PID if untreated
  6. Teenagers account for one-fifth of total cases
  7. Risk factors
     a. Sexually active females less than 20 years old
     b. Multiple sexual partners
     c. Previous episode of PID
     d. Presence of chlamydia, gonorrhea, and/or bacterial vaginosis
     e. Vaginal douching
  8. Oral contraceptive pill use is protective

- Signs and symptoms
  1. May be acute or mild
  2. Abdominal pain
  3. Vaginal discharge
  4. Fever
  5. Dysuria
  6. Dyspareunia
  7. Nausea/vomiting
  8. Vaginal spotting or bleeding (30%)

- Physical findings
  1. Lower abdominal tenderness, adnexal tenderness, and cervical motion tenderness of varying degrees—minimum criteria for empiric treatment of PID in sexually active young women and other women at risk for STD with complaint of pelvic or lower abdominal pain is presence of one or more of these three findings on pelvic examination

2. Adnexal mass
3. Fever of more than 101°F (> 38.4°C)
4. Mucopurulent cervical or vaginal discharge

- Differential diagnosis
  1. Ectopic pregnancy
  2. Appendicitis
  3. Ruptured ovarian cyst
  4. Torsion of adnexal mass
  5. Ulcerative colitis
  6. Degenerative leiomyoma
  7. Renal calculus

- Diagnostic tests/findings
  1. Testing to provide laboratory documentation of cervical infection with *C. trachomatis* or *N. gonorrhoeae*
  2. Sedimentation rate elevation and/or C-reactive protein
  3. Criteria for definitive diagnosis (in case of unsure diagnosis or poor response to treatment)
     a. Histologic evidence of endometritis on endometrial biopsy
     b. Sonography or other radiographic tests revealing tubo-ovarian abscess
     c. Laparoscopy—abnormalities consistent with PID

- Management/Treatment
  1. Regimen A—ceftriaxone IM once plus doxycycline orally bid for 14 days, with or without metronidazole orally bid for 14 days
  2. Regimen B—cefoxitin IM once with probenecid in a single dose plus doxycycline orally bid for 14 days, with or without metronidazole orally bid for 14 days
  3. Regimen C—other third-generation cephalosporin IM once plus doxycycline orally bid for 14 days, with or without metronidazole orally bid for 14 days
  4. Criteria for hospitalization
     a. Patient is pregnant
     b. Pelvic abscess is suspected
     c. When surgical emergency cannot be ruled out (ectopic pregnancy, appendicitis)
     d. Severe illness, high fever, nausea and vomiting
     e. Failure of outpatient therapy
  5. Follow-up, reexamine within 72 hours—if not significantly improved, review diagnosis and treatment; may need hospitalization
     a. Criteria for improvement—defervescence, reduction in direct or rebound abdominal tenderness; reduction in adnexal, uterine, and cervical motion tenderness
     b. Counsel on safer sexual practices

6. Partner treatment—treat if contact occurred with patient during the 60 days prior to onset of symptoms

☐ URINARY TRACT DISORDERS

Urinary Tract Infections (UTIs)

- Definition—a term that encompasses a broad range of clinical conditions affecting the urinary tract
  1. Cystitis—infection of the bladder
  2. Urethritis—infection of the distal urethra
  3. Acute pyelonephritis—infection of the kidney

- Etiology/Incidence
  1. *Escherichia coli* most common organism (80%), also *Staphyloccous saprophyticus* (15%), *Proteus mirabilis*, *Klebsiella pneumonia* (all reside in the GI tract)
  2. Colonization of bacteria in the vagina due to alterations in pH increase the risk of bladder colonization
  3. More common in women than men (ratio 1:8), with a 1–3% prevalence in nonpregnant women
  4. There are four major pathways of infection
     a. Ascending from urethra (> 90%)
     b. Hematogenous
     c. Lymphatic
     d. Direct extension from another organ
  5. Risk factors
     a. Neurologic disease
     b. Renal failure
     c. Diabetes
     d. Anatomic abnormalities
     e. Pregnancy
     f. Stones
     g. Instrumentation
     h. Poor success with medical regimen
     i. Poor hygiene
     j. Infrequent voiding
     k. Diaphragm, tampon, and spermicide use
     l. Sexual activity—coital frequency, new sexual partner
     m. Immunosuppression
     n. Sickle cell disease or trait
     o. Douching
     p. Catheterization
     q. Estrogen deficiency

- Signs and symptoms
  1. Range from mild to severe
     a. Acute cystitis
        (1) Abrupt onset
        (2) Dysuria
        (3) Frequency of urination

(4) Urgency of urination

(5) Suprapubic pain

(6) Nocturia

(7) Painful bladder spasms

(8) Pyuria

(9) Hematuria (gross)

    b. Pyelonephritis

      (1) Chills, fever

      (2) Dysuria

      (3) Frequency of urination

      (4) Urgency of urination

      (5) Cloudy malodorous urine

      (6) Nausea, vomiting

    c. Urethritis

      (1) Gradual onset

      (2) Frequency of urination

      (3) Malodorous vaginal discharge

- Physical findings
  1. UTI presentation inconsistent
  2. Pyelonephritis
     a. Unilateral or bilateral costovertebral angle tenderness
     b. Fever
     c. Flank or abdominal pain
     d. Vomiting

- Differential diagnosis
  1. Vaginitis
  2. Sexually transmitted infection
  3. Fungal infections of urethra or bladder
  4. Interstitial cystitis
  5. Infected calculus
  6. Fistula
  7. Obstructive uropathy
  8. Tuberculosis of bladder
  9. Malignancy
  10. Side-effects of chemotherapy or radiation

- Diagnostic tests/findings
  1. Urine microscopy on clean catch—test shows more than 5 WBC per high-powered field (HPF) and the presence of bacteria with few squamous cells
  2. Urine culture and sensitivity
     a. Traditional criterion for infection—a colony count of more than 100,000 organisms per milliliter
     b. As few as 10,000 colonies have been known to produce symptoms
     c. Evaluated for sensitivity to medications
  3. Enzymatic (dipstick) testing—less reliable (75% sensitivity)
     a. Indicates hematuria; nitrites indicate presence of bacteria; leukocyte esterase indicates presence of WBC

    b. Send urine for urinalysis and/or culture and sensitivity if dipstick is negative in symptomatic woman

  4. Test for vaginitis, and STD if indicated

  5. Cystoscopy if indicated

- Management/Treatment
  1. Uncomplicated UTI
     a. Treat even before tests results are available
     b. Use 3-day regimen—single dose treatment is less effective
     c. Suggested medical regimens for nonpregnant women:
        (1) Nitrofurantoin orally
        (2) Ciprofloxacin orally
        (3) Ofloxacin orally
        (4) Norfloxacin orally
        (5) Sulfamethoxazole-trimethoprim orally
  2. Recurrent infections—use above regimens for 7 days
  3. Pyelonephritis—use above regimens for 10 days
  4. Recurrent infection—retest and retreat
  5. Prevention/prophylaxis
     a. Void after intercourse
     b. Discontinue use of spermicides and diaphragm
     c. Intravaginal estrogen in women with atrophy of genitalia
     d. Avoid delay in emptying bladder
  6. Referral
     a. Patients with possible pyelonephritis
     b. Patients who experience relapse after complete course of antibiotics
     c. Pregnant women
     d. Women with history of pyelonephritis
     e. Chronic disease such as diabetes
     f. Suspected renal calculus, interstitial cystitis
     g. Women who frequently use catheters

Urinary Incontinence

- Definition—involuntary loss of urine

- Etiology/Incidence
  1. Etiologies alone or in combination
     a. Age-related genitourinary anatomic changes
     b. Medications, e.g., diuretics, antidepressants, antihistamines, sedatives
     c. Nerve damage from stroke, demyelinating disorders
     d. Infections, tumors, diabetes, herniated disc

e. Bladder neoplasm, fistulas, damage to urogenital structures, atrophy (decrease in estrogen)

f. Restricted mobility, cognitive and functional impairment

g. Multiparity, obesity, smoking, constipation, family history in first-degree relative are risk factors

h. Urge incontinence—most often associated with uninhibited detrusor contractions

2. 10–25% of women between 15 and 64 years will suffer from incontinence

3. 50% of nursing home population experience incontinence

4. Less than 50% of individuals seek help; most are silent sufferers

- Signs and symptoms
  1. Stress incontinence
     a. Loss of urine, usually in small amounts, with coughing, laughing, sneezing
     b. Vaginal dryness if atrophy present
  2. Urge incontinence
     a. Involuntary loss of urine preceded by a sudden, strong urge to urinate
     b. Usually voids large amounts
     c. Difficulty in controlling once flow begins
     d. Occurs without warning—cold weather, physical activity, laughing, sexual intercourse, or placing a key in a door lock
     e. Patient will often complain of frequent voiding, urgency, nocturnal enuresis, (10–30%)—overactive bladder
  3. Mixed urinary incontinence—presents with both symptoms of stress and urge incontinence

- Physical findings
  1. Urinary leakage with increased abdominal pressure
  2. Relaxed pelvic floor muscles—cystocele
  3. Vaginal atrophy, perineal irritation

- Differential diagnosis
  1. Urinary tract infection
  2. Prolapse of bladder
  3. Tumor compressing bladder
  4. Vaginal atrophy
  5. Stool impaction

- Diagnostic tests/findings
  1. Review prescription and nonprescription drugs for etiologic factors
  2. Voiding diary
  3. Urinary stress test to assess loss of urine when coughing and straining

4. Postvoid residual measurement using catheter or scan

5. Urinalysis/culture to evaluate for infection

6. Cystometry, urethroscopy, and cystoscopy may be useful

7. Urodynamic testing is confirmatory

- Management/Treatment
  1. Transient incontinence can usually be treated with identification and treatment of underlying medical problems, behavior therapy such as habit training and timed voiding
  2. Stress incontinence—pelvic muscle exercises/pelvic floor training with Kegel exercises and biofeedback, weight loss if obese, treatment for constipation, pessaries
  3. Urge incontinence—bladder retraining with scheduled voiding, biofeedback, Kegel exercises, avoiding bladder irritants, surgical removal of obstruction, anticholinergic agents (oxybutynin chloride, tolterodine tartrate)
  4. Mixed incontinence—combine measures for urge and stress incontinence
  5. Surgery according to diagnosis
  6. Referral to a urogynecologist

◻ BREAST DISORDERS

Fibrocystic Breast Changes

- Definition—"nondisease" that includes nonproliferative microcysts, macrocysts, and fibrosis; and proliferative changes such as hyperplasia and adenosis; hyperplasia with atypia is associated with a moderate risk for breast cancer
  1. Cystic changes—refers to dilatation of ducts; may regress with menses, may persist, or may disappear and reappear
  2. Fibrous change—mass develops following an inflammatory response to ductal irritation
  3. Hyperplasia—a layering of cells; has malignant potential if atypical
  4. Adenosis—related to changes in the acini in the distal mammary lobule; ducts become surrounded by a firm, hard, plaque like material

- Etiology/Incidence
  1. Etiology not understood; occurs in response to endogenous hormone stimulation, primarily estrogen
  2. Conflicting studies on association with ingestion of foods or beverages containing methylxanthines
  3. Most common benign breast condition in women

4. Palpable nodular changes observed in more than half of adult women 20 to 50 years of age; common ages 35 to 50
5. Detectable on radiography in 90% of women age 40 or older
6. Usually a regression of the signs after menopause

- Signs and symptoms
  1. Breast pain and nodularity; usually bilateral
  2. Frequently occurs or increases 1 to 2 weeks before menses
  3. May have clear or white nipple discharge

- Physical findings
  1. Multiple, usually cystic masses that are well-defined, mobile, and often tender
  2. Absence of breast skin changes
  3. Most common sites—upper outer quadrant and axillary tail
  4. May have clear-to-white nipple discharge

- Differential diagnosis
  1. Carcinoma
  2. Galactorrhea
  3. Mastitis
  4. Costochondritis

- Diagnostic tests/findings
  1. Mammography to identify and characterize masses
  2. Ultrasound to determine if mass is cystic
  3. Fine needle aspiration (FNA) if dominant mass; cytologic evaluation
  4. Biopsy or excision if dominant mass or following findings are present:
     a. Bloody fluid on aspiration
     b. Failure of mass to disappear after aspiration
     c. Recurrence of a cyst after two aspirations
     d. Solid mass not diagnosed as fibroma
     e. Bloody nipple discharge
     f. Nipple ulceration; presence of skin edema or erythema

- Management/Treatment
  1. Treatment not necessary
  2. Aspiration of palpable cysts may be curative
  3. Patients with symptomatic nodularity or with mastalgia are best treated medically
     a. Oral contraceptive pills; good first choice (improvement seen in 70–90% of women)
     b. Danazol
     c. Tamoxifen
     d. Bromocriptine
     e. Restriction of methylxanthines (caffeine, tea, cola, chocolate)
     f. Vitamin E to control breast pain (controversial; no more than 50 to 600 IU a day)
     g. Mild analgesics; supportive brassiere

Fibroadenoma

- Definition—benign breast mass derived from fibrous and glandular tissue

- Etiology/Incidence
  1. Etiology unknown; development soon after menarche—appears to be hormone related
  2. Most common benign, dominant mass in younger women
  3. Occurs most often in women 15 to 25 years of age
  4. Pregnancy may stimulate growth; may regress with menopause

- Signs and symptoms
  1. Painless, single, rubbery mass
  2. Round to lobular in shape
  3. May be from 2 to 4 cm in size to 15 cm tumors
  4. No nipple discharge
  5. Does not change with menstrual cycle

- Physical findings
  1. Firm, well delineated, freely movable, rubbery, round, nontender mass; usually unilateral
  2. No nipple discharge

- Differential diagnosis
  1. Carcinoma of the breast
  2. Cystosarcoma phyllodes
  3. Benign cyst

- Diagnostic tests/findings
  1. Fine needle aspiration (FNA) to determine whether cystic or solid
  2. Excisional biopsy
  3. Ultrasonography and/or mammography will help distinguish singular from multiple non-palpable masses (ultrasound best choice for young women)

- Management/Treatment
  1. Observation, if diagnosis is confirmed and younger than 25 years
  2. May be removed to alleviate patient anxiety or if diagnosis is uncertain
  3. Follow-up with monthly self-breast examinations and annual breast examination by clinician; annual mammograms if criteria of age and risk factors met
  4. Key points

a. No mass is obviously benign—each should be carefully evaluated to rule out carcinoma
b. Nipple discharge is seldom associated with carcinoma of the breast; when there is spontaneous clear, serous or bloody discharge or postmenopausal discharge present cancer should be ruled out with a thorough evaluation
c. Breast discomfort is usually associated with fibrocystic changes

Intraductal Papilloma

- Definition—benign lesion of the lactiferous duct, most common in the perimenopausal age group

- Etiology/Incidence
  1. Proliferation and overgrowth of epithelial tissue of the subareolar collection duct
  2. Occurs in the perimenopause, or menopausal woman 40 to 59 years of age
  3. Most common cause of pathologic nipple discharge

- Signs and symptoms
  1. Bloody, serous, or turbid discharge (not milk)—which may occur spontaneously
  2. Mass not usually palpable
  3. Feeling of fullness or pain beneath areola (possible)

- Physical findings
  1. Expression of serosanguineous nipple discharge from a single duct when pressure applied to affected duct
  2. Poorly delineated, soft mass may be palpated
  3. Papilloma are usually singular

- Differential diagnosis
  1. Intraductal carcinoma
  2. Multiple papillomatosis
  3. Galactorrhea

- Diagnostic tests/findings
  1. Microscopy of breast fluid to visualize fat globules
  2. Cytology of fluid—false negative rates of 20% for cancer
  3. Mammography
  4. Radiologic ductogram—use is controversial
  5. Excisional biopsy of duct

- Management
  1. Refer for surgical excision
  2. Excisional biopsy is curative

Breast Carcinoma

- Definition—malignant neoplasm of the breast

- Etiology/Incidence
  1. Possible interaction of ovarian estrogen and nonovarian estrogen; estrogen of exogenous origin with susceptible breast tissue
  2. Most common female malignancy—second to lung cancer as leading cause of cancer-related death; incidence is steadily increasing in US
  3. Incidence increases with age (75% are > 40 years of age)
  4. Cumulative lifetime risk is 10.2% or 1 in 9; increase in numbers may indicate better detection and larger numbers of women in their 40s and 50s
  5. Risk factors
     a. Women with BRCA1 and BRCA2
     b. Advancing age
     c. Mother and/or sister with breast cancer
     d. Previous breast cancer
     e. Perimenopausal status
     f. Previous endometrial or colon cancer
     g. Previous breast biopsy with atypical hyperplasia, lobular neoplasm
     h. Menarche before age 12; menopause after age 55
     i. Nulliparity, first pregnancy after 30
     j. Hormone replacement therapy, oral contraceptive pills (questionable)
     k. Obesity, environmental factors; exposure to radiation or pesticides
     l. Heavy alcohol use; fat in diet

- Signs and symptoms
  1. Breast mass—most often upper-outer quadrant
  2. May have spontaneous clear, serous, or bloody nipple discharge
  3. May have retraction, dimpling, skin edema, erythema
  4. Axillary, supraclavicular, or infraclavicular lymphadenopathy may be present

- Physical findings
  1. Mass fixed, poorly defined, irregular, usually nontender; palpable at 1 cm
  2. May have nipple discharge, irritation, retraction, edema
  3. Enlarged lymph nodes

- Differential diagnosis
  1. Fibroadenoma
  2. Fibrocystic breast changes
  3. Trauma
  4. Mastitis

- Diagnostic tests/findings
  1. Mammogram detects 30–50% of cancers
  2. Ultrasound to distinguish solid from cystic mass
  3. Histology for definitive diagnosis—specimen obtained through open biopsy, needle biopsy, fine needle aspiration (FNA), or stereotactic core needle biopsy
  4. CT scan of liver, lungs, bone to rule out metastasis
  5. Presence of estrogen receptors determined by assay
  6. Sentinel node biopsy
  7. Negative mammogram and negative aspiration cytology does not exclude malignancy

- Management/Treatment
  1. Referral to oncologist if malignancy is suspected; staging will determine appropriate treatment options
  2. Early breast cancer—surgery or surgery and radiation; 60–70% choose lumpectomy, axillary node dissection, and breast radiation
  3. Medical therapy for hormone receptor positive tumors—tamoxifen, aromatase inhibitors
  4. Radiotherapy and cytotoxic chemotherapy are adjuvant therapy in late disease

◘ CONGENITAL AND CHROMOSOMAL ABNORMALITIES

Müllerian Abnormalities

- Definition—congenital anomalies involving the uterus, fallopian tubes, and upper vagina resulting from absence of antimüllerian hormone (AMH)

- Etiology/Incidence
  1. Possible causes include teratogenesis, genetic inheritance, and multifactorial expression
  2. Occurs in up to 15% of women with recurrent spontaneous abortion and in 5–19% of infertile women

- Signs and symptoms
  1. History of pregnancy loss or infertility
  2. Amenorrhea, dysmenorrhea
  3. Dyspareunia

- Physical findings
  1. Many variations may occur
     a. Lack of development (agenesis); e.g., no vagina, uterus, tubes, uterine cavity
     b. Incomplete development (hypoplasia); e.g., partial vagina, bicornate uterus, partial uterine cavity
     c. Incomplete canalization (atresia); e.g., imperforate hymen, cervical atresia
     d. One-third have urinary tract abnormalities, e.g., ectopic kidney, renal agenesis, horseshoe shaped kidney, abnormal collecting ducts
  2. Ovaries may be developed, resulting in well-developed secondary sexual characteristics

- Differential diagnosis
  1. Various congenital anomalies
  2. Anomalies of urinary tract
  3. Primary amenorrhea

- Diagnostic tests/findings
  1. Structural abnormalities detected by ultrasonography, MRI, hysterosalpingogram, laparoscopy
  2. Chromosomal abnormalities ruled out with karyotyping (46XX)

- Management/Treatment
  1. Referral to reproductive endocrinologist
  2. Surgical intervention

Androgen Insensitivity/Resistance Syndrome

- Definition—genetically transmitted androgen receptor defect; individual is genotypic male (46XY) but phenotypic female; previously called testicular feminization

- Etiology/Incidence
  1. Individual has testes and a 46XY karyotype
  2. Transmitted by maternal X-linked recessive gene; a defect in androgen receptors; 25% risk of affected child, 25% risk of carrier
  3. Third most common cause of primary amenorrhea; represents 10% of all cases
  4. Risk of malignant transformation of gonads (5%); incidence of malignancy is rare before puberty

- Signs and symptoms
  1. Often not detected until puberty
  2. Primary amenorrhea
  3. Infertility

- Physical findings
  1. Uterus and ovaries are absent and a blind pouch vagina is present; labia underdeveloped; absent or scant pubic hair
  2. Normally developed breast with small nipples and pale areola

3. Inguinal hernias (50%) or labial masses in infant child due to partially descended testes; testes may be intra-abdominal
4. Scant body hair
5. Growth and development are normal; overall height usually greater than average
6. May have horseshoe kidneys

- Differential diagnosis
  1. Müllerian anomalies (agenesis)
  2. Incomplete androgen insensitivity

- Diagnostic tests/findings
  1. Karyotype reveals 46XY; phenotype normal female
  2. Testosterone greater than 3ng/mL and LH levels normal to slightly elevated

- Management/Treatment
  1. Once full development is attained (after puberty), gonads should be removed at about age 16 to 18
  2. Estrogen replacement therapy after gonads removed
  3. Evaluate other family members; sensitive counseling

Turner's Syndrome

- Definition—gonadal dysgenesis; an abnormality in, or an absence of one of the X chromosomes; phenotypically female; described by Turner in 1938

- Etiology/Incidence
  1. Usually a deficiency of paternal contribution of sex chromosomes reflecting paternal nondisjunction
  2. Occurs in 1 out of 2500 to 5000 liveborn girls
  3. Most common chromosomal abnormality found on spontaneous abortuses (45X)
  4. 60% of Turner's patients have a total loss of one X chromosome; 40% are mosaics or have structural aberrations in the X or Y chromosome

- Signs and symptoms
  1. Turner phenotype recognizable at any time of development
     a. Short stature, webbed neck, shield chest with widely spaced nipples, increased carrying angle of elbow, arched palate, low neck hairline, short fourth metacarpal bones, disproportionately short legs, lack of breast development, scant pubic hair
     b. Amenorrhea; lack of sexual development
     c. Autoimmune disorders; Hashimotos's thyroiditis (hypothyroidism [10%] with goiter

formation), Addison's disease (adrenal insufficiency), alopecia, and vitiligo
     d. Hearing loss
     e. Normal intelligence; may have difficulty with mathematical ability, visual–motor coordination, and spatial–temporal processing

- Physical findings
  1. No secondary sex characteristics
  2. Uterus present; absent or streak ovaries; infertile
  3. Congenital anomalies as described under signs and symptoms
  4. Renal (horseshoe kidney) and cardiac anomalies (coarctation of aorta, bicuspid aortic valves, mitral valve prolapse, aortic aneurysm)
  5. Hearing loss
  6. Hypothyroidism, adrenal insufficiency
  7. Alopecia, vitiligo

- Differential diagnosis—other forms of gonadal dysgenesis

- Diagnostic tests/findings
  1. FSH—if elevated need karyotype determination
  2. Ultrasonography or MRI scan
  3. Renal ultrasonography, cardiology consultation

- Management/Treatment
  1. Recognition of multisystem involvement and involvement of multiple medical specialists
  2. Refer to endocrinologist
  3. Estrogen and progesterone replacement
  4. Human growth hormone
  5. Participation in a genetic support group

☐ ADDITIONAL GYNECOLOGICAL DISORDERS

Chronic Pelvic Pain

- Definition—a nonspecific term associated with actual or potential tissue damage; noncyclic or cyclic pelvic pain that lasts longer than 6 months, is not relieved by nonnarcotic analgesics, and is of sufficient severity to cause functional disability and/or lead to seeking medical care

- Etiology/Incidence
  1. Gynecological, orthopedic, gastrointestinal, urologic, neurologic, and psychosomatic origin
  2. Relationship between pelvic pain and the underlying gynecological pathology is often inexplicable

3. Gynecological causes
   a. Endometritis
   b. Salpingo-oophoritis (PID)
   c. Adhesions
   d. Pelvic congestion syndrome
   e. Ovarian remnant syndrome
   f. Myomata uteri
   g. Endometriosis
   h. Adenomyosis
   i. Gynecological malignancies (especially late stage)
4. 48% associated with prior psychosexual trauma, including molestation, incest, and rape
5. Accounts for up to 10% of gynecological consultations, 10% of laparoscopies and 12% of hysterectomies in the US, costing $2 billion annually
6. Mean age is 28.6
7. 20% have coexistent psychological pathology
8. No significant differences by race, education, mean age of menarche, menstrual cycle, or gravidity and parity
9. Diagnosis is difficult and patients are often referred to many specialists while becoming frustrated, angry, and/or defensive

- Signs and symptoms
  1. Paroxysms of sharp, stabbing, sometimes crampy, or dull continuous pain, usually severe
  2. Dysmenorrhea, dysuria, or vaginal pain
  3. Pain may or may not be reproducible by manipulation of pelvic organs on bimanual examination

- Physical findings
  1. Physical and gynecological examination may be normal
  2. Findings consistent with specific medical, orthopedic, neurologic, gastrointestinal disorder
  3. Findings consistent with specific gynecological disorder

- Differential diagnosis
  1. Pregnancy, ectopic, spontaneous abortion, trophoblastic disease
  2. Gynecological disease—endometriosis, PID, cancer or torsion of ovaries, rupture of ovarian cyst
  3. Nongynecological disease—renal calculi, irritable bowel, appendicitis, urinary tract diseases including interstitial cystitis, orthopedic, neurologic, gastrointestinal disorders

- Diagnostic tests/findings
  1. Laboratory studies are of little value in the diagnosis of chronic pelvic pain
  2. Pregnancy test, CBC, erythrocyte sedimentation rate (ESR), urinalysis
  3. Pelvic ultrasonography, hysteroscopy
  4. If bowel or urinary symptoms; barium enema, upper GI series, IV pyelogram
  5. If musculoskeletal disease suspected; lumbosacral radiography and orthopedic consultation
  6. Diagnostic laparoscopy—ultimate method of diagnosis

- Management/Treatment
  1. Appropriate referral for treatment of organic pathology
  2. Referral for psychiatric evaluation if no physical causes found; counseling for prior sexual trauma or domestic violence
  3. May need both medical and psychological management
  4. Supplemental therapies may include biofeedback, acupuncture, transcutaneous nerve stimulation (TENS)

Pelvic Relaxation

- Definition—a nonspecific term denoting a condition occurring chiefly as weakness and defect in pelvic supporting tissues that includes:
  1. Cystocele—herniation of the bladder into the vaginal lumen
  2. Urethrocele—herniation of the urethra into the vagina
  3. Cystourethrocele—both urethra and bladder are herniated
  4. Rectocele—bulging or herniation of the anterior rectal wall and posterior vaginal wall into the opening of the vagina
  5. Enterocele—a portion of the large or small intestine herniates into the upper vagina or dissects into the rectovaginal space
  6. Vaginal prolapse—loss of support of the vaginal apex resulting in eversion toward the introitus
  7. Uterine prolapse—descent of the uterus and cervix into the vagina toward the introitus

- Etiology/Incidence
  1. Weakness in supporting structures include the pelvic diaphragm, ligaments, and fascia—commonly related to neuromuscular injury at childbirth, resulting in denervation injury of muscular floor

2. Other causes include conditions that cause chronic increase in abdominal pressure—obesity, straining, chronic lung disease (coughing); nerve function altered by diabetes, pelvic surgery, neurologic disorders, and hypoestrogenism

- Signs and symptoms
  1. May be asymptomatic and discovered during routine examination
  2. Pelvic, vaginal, and low back pain and pressure
  3. Bulging or mass in vagina; difficulty in walking
  4. Urinary incontinence, incomplete bladder emptying, difficulty in evacuation of feces
  5. Exposed vagina may become dry and ulcerated; purulent discharge

- Physical findings
  1. Descent of the anterior or posterior vaginal walls; various degrees of descent of the cervix into the vagina indicating uterine prolapse
  2. Poor muscle strength in pubococcygeal muscles
  3. Complete prolapse of uterus (prodentia); ulceration, purulent discharge, bleeding

- Differential diagnosis
  1. Tumors of pelvis or abdomen involving any abdominal structure
  2. Diverticulum of urethra

- Diagnostic tests/findings
  1. Rule out tumors with appropriate evaluation as indicated
  2. Valsalva to assess full extent of prolapse

- Management/Treatment
  1. Nonsurgical treatment—usually pessary
  2. Surgical treatment to correct vaginal anatomy (if severe)
  3. Kegel exercise to help improve muscle tone
  4. To avoid straining with bowel movements—use of stool softeners, dietary intervention, e.g., increase fluid intake, raw fruits and vegetables with skin, dried fruits, high fiber breakfast foods
  5. Use of biofeedback modalities

Toxic Shock Syndrome

- Definition—rare, potentially fatal, febrile condition affecting multiple systems

- Etiology/Incidence
  1. Associated with toxins produced by strains of *Staphylococcus aureus*

2. Occurs most often in Caucasian women under 30 years of age using tampons during menstruation; rarely associated with other articles placed in the vagina, such as diaphragms, sponges, and cervical caps
3. Incidence is 1 to 2 per 100,000 per year in women using tampons
4. 10% of population lacks sufficient antitoxin antibodies to *S. aureus*
5. Nonmenstruating associated cases (55%) are caused by puerperal sepsis, post-Cesarean endometritis, mastitis, PID, wound infection, insects

- Signs and symptoms
  1. Sudden onset fever, 102°F or greater
  2. Diffuse macular sunburn-like rash over face, trunk, and extremities that desquamates 1 to 2 weeks after onset
  3. Hyperemia of conjunctiva, oropharynx, tongue, vagina
  4. GI symptoms—nausea, vomiting, diarrhea, abdominal tenderness, dysphagia
  5. Genitourinary—vaginal discharge, adnexal tenderness
  6. Flulike symptoms—headache, sore throat, myalgia, rigors, photophobia, arthralgia
  7. Cardiorespiratory—symptoms of pulmonary edema, disseminated intravascular coagulation (DIC), endocarditis, acute respiratory distress syndrome (ARDS)
  8. Organ failure symptoms—renal, hepatic

- Physical findings
  1. Fever
  2. Diffuse macular erythematous rash and desquamation
  3. Hyperemia of conjunctiva, oropharynx, tongue, vagina
  4. Orthostatic hypotension
  5. Abdominal tenderness
  6. Vaginal discharge, adnexal tenderness
  7. Physical signs of pulmonary edema, disseminated intravascular coagulation, endocarditis, acute respiratory distress syndrome (ARDS)
  8. Altered sensorium

- Differential diagnosis
  1. Septic shock
  2. Rocky Mountain spotted fever
  3. Scarlet fever
  4. Staph food poisoning
  5. Meningococcemia (meningitis)
  6. Legionnaires's disease
  7. PID

- Diagnostic tests/findings
  1. Cultures to determine source of infection, e.g., throat, vagina, cervix, blood
  2. Serologic tests to rule out Rocky Mountain spotted fever, syphilis, rubeola
  3. Urinalysis
  4. Evaluation for presence of multiorgan involvement—serum multichemical analysis, clotting profile, blood gases, CBC with differential (platelets $\leq 100,000/mm^3$)
  5. Diagnostic criteria includes involvement of three or more organs or systems that include—cardiopulmonary, CNS, hematologic, liver, renal, mucous membranes, musculoskeletal, gastrointestinal

- Management/Treatment
  1. Refer immediately to hospital for emergency treatment in intensive care setting
  2. Prevention
     a. Avoidance of tampons or leave in place no longer than 4 hours; alternate with pads
     b. Educate regarding signs and symptoms and prompt treatment
     c. History of TSS—avoid tampons, cervical caps, diaphragms

Diethylstilbestrol (DES) in Utero

- Definition—a synthetic nonsteroidal estrogen approved by the FDA in 1942 to prevent abortion; prescribed for an estimated 2 million pregnant women for the purpose of preventing fetal wastage; did not prove to be effective; FDA withdrew approval for use in 1971

- Etiology/Incidence
  1. Vagina originally lined with columnar epithelium, which is eventually replaced with squamous epithelium; if DES is introduced that transformation is not completed; one-third of exposed patients will have columnar epithelium in the vagina (adenosis)
  2. Structural changes of the cervix and vagina occur in 25% of females exposed in utero to DES; transverse vaginal septum, cervical collar, uterine constriction band
  3. Occurrence of these abnormalities is related to the dose of medication and the first time exposed; risk is significant if administration was begun after the 18th week of gestation
  4. Increased incidence of preterm delivery, spontaneous abortion, and ectopic pregnancy
  5. Clear cell carcinoma of the vagina occurs rarely, a 1/1000 risk
  6. Columnar epithelium of vagina is especially susceptible to HPV
  7. 25% of male offspring may be affected with cryptorchidism, small testes, epididymal cysts

- Signs and symptoms
  1. May have discharge, postcoital bleeding, dyspareunia
  2. May report infertility; poor pregnancy outcomes

- Physical findings
  1. Vaginal adenosis (most common)
  2. Nodularity of cervix or vagina
  3. Visible cervical abnormalities, e.g., ridges, cockscomb, collar, hood on anterior cervix; pseudopolyps, hypoplasia
  4. Colposcopically resembles dysplasia; mosaic pattern, punctation
  5. Transverse or longitudinal vaginal septum
  6. Uterine abnormalities; T-shaped uterus, bicornate or didelphis uterus, septate uterus

- Differential diagnosis
  1. Congenital anomalies
  2. Genetic disorders

- Diagnostic tests/findings
  1. Pap test of squamocolumnar junction to rule out cancer
  2. Colposcopy and biopsy of suspicious areas
  3. Hysterosalpingogram or ultrasonography to evaluate structural anomalies

- Management/Treatment
  1. No current therapy
  2. Follow annually with Pap test/colposcopy
  3. Thorough palpation of vagina, cervix, and vaginal wall for masses
  4. Refer if abnormality suspected

Vulvar Dermatoses

- Definition—nonneoplastic disorders of vulvar epithelium growth and nutrition producing a number of gross changes; three major vulvar dermatoses: lichens sclerosus; lichens planus (other names include erosive lichens planus, erosive vaginitis, desquamative vaginitis); lichens simplex chronicus, (previously known as "nonneoplastic epithelial disorders"); may be seen on other parts of the body

- Etiology/Incidence
  1. Lichen sclerosus, lichen planus—etiology unknown; perianal involvement in 50% of patients, less than 20% have lesions on trunk; may be familial incidence and links with

certain histocompatibililty antigens (HLA) subtypes and autoimmune disease
2. Lichen simplex chronicus—thickening of skin in response to chronic rubbing or scratching; more common in people with hay fever or chronic inflammation; chronic candida often the initiating factor
3. Can occur at any age from early childhood to old age

- Signs and symptoms
  1. Lichen sclerosus
     a. Skin easily traumatized; bruises and purpura common; blisters, ulceration
     b. Severe itching and burning; lesions do not correlate with discomfort
     c. Skin of vulva thin and wrinkled
     d. Obliteration of clitoris
  2. Lichen planus
     a. May affect gingival and oral mucosa
     b. Untreated may cause vaginal adhesions
     c. Flares and remits spontaneously
     d. Secondary infection may occur
  3. Lichen simplex chronicus
     a. Can appear on any body surface
     b. Severe itching
     c. Thickening of vulvar skin

- Physical findings
  1. May be found on other parts of the body
  2. Lichen sclerosus
     a. Loss of pigmentation, symmetry of distribution, and loss of vulvar architecture with obliteration of the clitoris
     b. Thickened dermis; white, thin, wrinkled and scaly
     c. Bruises or purpura, blisters, ulcers
     d. Does not affect the vagina
     e. Confetti pattern of small dots can be confluent
  3. Lichen planus
     a. Shiny, smooth, flat topped papules, plaques on the skin and white patches of erosions on mucous membranes; may be widespread on vaginal mucosa
     b. Papules are purplish and range from pinpoint size to more than 1 cm in diameter; may scatter, coalesce into plaques, or become annular or linear along scars or scratch marks
     c. May be found on wrists, shins and buccal mucosa; occasional scarring and alopecia on scalp; nails—ridging, nail loss
     d. Superficial vaginal adhesions
     e. Flares and remits spontaneously—lasts from weeks to several years

4. Sometimes, autoimmune diseases are associated with lichen sclerosus and lichen planus—vitiligo, alopecia areata, ulcerative colitis, myasthenia gravis, and hypogammaglobulinemia
5. Lichen simplex chronicus
   a. Thickened, leathery, lichenified plaques on labia majora
   b. Other locations—nape of neck, ankle, forearm, antecubital and popliteal fossae; hair and scalp (excoriated papules)
   c. Pruritus especially with stress; scratching is sometimes violent, patient stops only when skin becomes eroded and painful

- Differential diagnosis
  1. Vitiligo
  2. Vulvar carcinoma
  3. Seborrheic dermatitis
  4. Psoriasis
  5. Tinea
  6. Vaginitis
  7. Sexually transmitted infection
  8. Parasitic infection

- Diagnostic tests/findings
  1. Colposcopy
  2. Biopsy is the gold standard for diagnosis
  3. Saline and KOH wet mount to rule out vaginitis
  4. STD testing if indicated

- Management/Treatment
  1. Lichen simplex chronicus—antifungal cream as directed (terconazole first choice)
  2. Superpotent topical steroids found to be best treatment for vulvar dermatoses that have thickened skin; clobetasol
  3. Apply sparingly
  4. Treatment may not be necessary in the absence of active disease—flares require initiation of topical steroid with a tapering regimen
  5. High-potency steroids should not be used for long periods of time (cause thinning of the skin and "rebound" dermatitis when discontinued)
  6. Should not be used when change in skin texture or thickness is absent
  7. Skin redness alone should not be treated with anything more potent than 1% hydrocortisone cream
  8. Testosterone ointment of no value
  9. Advise gentle soaps and cotton underwear
  10. Long-term/chronic conditions require patience on part of clinician and patient; counseling may be necessary; no overnight cure

11. May try Burow's solution soaks for relief of local irritation

Vestibulitis

- Definition—marked inflammation of the minor vestibular glands; reasons unclear

- Etiology/Incidence—may be bacterial, fungal, or viral agents; or unknown etiology

- Signs and symptoms
  1. Introital discomfort and dyspareunia of varying degrees; may be severe and incapacitating; dysuria
  2. Pain described as burning (most common)

- Physical findings
  1. Gross examination may be unremarkable
  2. Colposcopy or careful examination with a magnifying glass reveals tiny erythematous foci with mild edema around gland openings
  3. Hymen constricted, firm, and tender to palpation

- Differential diagnosis
  1. Vaginitis
  2. Sexually transmitted infection
  3. Lichen planus, sclerosus, or simplex chronicus
  4. Contact dermatitis
  5. Trauma

- Diagnostic tests/findings
  1. Colposcopy reveals classic inflammation of gland openings
  2. Pain can be reproduced by vestibule contact with a cotton-tipped applicator
  3. Wet mount and saline microscopic assessment; rule out vaginitis
  4. Testing for STD as indicated

- Management/Treatment
  1. Treat inflammation if cause is determined; frequently candidiasis
  2. Gabapentin or amitriptyline
  3. Surgery (laser) or excision may be useful; frequent recurrences
  4. Counseling or psychological support including antidepressants are useful to assist with chronic pain
  5. Expect long-term chronic therapy

Vulvodynia

- Definition—chronic vulvar discomfort, especially burning sensation

- Etiology/Incidence
  1. Constant pain usually means neurologic dysfunction of some kind (pudendal neuralgia, dyesethetic vulvodynia, "essential" vulvodynia, peripheral neuropathy, chronic local pain syndrome (CLPS), and others)
  2. May be related to urethral syndrome or interstitial cystitis

- Signs and symptoms
  1. Severe burning, stinging, irritation or "rawness"
  2. No visible dermatoses or intermittent symptoms
  3. Two major presentations
     a. Constant pain
     b. Pain with intercourse (dyspareunia)

- Physical findings—no visible lesions or dermatoses

- Differential diagnosis
  1. Vaginal infection
  2. Allergy/sensitivity
  3. Psychogenic disorder—history of sexual abuse, rape, incest

- Diagnostic tests/findings
  1. Colposcopy/biopsy to rule out dermatoses, pathology
  2. Testing to evaluate bladder—infection or other pathology
  3. Evaluate vaginal secretions as indicated

- Management/Treatment
  1. Treat infections as appropriate
  2. Amitriptyline, gabapentin, and/or clonazepam often helpful

Infertility

- Definition—inability to conceive after 1 year of unprotected coitus

- Etiology/Incidence
  1. Ovulatory dysfunction (15%)—poorly receptive cervical mucus due to estrogen levels, polycystic ovarian syndrome (PCOS), primary ovarian failure
  2. Tubal and pelvic pathology (35–40%)—fibroids, neoplasm, congenital anomalies, salpingitis, adhesions, endometritis, cervicitis, endometriosis
  3. Male factor (35–40%)
     a. Abnormal semen analysis, oligospermia, abnormal sperm penetration and sperm antibodies

b. Sperm exposure to heat, radiation, environmental toxins

c. Coital frequency, cannabis, cocaine, DES exposure

d. Anatomical abnormalities such as hypospadias, retrograde ejaculation (obstruction), varicocele

4. Aging women—increased incidence when oocytes are of advanced age

5. Cigarette and cannabis smoking (inhibits GnRH); greatest risk with smoking at an early age

6. Thyroid disease

7. Diethlystilbestrol exposure; also increases fetal wastage

8. Infrequent intercourse; possible sexual dysfunction

- Signs and symptoms—none specifically

- Physical findings—none specifically

- Differential diagnosis—none

- Diagnostic tests/findings
  1. Hysterosalpingogram
     a. Fluoroscopic radiography of the uterus and fallopian tubes to determine tubal patency and intrauterine/fallopian tube abnormalities; used to evaluate patients with history of infertility, spontaneous abortion, preterm delivery; contraindicated in patients allergic to radiopaque dye, pregnant, or with abnormal bleeding
     b. Dye is instilled in the uterus through the cervix; it then spreads through fallopian tubes; followed by radiographic assessment
  2. Hysteroscopy
     a. Minor operative procedure allows for inspection of endocervix and endometrial cavity; useful in the evaluation of infertility, abnormal bleeding, and endometrial cancer
     b. Under anesthesia, lighted hysteroscope is inserted through the cervix into the uterine cavity
  3. Postcoital testing (Huhner's test)
     a. Microscopic evaluation of sperm count and variability in cervical mucus following intercourse
     b. Instructions
        (1) No intercourse 48 hours prior to test
        (2) Intercourse during frame of ovulation
        (3) Evaluation within 6 to 24 hours
        (4) Specimen of mucus collected from cervix

(5) Sperm evaluation for normal characteristics

4. Basal body temperature
   a. Basal body temperature detects increase in body temperature in response to progesterone; indicates ovulation/anovulation; times ovulation for purpose of conception/contraception
   b. Procedure
      (1) Temperature reading each morning prior to arising/drinking/eating/activity
      (2) Recorded on graph
      (3) Normal value in follicular phase less than or equal to 98°F
      (4) Rises in luteal phase 0.4° to 0.6°F
      (5) Increase maintained until the next menses begins
      (6) This sustained increase indicates biphasic/ovulatory cycle

5. Ovulation prediction testing
   a. Urine test for LH
   b. Predicts ovulation within 24 to 26 hours

- Management/Treatment
  1. Female factors, ovulatory dysfunction—ovulation induction therapy
  2. Luteal phase defect—progesterone
  3. Infections/endometriosis—appropriate therapy
  4. Tubal occlusion/obstruction—surgery
  5. Male factor—antisperm antibodies treated by washing sperm or immunosuppressive drug therapy, varicocele repair, vasectomy reversal (50–60% success rate), nonreversible procedures require assisted reproductive technology
  6. Assisted reproductive technology (ART)—all the techniques used to achieve pregnancy that involve direct retrieval of oocytes from the ovary
     a. In vitro fertilization (IVF)—oocytes are extracted, fertilized in the laboratory, then transferred through the cervix into the uterus (most common procedure, success rate (15–20%)
     b. Gamete intrafallopian transfer (GIFT)—placement of oocytes into the fallopian tube (25% success rate)
     c. Zygote intrafallopian transfer (ZIFT)—placement of fertilized oocytes into the fallopian tube (18–20% successful)
     d. Tubal embryo transfer (TET)—placement of cleaving embryos into the fallopian tubes (not often used)
     e. Peritoneal oocyte and sperm transfer (POST)—placement of oocytes and sperm

in the pelvic cavity (play minimal role in treatment)

    f.   Subzonal insertion of sperm by microinjection (SUZI)—used for male factor

  7.   Sensitive counseling; infertility support groups

Abnormal Pap Test

- Definition—collection and microscopic evaluation of epithelial cells of the cervix and endocervix suggestive of future cervical cancer; results may range in degree from normal to atypical, mild, moderate, and severe abnormalities to invasive cancer

- Abnormalities may be reported in one or more of three synonymous terms
  1. Cervical dysplasia
  2. Cervical intraepithelial neoplasia (CIN)
  3. Squamous intraepithelial lesion (SIL)
  4. The most common nomenclature in use today is the Bethesda System (1988, revised 1991 and 2001)

- The 2001 Bethesda System for reporting results of cervical cytology includes
  1. Specimen adequacy
     a. Satisfactory for evaluation; will note presence/absence of endocervical/ transformation zone component
     b. Unsatisfactory for evaluation—specimen obscured by blood or inflammation, inadequate number of squamous cells, air dried slide, not processed because unlabeled
  2. Interpretation/Results
     a. General categorization
        (1) Negative for intraepitheal lesion or malignancy
        (2) Epithelial cell abnormality
        (3) Other
     b. Negative for intraepithelial lesion or malignancy
        (1) No epithelial abnormality
        (2) Will report presence of organisms
            (a) Trichomonas
            (b) Fungal organisms consistent morphologically with candida species
            (c) Shift in vaginal flora suggestive of bacterial vaginosis
            (d) Bacteria morphologically consistent with actinomyces species
            (e) Cellular changes consistent with herpes simplex virus
        (3) May report other nonneoplastic findings

        (a) Reactive cellular changes associated with inflammation, radiation, intrauterine device

        (b) Glandular cells status posthysterectomy

        (c) Atrophy

    c.   Epithelial cell abnormalities
      (1) Squamous cell abnormalities
         (a) Atypical squamous cells of undetermined significance (ASC-US)
         (b) Atypical squamous cells cannot exclude HSIL (ASC-H)
         (c) Low-grade squamous intraepithelial lesion (LSIL); encompasses human papillomavirus/mild dysplasia/cervical intraepithelial neoplasia 1(CIN 1)
         (d) High-grade squamous intraepithelial lesion (HSIL); encompasses moderate dysplasia/ carcinoma in situ/ CIN 2 and CIN 3
         (e) Squamous cell carcinoma
      (2) Glandular cell abnormalities
         (a) Atypical glandular cells (AGC) specified as endocervical, endometrial or glandular cells
         (b) Atypical glandular cells, favor neoplastic some features of neoplasm but not sufficient to reach interpretation of adenocarcinoma in situ
         (c) Endocervical adenocarcinoma in situ (AIS)
    d.   Other—endometrial cells in women 40 years of age or older

- Management/Treatment
  1. Specimen adequacy
     a. Satisfactory for evaluation—no action needed
     b. Unsatisfactory for evaluation—assess and treat as needed if inflammation is cause; repeat Pap test in 4–6 months; may defer to annual repeat if adequate history of normal Pap tests
  2. Organisms
     a. *Trichomonas vaginalis*—highly predictive but not 100%; treat if indicated
     b. Candida species—most are asymptomatic colonization and require no treatment; if symptomatic treat
     c. Bacterial vaginosis—correlate with clinical findings; treat if indicated
     d. Actinomyces—evaluate for signs/ symptoms of pelvic infection if intrauterine contraceptive (IUC) present; if has

pelvic infection remove IUC and treat with antibiotics, otherwise no treatment or IUC removal needed

    e. Herpes simplex virus—high predictive value; counsel client

3. Reactive changes associated with inflammation

    a. Examine—microscopy, STD tests as indicated

    b. Treat any identified cause

    c. It is of no value to treat empirically with topical sulfa cream

    d. Repeat Pap test if indicated

4. Endometrial cells in premenopausal woman with normal menstrual pattern—insignificant; must be evaluated with endometrial biopsy in postmenopausal woman or in premenopausal woman with abnormal bleeding

5. Atrophy—treat if symptomatic

6. Epithelial cell abnormalities

    a. ASC-US

      (1) Options include repeating Pap test at specified intervals, HPV-DNA testing for high-risk types, immediate colposcopy

        (a) Repeat Pap test at 6 months; if negative repeat again in 6 months; if second repeat is negative return to routine screening; any further ASC or greater do colposcopy

        (b) HPV-DNA testing for high-risk types; if positive refer for colposcopy; if negative repeat Pap test in 12 months

        (c) Immediate colposcopy

          i. No CIN/cancer and high-risk HPV either negative or unknown—repeat Pap test in 12 months

          ii. No CIN/cancer and positive for high-risk HPV—repeat Pap test at 6 and 12 months or repeat HPV-DNA testing in 12 months; repeat colposcopy for any abnormal findings in follow-up

          iii. CIN/cancer—refer to specialist

      (2) Postmenopausal women with clinical evidence of atrophy—treat with estrogen vaginal cream for 4–6 weeks and repeat Pap test; if negative repeat in 4–6 months; if negative at 4–6 months return to routine screening interval; if ASC-US or greater refer for colposcopy

      (3) Pregnant women—manage same as nonpregnant woman; acceptable to defer colposcopy until at least 6 weeks postpartum

      (4) Immunosuppressed; includes all infected with human immunodeficiency virus (HIV)—manage same as women who are not immunosuppressed

    b. ASC-H—colposcopic examination recommended

    c. LSIL

      (1) Colposcopic examination

        (a) No CIN2/3—repeat pap test at 6 and 12 months or HPV DNA testing at 12 months; if greater than or equal to ASC-US or HPV +, repeat colposcopy

        (b) CIN 2/3—refer to specialist

      (2) Postmenopausal women—options include repeating Pap test at 6 and 12 months, HPV-DNA testing for high-risk types, immediate colposcopy

      (3) Pregnant women—colposcopic examination by clinician familiar with cervical changes induced by pregnancy; endocervical curettage should not be done; acceptable to defer colposcopy until at least 6 weeks postpartum

      (4) Immunosuppressed; includes all infected with human immunodeficiency virus (HIV)—manage same as women who are not immunosuppressed

    d. HSIL—colposcopic examination is recommended; for women in whom future fertility is not an issue may consider immediate loop electrosurgical excision

    e. Squamous cell carcinoma—refer to specialist

    f. AGC—all subcategories except atypical endometrial cells

      (1) Colposcopic examination with endocervical sampling

      (2) Include endometrial sampling if 35 years of age or older, or abnormal bleeding

    g. AGC with atypical endometrial cells—include endometrial sampling regardless of age

    h. Adenocarcinoma—refer to specialist

◻ QUESTIONS

Select the best answer.

1. Premenstrual syndrome is suspected when a woman experiences symptoms only during:

    a. Ovulation

    b. The luteal phase

c. The LH surge

d. The follicular phase

2. Primary dysmenorrhea can best be treated with:

   a. Dopamine agonists

   b. GnRH agonists

   c. Prostaglandin inhibitors

   d. Tricyclic antidepressants

3. The most common cause for chronic pelvic pain in reproductive age women is:

   a. Adenomyosis

   b. Endometriosis

   c. Pelvic inflammatory infection

   d. Uterine fibroids

4. Which of the following contraceptive methods has also been FDA approved for treatment of endometriosis?

   a. Combination oral contraceptive pills

   b. Levonorgestrel IUS

   c. Progestin only contraceptive pills

   d. Sub Q 104 DMPA

5. A complication of pelvic inflammatory disease is:

   a. Adenomyosis

   b. Endometriosis

   c. Infertility

   d. Irritable bowel syndrome

6. The most common cause of urge urinary incontinence is:

   a. Detrusor irritability

   b. Neuromuscular injury

   c. Pelvic organ prolapse

   d. Sphincter incompetence

7. During a vaginal examination, you observe bulging of the anterior wall when you ask the patient to bear down. This is most likely a:

   a. Congenital abnormality

   b. Cystocele

   c. Rectocele

   d. Uterine prolapse

8. The definitive diagnosis of endometriosis is made with:

   a. CT scan

   b. Laparoscopy

   c. Serum CA 125

   d. Transvaginal ultrasound

9. Adenomyosis can be suspected when a woman has a/an:

   a. Boggy, tender uterus

   b. Enlarged irregularly shaped uterus

c. Fixed retroverted uterus

d. Prolapsed uterus

10. The most common benign neoplasm of the cervix is:

   a. Bartholin gland cyst

   b. Squamous papilloma

   c. Pedunculated myoma

   d. Polyp

11. A 22-year-old female presents with complaint of malodorous vaginal discharge and vulvar itching. On examination a watery, yellowish-green vaginal discharge is noted along with vulvar and vaginal erythema. The most likely findings on a wet mount examination will be:

   a. Clue cells

   b. Lactobacilli

   c. Pseudohyphae

   d. Trichomonads

12. Characteristics of Turner's syndrome include:

   a. Uterus absent, ovaries absent

   b. Uterus absent, ovaries present

   c. Uterus present, ovaries absent

   d. Uterus present, ovaries present

13. A 58-year-old woman complains of severe vulvar pruritus. On genital examination you note thin skin and purpura on the vulva. You suspect the diagnosis may be:

   a. Lichens sclerosus

   b. Local allergic reaction

   c. Lichen simplex chronicus

   d. Vulvodynia

14. A virginal 18-year-old presents for contraception, stating she plans to become sexually active. Upon examination you see an ulcerative, irregular lesion in the vaginal fornix. The lesion has a reddish appearing granular base. The lesion is likely:

   a. Genital herpes

   b. Lymphogranuloma venerum

   c. Toxic shock syndrome

   d. Ulceration from tampon injury

15. Which of the following is true concerning dysfunctional uterine bleeding?

   a. Appropriate diagnosis for bleeding until definitive diagnosis is made

   b. Most often occurs in women ages 20–40

   c. Usually associated with anovulatory cycles

   d. Usually associated with abnormal pelvic exam findings

16. Hirsutism is most commonly seen with:

    a. Androgen insensitivity syndrome
    b. Asherman's syndrome
    c. Polycystic ovarian syndrome
    d. Turner's syndrome

17. A 22-year-old experiences 6 months of amenorrhea. Laboratory test results include normal prolactin and thyroid stimulating hormone and negative pregnancy test. The next action will be to:

    a. Administer progestin challenge test
    b. Measure testosterone
    c. Order hysterosalpingogram
    d. Order MRI or CT scan of pituitary gland

18. The most common cause of menstrual abnormality in a reproductive age woman is:

    a. Adenomyosis
    b. Anovulation
    c. Coagulopathy
    d. Ectopic pregnancy

19. The pain of primary dysmenorrhea is:

    a. Always associated with pathology such as endometriosis
    b. Colicky, spasmodic, sometimes radiating up the back to the shoulders
    c. Colicky, spasmodic, sometimes radiating to the thighs and low back
    d. Dull ache associated with underlying pathology

20. A 16-year-old woman has not yet begun menstruating, but does have pubic hair. She is best described as having:

    a. Asherman's syndrome
    b. Oligomenorrhea
    c. Primary amenorrhea
    d. Secondary amenorrhea

21. Which of the following is the most accurate method to predict the occurrence of ovulation?

    a. Huhner's test
    b. Evaluation of cervical mucus
    c. LH surge test
    d. Basal body temperature

22. Toxic shock syndrome should be suspected in a woman presenting with sudden-onset fever, flulike symptoms, recent tampon use and:

    a. Dysuria
    b. Heavy vaginal bleeding
    c. Pale conjunctiva and vaginal walls
    d. Macular rash on face and trunk

23. A known risk factor for cancer of the cervix is:

    a. Cigarette smoking
    b. Early menarche
    c. Multiparity
    d. Uncircumcised partner

24. Polycystic ovarian syndrome predisposes to an increased incidence of:

    a. Adrenal tumors
    b. Endometriosis
    c. Endometrial cancer
    d. Ovarian cancer

25. In which of the following conditions would you expect to have a positive progestin challenge test?

    a. Androgen insensitivity syndrome
    b. Asherman's syndrome
    c. Polycystic ovarian syndrome
    d. Turner's syndrome

26. The most common presenting symptom of vulvar cancer is:

    a. Bleeding
    b. Pruritus
    c. Vaginal discharge
    d. Vaginal odor

27. A nonpregnant patient diagnosed with chlamydia is allergic to azithromycin. An alternative treatment is:

    a. Ciprofloxacin
    b. Doxycycline
    c. Penicillin
    d. Trimethoprim

28. A 26-year-old female has a Pap test report of ASC-US. This is her first abnormal Pap test. HPV-DNA testing is negative for high-risk HPV types. Recommended follow-up would include:

    a. Colposcopy in 6 months
    b. Repeat Pap smear in 4 to 6 months
    c. Repeat HPV-DNA testing in 1 year
    d. Repeat Pap test in 1 year

29. A treatment for atrophic vaginitis with the goal of prevention of recurrence is:

    a. Antifungal cream
    b. Low potency topical steroids
    c. Oral progestin therapy
    d. Topical estrogen cream

30. A 24-year-old woman presents with complaint of nontender mass in her left breast that does not change with menstrual cycle. On examination you note a freely moveable, 0.5 cm x 1 cm,

firm, rubbery nontender mass. The most likely diagnosis is:

a. Fibroadenoma
b. Fibrocystic breast changes
c. Intraductal papilloma
d. Cystosarcoma phyllodes

31. The Bethesda system equivalent for moderate dysplasia or CIN III on a Pap test is:

a. Atypical glandular cells of undetermined significance (AGS-US)
b. Carcinoma in situ
c. High grade squamous epithelial lesion
d. Low-grade squamous intraepithelial lesion

32. Potential causes for galactorrhea include all of the following except:

a. Heavy tobacco use
b. Hypothyroidism
c. Opiate use
d. Pituitary adenoma

33. Leiomyomata arising from tissue within the uterine wall are:

a. Interstitial
b. Pedunculated
c. Subserosal
d. Submucosal

34. The most common presenting symptom of leiomyomata uteri is:

a. Infertility
b. Menorrhagia
c. GI symptoms
d. Urinary frequency

35. Another name for a dermoid cyst is:

a. Benign cystic teratoma
b. Follicular cyst
c. Hyperplastic endometroma
d. Müllerian cyst

36. Your examination of a female patient indicates that she has external genital warts. You will want to explain to her that:

a. Her partner needs a blood test to see if he has subclinical infection.
b. She should have Pap tests every 6 months.
c. There is no therapy that will eliminate the HPV virus.
d. You cannot start treatment until you have her Pap test results.

37. A 36-year-old is seen in your office on day 18 of her cycle for her routine annual examination. She has no complaints. Pelvic exam reveals a 9 cm

firm pelvic mass anterior to the uterus. The most likely diagnosis is:

a. Benign cystic teratoma
b. Ectopic pregnancy
c. Endometrioma
d. Follicular cyst

38. Unopposed estrogen may predispose a 52-year-old woman to:

a. Endometrial hyperplasia
b. Fibrocystic breast changes
c. Follicular cysts
d. Ovarian carcinoma

39. A diagnosis of stress urinary incontinence is confirmed on the basis of:

a. Probable etiology
b. Pelvic muscle tone evaluation
c. Urodynamic testing
d. Symptom profile

40. The most common presenting symptom of cervical cancer is:

a. Dyspareunia
b. Lower abdominal pain
c. Irregular bleeding
d. Yellow vaginal discharge

41. The first step in the evaluation of HSIL Pap test result is:

a. HPV DNA testing
b. Colposcopic evaluation with endocervical biopsy
c. Endometrial biopsy
d. Repeat Pap test at 6 and 12 months

42. Persistent vague abdominal pain or discomfort in a 65-year-old woman may be an early sign of:

a. Choriocarcinoma
b. Benign cystic teratoma
c. Endometrial cancer
d. Ovarian cancer

43. A risk factor for endometrial cancer is:

a. DES exposure
b. Early menopause
c. Obesity
d. Multiparity

44. The most lethal gynecological malignancy is:

a. Cervical carcinoma
b. Choriocarcinoma
c. Endometrial carcinoma
d. Ovarian carcinoma

45. A positive "whiff" or amine test is suggestive of:

    a. Atrophic vaginitis
    b. Bacterial vaginosis
    c. Chronic lichens sclerosus
    d. Recurrent candidiasis

46. An indicator of loss of lactobacilli in the vagina is:

    a. Elevated pH
    b. Increased WBC on wet mount
    c. Malodorous vaginal discharge
    d. Vaginal itching

47. Trichomoniasis is best treated with:

    a. Oral fluconazole
    b. Oral metronidazole
    c. Topical clindamycin cream
    d. Topical metronidazole cream

48. Which of the following treatments for genital warts may be used during pregnancy?

    a. Imiquimod cream
    b. Podophyllin resin
    c. Podofilox gel
    d. Trichloracetic acid

49. A sexually active 18-year-old presents with post-coital spotting, dysuria, and a yellow discharge. On exam you find her cervix is erythematous and bleeds with contact. The most likely diagnosis is:

    a. Cervical cancer
    b. Chlamydia
    c. Primary syphilis
    d. Tampon injury

50. Risk factors for ovarian cancer include:

    a. Diabetes
    b. Late menopause
    c. History of human papillomavirus
    d. Oral contraceptive pill use for more than 5 years

51. Recommendations for repeat testing after treatment for chlamydia with doxycycline include:

    a. Test of cure 1 to 2 weeks after treatment if suspect noncompliance
    b. Test of cure 3 to 4 weeks after treatment for all patients
    c. Test for possible reinfection 1 month after treatment
    d. Test for possible reinfection 3 months after treatment

52. Effective treatment for the symptomatic relief of herpes genitalis is:

    a. Ceftriaxone
    b. Famcyclovir
    c. Silver nitrate
    d. Tetracycline

53. A lesion of secondary syphilis is:

    a. *Condyloma acuminata*
    b. *Condyloma lata*
    c. *Molluscum contagiosum*
    d. Inguinal bubo

54. Primary syphilis may be suspected when the patient presents with:

    a. A maculopapular rash
    b. An indurated, painless ulcer on the cervix
    c. Enlarged, tender inguinal lymph nodes
    d. Tender vesicles and papules on the vulva

55. Herniation of the bladder into the vagina is called:

    a. Cystocele
    b. Enterocele
    c. Urethrocele
    d. Vaginal prolapse

56. A 66-year-old woman with a history of pruritus presents with an ulceration of the vulva. The most likely diagnosis is:

    a. Chancroid
    b. Secondary trauma
    c. Syphilis
    d. Vulvar carcinoma

57. A 26-year-old woman presents with multiple, painless, umbilicated papules on her mons pubis. The most likely diagnosis is:

    a. *Condyloma acuminata*
    b. *Condyloma lata*
    c. Lymphogranuloma venereum
    d. *Molluscum contagiosum*

58. Which of the following statements concerning herpes genitalis is true?

    a. Suppressive therapy does not reduce viral shedding.
    b. Systemic symptoms are uncommon during recurrences.
    c. Topical acyclovir is as effective as oral acyclovir for recurrences.
    d. Transmission of the virus is unlikely to occur during the prodromal phase.

59. Disorders of pelvic support may be associated with all of the following *except*:

    a. Obesity
    b. Neuromuscular injury during childbirth

c. Pelvic surgery

d. Frequent urinary tract infections

60. A 58-year-old woman complains that she feels she's "sitting on a ball." She has significant constipation and rectal pressure. On examination you will most likely find:

a. Cystocele

b. Hemorrhoid

c. Rectocele

d. Urethrocele

61. Vaginal cancer is most commonly found in which part of the vagina?

a. The hymenal ring

b. Midway of the vagina

c. The posterior fourchette

d. The upper one-third of the vagina

62. Females exposed to DES in utero are at increased risk for:

a. Breast cancer

b. Ovarian cancer

c. Vaginal cancer

d. Vulvar cancer

63. Anticholinergic agents may be used in the treatment of:

a. Stress incontinence

b. Urge incontinence

c. Vestibulitis

d. Vulvodynia

64. The most common gynecological neoplasm is:

a. Adenocarcinoma

b. Adenosarcoma

c. Choriocarcinoma

d. Leiomyoma

65. The most common cause of pathologic nipple discharge in perimenopausal women is:

a. Breast cancer

b. Fibroadenoma

c. Intraductal papilloma

d. Prolactin secreting pituitary adenoma

66. The most common germ-cell tumor is:

a. Benign cystic teratoma

b. Choriocarcinoma

c. Embryonal carcinoma

d. Vaginal agenesis

67. An examination finding that is considered minimum criteria for empirical treatment of PID in a sexually active young woman presenting with lower abdominal or pelvic pain is:

a. Adnexal mass

b. Cervical motion tenderness

c. Fever higher than 101°F (> 38.4°C)

d. Vaginal discharge

68. Androgen insensitivity syndrome was previously known as:

a. Fragile X syndrome

b. Marfan's syndrome

c. Müllerian agenesis

d. Testicular feminization

69. The gonads should be removed after puberty in a person with androgen insensitivity syndrome to prevent:

a. Endometrial hyperplasia

b. Gonadal malignancies

c. Increased risk for breast cancer

d. Psychological trauma

70. The most common method of assisted reproductive technology is:

a. Gamete intrafallopian transfer (GIFT)

b. Intracytoplasmic sperm injection (ICZI)

c. In vitro fertilization (IVF)

d. Zygote intrafallopian transfer (ZIFT)

71. Turner's syndrome can be suspected when the patient has primary amenorrhea and:

a. Blind vaginal pouch with imperforate hymen

b. Low IQ and visual disturbances

c. Normal breast development but lack of pubic and axillary hair growth

d. Short stature and webbed neck

72. The most common chromosomal abnormality in spontaneous aborted fetuses is:

a. Fitz-Hugh-Curtis syndrome

b. Fragile X syndrome

c. Müllerian duct abnormalities

d. Turner's syndrome

73. Reactive cellular changes on a Pap test report are most likely the result of:

a. Inflammation

b. Low-grade epithelial lesion

c. Glandular cell abnormalities

d. Oral contraceptive use

74. A patient with latent syphilis may present with:

a. A maculopapular rash

b. An indurated painless ulcer

c. *Condyloma lata*

d. No signs of infection

75. CDC recommendations for follow up of female treated for PID with a recommended outpatient regimen is:

    a. Advise patient to return if pain and/or fever persists more than 5 days
    b. Reexamine patient within 72 hours after initiation of treatment
    c. Retest for chlamydia and gonorrhea in 2 weeks
    d. See patient in 1 week for second dose of ceftriaxone IM

76. Which of the following medications is most likely to cause a metallic taste?

    a. Acyclovir
    b. Azithromycin
    c. Fluconazole
    d. Metronidazole

77. A patient-applied treatment for human papillomavirus (HPV) is:

    a. Bichloracetic acid
    b. Clindamycin cream
    c. Imiquimod
    d. Podophyllin resin

78. Risk factors for breast carcinoma include:

    a. Early menopause
    b. History of endometrial cancer
    c. Multiparity
    d. History of intraductal papilloma

79. Characteristic "strawberry spots" on the cervix may be seen with:

    a. Bacterial vaginosis
    b. Chlamydia
    c. Herpes genitalis
    d. Trichamoniasis

80. Typical characteristics of vulvodynia include:

    a. Constant vulvar burning and discomfort
    b. Inflammation of the vestibular glands
    c. Thickened plaques on vulva
    d. Vulvovaginal edema and erythema

◻ ANSWERS

1. b		41. b	
2. c		42. d	
3. b		43. c	
4. d		44. d	
5. c		45. b	
6. a		46. a	
7. b		47. b	
8. b		48. d	
9. a		49. b	
10. d		50. b	
11. d		51. d	
12. c		52. b	
13. a		53. b	
14. d		54. b	
15. c		55. a	
16. c		56. d	
17. a		57. d	
18. b		58. b	
19. c		59. d	
20. c		60. c	
21. c		61. d	
22. d		62. c	
23. a		63. b	
24. c		64. d	
25. c		65. c	
26. b		66. a	
27. b		67. b	
28. d		68. d	
29. d		69. b	
30. a		70. c	
31. c		71. d	
32. a		72. d	
33. a		73. a	
34. b		74. d	
35. a		75. b	
36. c		76. d	
37. a		77. c	
38. a		78. b	
39. c		79. d	
40. c		80. a	

◻ BIBLIOGRAPHY

American College of Obstetricians and Gynecologists (ACOG). (2009). Cervical cytology screening. *Practice Bulletin, 109.* Washington, DC: Author.

American College of Obstetricians and Gynecologists (ACOG). (2008). Management of abnormal cervical cytology and histology. *Practice Bulletin, 99.* Washington, DC: Author.

American College of Obstetricians and Gynecologists (ACOG). (2008). Treatment of urinary tract infections in nonpregnant women. *Practice Bulletin, 91.* Washington, DC: Author.

American College of Obstetricians and Gynecologists (ACOG). (2005). Urinary incontinence in women. *Practice Bulletin, 63.* Washington, DC: Author.

American College of Obstetricians and Gynecologists (ACOG). (2004). Chronic pelvic pain. *Practice Bulletin, 51.* Washington, DC: Author.

Centers for Disease Control and Prevention (CDC). (2006). Guidelines for treatment of sexually transmitted diseases. *MMWR 2006, 55(No. RR-11).* Atlanta, GA: Author.

Chernecky, C., & Berger, B. (2008) *Laboratory tests and diagnostic procedures* (5th ed.). St. Louis: Saunders Elsevier.

Gibbs, R., Karlan, B., Haney, A., & Nygaard, I. (2008). *Danforth's obstetrics and gynecology* (10th ed.). Philadelphia, PA: Williams, Wilkins, and Wolters.

Ferri, F. F. (Ed.). (2008). *Ferri's clinical advisor: Instant diagnosis and treatment.* St. Louis: Mosby, Inc.

Katz, V., Lentz, G., Lobo, R., & Gershenson, D. (2007). *Comprehensive gynecology* (5th ed.). Philadelphia, PA: Mosby, Inc.

North American Menopause Society. (2007). *Menopause practice: A clinician's guide* (3rd ed.). Cleveland, OH: NAMS.

Schuiling, K., and Likis, F. (2006). *Women's gynecologic health.* Sudbury, MA: Jones and Bartlett.

Solomon, D., Davey, D., Kurman, R., Moriarty, A. et al. (2002). Consensus statement: The 2001 Bethesda system—terminology for reporting results of cervical cytology. *JAMA, 287*(16), 2114–2119.

Speroff, L., Glass, R. H., & Kase, N. G. (2005). *Clinical gynecologic endocrinology and infertility* (7th ed.). Baltimore, MD: Williams and Wilkins.

Tharpe, N., & Farley, C. (2009). *Clinical practice guidelines for midwifery and women's health* (3rd ed.). Sudbury, MA: Jones and Bartlett.

Wright, T., Massad, S., Dunton, J., Spitzer, M., Wilkinson, E., & Solomon, D. (2007). 2006 consensus guidelines for the management of women with abnormal cervical cancer screening tests. *American Journal of Obstetrics and Gynecology, 197*(4), 346–355.

Wynne, A., Woo, T., & Olyaei, A. (2007). *Pharmacotherapeutics for nurse practitioner prescribers* (2nd ed.). Philadelphia, PA: F. A. Davis.

8

Nongynecological Disorders/Problems

Sandra K. Pfantz

Beth M. Kelsey

Mary C. Knutson

◘ CARDIOVASCULAR DISORDERS

Hypertension

- Definition
    1. Systolic blood pressure (SBP) of 140 mm Hg or greater, or diastolic blood pressure (DBP) of 90 mm Hg or greater, as measured by at least two readings on two or more separate visits; or taking antihypertensive medication (NHBPEP, 1997)
    2. Classification of blood pressure (NHBPEP, 2003)

Classification	SBP		DBP
Normal	< 120	and	< 80
Prehypertension	120–139	or	80–90
Stage 1 hypertension	140–159	or	90–99
Stage 2 hypertension	≥ 160	or	≥ 100

    3. Evaluation of patients with documented hypertension has three objectives:
        a. To identify secondary causes
        b. To assess for target organ damage (TOD)—eye, brain, blood vessels, heart, and kidney
        c. To identify other cardiovascular risk factors or concomitant disorders that may define prognosis and guide therapy. Major cardiovascular risk factors include:
            (1) Smoking
            (2) Obesity (BMI ≥ 30)
            (3) Physical inactivity
            (4) Dyslipidemia
            (5) Diabetes mellitus
            (6) Microalbuminuria or estimated glomerular filtration rate (GFR) of less than 60 mL/min
            (7) Age older than 55 in men and older than 65 in women
            (8) Family history of premature cardiovascular disease (men < 55 and women < 65)

- Etiology/Incidence
    1. Etiology
        a. Primary or essential
            (1) No discernible cause; a complex polygenic and multifactorial disorder
            (2) Comprises 90–95% of diagnosed cases
        b. Secondary
            (1) Underlying disease or condition identified; requires separate treatment
            (2) Comprises 5–10% of adult cases
    2. Incidence
        a. 10–15% of Caucasian adults
        b. 20–30% of African-American adults
        c. Individuals normotensive at age 55 have a 90% lifetime risk (NHBPEP, 2003)

- Signs and symptoms
    1. Symptoms usually not present
    2. In cases of secondary hypertension, may be symptoms associated with secondary condition
        a. Weakness in primary aldosteronism
        b. Truncal obesity and purple striae in Cushing's syndrome

c. Palpitations, tremor and sweating in pheochromocytoma
3. In chronic hypertension, may be symptoms associated with TOD
   a. Symptoms associated with peripheral vascular disease, coronary artery disease and heart failure
   b. Symptoms associated with stroke or transient ischemic attack

- Physical findings
  1. Elevated blood pressure as noted in definition
  2. Findings associated with secondary causes or TOD
     a. Retinopathy
     b. S_4 gallop, S_3 gallop, precordial heave, and displaced point of maximal impulse
     c. Renal artery bruit in renal artery stenosis
     d. Delayed or absent femoral pulses and decreased blood pressure in lower extremities in coarctation of the aorta
     e. Diminished or absent peripheral pulses, edema
     f. Neurologic findings

- Differential diagnosis/Secondary causes
  1. Sleep apnea
  2. Chronic kidney disease
  3. Primary aldosteronism
  4. Renovascular disease
  5. Chronic steroid therapy and Cushing's syndrome
  6. Pheochromocytoma
  7. Coarctation of the aorta
  8. Thyroid or parathyroid disease
  9. Drug-induced or drug-related
     a. Drug abuse—cocaine, amphetamines, alcohol
     b. Combination hormonal contraception
     c. Sympathomimetics—OTC cold remedies

- Diagnostic tests/findings
  1. Recommended before initiating therapy to rule out secondary causes, determine the presence of risk factors, and assess for TOD
  2. Recommended initial laboratory tests
     a. Urinalysis
     b. CBC
     c. Blood glucose, serum potassium, creatinine or estimated GFR, calcium, lipid profile
        (1) Hypokalemia in primary aldosteronism
        (2) Elevated creatinine in renal disease
     d. Electrocardiogram (ECG) to assess evidence of ischemic heart disease or left ventricular hypertrophy (LVH)

3. Optional studies
   a. Measurement of urinary albumin excretion or albumin/creatinine ratio
   b. TSH
   c. Intravenous Pyelogram (IVP) to rule out renovascular disease
   d. 24-hour urine for metanephrines and catecholamines to rule out pheochromocytoma
   e. Chest radiograph to rule out cardiomegaly and coarctation of the aorta
   f. Echocardiogram is more sensitive study to detect LVH

- Management/Treatment (NHBPEP, 2003/JNC 7)
  1. Goals of therapy
     a. Prevent/minimize TOD
     b. Focus on achievement of systolic BP goal; most patients will achieve diastolic goal once systolic BP is at goal (< 140/90)
     c. BP goal in patients with coronary heart disease (CHD), diabetes, abdominal aortic aneurysm, peripheral arterial disease, carotid artery disease, 10-year Framingham risk score of 10% or greater, or renal disease is less than 130/80
  2. Nonpharmacologic—life style modifications recommended for all patients
     a. Weight reduction—maintain ideal body weight
     b. Adopt DASH eating plan—diet rich in fruits, vegetables, and low-fat dairy products with a reduced content of saturated and total fat
     c. Dietary sodium reduction—6 g NaCl
     d. Physical activity—engage in aerobic physical activity at least 30 minutes per day most days of the week
     e. Moderation of alcohol consumption
     f. Stop smoking
  3. Pharmacologic
     a. General principles of therapy
        (1) For most patients, thiazide-type diuretics should be used as initial therapy either alone or in combination with an agent from one of the following classes: ACE inhibitors, angiotensin-receptor blockers (ARBs), beta-blockers, or calcium channel blockers (CCBs)
           (a) Prehypertension—no drug therapy indicated
           (b) Stage 1 HTN—thiazide-type diuretic
           (c) Stage 2 HTN—two drug regimen for most; usually thiazide diuretic plus ACE inhibitor, ARB, beta-blocker, or CCB

(2) Compelling indications requiring the use of other agents as initial therapy
  (a) Ischemic heart disease
    i. Stable angina—beta-blocker; long-acting CCB as an alternative
    ii. Post-MI—ACE inhibitors, beta-blockers, aldosterone antagonist
  (b) Diabetes—ACE inhibitors or ARBs favorably affect progression of nephropathy
(3) Most patients will require two or more antihypertensive agents to reach their BP goal
  b. Classification of drugs for hypertension by drug action (see **Table 8-1**)
    (1) Diuretics
      (a) Commonly employed as initial therapy
      (b) Blacks and elderly respond well; drug of choice isolated systolic hypertension
    (2) Sympatholytic agents
      (a) Beta adrenergic blockers
      (b) Peripheral alpha 1 blockers
      (c) Central alpha 2 receptor agonists
    (3) Calcium channel blockers
      (a) Dihydropyridines
      (b) Diltiazem, Verapamil
    (4) ACE inhibitors
      (a) Indicated in diabetics with proteinurea
      (b) Blacks and elderly respond less well; use with diuretic
    (5) Angiotensin-receptor blockers
    (6) Direct vasodilators
  4. Patient education
    a. Lifelong nature of hypertensive condition
    b. Asymptomatic nature of hypertension
    c. Adherence to treatment regimens reduces complications and deaths
    d. Critical to comply with recommended follow-up and monitoring schedule

- Referral
  1. Evaluation and management of secondary causes
  2. Resistance to drug therapy; failure to respond to three-drug regimen that includes a diuretic

Heart Murmurs

- Definition
  1. Prolonged extra heart sounds heard during either systole or diastole; commonly associated with dynamics of regurgitation or stenosis

  2. Classification
    a. Innocent or functional murmurs
      (1) Transient; pose no direct threat to health
      (2) Most frequently heard during systole
      (3) No structural or functional cardiac abnormality
      (4) Often noted in pregnancy due to increased cardiac output
    b. Pathologic murmurs are indicative of heart or valvular disease, e.g., aortic or pulmonary stenosis, atrial septal defect, rheumatic heart disease

- Etiology/Incidence
  1. Etiology
    a. Turbulent blood flow into, through, or out of the heart can result in audible murmur
    b. Characteristics of sound depend upon the following factors:
      (1) Size of valve opening
      (2) Integrity of valve
      (3) Vigor of contraction
      (4) Rate of flow
      (5) Thickness of chest wall
  2. Incidence
    a. Innocent systolic murmurs occur in 50–70% of children and up to 50% of adults at some time
    b. Pathologic murmurs are less common but incidence increases with age
      (1) Congenital—Marfan's syndrome, valve malformation
      (2) Acquired—Rheumatic heart disease, mitral valve prolapse (MVP)

- Signs and symptoms
  1. Innocent murmurs—not symptomatic
  2. Pathologic
    a. Possible chest pain
    b. Shortness of breath on exertion
    c. Orthopnea
    d. Cough or wheeze
    e. Paroxysmal nocturnal dyspnea
    f. Growth failure

- Physical findings
  1. Innocent
    a. Usually none except audible murmur
    b. Soft (grade 1 or 2 intensity), medium pitch, systolic murmur
    c. Heard best when patient is supine
    d. Disappears with standing or straining
    e. Increases with increased cardiac output, e.g., fever, exercise

■ **Table 8-1** Hypertension Pharmacology (representative list)

Drug Name	Action	Side-effects	Interactions	Contraindications
Diuretics				
Thiazides Hydrochlorothiazide Indapamide	Inhibits sodium reabsorption from distal renal tubules; reduced sodium results in decreased vascular tone	Increases cholesterol and glucose levels; decreases potassium, sodium, magnesium levels; increases uric acid, calcium levels; rarely, blood dyscrasias	Enhances other classes of antihypertensives; may decrease oral sulfonylurea drug efficacy; raises serum lithium levels	Anuria; sulfonamide allergy; pregnancy category B/C; not recommended for nursing mothers
Loop diuretics Ethacrynic acid Furosemide	Inhibits sodium reabsorption from ascending Loop of Henle	Dehydration, electrolyte imbalance	Ototoxicity with aminogylcosides	Anuria, hepatic coma, lactation; pregnancy category C; caution in nursing mothers
Potassium-sparing agents Spironolactone Triamterene	Inhibits sodium exchange for potassium in distal tubule	Hyperkalemia, hyponatremia GI disturbances, rash, gynecomastia	May exacerbate hyperkalemia with ACE inhibitors	Renal impairment, anuria, hyperkalemia; caution in pregnancy; not recommended for nursing mothers
Sympatholytic agents				
Beta-adrenergic blockers Propranolol Atenolol	Inhibits sympathetic stimulation of the heart; blocks renin release from kidney	Bronchospasm, bradycardia, heart failure, may mask insulin-induced hypoglycemia, insomnia, fatigue, decreased exercise tolerance	Effects blunted by NSAIDs; masks/prolongs insulin-induced hypoglycemia	Asthma, congestive heart failure, type 1 diabetes, Raynaud's disease; pregnancy category C; not recommended while nursing
Alpha-adrenergic blockers Prazosin Terazosin	Inhibits stimulation of alpha$_1$ receptors on arterioles and veins	Orthostatic hypotension, syncope with first dose	Hypotension with other antihypertensives	Precaution in pregnancy and nursing mothers

Drug	Mechanism	Side effects	Drug interactions	Comments
Central alpha adrenergic agonists Clonidine Methyldopa	Decreases sympathetic outflow; results in decreased cardiac output and PVR	Dry mouth, sedation	Antagonized by tricyclic antidepressants	Pregnancy category B; not recommended nursing mothers
Calcium antagonists Nifedipine Diltiazem Verapamil	Decreases myocardial contractility and peripheral resistance	Tachycardia, dizziness, headache, edema, conduction defects, heart failure	Verapamil & beta-adrenergic blockers have additive cardiodepressive effects	Congestive heart failure, A-V block, pregnancy category C; do not use while nursing
ACE inhibitors Captopril Enalapril	Inhibits angiotensin-converting enzyme; prevents conversion of angiotensin I to angiotensin II; a potent vasoconstrictor	Common: cough; rare: angioedema, hyperkalemia, rash, loss of taste	Antacids reduce bioavailability; effects blunted by NSAIDs	Bilateral renal artery stenosis, pregnancy category C (1st trimester), D (2nd & 3rd trimester); use with caution while nursing
Angiotensin II receptor blockers Losartin, Valsartan	Block binding of angiotensin II to receptor	Similar to ACE inhibitors, but do not cause cough; rare: angioedema.	Hyperkalemia with potassium sparing diuretics, potassium supplements	Pregnancy category C (1st trimester), D (2nd & 3rd trimester); not recommended while nursing
Minoxidil Hydralazine	Act on vascular smooth muscle to cause dilation of arterioles	Tachycardia, headache aggravation of angina, fluid retention	Guanethidine	Pheochromocytoma; pregnancy Category C; not recommended while nursing

2. Pathologic
   a. Diastolic murmur or any murmur above grade 3
   b. Intensifies with exercise or Valsalva maneuver
   c. Click, associated with MVP, pulmonic stenosis, aortic stenosis
   d. Cyanosis
   e. Jugular vein distension
   f. Hepatomegaly
   g. Pedal edema
   h. Diminished femoral pulses or unequal blood pressure in left and right arms

- Differential diagnosis—focused on differentiating innocent versus pathologic murmur

- Diagnostic tests/findings—indicated only if pathologic murmur suspected
  1. Echocardiography—confirms severity, location of clinically detected lesions
  2. Chest radiograph—suspected cardiac enlargement
  3. CBC—rule out anemia
  4. Thyroid function tests—rule out hyper- or hypothyroidism

- Management/Treatment
  1. Low-grade, asymptomatic systolic murmur with low-risk history can be assumed innocent and followed up at next visit
  2. Pharmacologic—bacterial endocarditis prophylaxis for susceptible patients
     a. Patients with valvular heart disease, prosthetic heart valves, or other structural cardiac abnormalities
     b. Indicated dental, upper respiratory, gastrointestinal, and genitourinary procedures
     c. Give oral amoxicillin 2 g 1 hour before procedure
  3. Patient education
     a. Self-knowledge and self-disclosure in future encounters
     b. Follow-up schedule if indicated

- Referral
  1. Diastolic murmurs
  2. Suspected pathologic systolic murmurs

Thromboembolic Disease

- Definition
  1. Occlusion or obstruction of venous flow by concomitant inflammation and clotting
  2. Classifications

   a. Deep vein thrombosis (DVT), acute or recurrent
   b. Superficial thrombophlebitis

- Etiology/Incidence/Risk factors
  1. Etiology
     a. Origin of most venous thrombi lie in Virchow's triad—endothelial damage, stasis, hypercoagulability
        (1) Endothelial damage secondary to trauma
        (2) Stasis secondary to immobility
        (3) Hypercoagulability secondary to protein deficiency states such as protein C or S, antithrombin III; nephrotic syndrome, chronic liver disease, and certain malignancies
     b. DVT occurs as blood clots form within the deep venous plexus of the calf or within the popliteal, femoral, iliac veins
     c. Approximately 40% of DVTs embolize to pulmonary circulation when thigh veins involved; risk minimal when only calf veins involved
     d. Prevention of pulmonary embolus (PE) necessitates prompt diagnosis and treatment of DVT
     e. Superficial thromboses usually occur in varicose veins
  2. Incidence
     a. DVT/pulmonary emboli—500,000 cases annually
     b. Superficial thrombophlebitis—125,000 cases annually
  3. Risk factors
     a. Recent surgery—gynecological or orthopedic procedures of the hip, knee
     b. Immobility
     c. Advancing age—mean age for DVT is age 60
     d. Cancer—especially adenocarcinomas
     e. Pregnancy and early postpartum
     f. Oral estrogen use—contraceptives and hormone therapy
     g. Congestive heart failure or recent MI
     h. Prior history of thromboembolic disease
     i. Obesity

- Signs and symptoms
  1. DVT/superficial thrombophlebitis
     a. Acute onset of unilateral leg pain
     b. Local swelling, erythema, warmth
  2. PE
     a. Unilateral chest pain
     b. Anxiety, restlessness
     c. Dyspnea

- Physical findings
  1. DVT—often no findings
     a. Calf tenderness to compression; pain elicited with dorsiflexion of foot (Homan's sign)
     b. Palpable venous cord
     c. Unilateral leg edema; skin may be warm and erythematous
  2. PE
     a. Cyanosis
     b. Diminished breath sounds over involved area
     c. Tachypnea
     d. Cough with hemoptysis
     e. Tachycardia
     f. Fever
  3. Superficial thrombophlebitis
     a. Localized area of edema, erythema and tenderness over a superficial vein
     b. Increased temperature in surrounding skin

- Differential diagnosis
  1. DVT
     a. Muscle strain or contusion
     b. Cellulitis—more diffuse redness
     c. Popliteal (Baker's) cyst
  2. PE
     a. Myocardial infarction
     b. Pneumothorax
     c. Pneumonia

- Diagnostic tests/findings
  1. Superficial thrombophlebitis—usually none indicated
  2. DVT
     a. Duplex ultrasound
     b. Plasma D-dimer ELISA
        (1) Measures active breakdown of thrombi
        (2) Elevated in 95–98% of DVT
        (3) Best used for confusing diagnoses, recurrent diagnoses
     c. Contrast venography—best used for suspected calf vein thrombus or when clinical findings conflict with ultrasound
  3. PE
     a. Ventilation-perfusion (V/Q) lung scan
     b. Arterial blood gases
     c. ECG and chest radiograph
     d. Plasma D-dimer ELISA
     e. Pulmonary angiogram
  4. Hypercoagulation states
     a. Test for protein C or S deficiency
     b. Antithrombin III deficiency

- Management/Treatment
  1. Refer suspected DVT or PE for immediate medical management
  2. Superficial thrombophlebitis
     a. Nonpharmacologic—elevation of leg and compression with an ace wrap
     b. Pharmacologic—nonsteroidal anti-inflammatory drugs (see Acute Otitis Media this chapter)
  3. Patient education
     a. Avoid prolonged standing
     b. Use of support hose

Dyslipidemia

- Definition
  1. Increased levels of total blood cholesterol, and low-density lipoproteins (LDL) or triglycerides; suppressed high-density lipoproteins (HDL), or any combination; risk factor for the development of coronary heart disease in adults
  2. Classifications using National Cholesterol Education Program (NCEP) Adult Treatment Panel III (ATP III) Guidelines (NHLBI, 2001)
     a. Elevated LDL-C greater than 130 mg/dL
     b. Hypertriglyceridemia greater than 200 mg/dL
     c. Low HDL-C less than 40 mg/dL
     d. Combined dyslipidemia
     e. Metabolic syndrome—any three risk factors
        (1) Abdominal obesity/waist circumference
           (a) Men, greater than 40 inches
           (b) Women, greater than 35 inches
        (2) Triglycerides greater than 150 mg/dL
        (3) HDL-C
           (a) Men, less than 40 mg/dL
           (b) Women, less than 50 mg/dL
        (4) Blood pressure 130/85 or greater
        (5) Fasting glucose 110 or greater

- Etiology/Incidence
  1. Etiology
     a. Genetic predisposition
     b. Secondary causes
        (1) Obesity
        (2) Disease processes, e.g., endocrine and metabolic disorders, obstructive liver disease, renal disorders
        (3) Drugs, e.g., corticosteroids, thiazide diuretics, beta-blockers
  2. Incidence—estimated 65 million Americans have high cholesterol
  3. Risk factors that modify LDL goals
     a. Cigarette smoking

b. Hypertension (BP > 140/90 or on antihypertensive medication)

c. Low HDL cholesterol (< 40 mg/dL; > 60 mg/dL counts as a negative risk factor)

d. Family history of premature coronary heart disease (CHD)
    (1) CHD in male first-degree relative at younger than 55 years
    (2) CHD in female first-degree relative at younger than 65 years

e. Age (men ≥ 45 years; women ≥ 55 years)

- Signs and symptoms—None except those associated with CHD

- Physical findings
    1. Xanthomas
    2. Arcus senilis
    3. Central obesity

- Differential diagnosis—focused on ruling out secondary causes

- Diagnostic tests/findings
    1. Screening schedule
        a. A fasting lipoprotein profile (total cholesterol, LDL-C, HDL-C, TG) should be obtained every 5 years in patients 20 years or older (NHLBI, 2001)
        b. If fasting opportunity not available at initial screen, obtain total cholesterol and HDL-C; if total cholesterol is greater than 200 or HDL-C is less than 40, have patient return for fasting profile
    2. Cholesterol classification mg/dL-ATP III
        a. Total cholesterol
            (1) Less than 200—desirable
            (2) 200–239—borderline high
            (3) Greater than 240—high
        b. LDL cholesterol
            (1) Less than 100 optimal
            (2) 100–129—near or above optimal
            (3) 130–159—borderline high
            (4) 160–189—high
            (5) 190 or greater—very high
        c. HDL cholesterol
            (1) Less than 40—low
            (2) 60 or greater—high

- Management/Treatment
    1. Treatment of dyslipidemia is based on risk of CHD events
        a. Determine if patient has clinically manifested CHD or CHD risk equivalents—peripheral vascular disease, abdominal aortic aneurysm, symptomatic carotid artery disease, diabetes, or Framingham risk of greater than 20%
        b. If not, count number of CHD major risk factors
        c. If patient has two or more risk factors, determine the 10-year risk of a CHD event with the Framingham risk tool
            (1) Framingham risk tool calculates 10-year risk of CHD event
            (2) Website for CHD risk assessment tool—http://www.nhlbi.nih.gov/guidelines/cholesterol
        d. Assign a treatment goal for LDL-C based on number of risk factors or risk equivalents for CAD
            (1) LDL-C goal of less than 100—CHD or CHD risk equivalents
            (2) LDL-C goal of less than 130—No CHD with 2 or more risk factors (10-year risk of CHD ≤ 20%)
            (3) LDL-C goal of less than 160—No CHD and 0–1 risk factors
    2. Nonpharmacologic/Therapeutic life style changes
        a. Dietary modification
            (1) Cholesterol reduction from diet modification and dietary supplements can average 10–15%
            (2) Nutrition recommendations from NCEP
                (a) Total fat 25–35% of total calories/day; less than 7% from saturated fat, 20% or less from monounsaturated fat, 10% or less from polyunsaturated fat
                (b) Carbohydrate 50–60% of total calories/day
                (c) Protein 15 g/day
                (d) Cholesterol less than 200 mg/day
            (3) Foods/supplements
                (a) Fiber 20–30 g/day; 10–25 g/d soluble fiber
                (b) Plant stanols/sterols 2–3 g/d available in margarines and salad dressings
                (c) Nuts as a snack—walnuts, almonds
                (d) Substitute soy protein
                (e) Omega-3 fish oil capsules
        b. Encourage exercise for 30 min/day—this can be walking
        c. Aggressive smoking cessation program
        d. Weight loss for overweight and obese patients (goal BMI < 25); initial weight loss goal of 5–10% of current weight

3. Pharmacologic
   a. For most patients at moderate risk, lifestyle changes should be prescribed and followed for 3 months before initiating drug therapy; early drug therapy indicated for high-risk patients
   b. Pattern of dyslipidemia directs drug choice
      (1) Elevated LDL-C—statins with niacin and bile acid resins as alternatives
      (2) Hypertriglyceridemia—niacin and fibrates
      (3) Low HDL-C—niacin
      (4) Combined dyslipidemia—statins, niacin, fibrates
   c. Pharmacologic agents
      (1) Statins/HMG-CoA reductase inhibitors
         (a) Atorvastatin (Lipitor), fluvastatin (Lescol), lovastatin (Mevacor), pravastatin (Pravachol), rosuvastatin (Crestor), simvastatin (Zocor)
         (b) Drug action—inhibits HMG-CoA reductase, the enzyme that controls cholesterol biosynthesis in cells
         (c) Side-effects—elevated liver enzymes and myopathy; monitor liver function
         (d) Drug interactions—combined with fibrates or niacin may increase risk of myopathy
         (e) Contraindications/precautions—severe liver disease; pregnancy category X; not recommended while nursing
      (2) Nicotinic acid
         (a) Niacin/immediate release; Niaspan/extended release
         (b) Drug action—decreases synthesis of LDL-C by reducing hepatic synthesis of VLDL cholesterol; increases HDL by decreasing its catabolism
         (c) Side-effects—flushing, pruritus/decreased when premedicated with ASA; dyspepsia, hyperglycemia, hyperuricemia, hepatotoxicity
         (d) Drug interactions—additive hypotensive effect with antihypertensives; monitor for myopathy if used with statins
         (e) Contraindications/precautions—liver disease, severe gout, peptic-ulcer; pregnancy category C; not recommended in nursing mothers
      (3) Bile acid sequestrants
         (a) Cholestyramine (Questran), colestipol (Colestid), colesevelam (Welchol)
         (b) Drug action—binds cholesterol-containing bile acids in intestines forming insoluble complex that is excreted
         (c) Side-effects—gastrointestinal effects, e.g., constipation, bloating, nausea, cramping; no systemic toxicity
         (d) Drug interactions—may interfere with absorption of other medications; administer other drugs 1 hour before or 3 hours after resin
         (e) Contraindications/precautions—patients with triglycerides greater than 500 mg/dL and patients with low HDL-C; pregnancy category C; caution while nursing
      (4) Fibric acid derivatives
         (a) Gemfibrizil (Lopid), fenofibrate (Tricor)
         (b) Drug actions—acts primarily on triglyceride-rich lipoproteins, resulting decrease in plasma triglycerides, a moderate decrease in LDL-C, and an increase in HDL-C
         (c) Side-effects—dyspepsia, gallstones, myopathy
         (d) Drug interactions—may increase risk of myopathy when combined with statins; may potentiate effect of warfarin
         (e) Contraindications/precautions—severe renal or hepatic disease; pregnancy category C; not recommended while nursing
      (5) Ezetimibe (Zetia)
         (a) Drug action—cholesterol absorption inhibiter, use alone or in combination with a statin
         (b) Side-effects—back pain, arthralgia, diarrhea, abdominal pain; with statin, increase in serum transaminases
         (c) Drug interactions—not recommended for use with fibrates; separate dosing bile acid sequestrants
         (d) Contraindications/precautions—liver disease; pregnancy category C; not recommended in nursing mothers

(6) Combination medications
    (a) Statin plus aspirin
    (b) Statin plus calcium channel blocker
    (c) Statin plus cholesterol absorption inhibitor
    (d) Statin plus niacin
4. Patient education
    a. Therapeutic life style changes
    b. Monitoring schedule

- Referral
1. Nutritional consultation
2. Lipid specialist with unusually severe, refractory, or complex disorders

Coronary Artery Disease

- Definition—atherosclerotic changes to coronary vasculature; decreased blood flow through coronary arteries due to partial obstruction or vasospasm

- Etiology/Incidence/Risk factors
1. Etiology
    a. Atherosclerosis develops with the formation of fatty streaks, fibrous plaques, and complicated lesions that narrow the lumen of the coronary arteries
    b. Angina pectoris—myocardial ischemia secondary to inability of the coronary arteries to supply oxygenated blood to meet myocardial oxygen demands
    c. Acute coronary syndromes—a plaque may rupture with thrombus formation that impedes/completely occludes the coronary lumen
        (1) Unstable angina
        (2) Acute myocardial infarction
2. Cardiovascular disease is the leading killer of women; one of every two women will die from coronary artery disease or stroke
3. Risk factors include
    a. Cigarette smoking
    b. Hypertension
    c. Dyslipidemia
    d. Diabetes mellitus
    e. Genetic predisposition
    f. Obesity
    g. Sedentary lifestyle

- Signs and symptoms
1. May be asymptomatic
2. Angina pectoris
    a. Clinical syndrome characterized by discomfort in the chest, jaw, shoulder, back, or arm
    b. Precipitated by exertion or emotional stress and relieved by nitroglycerin
    c. Chronic stable angina is predictable; no change in pattern or frequency of episodes
3. Palpitations

- Physical findings
1. May be no specific findings
2. Elevated blood pressure
3. Dyspnea, tachycardia, pallor, diaphoresis during acute angina episode

- Differential diagnosis
1. Unstable angina
2. Myocardial infarction
3. Pulmonary disease—pulmonary embolism, pneumothorax, pneumonia
4. GI disorders—gastroesophageal reflux, cholecystitis, peptic ulcer
5. Musculoskeletal conditions—costochondritis, muscle strain
6. Anxiety disorders
7. Acute aortic dissection
8. Herpes zoster

- Diagnostic tests/findings
1. Electrocardiogram—may show transient T-wave inversion or ST segment depression or elevation during acute angina episode
2. Exercise or pharmacologic stress testing—ischemic changes or angina during test is clinically diagnostic
3. Myocardial perfusion imaging—used to confirm and assess extent and location of coronary artery disease
4. Coronary angiography—definitive test for coronary artery disease

- Management/Treatment
1. Nonpharmacologic
    a. Primary prevention—smoking cessation; dietary management of hypertension, dyslipidemia, diabetes, obesity; regular aerobic exercise
    b. Secondary prevention—surgical revascularization
        (1) PCTA/percutaneous transluminal angioplasty
        (2) CABG/coronary artery bypass graft
2. Pharmacologic—the treatment of stable angina has two major purposes: to prevent myocardial infarction and to reduce the symptoms of angina
    a. Primary prevention
        (1) Medications for treatment of hypertension, diabetes, hyperlipidemia, and smoking cessation

(2) Aspirin 81–325 mg

b. Secondary management of angina—may use a combination of medications for increased effectiveness

  (1) Sublingual nitroglycerine 0.4 mg as needed for symptomatic relief of anginal episodes (see Long acting nitrates section)

  (2) Beta adrenergic blockers—metoprolol, propranolol, atenolol; preferred initial therapy in absence of contraindications

    (a) Drug action—decrease myocardial demand by decreasing heart rate, systolic blood pressure, and contractility

    (b) Side-effects—fatigue, dizziness, depression, bradycardia, hypotension, nausea, diarrhea, dyspnea, bronchospasm, rash

    (c) Drug interactions—may potentiate other antihypertensives, may antagonize effects of sympathomimetic drugs

    (d) Contraindications—sinus bradycardia, heart block greater than one degree, heart failure, cardiogenic shock; pregnancy category C

  (3) Calcium channel blockers—verapamil, amlodipine/long acting formulations only

    (a) Drug action—promote peripheral arterial vasodilation, which decreases oxygen demand by decreasing afterload, also decrease coronary vasospasm

    (b) Side-effects—hypotension, edema, bradycardia, constipation, dizziness, headache, fatigue, nausea, dyspnea, rash

    (c) Drug interactions—may potentiate beta blockers, other antihypertensives, digitalis; antagonized by rifampin, phenobarbital

    (d) Contraindications—severe left ventricular dysfunction, hypotension, heart block greater than one degree, cardiogenic shock; pregnancy category C

  (4) Long acting nitrates—nitropaste, nitropatches, isosorbide dinitrate

    (a) Drug action—cause venous dilation, which decreases venous return to the heart and modest arterial vasodilation; results in decreased myocardial oxygen demand

    (b) Side-effects—headache, dizziness, flushing, orthostatic hypotension, tachycardia, nausea, rash

    (c) Drug interactions—hypotension potentiated with alcohol, other vasodilators, calcium channel blockers

    (d) Contraindications—acute myocardial infarction; pregnancy category C

3. Patient education

  a. Instructions on use and side-effects of medications

  b. Education and support for life style changes

- Referral
  1. Patients with unstable angina
  2. Patients with stable angina who cannot be controlled with medication

◘ EYE, EAR, NOSE, AND THROAT DISORDERS

Allergic Rhinitis

- Definition—inflammation of mucous membranes of nose in response to contact with specific allergens, triggering production of IgE antibodies, causing histamine release and subsequent edema, itching, discharge, and sneezing

- Etiology/Incidence
  1. Seasonal—occurs at specific times of year when pollens/allergens are present (hay fever)
     a. Trees—April to July
     b. Grasses—May to July
     c. Ragweed—August to October
  2. Perennial—year-round symptoms usually related to dust mites, mold, cockroaches, and animal dander
  3. Affects approximately 10% of adults; onset typically between ages 10–20

- Signs and symptoms
  1. Nasal congestion, clear rhinorrhea, sneezing
  2. Pruritus of nose, throat, eyes
  3. Sore throat and cough from postnasal drip

- Physical findings
  1. Pale, boggy nasal mucosa
  2. Clear, thin rhinorrhea
  3. Injected conjunctiva, tearing
  4. "Allergic shiners" or dark discoloration beneath both eyes

■ **Table 8-2** Antihistamines, Decongestants and Anti-inflammatory Medications for Respiratory Disorders (representative list)

Drug	Action	Side-effects	Interactions	Contraindications
Antihistamines				
1st generation Chlorpheniramine (Chlor-Trimeton) Diphenhydramine (Benadryl)	Block action of histamine; anticholinergic effects	Drowsiness, dry mucous membranes, blurred vision	Additive effects with alcohol, sedatives, anti-anxiety agents	Pregnancy category B; caution nursing mothers
2nd generation Loratidine (Claritin) Desloratidine (Clarinex) Fexofenadine (Allegra) Cetirizine (Zyrtec)	Selective peripheral histamine receptor antagonist; no anticholinergic effects	Fewer sedating effects (with exception of cetirizine)	Zyrtec—potentiates other CNS depressants	Caution in patients with renal or hepatic dysfunction. Pregnancy categories B/C; not recommended while nursing
Azelastine HCL (Astelin)	Topical antihistamine	Bitter taste, somnolence, headache	Potentiates other CNS depressants	Pregnancy category C; caution nursing mothers
Decongestants				
Pseudoephedrine	Alpha-adrenergic agonists; vasoconstriction reduces engorgement of mucosa	Increases heart rate and BP. CNS stimulation. Use with caution in hypertensive patients	Hypertensive crisis with MAO inhibitors	Severe hypertension or cardiovascular disease. Pregnancy category C; not recommended while nursing
Nasal corticosteroids				
Budesonide (Rhinocort) Fulticasone (Flonase)	Anti-inflammatory effects; therapeutic benefit not immediate	Local irritation, epistaxis, headache. Systemic absorption at recommended doses minimal	Cytochrome P450 effect	Pregnancy category C; not recommended while nursing
Mast cell stabilizers				
Cromolyn (Nasalcrom)	Prevents degranulation of mast cells; prophylactic drug	Local reactions: burning, stinging, sneezing	None known	Precautions for pregnancy/nursing mothers

- Differential diagnosis
  1. Vasomotor rhinitis
  2. Atrophic rhinitis
  3. Secondary to selected medications—antihypertensive agents
  4. Rhinitis medicamentosa—excessive topical use of topical vasoconstrictors
  5. Nasal polyps

- Diagnostic tests/findings
  1. Usually none indicated
  2. Nasal smear for eosinophils—eosinophils present in 65–75% of cases
  3. Skin tests to determine specific allergens; gold standard test
  4. In vitro serum allergy tests—RAST; expensive and not as sensitive as specific skin testing

- Management/Treatment
  1. Nonpharmacologic—allergen avoidance
     a. Bedroom must be the most allergen free
     b. Environmental control—vacuum, dust, remove carpeting, feather pillows, stuffed animals
     c. Eliminate or restrict exposure to pets; pets should not be in bedroom
     d. Air conditioning/air filters
  2. Pharmacologic (see **Table 8-2**)
     a. Antihistamines
        (1) Generally considered first line therapy
        (2) Highly effective in reducing itching, sneezing, rhinorrhea; minimal effect on nasal congestion
        (3) More effective if given before onset of symptoms
     b. Decongestants
     c. Topical corticosteroids
        (1) Given their effectiveness, increased use as first line treatment
        (2) Not helpful with ocular symptoms
        (3) Slow onset of effect; must be used on regular basis to be effective
     d. Mast cell stabilizers
     e. Montelukast (see **Table 8-3**)
  3. Patient education
     a. Identify and eliminate or avoid allergens, e.g., remove carpeting, pets, install air filters
     b. Appropriate use of medications, combinations, side-effects, and overuse syndromes

- Referral—refer for skin tests to determine specific allergens

Conjunctivitis

- Definition—encompasses a broad group of conditions presenting as inflammation of the conjunctiva

- Etiology/Incidence
  1. Viral conjunctivitis—adenovirus most common; herpes simplex and herpes zoster
  2. Bacterial conjunctivitis—*Staphylococcus aureus* (adults), *Streptococcus pneumoniae* and *Haemophilus influenzae* (children)
  3. Allergy—type I, IgE mediated hypersensitivity reaction precipitated by small airborne allergens, e.g., pollen, animal dander, dust
  4. Most common eye complaint in primary care

- Signs and symptoms
  1. Sensation of grit in eye, "scratchy"; mild discomfort
  2. Pain, photophobia, blurred vision that fails to clear with blink are not typical features of primary conjunctival process
  3. Viral conjunctivitis
     a. Acute onset; may be unilateral or bilateral with a watery discharge
     b. Preauricular adenitis
     c. May be associated with upper respiratory infection
  4. Bacterial conjunctivitis
     a. Acute onset; symptoms begin in one eye and spread to other eye
     b. Mucopurulent discharge; patient reports eyelids are matted together on awakening
     c. Marked conjunctival injection of abrupt onset with copious purulent discharge associated with gonococcal infection; sight-threatening ocular infection
  5. Allergic conjunctivitis
     a. Major cause of chronic conjunctivitis
     b. Complaints of bilateral itching, tearing, redness, and mild eyelid swelling
     c. Discharge is clear and watery or stringy and mucoid
     d. Personal or family history of atopic disease

- Physical findings
  1. Characterized by dilation of superficial conjunctival blood vessels, resulting in hyperemia; hyperemia greatest at the periphery of the bulbar conjunctiva
  2. Discharge (see Signs and symptoms)
  3. Cornea clear; PERRL
  4. Visual acuity with no acute change
  5. Preauricular adenopathy

■ **Table 8-3** Asthma Quick-Relief and Long-Term-Control Medications (representative list)

Drug	Action	Side-effects	Interactions	Contraindications/ Precautions
Short acting inhaled B_2-agonists				
Albuterol (MDI and Nebulizer soln)	Relaxes bronchial smooth muscle by selective action on B_2-receptors	Tachycardia, nervousness, skeletal muscle tremor	MAO inhibitors, tricyclic antidepressants, sympathomimetic agents; antagonized by beta-blockers	Cardiovascular disease; pregnancy category C; not recommended for nursing mothers
Inhaled corticosteroids				
Fluticasone MDI/DPI* Budesonide DPI	Inhibits inflammatory response	Minimal systemic effects; oropharyngeal candidiasis, dysphonia	Cytochrome P450 effect; caution with CYP3A4 inhibitors, e.g., ketoconazole	Not for treatment of acute attack; pregnancy category C; use caution with nursing mothers
Oral steroids				
Prednisone		Adrenal suppression; masks infection	NSAIDs	Systemic mycoses; live vaccination
Long acting inhaled B_2-agonists				
Salmeterol DPI (Diskus)	Relaxes bronchial smooth muscle by selective action on B_2-receptors	Headache, pharyngitis, URI, tachycardia, tremor	MAO inhibitors, tricyclic antidepressants, sympathomimetic agents; antagonized by beta-blockers	Should not be used for symptom relief or acute exacerbation; cardiovascular disease; pregnancy category C; not recommended for nursing mothers

	Action	Side Effects	Drug Interactions	Notes
Combined medication				
Fluticasone (Salmeterol)	Combined anti-inflammatory/ broncho-dilating effects	Respiratory tract infection, laryngeal spasm/swelling, headache, hoarseness	MAO inhibitors, tricyclic antidepressants, sympathomimetic agents; antagonized by beta-blockers	Not for treatment of acute attack; pregnancy category C; use caution with nursing mothers
Leukotriene modifiers				
Montelukast	Leukotriene receptor antagonist	Headache, fatigue, fever, GI upset	Monitor with drugs that induce Cytochrome P450 enzymes, e.g., rifampin	Pregnancy category B; use caution with nursing others
Mast cell stabilizers				
Cromolyn (Nedocromil)	Prevents mast cell release of histamine, leukotrienes, slow-reacting substance of anaphylaxis	Bronchospasm, throat irritation, bad taste, cough	None identified	Not for treatment of acute attacks; pregnancy category B; caution with nursing mothers
Methylxanthines				
Theophylline	Relaxes bronchial smooth muscle	GI upset, headache, CNS stimulation, diuresis, arrhythmias, seizures	Cytochrome P450 effect; numerous drugs may effect serum concentration via induction or inhibition of P450 enzymes	Peptic ulcer disease, arrhythmias, seizure disorders; pregnancy category C; not recommended for nursing mothers

*Metered-dose inhaler/Dry-powdered inhaler

- Differential diagnosis
  1. Foreign body
  2. Subconjunctival hemorrhage
  3. Blepharitis
  4. Episceritis/scleritis
  5. Keratitis
  6. Uveitis
  7. Acute angle closure glaucoma

- Diagnostic tests/findings
  1. Fluorescein stain—stain uptake suggests corneal involvement
  2. Diagnostic testing if gonococcal, chlamydial infection, chronic or recurrent infection suspected, or failure to respond to treatment

- Management/Treatment
  1. Viral
     a. Self-limited; topical antibiotics often prescribed
     b. Avoid touching eyes; avoid close contact for approximately 2 weeks
  2. Bacterial
     a. Broad spectrum topical antibiotic—sodium sulfacetamide (Sulymid); polymixin B/trimethoprim (Polytrim); tobramycin (Tobrex)
     b. Reserve fluoroquinolones for severe infections
  3. Allergic
     a. Removal of offending allergen if possible
     b. Topical antihistamine—levocabastine (Livostin)
     c. Mast cell stabilizer—cromolyn (Crolom)
     d. Mast cell stabilizer/antihistamine—olopatadine HCL (Patanol)
     e. Topical NSAIDs—ketorolac (Acular)

- Referral
  1. Patients with pain, photophobia, blurred vision; circumcorneal erythema/ciliary flush
  2. No improvement after 48 hours of treatment

Acute Otitis Media

- Definition—infection of the middle ear that is often preceded by upper respiratory infection or allergies

- Etiology/Incidence/Risk factors
  1. Etiology
     a. Eustachian tube dysfunction secondary to URI or allergies causes edema and congestion that impedes flow of middle ear secretions; accumulation of secretions promotes growth of pathogens

  b. Common pathogens—*Streptococcus pneumoniae, Haemophilus influenzae, Moraxella catarrhalis*, viruses
  2. Highest incidence in childhood, younger than age 10
  3. Risk factors
     a. Recent/current URI
     b. Exposure to cigarette smoke, active or passive

- Signs and symptoms
  1. Ear pain, decreased hearing, fever
  2. Aural pressure
  3. Vertigo, nausea and vomiting

- Physical findings
  1. Full or bulging tympanic membrane (TM) with absent or obscured landmarks
  2. Distorted light reflex
  3. Decreased/absent mobility of TM on pneumatic otoscopy
  4. Erythema of TM is an inconsistent finding
  5. Bullae on TM; often associated with *Mycoplasma pneumoniae*
  6. Preauricular or cervical lymphadenopathy

- Differential diagnosis
  1. Otitis externa
  2. Otitis media with effusion
  3. Temporomandibular joint (TMJ) syndrome
  4. Dental abscess
  5. Mastoiditis

- Diagnostic tests/findings
  1. Usually none indicated
  2. Tympanometry for recurrent infections; indicator fluid posterior to TM

- Management/Treatment
  1. Pharmacologic
     a. Antibiotics
        (1) Amoxicillin; for penicillin-allergic patients, trimethoprim/sulfamethoxazole or erythromycin; if inadequate response, change to amoxicillin-clavulanate
        (2) Side-effects
            (a) GI upset, nausea, vomiting, diarrhea
            (b) Rashes, urticaria
        (3) Drug interactions—trimethoprim/sulfamethoxazole may potentiate oral anticoagulants, hypoglycemics
        (4) Contraindications/precautions
            (a) Hepatic impairment

(b) Pregnancy category B except sulfa drugs, which are category C; sulfa not recommended while nursing

b. No demonstrated benefit with use of decongestants

c. Analgesics/antipyretics

(1) Acetaminophen

(a) Drug action—inhibits CNS prostaglandin synthesis

(b) Side-effects—can cause serious or fatal hepatic injury

(c) Drug interactions—increased risk of hepatotoxicity with chronic, heavy alcohol use

(d) Contraindications/precautions—pregnancy category B; use with caution while nursing

(2) Nonsteroidal anti-inflammatory drugs (NSAIDs)

(a) Ibuprofen, naproxen, ketoprofen

(b) Drug action

i. Inhibits cyclooxygenase, the enzyme that catalyzes the synthesis of prostaglandins and thromboxane from arachidonic acid

ii. Analgesic, anti-inflammatory and antipyretic effects

(c) Side-effects

i. Hypersensitivity

ii. Dyspepsia, GI bleeding

iii. Tinnitus, drowsiness, headache

iv. Nephrotoxiciy

v. Hepatotoxicity

(d) Interactions

i. Decreased antihypertensive effect of ACE inhibitors, beta-blockers, diuretics

ii. Potentiates anticoagulants

(e) Contraindications/precautions

i. Aspirin allergy

ii. Pregnancy C, but contraindicated in third trimester; not recommended while nursing

2. Patient education

a. Appropriate ear canal hygiene

b. Antibiotic use and side-effects

c. Need for additional care if no improvement in 2 to 3 days

• Referral

1. For suspected extension of infection, mastoiditis, or perforation of tympanic membrane

2. Persistent hearing loss after adequate treatment

3. Recurrent infections; patient may require consideration for myringotomy

Sinusitis

• Definition—inflammation of the mucosal surface of the paranasal sinuses

• Etiology/Incidence

1. Etiology

a. Acute sinusitis—caused by viral or bacterial infections and allergies; bacterial causes include *Streptococcus pneumoniae, Haemophilus influenzae, Moraxella catarrhalis*

b. Infection usually involves maxillary and ethmoid sinuses

c. Chronic sinusitis occurs with episodes of prolonged infection that resist treatment and/or repeated or inadequately treated acute infection; treatment failure secondary to failure of sinuses to drain, which may be associated with anatomic defect

2. Incidence–accounts for 6% of primary care office visits

• Signs and symptoms

1. Acute sinusitis

a. Nasal congestion, facial pain, toothache, headache, fever, yellow/green nasal drainage

b. Increased pain with bending over or sudden head movement

c. Common cold and allergic/vasomotor rhinitis may precede infection

d. "Double sickening"—URI symptoms with initial improvement followed by increasing nasal symptoms

2. Chronic sinusitis

a. Nasal congestion, discharge, and cough that last longer than 30 days

b. Dull ache or pressure across forehead and/or midface

c. Constant postnasal drip and chronic cough

• Physical findings

1. Afebrile or low-grade fever

2. Mucopurulent nasal discharge; postnasal discharge

3. Nasal mucosa swollen, pale, dull red to gray

4. Pain on firm palpation over sinus areas

• Differential diagnosis

1. Uncomplicated URI

2. Migraine headaches

3. Allergic/vasomotor rhinitis

4. Nasal polyps
5. Dental abscess

- Diagnostic tests/findings
  1. None for typical presentation
  2. Sinus radiography
     a. Confirmed by mucosal thickening, sinus opacity, air–fluid levels
     b. Normal sinus radiography to exclude maxillary and frontal disease; ethmoid involvement more difficult to exclude
  3. CT scan—reserved for complicated disease and search for ethmoidal disease in patients with refractory symptoms and negative conventional radiographs

- Management/Treatment
  1. Nonpharmacologic
     a. Saline nasal spray
     b. Steam inhalation
     c. Warm compresses
     d. Hydration—2000 to 3000 mL daily
  2. Pharmacologic
     a. Antibiotics (see Acute Otitis Media this chapter)
        (1) If signs and symptoms are present 10 or more days after onset of upper respiratory symptoms
        (2) If signs and symptoms of acute sinusitis worsen with 10 days of initial improvement
     b. Oral/topical decongestants
        (1) Oral decongestants (see Table 8-2)
        (2) Topical decongestant/oxymetazoline spray 0.05%
            (a) Provides rapid relief
            (b) Should not be used for longer than 3–5 days to prevent rebound congestion
     c. Nasal steroids—to reduce mucosal inflammation (see Table 8-2)
     d. Antihistamines not recommended unless patient has allergies
     e. Pain management as needed with acetaminophen, NSAIDS, opioids if severe
  3. Patient education
     a. Avoidance of allergens, environmental irritants, e.g., cigarette smoke
     b. Importance of maintaining adequate hydration

- Referral
  1. Severe facial pain, periorbital swelling
  2. Failure to respond to two courses of antibiotic
  3. Suspected anatomic abnormality
  4. Chronic sinusitis or more than three episodes of acute sinusitis per year

Common Cold

- Definition—an acute, mild, self-limited viral infection of the upper respiratory tract mucosa

- Etiology/Incidence/Risk factors
  1. Etiology
     a. Inflammation of the mucosal membranes from the nasal mucosa to the bronchi
     b. Rhinovirus, coronavirus, adenovirus
     c. Spread by airborne droplets and contact with infectious secretions on hands and environmental surfaces
     d. Incubation period 48–72 hours
  2. Incidence
     a. Peaks in winter months
     b. Children—6 to 8 infections per season
     c. Adults—2 to 4 per season
  3. Risks
     a. Repeated exposure to groups of children
     b. Close quarters, contact

- Signs and symptoms
  1. General malaise
  2. Nasal congestion and clear rhinorrhea
  3. Sneezing, coughing, sore throat, hoarseness
  4. Tearing, burning sensation of eyes

- Physical findings
  1. Low-grade fever
  2. Nasal mucosa swollen and erythematous
  3. Conjunctiva slightly red
  4. Throat erythematous with cervical lymphadennopathy

- Differential diagnosis
  1. Allergic rhinitis
  2. Streptococcal pharyngitis
  3. Influenza
  4. Otitis media

- Diagnostic tests/findings
  1. Generally none recommended
  2. Rapid strep screen/throat culture if streptococcal pharyngitis suspected

- Management/Treatment
  1. Nonpharmacologic
     a. Inhalation of warm vapors
     b. Saline nasal drops or sprays
     c. Saline gargles/throat lozenges
     d. Increase fluids
  2. Pharmacologic
     a. Acetaminophen or NSAIDs (see Acute Otitis Media this chapter)
     b. Topical/oral decongestants (see Table 8-2)

c. Cough suppressants—e.g., dextromethorphan
  (1) Drug action—depresses cough reflex by direct inhibition of cough center in the medulla
  (2) Side-effects—minimal CNS depressant action
  (3) Drug interactions—hyperpyretic crisis with MAOIs
  (4) Contraindications/precautions
    (a) Persistent or chronic cough
    (b) First trimester of pregnancy; caution while nursing
d. Expectorants—e.g., guaifenesin
  (1) Drug action—may increase output of respiratory tract secretions facilitating removal of mucus
  (2) Side-effects—GI upset, drowsiness, headache
  (3) Drug interactions—may increase toxicity/effect of disulfiram, MAOIs, metronidazole, procarbazine
  (4) Contraindications/precautions—pregnancy category C; use with caution while nursing
3. Patient education
  a. Infection control
  b. Self-limited nature of infection
  c. Symptoms of complications; secondary bacterial infection

Pharyngitis

- Definition—inflammation of the pharynx and tonsils

- Etiology/Incidence
  1. Etiology
    a. Viral—most common cause is rhinovirus and adenovirus
    b. Bacterial
      (1) Group A β-hemolytic streptococci (GABHS)
      (2) *Neisseria gonorrhea*
    c. Noninfectious causes—allergic rhinitis or postnasal drip
  2. Incidence
    a. One of the most frequent reasons for outpatient care in US
    b. Accounts for 16 million office visits per year; 2.5% of visits to primary care providers

- Risks—crowded work or living conditions

- Signs and symptoms
  1. Viral pharyngitis
    a. Sore throat, fever, malaise, cough, headache, myalgias, and fatigue
    b. May also complain of rhinitis, congestion, conjunctivitis
  2. GABHS
    a. Sudden onset of sore throat, fever, chills, headache, nausea/vomiting
    b. Rhinitis, cough, conjunctivitis not typically present

- Physical findings
  1. Viral pharyngitis—mild erythema of the pharynx with little or no exudates
  2. Bacterial pharyngitis
    a. Marked erythema of the throat, exudates, tender anterior cervical lymphadenopathy
    b. Erythematous "sandpaper" rash/accentuation in groin and axillae with scarlet fever

- Differential diagnosis
  1. Peritonsillar abscess
  2. Infectious mononucleosis
  3. Pharyngeal candidiasis
  4. Diphtheria
  5. Epiglottitis

- Diagnostic tests/findings
  1. Rapid strep antigen test—detects only GABHS (5–10% false negatives); throat culture if negative rapid strep test
  2. Throat culture for suspected gonococcal infection

- Management/Treatment
  1. Nonpharmacologic
    a. Adequate hydration
    b. Saline gargles
    c. Topical anesthetics, e.g., lozenges, sprays
  2. Pharmacologic
    a. GABHS
      (1) Penicillin V PO/benzathine pencillin IM
        (a) Drug action—bactericidal
        (b) Side-effects—hypersensitivity reactions
        (c) Contraindications/precautions—penicillin allergy; pregnancy category B
      (2) Erythromycin if penicillin allergy
    b. Gonococcal pharyngitis—Ceftriaxone IM
      (1) Drug action—bactericidal
      (2) Side-effects—injection site reaction, hypersensitivity reactions
      (3) Drug interactions—potentiated by probenecid
      (4) Contraindications/precautions—penicillin allergy; pregnancy category B

(5) Alternative agents—azithromycin, spectinomycin—obtain pharyngeal culture 3–5 days after treatment if use alternative regimen

- Referral
  1. Suspected peritonsillar abscess
  2. Epiglottitis

Infectious Mononucleosis (IM)

- Definition—an acute viral syndrome secondary to Epstein-Barr virus characterized by fever, pharyngitis, and lymphadenopathy

- Etiology/Incidence
  1. Etiology
     a. Causal agent is Epstein-Barr virus (EBV)
     b. Mode of transmission is oropharyngeal route via saliva
  2. Incidence—rarely symptomatic in children younger than 5 years; most clinically apparent infections occur in individuals 10–35 years old

- Signs and symptoms
  1. Prodrome of headache, malaise, fatigue, anorexia
  2. Fever, sore throat, swollen lymph nodes

- Physical findings
  1. Tonsillar enlargement with exudate
  2. Palatal petecchiae at junction of hard and soft palates (25% of cases)
  3. Lymphadenopathy; particularly posterior cervical
  4. Fever compatible with severity of infection
  5. Hepatomegaly (25% cases)
  6. Splenomegaly (50% cases)

- Differential diagnosis
  1. Streptococcal pharyngitis
  2. Other viral causes of pharyngitis
  3. Hepatitis
  4. HIV infection

- Diagnostic tests/findings
  1. Monospot/heterophile antibody test
     a. Up to 86% specific; 99% sensitive
     b. Initially negative, usually positive by 1 to 2 weeks after onset of symptoms
  2. CBC—lymphocytic leukocytosis with 10% of cells atypical
  3. Elevated aminotransferases (AST, ALT), bilirubin
  4. Throat culture—frequent secondary infection with GABHS

- Management/Treatment
  1. Nonpharmacologic—lozenges, gargles for relief of pharyngitis; treatment largely supportive
  2. Pharmacologic
     a. Fever—acetaminophen, NSAIDs to reduce fever, aches (see Acute Otitis Media this chapter)
     b. Corticosteroids—prescribed for significant pharyngeal edema and obstructive tonsillar enlargement
  3. Patient education
     a. Rest during acute phase of illness; activity as tolerated
     b. Contact sports, heavy lifting, and strenuous activity should be avoided for at least 1 month
     c. Avoid alcohol for at least 1 month
     d. Seek immediate care with sudden onset of severe abdominal pain

- Referral
  1. Onset of abdominal pain—possible ruptured spleen
  2. Airway obstruction from pharyngeal edema

◘ LOWER RESPIRATORY DISORDERS

Community-Acquired Pneumonia

- Definition—acute infection of the lower respiratory tract that is associated with symptoms of acute infection, altered breath sounds or rales on physical examination and acute infiltrate on chest radiograph in a patient who has not been hospitalized or resided in a long-term care facility for 14 days before the onset of symptoms.

- Etiology/Incidence/Risk factors
  1. Etiology
     a. Bacterial—*Streptococcus pneumoniae, Haemophilus influenzae, Legionella pneumophila*
     b. Nonbacterial—*Mycoplasma pneumoniae, Chlamydia pneumoniae*
     c. Viral—Influenza, adenovirus
  2. Incidence—sixth leading cause of death; leading cause of death from infectious disease
  3. Risk factors
     a. Preceding viral URI
     b. Cigarette smoking
     c. Age older than 50
     d. Chronic lung disease
     e. Corticosteroid use
     f. Immunosuppression

- Signs and symptoms
  1. May be masked or absent in very young, elderly, immunosuppressed, coexisting chronic disease
  2. Fever, chills, sweats
  3. Cough with/without sputum production
  4. Dyspnea, pleuritic chest pain
  5. Associated symptoms—lethargy, headache, anorexia, nausea, vomiting

- Physical findings
  1. Tachycardia
  2. Tachypnea, dyspnea
  3. Percussion
     a. Often normal in early disease
     b. Dullness over area of consolidation
  4. Auscultation
     a. Coarse rhonchi may clear or shift with cough
     b. Nonclearing rales
     c. Diminished breath sounds over consolidation
  5. Fever with chills, high spikes (102.2°F or above) especially if bacterial etiology
  6. Small areas of pneumonia cannot always be detected by physical examination

- Differential diagnosis
  1. Bronchitis
  2. Atelectasis
  3. Chronic obstructive pulmonary disease
  4. Congestive heart failure
  5. Malignancy
  6. Tuberculosis
  7. Pulmonary embolism

- Diagnostic tests/findings
  1. Chest radiograph
     a. Establishes diagnosis by revealing an infiltrate; helps distinguish pneumonia from acute bronchitis
     b. Demonstrates the presence of complications such as pleural effusion and multilobar disease
  2. Value of sputum collection for Gram's stain and culture is controversial
  3. CBC with differential—white blood cell (WBC) elevation (10,000/mm³ to 25,000/mm³) with a shift to left, e.g., bandemia, neutrophilia, especially if bacterial etiology

- Management/Treatment
  1. Nonpharmacologic
     a. Oral hydration and humidification
     b. Improve oxygenation, e.g., smoking cessation

  2. Pharmacologic
     a. Empiric antimicrobial therapy
        (1) Patients without comorbidity and less than 60 years—azithromycin or clarithromycin (MACROLIDE)
           (a) Drug action—inhibits bacterial protein synthesis
           (b) Side-effects—GI effects
           (c) Drug interactions—inhibits cytochrome P450 enzymes; may inhibit metabolism of other drugs
           (d) Contraindications/precautions—hypersensitivity to macrolide antibiotics; pregnancy category B; enters human milk/use caution
           (e) Alternative agents include doxycycline, levofloxacin
        (2) Patients with comorbidity or over 60 years—levofloxacin
           (a) Drug action—inhibits bacterial DNA synthesis
           (b) Side-effects—GI upset, CNS toxicity
           (c) Drug interactions—avoid drugs that prolong QT interval; increased risk of tendon rupture with corticosteroids; inhibits cytochrome P450 enzymes; may inhibit metabolism of other drugs
           (d) Contraindications/precautions—pregnancy category C; not recommended for nursing mothers
           (e) Alternative agents include beta-lactam/macrolide combination
     b. Antipyretics—acetaminophen, NSAIDs (see Acute Otitis Media this chapter)
  3. Patient education
     a. Infection containment principles
     b. Need for hydration
     c. Rest
     d. Increased caloric requirements with fever
     e. Medication schedules and side-effects

- Referral/MD consult
  1. Base decision to hospitalize on age, comorbid illness, physical examination, and laboratory findings
  2. No improvement in 24 to 36 hours
  3. Fever over 102°F, pallor or cyanosis, nasal flaring
  4. Mental confusion

Asthma

- Definition
  1. A chronic inflammatory disorder of the airways in which many cells and cellular

elements play a role, in particular, mast cells, eosinophils, T lymphocytes, neutrophils, and epithelial cells; in susceptible individuals, this inflammation causes recurrent episodes of wheezing, breathlessness, chest tightness and cough, particularly at night and the early morning; these episodes are associated with airflow obstruction that is often reversible; the inflammation also causes an associated increase in existing bronchial hyperresponsiveness to a variety of stimuli (NHLBI, 2007)

2. Classification correlates to treatment recommendations
   a. Intermittent—step 1
      (1) Symptoms 2 times/week or less; nocturnal symptoms 2 times/month or less
      (2) PEF/FEV$_1$ greater than 80% of predicted value; variability less than 20%; normal between exacerbations
   b. Mild persistent—step 2
      (1) Symptoms 3–6 times/week; nocturnal symptoms 3–4 times/month
      (2) PEF/FEV$_1$ greater than 80% of predicted value; variability 20–30%
   c. Moderate persistent—step 3
      (1) Daily symptoms; nocturnal symptoms more than 1 time/week but not nightly
      (2) PEF/FEV$_1$ greater than 60% but less than 80%; variability greater than 30%
   d. Severe persistent—step 4
      (1) Continual daily symptoms; frequent nocturnal symptoms
      (2) PEF/FEV$_1$ less than 60%; variability greater than 30%

- Etiology/Incidence
  1. Etiology
     a. Caused by single or multiple triggers
        (1) Allergic triggers
            (a) Airborn pollens, molds, dust mites, cockroaches, animal dander
            (b) Food additives or preservatives
            (c) Feather pillows
        (2) Nonallergic triggers
            (a) Smoke and other pollutants
            (b) Viral respiratory infections
            (c) Medications—ASA, NSAIDs, beta-blockers
            (d) Exercise
            (e) Gastroesophageal reflux
            (f) Emotional factors
            (g) Menses, pregnancy
     b. In children there is generally a strong history of atopy; adult-onset asthma may be related to allergens, but nonallergic triggers likely to be a factor
  2. Incidence
     a. Occurs in approximately 3% of the general population
        (1) Affects approximately 10% of children
        (2) Affects approximately 5% of adults
     b. Can occur at any age; increasing in prevalence in US

- Signs and symptoms
  1. Episodic wheeze, chest tightness, shortness of breath or cough; cough may be sole symptom
  2. Symptoms worsen in presence of aeroallergens, irritants, and exercise
  3. Symptoms occur or worsen at night; cause nighttime awakening
  4. History of allergic rhinitis or atopic dermatitis; family history of asthma, allergic rhinitis or atopic dermatitis

- Physical findings
  1. Hyperexpansion of thorax; hyperresonance with percussion
  2. Wheezing; prolonged expiratory phase
  3. Diminished breath sounds
  4. Tachypnea, dyspnea
  5. Atopic dermatitis/eczema or other skin manifestations of allergic skin disorders
  6. Increased nasal secretions, mucosal swelling, nasal polyps

- Differential diagnosis
  1. Acute infection—bronchitis, pneumonia
  2. Chronic obstructive pulmonary disease (COPD); may overlap with asthma
  3. Heart disease—heart failure
  4. Foreign body aspiration
  5. Pulmonary emboli
  6. Cough secondary to drugs such as ACE inhibitors

- Diagnostic tests/findings
  1. Pulmonary function tests/spirometry—to establish airway obstruction
     a. FEV$_1$ (forced expiratory volume in 1 second) less than 80% of predicted; FEV$_1$/FVC (forced vital capacity) less than 65% or below limit of normal
     b. Spirometry and peak flow rates improve with bronchodilator challenge; FEV$_1$ increases 12% and at least 200 mL after use of inhaled short acting B$_2$-agonist
  2. If normal spirometry, assess diurnal variation in PEF (peak expiratory flow); 20% difference between two measures/PEF variability supports diagnosis of asthma

3. Bronchoprovocation with methacholine, histamine, or exercise if diagnosis in question; negative test helps exclude diagnosis of asthma
4. Chest radiograph if infection, large airway lesions, heart disease, or foreign body obstruction suspected

- Management/Treatment
  1. Goals
     a. Minimize symptoms, normalize daily activity
     b. Maintain near-normal pulmonary function
     c. Minimal use of short acting B_2-agonist
  2. Nonpharmacologic
     a. Peak flow monitoring
        (1) Establish patient's "personal best" and develop "Asthma Action Plan"
        (2) A drop in peak flow below 80% indicates an acute exacerbation and need to contact clinician for medication adjustment
        (3) A drop in peak flow below 50% indicates need for emergency treatment
     b. Avoidance of known allergens, triggers
     c. Adequate hydration and humidity
     d. Annual influenza vaccine and pneumococcal vaccine
  3. Pharmacologic—stepwise approach (see Table 8-3)
     a. Intermittent—step 1
        (1) No daily medications
        (2) Short acting inhaled B_2-agonist as needed for symptoms
        (3) Course of systemic corticosteroids recommended for severe exacerbations
     b. Mild persistent—step 2
        (1) Low-dose inhaled corticosteroids
        (2) Alternative treatments—mast-cell stabilizer, leukotriene modifier, or theophylline
        (3) Short acting inhaled B_2-agonist as needed for symptoms
     c. Moderate persistent—step 3
        (1) Low-medium dose inhaled corticosteroids and long acting inhaled B_2-agonist
        (2) Alternative treatments: add leukotriene or theophylline; increase inhaled corticosteroid within medium dose range
        (3) Short acting inhaled B_2-agonist as needed for symptoms
     d. Severe persistent—step 4
        (1) High-dose inhaled corticosteroids and long acting inhaled B_2-agonist; oral corticosteroid if needed
        (2) Short acting inhaled B_2-agonist as needed for symptoms
     e. Severe exacerbation (peak flow < 60%) can occur with any category of asthma; consider short course of oral steroids 40–60 mg/d for 5–10 days (NHLBI, 2007)
  4. Patient education
     a. How to recognize signs of worsening asthma
     b. Use of peak flow meter
     c. Clear instructions on use of written "Asthma Action Plan"
     d. Proper use of inhaler for effective dosing
     e. Prophylactic medication, e.g., pre-exercise dosing
     f. Control of environmental factors, e.g., allergens and irritants

- Referral
  1. Failure to respond to emergency treatment; arrange for emergency room treatment if signs of severe obstruction present—peak flow reduced by 50%, pulsus paradoxus, use of accessory muscles of respiration
  2. Difficulty controlling asthma or if step 4 is required

Tuberculosis (TB)

- Definition—necrotizing bacterial infection caused by *Mycobacterium tuberculosis;* most commonly infects the lungs, but any organ can be affected
  1. Active TB disease/ATBD—signs, symptoms, and radiographic findings secondary to *M. tuberculosis;* disease may be pulmonary or extrapulmonary
  2. TB infection/Latent TB infection (LTBI)
     a. Positive tuberculin skin test with no signs or symptoms of disease
     b. Chest radiograph negative or only granulomas/calcifications in lungs and/or regional lymph nodes

- Etiology/Incidence/Risk factors
  1. Etiology—*Mycobacterium tuberculosis;* spread by small airborne particles
  2. Incidence
     a. 10 to 15 million infected in US; 90–95% of primary TB infections remain in a latent or dormant stage
     b. Incidence rising due to HIV infection
  3. Risk factors
     a. HIV-infected individuals

b. Incarceration, crowding, or institutional living
c. Intravenous drug use, alcoholism
d. Racial or ethnic groups at risk—Hispanic, Native American, African American
e. Healthcare workers in hospitals, clinics, daycare, long-term care, correctional facilities
f. Household contacts of diagnosed cases

- Signs and symptoms
  1. TB infection/LTBI
     a. Asymptomatic state may last months to years
     b. 10% go on to develop active TB
  2. Active TB/ATBD
     a. Generalized symptoms
        (1) Night sweats, fever
        (2) Malaise, weakness
        (3) Anorexia
        (4) Weight loss
     b. Pulmonary symptoms
        (1) Productive cough, possible hemoptysis
        (2) Chest pain
        (3) Dyspnea
     c. Systemic symptoms (extrapulmonary sites)
        (1) Pelvic pain
        (2) Flank pain

- Physical findings
  1. Generally normal appearance in early disease, progressing to cachectic
  2. Unexplained fever
  3. Lung findings—increased tactile fremitus and dullness to percussion over consolidated areas; apical rales and whispered pectoriloquy
  4. Advanced disease—purulent green or yellow sputum
  5. Hemoptysis

- Differential diagnosis
  1. Pneumonia
  2. Malignancy
  3. Chronic obstructive pulmonary disease
  4. Silicosis
  5. Sarcoidosis

- Diagnostic tests/findings
  1. Purified protein derivative (PPD) skin test (antigen response) recommended for routine screening of individuals at risk of infection
     a. Positive test indicates exposure, not active disease
     b. PPD interpretation
        (1) A reaction of 5 mm or greater is considered positive in patients with
            (a) HIV infection, immunocompromised/immunosuppressed individuals
            (b) Those with abnormal chest radiographs consistent with healed TB lesions
            (c) Recent close contact with infected person
        (2) A reaction of 10 mm or greater is considered positive among
            (a) Recent arrivals (< 5 years) from high prevalence areas
            (b) Low socioeconomic status, homeless
            (c) Aged, nursing home resident, incarcerated individual
            (d) Individuals with chronic disease or predisposing conditions, e.g. gastrectomy, diabetes mellitus, or corticosteroid therapy
        (3) A reaction of 15 mm or greater is considered positive among individuals without risk factors
     c. False-negative
        (1) PPD administered after live virus vaccine
        (2) Immunosuppressed
        (3) Elderly
     d. False-positive
        (1) Recent BCG vaccine
        (2) Nontuberculosis mycobacterium
     e. "Positive converter"—previous negative PPD
  2. QuantiFERON-TB Gold blood test also used for routine screening
     a. Less false positives than skin test
     b. More convenient—1 office visit, results within 24 hrs
     c. Not affected by prior BCG vaccination
     d. Some follow-up as for positive skin test
     e. More expensive
  3. Chest radiography, both antero-posterior and lateral views, indicated with positive PPD result
     a. Identifies active pulmonary disease; negative chest radiograph rules out active TB
     b. Radiologic findings include apical scarring, hilar adenopathy with peripheral infiltrate and upper lobe cavitation
  4. Three sputum samples required for both smear and culture in patients suspected of pulmonary TB
     a. A presumptive diagnosis of TB can be made with detection of acid-fast bacilli in sputum smear
     b. A positive culture for *M. tuberculosis* is essential to confirm diagnosis

- Management/Treatment
  1. LTBI
     a. Nonpharmacologic—not applicable
     b. Pharmacologic
        (1) Treatment goal—stop progression to active disease state
        (2) Recommended for individuals at high risk of exposure and those at high risk of progression from latent TB infection to active disease
            (a) Close contact of confirmed active TB
            (b) Foreign-born persons from endemic countries and in US for 5 years or less
            (c) Residents and employees of congregate settings
            (d) Healthcare workers with high-risk patients
            (e) Persons with HIV or otherwise immunosuppressed
            (f) Others on a case-by-case basis assessment of risk for developing active disease
        (3) Screening procedures to identify appropriate individuals for preventive treatment
            (a) Exclude active disease with chest radiograph
            (b) Exclude individuals who have already been adequately treated
            (c) Identify contraindications to isoniazid
            (d) Identify individuals needing special consideration, e.g., pregnant, older than 35
        (4) Treatment with isoniazid for 9 months
            (a) Drug action—inhibition of myocolic acid synthesis resulting in disruption of bacterial cell wall
            (b) Side-effects—GI symptoms; hepatitis/monitor transaminase levels at baseline, 3, 6, and 9 mos; peripheral neuropathy/dose with vitamin B_6 (pyridoxine)
            (c) Drug interactions—alcohol increases risk of hepatitis; pyridoxine deficiency increases risk of peripheral neuropathy
            (d) Drug contraindications/precautions—acute hepatic disease; pregnancy category C
  2. Active disease treatment—consult/referral to specialist
     a. Nonpharmacologic
        (1) Well-balanced diet; additional caloric intake may be needed to maintain or gain weight
        (2) Outdoor exercise
     b. Pharmacologic
        (1) Typical regimen includes isoniazid, rifampin, pyrazinamide for 2 months; isoniazid and rifampin for 4 months; given resistance concerns include ethambutol in initial regimen until drug susceptibility tests are known
        (2) Directly observed therapy (DOT) is one method to ensure compliance; healthcare provider/designee observes patient ingest medications
  3. Patient education
     a. Importance of continuous treatment
        (1) Possibility of microbial resistance
        (2) Signs of developing side-effects, drug interactions
     b. Infection control principles
        (1) Reducing respiratory droplet broadcast
        (2) Care with disposal of infected wastes, tissues
        (3) Avoiding crowded conditions, contact with susceptible individuals while infectious
     c. Follow-up requirements, liver function monitoring
     d. Necessity for contact evaluation and treatment
     e. Importance of general health maintenance

- Referral
  1. Patients with ATBD
  2. Report all cases to health department for monitoring, strain identification
  3. Health department follow-up for contact tracing, risk assessment

☐ GASTROINTESTINAL DISORDERS

Constipation

- Definition—constipation is a symptom rather than a disease
  1. Decreased frequency of defecation
  2. May also include complaints of straining at stool, hard or small stools, sense of incomplete evacuation, abdominal pain or bloating, or need for digital manipulation to enable defecation

- Etiology/Incidence
  1. Etiology
     a. Functional causes—low-fiber diet, motility disorders (irritable bowel syndrome), sedentary life style, dehydration

b. Structural abnormalities—anal disorders (anal fissure), colonic mass with obstruction (adenocarcinoma)

c. Systemic disease or condition—hypothyroidism, pregnancy

d. Neurologic, neuromuscular disorder—multiple sclerosis, spinal cord disorders

e. Psychogenic disorders—depression

f. Medications—laxative overuse, anticholinergics, narcotics, calcium channel blockers

2. Prevalence—unknown due to frequent self-treatment; commonly reported by patients, especially elderly

3. Risks
   a. Female gender/pregnancy
   b. Older age
   c. Low-fiber diet
   d. Immobility

- Signs and symptoms
  1. Typically fewer than three bowel movements per week
  2. Hard feces, difficult to pass
  3. Abdominal bloating or pain
  4. Hemorrhoids

- Physical findings
  1. Firm-to-hard stool in rectum
  2. Fecal impaction
  3. Abdomen
     a. Normal bowel sounds
     b. Nontender with simple constipation

- Differential diagnosis (see also Etiology)
  1. Irritable bowel syndrome
  2. Obstruction
  3. Chronic/systemic disease
  4. Medication/drug use

- Diagnostic tests/findings—indicated when "red flags" identified, constipation is persistent or fails to respond to treatment, or particular disorder suspected
  1. Red flags
     a. Abdominal pain, nausea/vomiting
     b. Weight loss
     c. Melena, rectal bleeding
     d. Rectal pain
     e. Fever
     f. New onset over age 50
  2. Diagnostic tests
     a. CBC, TSH, glucose
     b. Stools for hemoccult
     c. Flexible sigmoidoscopy/colonoscopy

- Management/Treatment
  1. Nonpharmacologic
     a. Increased fluid intake
     b. Exercise
     c. High-fiber diet—bran, fruits, vegetables, whole grain cereals and bread
  2. Pharmacologic
     a. Bulk-forming agents—psyllium husk, methylcellulose, calcium polycarbophil
        (1) Drug action
            (a) Increased stool bulk, retention of stool water, reduces transit time
            (b) Used to prevent constipation, not useful treatment of acute constipation
        (2) Side-effects
            (a) Must be taken with ample fluid to prevent esophageal/intestinal obstruction or fecal impaction
            (b) Abdominal distention and flatus
        (3) Drug interactions—decreased absorption of digitalis, salicylates, tetracyclines, nitrofurantoin, and others
        (4) Contraindications/precautions
            (a) Signs of fecal impaction
            (b) GI obstruction
            (c) Pregnancy category B
     b. Stool softeners—docusate sodium
        (1) Drug action
            (a) Act as surfactants; lower surface tension, which facilitates penetration of water into stool
            (b) Useful for patients complaining of hard stools and those for whom straining at stool should be avoided
        (2) Side-effects
            (a) Bitter taste, throat irritation
            (b) Mild abdominal cramping, diarrhea
        (3) Drug interactions—may increase absorption of mineral oil
        (4) Contraindications/precautions
            (a) Acute abdominal pain, intestinal obstruction
            (b) Pregnancy category C
            (c) Because absorption minimal, should pose no risk to breast-feeding infant
     c. Hyperosmolar laxatives—sorbitol, lactulose, polyethylene glycol
        (1) Drug action
            (a) Nonabsorbable disaccharide that acts as osmotic diuretic
            (b) Drug of choice after bulk forming laxatives for chronic constipation

(2) Side-effects
    (a) Flatulence
    (b) Intestinal cramps, diarrhea
(3) Drug interactions—antacids
(4) Contraindications/precautions
    (a) Acute surgical abdomen, intestinal obstruction, fecal impaction
    (b) Galactose restricted diets
    (c) Pregnancy category B; caution in nursing mothers

d. Saline laxatives—magnesium hydroxide/milk of magnesia
  (1) Drug action
    (a) Variety of poorly absorbed salts that draw water into intestinal lumen causing fecal mass to soften and swell; swelling stretches intestinal lumen and stimulates peristalsis
    (b) Treatment of acute constipation
  (2) Side-effects
    (a) Diarrhea, abdominal cramps
    (b) Fluid and electrolyte disturbances
  (3) Drug interactions
    (a) Decreased absorption of quinolones and tetracyclines
    (b) Premature absorption of enterically coated drugs
  (4) Contraindications/precautions
    (a) Renal failure
    (b) Acute surgical abdomen, intestinal obstruction, fecal impaction
    (c) Pregnancy category B; no problems reported in nursing mothers

3. Patient education
  a. Emphasize importance of prompt response to defecation signal
  b. Judicious use of laxatives
  c. Adequate fluid intake (6–8 glasses of water)
  d. Increased fiber in diet

- Referral—any suspected obstructive or serious systemic pathology

Diarrhea

- Definition—defecation characterized by increased frequency, fluidity, or volume
  1. Acute—less than 1–2 weeks duration
  2. Chronic—more than 3 weeks duration

- Etiology/Incidence/Risk factors
  1. Etiology
    a. Acute
      (1) Viral—Norwalk
      (2) Bacterial—Salmonella, Shigella, *E. coli* (traveler's diarrhea)
      (3) Protozoa—*Giardia lamblia, E. histolytica*
      (4) Bacterial toxins—Staphylococcus, Clostridium
      (5) Medications—antibiotics, laxatives, antacids, alcohol
    b. Chronic or recurrent
      (1) Protozoa—*Giradia lamblia, E. histolytica*
      (2) Inflammatory—ulcerative colitis, Crohn's disease, ischemic colitis
      (3) Drugs
      (4) Functional—irritable bowel syndrome
      (5) Malabsorption—sprue, pancreatic insufficiency, lactase deficiency
      (6) Postsurgical—postgastrectomy dumping syndrome
      (7) Systemic diseases—diabetes, hyperthyroidism
  2. Incidence—estimated that the average adult in the United States experiences 1–2 acute diarrheal episodes per year
  3. Risk factors
    a. Travel
    b. Close contact with infected persons, e.g., daycare, institutionalization
    c. Decreased immunity—renders individuals more susceptible to organisms that generally do not cause symptoms in immunocompetent hosts

- Signs and symptoms
  1. Abrupt onset
  2. Increased frequency and volume of stools
  3. Crampy abdominal pain
  4. May be associated with nausea and vomiting
  5. Dehydration if severe

- Physical findings
  1. Acute
    a. Occasionally—low-grade fever; postural changes in pulse, blood pressure
    b. Abdominal examination—hyperactive bowel sounds; diffuse tenderness to palpation
  2. Chronic—signs associated with specific causes, e.g., thyromegaly, lymphadenopathy, cachexia, rectal mass, impaction

- Differential diagnosis—diarrhea is a symptom (see Etiology)

- Diagnostic tests/findings
  1. Usually none indicated for symptoms lasting less than 72 hours unless associated with bloody diarrhea or patient appears ill

2. If persistent or chronic
    a. Stool evaluation
        (1) For fecal leukocytes
        (2) For occult blood
        (3) For culture for bacterial pathogens
        (4) For ova and parasites × 3
        (5) Giardia antigen assay
        (6) *Clostridium difficile* toxin assay
        (7) Qualitative fat (sudan stain)—fat content increased in presence of small bowel disease or pancreatic insufficiency
    b. HIV testing
    c. Hematologic evaluation for indications of underlying disease
        (1) CBC, electrolytes, and sedimentation rate for indications of infection, dehydration
        (2) TSH low in hyperthyroidism
        (3) Hyperglycemia in diabetes mellitus

- Management/Treatment
    1. Nonpharmacologic
        a. Observation—acute attacks usually self-limited
        b. Hydration/electrolyte replacement
        c. Normal diet as soon as patient able to tolerate
        d. For lactase deficiency, limit milk products and consider exogenous lactase
    2. Pharmacologic
        a. Antimotility agents—use is controversial; avoid use in patients with bloody diarrhea and severe systemic illness
            (1) Agents
                (a) Loperamide
                (b) Diphenoxalate-atropine
            (2) Drug action—slows intestinal transit, allowing more time for absorption
            (3) Side-effects
                (a) Abdominal pain
                (b) Distention
                (c) Dizziness, fatigue
                (d) Rash
                (e) Anticholinergic effects
            (4) Drug interactions—diphenoxylate/atropine
                (a) Potentiates MAOIs
                (b) CNS depressant effects with alcohol use
            (5) Contraindications/precautions
                (a) Acute dysentery
                (b) Pseudomembranous, ulcerative colitis
                (c) Pregnancy category B/C; not recommended while nursing
        b. Antisecretory agents/bismuth subsalicylate
            (1) Drug action—may involve adsorption of bacterial toxins and/or local anti-inflammatory effect
            (2) Side-effects—darkened tongue or stool
            (3) Drug interactions—potentiates oral anticoagulants; salicylism with aspirin
            (4) Contraindications/precautions—hypersensitivity to salicylates; influenza or varicella; pregnancy category C/D (third trimester); not recommended in nursing mothers
        c. Antibiotics
            (1) Indicated only when pathogen identifiable
            (2) May exacerbate simple episode
            (3) Traveler's diarrhea—ciprofloxacin or trimethoprim-sulfamethoxazole for 3 days
    3. Patient education
        a. Maintain fluid intake
        b. Normal diet when tolerated
        c. Use of antidiarrheal agents

- Indications for referral
    1. Blood in stools
    2. Diarrhea accompanied by severe abdominal pain
    3. Irreversible or progressive symptoms
    4. Definitive diagnosis and management of underlying disease

Hemorrhoids

- Definition
    1. Varicosities of the hemorrhoidal plexus in the lower rectum or anus
    2. Internal
        a. Originate above the anorectal line
        b. Covered by nonsensitive rectal mucosa
    3. External
        a. Originate below the anorectal line
        b. Covered by well-innervated epithelium

- Etiology/Incidence/Risk factors
    1. Etiology
        a. Thin-walled, dilated vessels; engorge with increased intra-abdominal pressure
        b. Prolapse may be secondary to passage of a large, hard stool; increase in venous pressure from pregnancy or heart failure; or straining due to lifting or defecation
    2. One of the most commonly encountered anorectal conditions in general practice

3. Risk factors
   a. Constipation, straining at stool
   b. Pregnancy
   c. Low-fiber diet
   d. Pelvic congestion
   e. Poor pelvic musculature
   f. Loss of muscle tone with advanced age

- Signs and symptoms
  1. Internal—painless, bright red bleeding with defecation
  2. External—itching, pain, and bleeding with defecation

- Physical findings
  1. Internal
     a. Usually not palpable unless thrombosed
     b. Usually not visible unless prolapsed
  2. External
     a. Protrude with straining or standing
     b. Blue, shiny masses at the anus if thrombosed
     c. Painless, flaccid skin tags (resolved thrombotic hemorrhoids)

- Differential diagnosis
  1. Condyloma accuminata
  2. Rectal prolapse
  3. Rule out other causes for bleeding
     a. Colorectal cancer
     b. Polyps
     c. Anal fissures
     d. Inflammatory bowel disease
     e. Colonic diverticulitis

- Diagnostic tests/findings
  1. Anoscopic examination—with internal hemorrhoids bright red to purplish bulges
  2. Additional testing if underlying pathology suspected

- Management/Treatment—no treatment necessary if asymptomatic
  1. Nonpharmacologic
     a. Increase bulk/fiber/fluids in diet
     b. Sitz baths
     c. Witch hazel pads or gel—may provide transient relief and help reduce inflammation
  2. Pharmacologic
     a. Topical anesthetic/steroid suppositories and ointments
        (1) Drug action—anesthetic and anti-inflammatory action
        (2) Side-effects
            (a) Local irritation, contact dermatitis, folliculitis
            (b) Dermal atrophy with topical steroid; possibility of systemic absorption
        (3) Drug interactions—none
        (4) Contraindication/precautions—some are pregnancy category C; not recommended while nursing
     b. Bulk-forming agents (see Constipation this chapter)
     c. Stool softeners (see Constipation this chapter)
  3. Patient education
     a. Regulation of bowel habits
     b. Dietary changes to maintain hydration, bulk
     c. Appropriate use of bulk laxatives, stool softeners, hemorrhoidal preparations

- Referral
  1. Acute thrombosis of an external hemorrhoid
  2. Failure to respond to conservative management

Irritable Bowel Syndrome (IBS)

- Definition
  1. A functional disorder characterized by altered bowel habits and abdominal pain
  2. Rome criteria helpful in establishing diagnosis (Thompson, Longstretch, and Drossman, 1999)
     a. Presence for at least 12 weeks in the preceding 12 months of continuous or recurrent abdominal pain that cannot be explained by structural/biochemical abnormalities
     b. Associated with at least two of the following:
        (1) Abdominal pain relieved with defecation
        (2) Onset associated with change in stool frequency—diarrhea or constipation
        (3) Onset associated with change in form of stool

- Etiology/Incidence/Risk factors
  1. Etiology—proposed
     a. Altered bowel motility
     b. Visceral hypersensitivity
     c. Imbalance of neurotransmitters
     d. Infection
  2. Prevalence—as high as 15% in general population; only 25% of persons with symptoms consistent with IBS seek care
  3. Risk factors—female to male ratio of 2:1; late teens early adulthood

- Signs and symptoms
    1. Refer to Rome criteria
    2. May also report bloating, fecal urgency, incomplete evacuation
    3. Presence of the following symptoms suggest organic disease (alarm symptoms)
        (a) New onset over 50
        (b) Pain/diarrhea that interferes with sleep
        (c) Fever
        (d) Rectal bleeding, anemia
        (e) Weight loss
        (f) Persistent diarrhea or severe constipation

- Physical findings—left-lower quadrant tenderness on abdominal examination

- Differential diagnosis
    1. Lactose intolerance
    2. Colon cancer
    3. Infectious disease/parasitic infestation (Giardia)
    4. Inflammatory disease (ulcerative colitis, Crohn's disease)
    5. Laxative abuse

- Diagnostic tests/findings
    1. Limited work-up in patients lacking alarm symptoms
        a. CBC, chemistry panel, sedimentation rate
        b. Stool studies including fecal leukocytes, occult blood, ova, and parasites
        c. Flexisigmoidoscopy
        d. If patient is 50 years old or older, colonoscopy or barium enema and flexisigmoidoscopy

- Management/Treatment
    1. Nonpharmacologic
        a. Effective patient–provider relationship; reassurance of benign nature of disease
        b. Diet
            (1) Decrease caffeine, alcohol, fatty foods, gas forming foods, or products containing sorbitol; limit milk products if lactose intolerance suspected
            (2) Increase fiber in diet or in the form of supplements
        c. Stress management, relaxation techniques, identify "triggers"
        d. Exercise
    2. Pharmacologic—use patient's symptoms as a guide
        a. Pain predominant
            (1) Antispasmodic/anticholinergic—dicyclomine hydrochloride, *L*-hyoscyamine sulfate

[handwritten: Bentyl]

(a) Drug action—selectively inhibits gastrointestinal smooth muscle and may reduce pain and bloating
(b) Side-effects—drowsiness, anticholinergic effects
(c) Drug interactions—alcohol, CNS depressants, additive anticholinergic effects with other anticholinergics
(d) Contraindications/precautions
    i. Glaucoma
    ii. Unstable cardiovascular disease
    iii. GI or urinary tract obstruction
    iv. Pregnancy category B/C; contraindicated in nursing mothers
(2) Tricyclic antidepressants—amitryptyline, nortriptyline, desipramine
(a) Drug action—analgesic and mood-enhancing properties; anticholinergic effects
(b) Side-effects—drowsiness, anticholinergic effects
(c) Drug interactions—fluoxetine, MAO inhibitors, alcohol, CNS depressants
(d) Contraindications/precautions
    i. During or within 14 days of MAO inhibitors; postacute MI
    ii. Pregnancy category C; not recommended in nursing mothers

b. Diarrhea predominant
(1) Loperamide, diphenoxylate/atropine (see Diarrhea this chapter)
(2) Alosetron
(a) Drug action—a 5-HT3 receptor antagonist, decreases intestinal secretion, motility, and afferent pain signals
(b) Limited use for women with severe chronic diarrhea predominant IBS; unresponsive to conventional therapy and not caused by anatomic or metabolic abnormality
(c) Side-effects—possible severe adverse GI effects including ischemic colitis and serious complications of constipation resulting in hospitalization, and rarely blood transfusion, surgery, and death
(d) Contraindications/precautions—only healthcare providers enrolled in Lotronex (alosetron)

prescribing program should prescribe; discontinue immediately in patients who develop constipation or symptoms of ischemic colitis

    c. Constipation predominant
- (1) Fiber supplements—psyllium, polycarbophil, methylcellulose (see Constipation this chapter)
- (2) Osmotic laxative—lactulose, sorbitol, polyethylene glycol, magnesium hydroxide (see Constipation this chapter)
- (3) Lubiprostone
  - (a) Drug action—chloride channel activator, enhances GI motility
  - (b) Indicated only for adult women with constipation-predominant IBS
  - (c) Side-effects—nausea, headache, diarrhea, abdominal pain
  - (d) Contraindications/precautions—younger than 18 years of age; renal or hepatic impairment; pregnancy category C; not recommended in nursing mothers; discontinue if diarrhea occurs

3. Patient education
   - a. Appropriate implementation of the non-pharmacologic measures
   - b. Reassurance of the relative benign nature of disorder
   - c. Need for reevaluation if symptoms progress or change

- Referral—onset in those older than 50; presence of symptoms suggestive of organic disease/alarm symptoms

Appendicitis

- Definition—inflammation of the wall of the vermiform appendix that may result in perforation with subsequent peritonitis

- Etiology/Incidence
  1. Etiology
     - a. Based on operative findings, classified as simple, gangrenous, or perforated
     - b. Acute appendicitis secondary to obstruction due to fecal material, lymphoid hyperplasia, foreign bodies, or parasites with secondary bacterial infection
     - c. Gangrene and perforation develop within 24–36 hours; perforation results in release of luminal contents into peritoneal cavity
  2. Incidence—occurs in all age groups; highest incidence in males 10–30 years of age

- Signs and symptoms—classic sequence of symptoms
  1. Pain is initial symptom; begins in epigastrum or periumbilical area
  2. Anorexia, nausea, or vomiting
  3. Pain localizes to RLQ after several hours
  4. Sense of constipation; infrequently diarrhea

- Physical findings
  1. Fever of 99–100°F (> 100° F may indicate peritonitis)
  2. Tenderness localized to McBurney's point; pain worsened and localized with cough
  3. Signs of peritoneal irritation—guarding, rigidity, and rebound tenderness RLQ
  4. Absent bowel sounds
  5. Positive psoas sign—pain with flexion at the hip against resistance or hyperextension
  6. Positive Rovsing's sign—RLQ pain elicited when LLQ is deeply palpated and pressure is released
  7. Positive obturator sign—pain with passive internal rotation of flexed right hip/knee
  8. Rectal examination may reveal tenderness/mass

- Differential diagnosis
  1. Ovarian, e.g., mittelschmerz, cyst
  2. Ectopic pregnancy
  3. Pelvic inflammatory disease
  4. Pyelonephritis, calculi
  5. Gallbladder or pancreatic inflammation
  6. Gastroenteritis

- Diagnostic tests/findings
  1. White blood cell count—moderate leukocytosis 10,000–18,000/mm^3
  2. Urinalysis may demonstrate hematuria and pyuria
  3. Pregnancy test
  4. Ultrasound diagnostic in 85% of patients
  5. Focused appendix computerized tomography (FACT)—highly specific and sensitive but time and expense limits usefulness in routine diagnosis

- Management/Treatment
  1. Nonpharmacologic—none
  2. Pharmacologic—none
  3. Patient education
     - a. Need for emergency care if pain or other symptoms change during observation, evaluation period
     - b. Postoperative care instructions

- Referral—immediate surgery consult for acute abdomen

Peptic Ulcer Disease (PUD)

- Definition—group of ulcerative disorders involving the upper GI tract that requires acid and pepsin and/or abnormal mucosal resistance for their formation

- Etiology/Incidence/Risk factors
  1. Etiology
     a. Acid and pepsin activity overpower mucosal defenses to produce ulcers when mucosal defense is impaired by exogenous factors/*Helicobactor pylori* and NSAIDs
     b. *H. pylori* is an established causative factor; 90–95% of duodenal ulcer patients and 70–80% of gastric ulcer patients infected with *H. pylori*
     c. *H. pylori* is a gram-negative bacterium; produces urease that breaks down urea-forming ammonia and CO_2 allowing organism to control pH of its environment
     d. NSAIDs damage mucosa through a direct action and systemically by inhibiting endogenous prostaglandin synthesis; NSAID-related ulcers more likely to be gastric
  2. Incidence
     a. Estimated 5–10% of the general population
     b. Male/female ratio nearly equal
     c. Duodenal ulcers more common; peak incidence of gastric ulcers ages 55–65
  3. Risk factors
     a. Family history—likely due to familial transmission of *H. pylori*
     b. Cigarette smoking—delays healing and increases risk of recurrence
     c. Steroids

- Signs and symptoms
  1. Burning or deep epigastric pain that occurs 1–3 hours after meals; relieved by ingestion of food or antacids
  2. Pain commonly causes early morning awakening
  3. Other dyspeptic symptoms—nausea, vomiting, belching, bloating
  4. Symptomatic periods occur in clusters lasting a few weeks followed by symptom-free periods for weeks/months
  5. Gastric ulcer presentation more variable; food may make symptoms worse
  6. Complications—hemorrhage, perforation, obstruction
  7. Alarm symptoms for gastric cancer or complicated PUD
     a. Older than 45 years
     b. Rectal bleeding or melena; anemia
     c. Weight loss, dysphagia
     d. Abdominal mass, jaundice
     e. Family history of gastric cancer
     f. Anorexia/early satiety

- Physical findings
  1. Usually none in uncomplicated peptic ulcer disease
  2. Occasionally, well localized epigastric tenderness

- Differential diagnosis
  1. Gastroesophageal reflux disease
  2. Nonulcer dyspepsia
  3. Gastric carcinoma
  4. Angina

- Diagnostic tests/findings
  1. Stool for occult blood
  2. *H. pylori* testing
     a. Noninvasive—unless indications for endoscopy, use serology to identify infection and stool antigen test or urea breath test to determine cure, if indicated
        (1) Serologic test—ELISA detects IgG antibodies indicating current or past infection; may or may not revert to negative after treatment
        (2) Stool antigen test—reverts to negative within 5 days/few months after eradication of organism
        (3) Urea breath test—detects presence or absence of active infection
     b. Invasive testing—mucosal biopsy during endoscopy
        (1) Histologic testing
        (2) Rapid urease testing
        (3) Culture

- Management/Treatment
  1. Nonpharmacologic
     a. Avoid aspirin and NSAIDs
     b. Smoking cessation if appropriate
     c. Decreased intake of coffee and other caffeine-containing beverages
     d. Attend to stress-related issues
  2. Pharmacologic
     a. Disease not due to *H. pylori*
        (1) Histamine (H_2RA) receptor antagonists—cimetidine, ranitidine, nizatidine, famotidine
           (a) Drug action—inhibits acid secretion by blocking H_2 receptors in parietal cell
           (b) Side-effects
              i. Headache, fatigue, dizziness

ii.   Minimal GI upset
(c) Drug interactions—may alter absorption of certain drugs secondary to changes in gastric pH
(d) Contraindications/precautions
   i.   Severe renal insufficiency
   ii.   Pregnancy category B; not recommended while nursing
(2) Proton pump inhibitors (PPIs)—omeprazole, lansoprazole, rabeprazole, pantoprazole, esomeprazole
(a) Drug action—inhibits gastric acid secretion by inhibiting the final step in acid secretion by altering the activity of the proton pump; virtual cessation of acid production
(b) Side-effects
   i.   Headache
   ii.   Nausea, abdominal pain, flatulence, constipation, diarrhea
(c) Drug interactions—may interact with drugs that depend on gastric pH for absorption
(d) Contraindications/precautions
   i.   Omeprazole—pregnancy category C; not recommended while nursing
   ii.   Lansoprazole—pregnancy category B; caution while nursing
b.   Ulcers caused by *H. pylori*—eradication of *H. pylori* to reduce risk of recurrent duodenal ulcer
(1) PPI triple therapy—lansoprazole, amoxicillin, clarithromycin
(2) Bismuth quadruple therapy—bismuth, metronidazole, tetracycline, plus PPI or H$_2$RA
(3) Persistent *H. pylori* infection—retreat with alternative combination
3.   Patient education
a.   Importance of positive life style changes, e.g., smoking cessation, decreased alcohol consumption
b.   Purpose, dosage, side-effects of medications
c.   Importance of compliance with medication regimen

- Referral
1.   Patients with weight loss, dysphagia, anorexia, vomiting, hematemesis/melena; new onset pain in patient over 45
2.   If treatment for *H. pylori* fails second time, referral indicated

3.   Obtain surgical consultation for patients with evidence of bleeding, gastric outlet obstruction, or perforation

Viral Hepatitis

- Definition—a group of systemic infections involving the liver with common clinical manifestations caused by different viruses with distinctive epidemiologic patterns

- Etiology/Incidence/Risk factors
1.   Hepatitis A virus (HAV)
a.   Spread via fecal–oral route; spreads readily in households and child care centers
b.   Mean incubation time 25 days; range 15 to 60 days; maximum infectivity 2 weeks before jaundice; acute onset
c.   Infections in infancy/childhood generally mild without jaundice; adult infections can be severe
d.   Self-limited; no carrier state or chronic liver disease results
e.   Accounts for more cases of acute viral hepatitis than all other hepatotropic viruses combined
2.   Hepatitis B virus (HBV)
a.   Transmitted in blood, blood products, and infected body fluids (saliva, vaginal secretions, semen) by parenteral, sexual, perinatal exposure
b.   Mean incubation time 75 days; range 28 to 160 days
c.   Spectrum of illness ranging from asymptomatic seroconversion to acute illness; fulminant hepatitis results in less than 1%
d.   Up to 10% infected as adults and 90% infected as neonates become chronic carriers; increased risk of cirrhosis, hepatocellular carcinoma
3.   Hepatitis C virus (HCV)
a.   Associated with IV drug use and blood transfusion before 1992; other risks include drug inhalation, multiple sex partners, body piercing/tattooing, needle stick injuries, hemodialysis; sexual transmission accounts for less than 5% of cases; perinatal transmission occurs in 3–5% of infants born to infected mothers
b.   Mean incubation time 50 days; range 2 to 22 weeks; onset insidious
c.   Acute disease often mild in adults; asymptomatic in children
d.   Up to 80% of patients develop chronic hepatitis; 20–30% eventually develop cirrhosis or hepatocellular carcinoma

4. Hepatitis D virus (HDV)
   a. A defective virus that requires co-infection with HBV; may be transmitted with HBV or as superinfection in established chronic HBV infection
   b. Transmitted through blood/blood products, IV drug use, or sexual contact
   c. Incubation period for superinfection is 2–8 weeks
   d. Contributes to severity of HBV infection
   e. Suspect superinfection with HDV in patient who presents with fulminant hepatitis and chronic HBV
5. Hepatitis E virus (HEV)
   a. Spread via fecal–oral route
   b. Endemic in developing countries
   c. Mean incubation time 27 days; range 2 to 9 weeks
   d. More common in children and young adults; infection during pregnancy can lead to liver failure
   e. No risk of chronicity or carcinoma
6. Miscellaneous viral causes
   a. Herpes simplex virus
   b. Epstein-Barr virus
   c. Cytomegalovirus

• Signs and symptoms—all viral types produce very similar syndromes; severity of illness can vary widely
1. Phase 1—incubation
   a. Asymptomatic
   b. Weeks to months
2. Phase 2—pre-icteric (prodromal)
   a. 3 to 10 days in length
   b. Malaise, fatigue
   c. Anorexia, nausea, vomiting
   d. "Flu-like" aches, headache
   e. Skin rash
   f. Change in sense of smell or taste; aversion to cigarettes
3. Phase 3—icteric
   a. 1 to 4 weeks in length
   b. RUQ pain
   c. Dark-colored urine
   d. Clay-colored stools
   e. Jaundice of skin, sclera, nail beds
4. Phase 4—convalescence
   a. May last weeks to months
   b. Chronic disease develops in certain types
   c. Hepatitis B, C, D may be fatal; HEV 30% mortality rate in pregnant women

• Physical findings
1. Rash—maculopapular and urticarial lesions
2. Low-grade fever

3. Jaundice
4. Hepatomegaly
5. Splenomegaly

• Differential diagnosis—noninfectious causes of hepatitis, e.g., hepatotoxic drugs, alcohol

• Diagnostic tests/findings
1. Viral serologies (see **Table 8-4**)
2. Urinalysis—positive for protein, bilirubin
3. Liver function tests
   a. Marked elevation—alanine aminotransferase (ALT) and aspartate aminotransferase (AST)
   b. Mild elevation of alkaline phosphatase
   c. Normal serum bilirubin or mild bilirubinemia

• Management/Treatment
1. Nonpharmacologic
   a. Activity as tolerated; avoid strenuous activities or contact sports
   b. Hydration
   c. Maintain adequate caloric intake and balanced diet; small feedings may be better tolerated
   d. Discontinue all but essential medications
   e. Avoid alcohol
2. Pharmacologic
   a. Antiemetics if indicated for nausea—trimethobenzamide (Tigan)
      (1) Drug action—acts centrally to inhibit the medullary chemoreceptor trigger zone
      (2) Side-effects—drowsiness, dizziness, blurred vision, hypotension
      (3) Drug interactions—potentiates alcohol, other CNS depressants
      (4) Contraindications/precautions—pregnancy category C; not recommended while nursing
   b. Chronic hepatitis B
      (1) Antiviral treatment indicated for active viral replication (sustained presence of HBeAg and HBV DNA), elevated ALT levels, and histologic evidence of chronic liver injury
      (2) Agents approved for treatment of chronic HBV—interferon alfa, lamivudine, entecavir, adefovir dipivoxil, telbivudine
   c. Chronic hepatits C—peginterferon in combination with ribavirin
   d. Prevention
      (1) HAV
         (a) Immune globulin
         (b) HAV vaccine

■ **Table 8-4** Serologic Diagnosis and Markers of Active or Chronic Hepatitis

Test Name	HAV	HBV	HCV	HDV	HEV
IgM anti-HAV	+ acute stage & up to 12 months	N.A.	N.A.	N.A.	N.A.
IgG anti-HAV	Remote infection/ immunity	N.A.	N.A.	N.A.	N.A.
HbsAg	N.A.	+ acute & chronic infection	N.A.	Positive	N.A.
Anti-HBs	N.A.	+ resolution	N.A.	Negative	N.A.
IgM anti-HBc	N.A.	+ acute stage, resolves 3-12 mos	N.A.	+ co-infection HBV	N.A.
IgG anti-HBc	N.A.	Remote/resolved inf.	N.A.	+ superinfection	N.A.
HBeAg	N.A.	+ active viral replication	N.A.	+ active viral replication	N.A.
HBV DNA		+ active viral replication	N.A.	+ active viral replication	N.A.
Anti-HCV	N.A.	N.A.	+ late in acute & in chronic infection	N.A.	N.A.
HCV RNA	N.A.	N.A.	+ confirms	N.A.	N.A.
Anti-HDV	N.A.	N.A.	N.A.	Positive	N.A.

KEY: IgM anti-HAV = immune globulin M class, HAV antibody
IgG anti-HAV = immune globulin G class, HAV antibody
HBsAg = hepatitis B surface antigen
Anti-HBs = HBV surface antibody
IgM anti-HBc = immune globulin M class, HBV core antibody
IgG anti-HBc = immune globulin G class, HBV core antibody
HBeAg = HBV e antigen
Anti-HCV = hepatitis C antibody
Anti-HDV = hepatitis D antibody
HEV = no commercially available serologic test
HBV DNA = hepatitis B deoxyribonucleic acid
HCV RNA = hepatitis C ribonucleic acid
N.A. = Not Applicable

(2) HBV
  (a) HBIG
  (b) HBV vaccine
3. Patient education
  a. Careful disposal of infected wastes
  b. Scrupulous hand-washing, food-handling techniques
  c. Need for prophylactic immunization of contacts, household members
  d. Safer sexual practices
  e. Avoidance of blood contamination—no sharing toothbrushes, razors, needles
  f. Laboratory follow-up
    (1) Monitor aminotransferase at 1–4 week intervals during acute illness
    (2) Monitor HBsAg and anti-HBsAg until anti-HBs present

- Referral
1. Fulminant disease—patients presenting with altered mental state
2. Chronic HBV patients who require treatment
3. HCV—early identification/referral important because evidence suggests that early treatment reduces risk of chronic infection

Cholecystitis

- Definition
1. Gallstones/cholelithiasis
2. Biliary colic is most common symptom of cholelithiasis and results from transient obstruction of the cystic duct by a stone
3. Acute cholecystitis is the most common complication of cholelithiasis and develops when gallstone(s) obstruct the cystic duct resulting in distention and inflammation of the gallbladder; secondary bacterial infection occurs in about 50% of cases
4. Choledocholelithiasis is the presence of stones in the common bile duct and occurs in 10–15% of patients with cholelithiasis; associated with high rate of complications—jaundice, acute cholangitis, gallstone pancreatitis
5. Acute acalculous cholecystitis occurs in seriously ill hospitalized patients; probably associated with biliary "sludge"

- Etiology/Incidence/Risk factors
1. Etiology
  a. Gallstones may be result of imbalance in bile components
  b. About 85–95% of gallstones are composed primarily of cholesterol
  c. Pigment stones are composed of calcium bilirubinate; less common

2. Incidence—gallstones occur in 10–15% of the US population
  a. Majority of patients with gallstones have asymptomatic disease
  b. About 20% of asymptomatic patients develop symptoms over a period of 20 years; majority present with biliary pain rather than biliary complication
3. Risk factors for cholethiasis
  a. Female gender
  b. Advanced age
  c. Obesity
  d. Multiparity, pregnancy
  e. Rapid weight loss
  f. Hypertriglyceridemia
  g. Medications/oral contraceptives

- Signs and symptoms
1. Biliary colic—presenting symptom in more than 90% of patients
  a. Severe, steady pain localized to the epigastrum or RUQ; may radiate to back or scapula
  b. Pain is precipitated by spasm of a dilated cystic duct obstructed by gallstone(s)
  c. Attacks of biliary colic more common at night
  d. Pain typically has a sudden onset and may last 3 hours; may be accompanied by nausea/vomiting
2. Acute cholecystitis
  a. Pain similar to biliary colic but lasts longer; associated with nausea/vomiting and fever
  b. Symptoms of local inflammation and systemic toxicity
  c. Pain shifts from epigastrum to RUQ; sequence secondary to visceral pain from ductal impaction by stones progressing to inflammation of the gall bladder with parietal pain
  d. Most patients have had previous attacks of biliary colic
3. Choledocholithiasis—stones in the common bile duct
  a. May remain asymptomatic
  b. May result in biliary pain, obstructive jaundice, ascending cholangitis (bacterial infection of biliary tract), or biliary pancreatitis
4. Acute suppurative cholangitis—pain, jaundice, chills/Charcot's triad
5. Pancreatitis—upper abdominal pain radiating to the back

- Physical findings—acute cholecystitis
  1. Fever
  2. Murphy's sign—inspiratory arrest secondary to pain during deep palpation of right subcostal region; relatively specific finding
  3. Gallbladder distended and palpable
  4. Jaundice
  5. Localized tenderness may be only finding in elderly patients; pain and fever may be absent

- Differential diagnosis
  1. Appendicitis
  2. Pancreatitis
  3. Ruptured ectopic pregnancy or ovarian cyst
  4. Peptic ulcer disease

- Diagnostic tests/findings
  1. Ultrasound
     a. Has a 95% sensitivity for detecting stones in the gallbladder; detects bile duct stones in only 50% of cases
     b. Best noninvasive imaging technique to diagnose acute cholecystitis; findings include thick gallbladder wall, gallbladder distension, sludge in the lumen, pericholecystic fluid
  2. Heptatobiliary scintigraphy—can confirm/exclude diagnosis of acute cholecystitis with high degree of sensitivity/specificity
  3. Endoscopic retrograde cholangiopancreatography (ERCP)—best study for diagnosis of choledocholithiasis
  4. Computerized tomography (CT)/MRI—comparable to ERCP in terms of diagnostic accuracy
  5. Leukocytosis with a "left shift" observed in acute cholecystitis; serum aminotranferases, alkaline phosphatase, bilirubin, and amylase may also be elevated
  6. Elevation of serum bilirubin and alkaline phosphatase in choledocholithiasis
  7. Amylase greater than 1000 U/dL indicates acute pancreatitis

- Management/Treatment
  1. Expectant management for patients with asymptomatic gallstones
  2. Elective cholecystectomy for most patients with symptomatic cholelithiasis
  3. Acute cholecystitis managed with hospital admission; early cholecystectomy once patient is stable
  4. Bile duct stones should be removed whether symptomatic or not because of high rate of complications

Gastroesophageal Reflux Disease (GERD)

- Definition
  1. Gastroesophageal reflux refers to movement of gastric contents from the stomach into the esophagus
  2. GERD refers to symptomatic clinical condition or histologic alteration that results from episodes of reflux
  3. When esophagus is repeatedly exposed to refluxed material for prolonged periods of time, inflammation of esophagus can occur
  4. Complications—esophagitis; strictures; Barrett's esophagus, which carries a 10% risk of progression to adenocarcinoma

- Etiology/Incidence/Risk factors
  1. Etiology
     a. Contributing factors include reflux of caustic gastric contents, a breakdown in defense mechanism of esophagus, and a functional abnormality that results in reflux
     b. Most common etiology is prolonged esophageal acid exposure due to transient lower esophageal relaxations
     c. Less common mechanisms include pathologically weak lower esophageal sphincter (LES) tone, hiatal hernia, esophageal motility disorder, Zollinger-Ellison syndrome, and delayed gastric emptying
  2. Incidence
     a. Physiologic reflux occurs in normal individuals
     b. Reflux occurs regularly in up to 40% of healthy individuals who do not seek treatment
  3. Risk factors
     a. Foods that lower LES pressure—high fat, chocolate, peppermints
     b. Foods that irritate esophageal mucosa—citrus fruits, spicy tomato drinks
     c. Drugs that lower LES pressure—calcium channel blockers, progesterone
     d. Cigarette smoking, alcohol
     e. Pregnancy
     f. Obesity

- Signs and symptoms
  1. "Heartburn"—retrosternal burning sensation radiating upward
  2. Acid regurgitation—effortless return of gastric contents into pharynx
  3. Symptoms usually occur postprandially
  4. Symptoms aggravated by reclining, straining, bending, or stooping

5. Atypical symptoms
   a. Odynophagia—burning, squeezing pain with swallowing
   b. Dysphagia—sensation of food lodged in the chest secondary to stricture
   c. Globus sensation—sensation of lump in the throat
6. Extraesophageal symptoms
   a. Hoarseness
   b. Chronic cough
   c. Asthma/reactive airway disease
   d. Hiccups
   e. Dental disease
   f. Nausea

- Physical findings
  1. Usually normal examination
  2. Occasionally epigastric tenderness with palpation

- Differential diagnosis
  1. Cardiac chest pain
  2. Peptic ulcer disease
  3. Infectious esophagitis—viral, fungal
  4. Medication-induced esophagitis—antibiotics
  5. Esophageal/gastric malignancy
  6. Hepatobiliary disease

- Diagnostic tests/findings
  1. Diagnosis of GERD based on clinical findings and confirmed by response to therapy
  2. Diagnostic evaluation if symptoms chronic or refractory to therapy or if esophageal complications suspected
     a. Endoscopy
        (1) Useful for diagnosis of complications—esophagitis, strictures, Barrett's esophagus
        (2) Indications
            (a) Dysphagia or odynophagia
            (b) Weight loss
            (c) Evidence of GI bleeding or iron deficiency anemia
            (d) Screen for Barrett's if 10 years or more of GERD symptoms
     b. Upper GI may demonstrate structural problems; evaluation of dysphagia
     c. Ambulatory esophageal pH monitoring—best test to establish abnormal acid reflux

- Management/Treatment
  1. Nonpharmacologic
     a. Weight loss
     b. Smoking cessation
     c. Elevate head of bed (HOB); sleep on wedge-shaped bolster
     d. Avoid recumbency for 3 hours postprandially
     e. Reduce fat to no more than 30% of calories
     f. Reduce consumption of alcohol, chocolate, colas, coffee, peppermint, citrus juices, tomato products
  2. Pharmacologic
     a. Commercially available antacids and anti-refluxants/alginic acid are useful for mild symptoms
        (1) Drug action
            (a) Neutralizes acids
            (b) Produces foaming neutral barrier to reflux
        (2) Side-effects—diarrhea, constipation
        (3) Drug interactions—reduces absorption of tetracycline, possibly other drugs
        (4) Contraindications/precautions—impaired renal function
     b. H_2-receptor antagonists (acid reducers)—effective treatment for less severe GERD (see PUD this chapter)
     c. Proton pump inhibitors (acid suppressant agents)—most effective agents for healing esophagitis and preventing complications (see PUD this chapter)
  3. Patient education—life style modifications

- Referral
  1. Symptoms of dysphagia, weight loss, blood loss, obstructive symptoms including nausea/vomiting, early satiety, anorexia
  2. Long-standing or refractory cases
  3. Candidates for surgical intervention

◘ HEMATOLOGIC DISORDERS

Anemias

- Definition
  1. Abnormally low hemoglobin concentration (< 12 g/dL for women 13 g/dL for men) or inadequate red blood cell population (RBC)
  2. Numerous diverse causes
  3. Usually classified according to RBC size—mean corpuscular volume/MCV
     a. Microcytic anemia (MCV < 80 fL), e.g., iron deficiency anemia, thalassemia trait
     b. Macrocytic anemia (MCV > 100 fL), e.g., B_{12} deficiency, folate deficiency, liver disease
     c. Normocytic anemia (MCV 80–100 fL), e.g., anemia of chronic disease, hemolysis/hemoglobinopathy/sickle cell disease, renal failure

- Etiology/Incidence—commonly encountered anemias
  1. Iron deficiency anemia (IDA)
     a. Etiology
        (1) Blood loss—GI overt/occult, menorrhagia
        (2) Inadequate dietary intake—most common in infants and adolescents
        (3) Metabolic demands in excess of intake—pregnancy, lactation
     b. Incidence
        (1) Most common form of anemia; represents 25% of all anemia cases
        (2) Affects 10–15% of premenopausal women
     c. Risk factors
        (1) Female gender
        (2) Menorrhagia
        (3) Pregnancy
  2. Anemia of chronic disease
     a. Etiology
        (1) A hypoproliferative anemia associated with underlying chronic disorders such as infections, inflammatory disorders, and malignancy
        (2) Reduced production and response to erythropoietin; decreased RBC life span
        (3) Defect in iron-reutilization
     b. Incidence—second most common anemia
  3. Vitamin B_{12} deficiency anemia
     a. Etiology
        (1) B_{12} deficiency alters DNA synthesis
        (2) B_{12} deficiency develops secondary to lack or relative deficiency of intrinsic factor that leads to impaired vitamin B_{12} absorption (pernicious anemia)
           (a) Autoimmune reaction involving gastric parietal cells
           (b) History of gastrectomy
        (3) Rarely secondary to nutritional deficiency of vitamin B_{12}
     b. Incidence—regarded as a disorder affecting older persons of northern European descent; likely underrecognized in other populations
     c. Risk factors
        (1) Usually presents around age 60, familial tendency
        (2) Both sexes equally affected
        (3) Strict vegan diet
        (4) Recent gastric surgery
  4. Folic acid deficiency anemia
     a. Etiology
        (1) Folic acid deficiency alters synthesis of DNA and RBC maturation
        (2) Folic acid deficiency due to
           (a) Malabsorption syndromes
           (b) Increased demand—pregnancy, infancy
           (c) Inadequate intake—alcoholics, elderly
        (3) Certain drugs decrease folic acid levels—oral contraceptives, dilantin
     b. Incidence
        (1) Found in all races and age groups
        (2) Most common megaloblastic anemia in pregnancy
     c. Risk factors
        (1) Pregnancy
        (2) Alcoholism
  5. Sickle cell anemia
     a. Etiology
        (1) A chronic hemolytic anemia characterized by sickle-shaped RBC
        (2) Autosomal recessive genetic disorder
           (a) Hgb S develops instead of Hgb A
           (b) Individual is homozygous for Hgb S
     b. Incidence
        (1) Homozygous Hgb S in an estimated 0.5% African Americans
        (2) Heterozygous trait in an estimated 8% of African Americans; essentially asymptomatic carrier state
        (3) Most common hemoglobinopathy in the US
     c. Risk factors
        (1) African-American race
        (2) Lower frequency in persons of Mediterranean ancestry

- Signs and symptoms
  1. Iron deficiency anemia
     a. Asymptomatic unless severe, then nonspecific
     b. Fatigue, generalized weakness
     c. Dyspnea on exertion
     d. Headaches
     e. Pica
  2. Anemia of chronic disease
     a. Symptoms common to all anemias—fatigue, weakness, exertional dyspnea, lightheadedness, anorexia
     b. Other signs and symptoms related to specific underlying disease
  3. Vitamin B_{12} deficiency
     a. None at first, insidious onset
     b. Fatigue, weakness, lightheadedness
     c. Dyspnea, palpitations
     d. GI disturbances—anorexia, bloating, diarrhea

e. Sore tongue
f. Neurologic—paresthesias, ataxia
g. Loss of taste and smell
4. Folate deficiency—signs and symptoms similar to vitamin B_{12} deficiency, except there is no neurologic involvement
5. Sickle cell
a. Often none during remissions
b. Vaso-occlusvie crises—precipitating factors include infection, physical or emotional stress, blood loss
(1) Malaise, chills
(2) Pain, especially in bones, abdomen, chest, lower legs
(3) Headaches, epistaxis, vomiting
(4) Difficulty or refusal to walk

- Physical findings
1. Iron deficiency anemia
a. Often none
b. Skin or conjunctival pallor
c. Glossitis, stomatitis
d. Tachycardia with/without systolic flow murmur
e. Tachypnea
f. Nail changes
(1) Spoon shaped (koilonychia)
(2) Brittle, easily split
g. Hair thinning, breaking
2. Anemia of chronic disease
a. Ill appearance
b. Signs of precipitating illness
3. Vitamin B_{12} deficiency
a. Skin pale, occasionally jaundiced
b. Stomatitis, glossitis, smooth beefy red tongue
c. Tachycardia, arrhythmias, systolic flow murmur
d. Organomegaly—hepatomegaly, splenomegaly
e. Neurologic
(1) Ataxia, positive Romberg test
(2) Hyperactive reflexes
(3) Peripheral loss of sensation, decreased vibratory sense, impaired proprioception
(4) Changes in mental state with possible wide range of expression—mild confusion to acute psychosis
4. Folate deficiency
a. Pallor
b. Tachycardia, tachypnea
c. Malnourished appearance
d. No neurologic findings
5. Sickle cell
a. In crises

(1) Temperature, pulse, respirations elevated
(2) Hypotension
(3) Pallor, cyanosis secondary to poor oxygenation
(4) Scleral jaundice
(5) Decreased skin turgor
b. Chronic findings due to anemia, vaso-occlusive events, end-organ damage
(1) Cardiomegaly
(2) Skin ulcers, especially on lower extremities
(3) Osteomyelitis
(4) Retinopathy
(5) Renal disease—hematuria

- Differential diagnosis
1. Iron deficiency anemia
a. Anemia of chronic disease
b. Thalassemia trait
c. Sideroblastic anemia
2. Anemia of chronic disease—diagnosis of exclusion
a. Iron deficiency anemia
b. Anemia of renal disease
3. Vitamin B_{12} deficiency
a. Nutritional deficiency
b. Malabsorption
c. Chronic alcoholism
d. Chronic gastritis (*H. pylori* infection)
e. Folic acid deficiency
4. Folate deficiency
a. Pernicious anemia
b. Medication, toxins
5. Sickle crises
a. Appendicitis
b. Acute cholecystitis
c. Pneumonia

- Diagnostic tests/findings
1. World Health Organization standard for anemia diagnosis
a. Hemoglobin 13 g/dL or less in men (approximately 38% hematocrit)
b. Hemoglobin 12 g/dL or less in women (approximately 35% hematocrit)
2. Severe anemia (symptomatic) generally less than 25% Hct
3. Iron deficiency anemia—hypochromic microcytic RBCs
a. RBC changes in early disease may be mild
b. MCV less than 80 fL
c. Increased red cell width (RDW)
d. Serum ferritin less than 10 μg/L
(1) Levels reflect iron stores; single most useful test for diagnosing IDA

(2) Ferritin is an acute-phase reactant; may be elevated in inflammatory disease

   e. Decreased reticulocyte count

4. Anemia of chronic disease—normochromic-normocytic early in course, becomes microcytic
   a. Anemia is typically mild; hematocrit remains around 30%
   b. Low serum iron levels; normal or increased TIBC
   c. Normal or increased serum ferritin

5. Vitamin B_{12} deficiency—megaloblastic-macrocytic anemia
   a. MCV greater than 100 fL
   b. Serum B_{12} decreased, less than 100 pg/mL
   c. Peripheral blood smear—RBCs of widely varying size (anisocytosis) and shape (poikilocytosis)
   d. Serum methylmalonic acid and homocysteine levels elevated
   e. Schilling test or assay for anti-intrinsic factor antibody
      (1) Obtain if vitamin B_{12} deficiency detected
      (2) Helps distinguish lack of intrinsic factor from malabsorption

6. Folate deficiency—megaloblastic-macrocytic anemia
   a. MCV greater than 100 fL
   b. Serum folate less than 3 ng/mL; normal serum B_{12}
   c. Elevated homocysteine level; normal methylmalonic acid level

7. Sickle cell anemia
   a. Hgb of 7–9 g/dL; hematocrit 20–30%
   b. Mild leukocytosis—12,000 to 15,000/mm^3
   c. Reticulocytosis 10–25%
   d. Irreversibly sickled cells on peripheral smear
   e. Platelets maybe elevated
   f. Sickledex used for screening—sickle cells present in patients with disease and trait
   g. Hemoglobin electrophoresis—Hgb S/85–95% in sickle cell anemia; Hgb S/40% in sickle cell trait

- Management/Treatment
  1. Iron deficiency anemia—identify the cause of iron deficiency and correct it
     a. Nonpharmacologic
        (1) Diet with increased iron content
        (2) Hemoglobin monitoring schedule
           (a) Check 3 weeks after initiation of treatment; recheck in 6–8 weeks
           (b) Ongoing monitoring every 3 months until stable
     b. Pharmacologic
        (1) Ferrous sulfate—may need to continue therapy 4–6 months to replenish iron stores; may discontinue when serum ferritin exceeds 50 µg/L
           (a) Drug action—replenishes depleted iron stores; incorporated into hemoglobin; allows the transportation of oxygen via hemoglobin
           (b) Side-effects
              i. Nausea, vomiting, GI upset
              ii. Black stools
              iii. Constipation
           (c) Drug interactions
              i. Antacids, calcium supplements inhibit iron absorption
              ii. Inhibits tetracycline absorption
           (d) Contraindications/precautions
              i. Hemochromocytosis
              ii. Caution in elderly
              iii. Caution with peptic ulcer

  2. Anemia of chronic disease
     a. Nonpharmacologic—treatment of underlying disorder; transfusion if severe anemia
     b. Pharmacologic—none; iron, folate and B_{12} have not been shown to be effective

  3. Vitamin B_{12} deficiency
     a. Nonpharmacologic—none
     b. Pharmacologic
        (1) B_{12}/cyanocobalamin—dose IM daily for one week, then weekly until Hct is normal, then monthly for life
        (2) Cyanocobalamin nasal gel—weekly dosing; alternate maintenance therapy
        (3) Drug action—required for hematopoiesis
        (4) Side-effects
           (a) Manifested with parenteral use—local stinging, burning at injection site; urticaria, itching; pulmonary edema, anaphylaxis
           (b) Manifested with intranasal use—headache, nausea, rhinitis
        (5) Drug interactions—ethanol decreases B_{12} absorption; decreased response with concomitant chloramphenicol, neomycin
        (6) Contraindications/precautions—hypersensitivity to cobalt

4. Folate deficiency
   a. Nonpharmacologic—increased dietary sources of folic acid/legumes, leafy green vegetables, fruits and liver
   b. Pharmacologic—folic acid
      (1) Drug action—cofactor in biosynthesis of nucleic acids needed for RBC synthesis
      (2) Side-effects
         (a) Allergic reactions—skin rash, urticaria, itching
         (b) Gastrointestinal—nausea, bloating, flatulence, foul taste in mouth
         (c) CNS—sleep disturbances, irritability, confusion
      (3) Drug interactions
         (a) Oral contraceptives increase risk of folic acid deficiency
         (b) Corticosteroids increase folic acid requirements
         (c) Sulfonamides decrease absorption of folic acid
5. Sickle cell
   a. Nonpharmacologic
      (1) Treat all infections aggressively
      (2) Maintain hydration, oxygenation
   b. Pharmacologic—maintained continuously on folic acid supplement
   c. Therapy during crisis
      (1) Hydration and adequate oxygenation
      (2) Analgesics for pain control
      (3) Antibiotics for associated infections
6. Patient education
   a. Iron deficiency anemia
      (1) Take iron with meals to alleviate GI distress; taking with orange juice or other vitamin C source will enhance absorption
      (2) Dietary counseling to improve iron intake and overall nutrition
      (3) Need for follow-up blood monitoring
   b. Vitamin B_{12} deficiency—need for monthly supplementation
   c. Folate deficiency
      (1) Folate maintenance dosage
      (2) Avoid overcooking folate-rich foods
   d. Sickle cell
      (1) Consider genetic counseling
      (2) Crises avoidance
         (a) Maintain good nutrition
         (b) Avoid temperature extremes
         (c) Immunizations for pneumococcus and influenza
      (3) Routine evaluation of body systems every 3 to 6 months

- Referral
  1. Evaluation of suspected GI blood loss
  2. Sickle cell crisis
  3. Evaluation of resistant cases

◘ IMMUNOLOGIC DISORDERS

Human Immunodeficiency Virus (HIV) Infection

- Definition
  1. HIV infection produces a spectrum of disease progressing from a clinically latent or asymptomatic state to a state of profound immunosuppression with acquired immune deficiency syndrome (AIDS) as a late manifestation
  2. Stages of HIV infection
     a. Transmission/primary HIV infection
     b. Acute HIV infection/seroconversion
     c. Asymptomatic infection/clinically latent period with or without persistent generalized lymphadenopathy (PGL)
     d. Early symptomatic infection; previously referred to as "AIDS-related complex"
     e. AIDS, specific clinical conditions present or CD4+ cell count less than 200/mm³
     f. Advanced HIV infection, characterized by CD4+ cell count less than 50/mm³

- Etiology/Incidence
  1. Etiology
     a. HIV virus transmitted through direct contact with blood, blood products, other body fluids
     b. Methods of transmission include—sexual contact, sharing needles, blood transfusions, babies born to HIV-infected mothers, occupational exposure
  2. Incidence
     a. Prevalence of HIV infection in general population unknown due to reluctance to disclose HIV status; reluctance to seek testing; long asymptomatic interval after infection
     b. 56,000 new HIV infections reported in US in 2006; prevalence estimated to be 1 to 2 million cases at end of 2003
     c. Diagnosed AIDS rising faster among women than in other groups
     d. 27% of new HIV infections reported in 2006 were female
     e. Black females disproportionately affected—rate of infection is 19 times higher than in white females
     f. Hispanic females have rate of infection five times higher than white females

3. Risk factors
   a. Unprotected or traumatic sexual activity, e.g., multiple partners or partners with other partners, anal intercourse, use of nonbarrier contraception
   b. Heterosexually acquired HIV infection rising rapidly, especially among women
   c. Intravenous drug use, sharing needles
   d. Infant of HIV-positive mother (vertical transmission)—15–25% if woman does not receive antiretroviral therapy during pregnancy
      (1) Risk of transmission may be reduced to less than 1% if pregnant woman receives multi-agent antiretroviral therapy and has undetectable viral load at delivery
      (2) Risk of transmission greater with maternal CD4+ counts of less than 200/mm³
   e. Transfusion of blood or blood products, artificial insemination, organ transplant recipient prior to 1985
   f. Healthcare worker or service worker exposed to blood or body fluids, e.g., needle stick injury, splash

- Signs and symptoms
  1. Acute HIV infection and seroconversion
     a. Moderate "flu-like" syndrome 2 to 4 weeks after inoculation
     b. Fever, diarrhea, headache, oral lesions on palate, lethargy, muscle/joint pain, rash lasting 2 to 4 weeks
     c. Self-limited; patients who seek care often misdiagnosed
     d. Seroconversion usually in 6–12 weeks; may take up to 6 months
  2. HIV disease progression—asymptomatic infection
     a. 12 weeks to 8 or more years; period of intense battle by immune system
     b. Influenced by general physical condition, age, mitigating drug therapy
        (1) Risk of progression correlates with length of seroconversion illness
        (2) Earliest HIV detection improves opportunity for successful antiviral therapy
  3. Early symptomatic HIV infection
     a. Usually occurs in 8 to 10 years; immune system begins to weaken
     b. Constitutional symptoms
        (1) Fatigue, headache, arthralgia, myalgia
        (2) Weight loss, anorexia, diarrhea
        (3) Fevers, night sweats, chills
     c. Occurrence of opportunistic infections

4. Advanced Disease/AIDS
   a. Usually occurs in 10 to 11 years
   b. Severe infections
5. Opportunistic infections
   a. Caused by a spectrum of pathogens that rarely cause disease in healthy people; most occur when CD4+ count is less than 200
   b. May be the reactivation of a previous pathogen; may have atypical presentation
   c. Causative agents include bacterial, fungal, viral, and parasitic infections
      (1) Candidiasis—mouth, vagina, penis, esophagus, large intestine, skin
      (2) Toxoplasmosis
      (3) Malignancies
      (4) Kaposi's sarcoma
      (5) Lymphoma—late manifestation of HIV
      (6) Invasive squamous cell carcinoma—cervix, vulva, anus secondary to human papillomavirus (HPV)
      (7) Pneumocystis carinii pneumonia—major AIDS defining diagnosis
      (8) Tuberculosis
      (9) Mycobacterium avium complex/MAC—occurs in late stage HIV infection

- Physical findings—related to immunocompromised status
  1. Early findings
     a. Lymphadenopathy
     b. Dermatologic abnormalities—seborrheic dermatitis, folliculitis
     c. Oral lesions—aphthous ulcers, herpes simplex labialis, thrush, oral hairy leukoplakia
  2. As disease progresses, more frequent skin disorders, oral lesions, infections

- Differential diagnosis
  1. Lymphomas
  2. Pneumonia
  3. Tuberculosis
  4. Chronic fatigue syndrome
  5. Mononucleosis

- Diagnostic tests/findings
  1. Diagnosis
     a. Enzyme-linked immunosorbant assay (ELISA)—positive for HIV antibodies (highly sensitive)
     b. Western Blot—confirms ELISA, detects HIV (highly specific)
     c. Oral fluid, urine, and home kits also available
     d. Antigen tests—can directly detect virus

(1) Nucleic acid testing—use in patients suspected of having acute retroviral syndrome

(2) HIV blood culture

(3) p24 antigen detects presence of HIV protein

(4) RNA PCR assay and branched DNA (bDNA) assay; measure amount of HIV RNA in plasma

2. Screening battery for women with established HIV infection

   a. Complete blood count every 3 months
   b. Chemistry panel every 6 months
   c. RPR or VDRL every 6–12 months
   d. Varicella, cytomegalovirus serology—baseline
   e. Hepatitis A, B, C—baseline and as indicated
   f. Toxoplasmosis—as indicated
   g. Chest radiography—as indicated
   h. PPD skin testing every 6 months
   i. Pap test—every 6 months first year after diagnosis and annually thereafter
   j. Quantitative plasma HIV ribonucleic acid (RNA) every 3 months
      (1) Useful for predicting progression of disease by indicating viral load
      (2) Monitoring response to antiviral therapy
   k. CD4+ cell count every 3 months
      (1) Indicative of immune status, predictor of disease progression
      (2) Complements viral load assay
      (3) Normal is 800 to 1050 cells/mm^3
      (4) Patients with CD4+ of 200 cells/mm^3 or less are likely to have symptoms or an AIDS defining condition

- Management/Treatment
  1. Nonpharmacologic
     a. Symptomatic treatment for fever, diarrhea
     b. Laboratory monitoring
     c. Maintain optimum nutrition, extra calories
  2. Pharmacologic (see **Table 8-5**)
     a. Antiretroviral therapy for HIV suppression
        (1) Highly active antiretroviral therapy (HAART)—combining three or four drugs is the standard of care for treatment of HIV infection
        (2) Goal to reduce HIV RNA to minimal levels for as long as possible (undetectable level < 500 copies/mL)
        (3) Decisions regarding need to change therapy based on measured antiviral effect per HIV RNA levels
        (4) HIV mutates rapidly

(a) HIV can mutate rapidly from a drug-sensitive form to a drug-resistant form

(b) Treatment with a combination of drugs to minimize development of resistance

(5) Treatment modification called for when HIV RNA levels fail to reach less than 500 copies/mL after 6 months of therapy

   b. Antiretroviral drug classes
      (1) Nucleoside reverse transcriptase inhibitors (NRTIs)
      (2) Nonnucleoside reverse transcriptase inhibitors (NNRTIs)
      (3) Protease inhibitors (PIs)
      (4) Nucleotide reverse transcriptase inhibitors

3. Patient education
   a. Natural history of HIV infection
   b. Explain modes of transmission
      (1) Discuss lifelong ability to transmit virus
      (2) Teach effective ways to reduce fluid exchange
         (a) Breastfeeding contraindicated
         (b) Encourage "safe sex" practices; condom use, limiting number of partners
         (c) Eliminate needle sharing
   c. Emphasize behaviors that protect/enhance immune system
      (1) Current immunizations
         (a) Hepatitis B and A
         (b) Pneumococcal vaccine (every 5 years)
         (c) Influenza (annually)
         (d) Tetanus vaccine
         (e) Live vaccines contraindicated
      (2) Stop tobacco, alcohol, street drug use
      (3) Nutritious diet, clean food preparation techniques
      (4) Reduce/manage stress
      (5) Exercise as tolerated
      (6) Avoid infectious individuals, and high-risk environments, e.g, child care settings, work settings such as hospitals
      (7) Avoid or eliminate exposure to pets, especially dogs, cats, or birds
      (8) Control travel exposures
   d. Drug regimens, interactions, and resistance—importance of adherence to medication schedule, CD4+ monitoring
   e. HIV and pregnancy implications—encourage antiviral medication to reduce vertical transmission
   f. Contraception

■ **Table 8-5** Antiretroviral Therapy for HIV Suppression (representative list)

Drug	Side-effects	Interactions	Contraindications
Nucleoside reverse transcriptase inhibitors zidovudine (AZT, ZDV) didanosine (ddI) zalcitabine (ddC) stavudine (d4T) lamivudine (3TC) abacavir	AZT—bone marrow suppression, GI effects Ddl—pancreatitis d4T/ddC—peripheral neuropathy 3TC—minimal toxicity	Caution with other nephrotoxic, cytotoxic myelosuppressive drugs; antagonized by rifampin	Monitor closely for hematologic toxicity and opportunistic infections; pregnancy category C; not recommended while nursing
Nonnucleoside reverse transcriptase inhibitors (NNRTI)—efavirenz, nevirapine, delavirdine	Mild to moderate skin rash, nausea, dizziness, headache, impaired concentration, vivid dreams, insomnia (efavirenz)	Metabolized by and can induce/inhibit cytochrome P450 enzymes; drug interactions can occur with PIs and many other drugs	Monitor liver, renal functions; pregnancy category C; not recommended while nursing
Nucleotide reverse transcriptase inhibitor Tenofovir	GI effects, headache	Do not dose with ddI	Renal insufficiency; pregnancy category B; not recommended for nursing mothers
Protease inhibitors (PIs)—amprenavir, indinavir, nelfinavir ritonavir, saquinavir, lopinavir/ritonavir	GI effects; hyperlipidemia Indinavir—kidney stones	Metabolized by cytochrome P450 enzymes; drug interactions common; avoid rifampin	Impaired hepatic function; monitor blood, liver and hyperglycemia; pregnancy category B; not recommended while nursing

(1) Barrier methods reduce transmission
    (a) Condoms—male or female for vaginal or anal penetrative acts
    (b) Dental dams or plastic film for oral contact
    (c) Stress need for consistent barrier use in addition to other contraception
(2) Oral contraceptives and depomedroxyprogesterone acetate (DMPA) injections—not contraindicated; limited data indicate antiretroviral drugs have potential to either increase or decrease bioavailability of contraceptive hormones
(3) Spermicides—controversy regarding role in possible increase in vaginal susceptibility
(4) IUC—not contraindicated if HIV positive or if has AIDS but is clinically well on antiretroviral therapy

- Referral
  1. All cases initially for full evaluation
  2. Monitoring and titration of medications
  3. Evaluation of new symptomatology

Systemic Lupus Erythematosus (SLE)

- Definition—chronic, inflammatory, multisystem disorder of the immune system characterized by periods of remission and exacerbation; course of disease unpredictable and highly variable

- Etiology/Incidence/Risk factors
  1. Etiology
     a. An autoimmune disorder—abnormal immune response creates antibodies to normal tissue
     b. Associated with reaction to some medications—chlorpromazine, hydralazine, isoniazid, methyldopa
     c. Criteria for diagnosis; 4 of 11 criteria to make diagnosis (American College of Rheumatology)
        (1) Malar rash
        (2) Discoid rash
        (3) Photosensitivity
        (4) Oral ulcers
        (5) Arthritis involving two or more peripheral joints
        (6) Serositis—pleuritis, pericarditis, or peritonitis
        (7) Renal disorder involving proteinuria or cellular casts
        (8) Neurologic disorder involving seizures or psychoses
        (9) Hematologic disorders—hemolytic anemia, leukopenia, thrombocytopenia
        (10) Positive ANA (antineutrophil antibody) test
        (11) Positive other immunologic test—antidouble stranded DNA (anti-dsDNA), anti-Smith (anti-Sm), LE (lupus erythematosus) cell preparation, false-positive syphilis serology
  2. Incidence
     a. 4–6 individuals/100,000/year
     b. Primarily affects women of childbearing age
  3. Risk factors
     a. African-American or Hispanic descent
     b. First-degree relative with SLE

- Signs and symptoms
  1. Early symptoms—vague, nonspecific, frequently misdiagnosed
  2. Fever, fatigue
  3. Arthralgia, arthritis
  4. Photosensitivity
  5. Headache, depression
  6. Seizures

- Physical findings
  1. Malar rash—erythematous, flat or raised rash over malar eminences
  2. Discoid rash—erythematous raised patches with scaling
  3. Alopecia
  4. Oral ulcers
  5. Pleurisy
  6. Pericarditis

- Differential diagnosis
  1. Contact dermatitis, eczema
  2. Rheumatoid arthritis
  3. Infectious processes
  4. Chronic fatigue syndrome

- Diagnostic tests/findings
  1. Positive ANA
  2. Anti-dsDNA, anti-Sm, LE cell prep, false-positive VDRL
  3. CBC—anemia, leukopenia, lymphopenia, thombocytopenia
  4. Serum creatinine to assess kidney function
  5. Urinalysis to determine presence of hematuria, cellular casts, and proteinuria

- Management/Treatment
  1. Nonpharmacologic
     a. Physical rest
     b. Protection from direct sunlight

    c. Proper diet and nutrition
2. Pharmacologic
    a. Some drugs may induce or aggravate symptoms
    b. Treatment is generally symptomatic and variable
    c. Nonsteroidal anti-inflammatory drugs (NSAID)—may control associated fever, arthralgias but not fatigue, malaise, major organ system involvement
    d. Corticosteroids indicated for life-threatening manifestations
    e. Hydroxychloroquine
      (1) Drug action—antimalarial drug; may help treat lupus rashes and joint symptoms
      (2) Side-effects
        (a) Irreversible retinopathy, corneal edema
        (b) Neuromuscular dysfunction
        (c) Pruritus, rash, skin pigmentation
        (d) Blood dyscrasias
      (3) Drug interactions
        (a) Hepatotoxic drugs
        (b) Dermatotoxic drugs
      (4) Contraindications/precautions
        (a) Hepatic dysfunction, alcoholism
        (b) Psoriasis
        (c) Pregnancy category C; not recommended while nursing
3. Patient education
    a. Sunscreen, protective clothing to avoid UV light
    b. Relaxation, stress reduction
    c. Individualized exercise/rest program
    d. Prompt treatment of infections
    e. Avoidance of pregnancy
      (1) Effective contraception
        (a) Controversy regarding oral contraceptive (OC) effect on SLE, but considered safe relative to pregnancy with SLE
          i. Trial on OC warranted
          ii. May increase symptoms
        (b) Progestin-only methods may be used
        (c) Intrauterine contraception (IUC)—may use if not severely immunocompromised
      (2) Careful supervision of obstetric care
        (a) Increased risk for premature delivery, spontaneous abortion, intrauterine fetal death, intrauterine growth restriction, and preeclampsia
        (b) Exacerbation of symptoms likely—usually mild to moderate in severity
        (c) Pregnancy outcomes best when mother has been in remission for at least 6 months prior to pregnancy and has normal renal function
    f. Avoidance of surgery, dental procedures when SLE symptoms present
    g. Immunizations
      (1) Live vaccines not advisable
      (2) Killed vaccines generally do not exacerbate SLE

- Referral
1. Evaluation of new symptoms, exacerbations
2. When invasive procedures are indicated
3. Social services, family or individual counseling regarding chronic disease coping strategies

Rheumatoid Arthritis

- Definition—an autoimmune disorder characterized by symmetric, erosive destruction of synovial tissues resulting in deformity and loss of joint function; may involve extra-articular manifestations

- Etiology/Incidence
1. Etiology
    a. Exact etiology unknown
    b. Complex of factors likely
      (1) Genetic
      (2) Environmental—viral, bacterial trigger suspected
      (3) Hormonal—controversial
    c. Criteria for diagnosis; 4 of 7 criteria, with criteria 1–4 present for at least 6 weeks (American College of Rheumatology)
      (1) Morning stiffness for more than 1 hour
      (2) Involvement of at least three joint groups with soft tissue swelling
      (3) Swelling involving at least one of the following joint groups—proximal interphalangeal (PIP), metacarpophalangeal (MCP), or wrists
      (4) Symmetrical joint swelling
      (5) Subcutaneous nodules
      (6) Positive rheumatoid factor
      (7) Radiographic changes consistent with rheumatoid arthritis (RA)
2. Incidence
    a. Prevalence—approximately 1% of the population

b. Occurs twice as often in women; third to sixth decades

c. Increased incidence among family groups

- Signs and symptoms
  1. Morning stiffness in joints lasting more than 1 hour
  2. Joint pain, constant or recurring; insidious development over weeks to months
  3. Joint warmth and redness; functional impairment
  4. Fatigue, depression
  5. Malaise, low-grade fever

- Physical findings
  1. Soft tissue swelling—most frequently in metacarpophalangeal (MCP) and proximal interphalangeal (PIP) joints; usually symmetric
  2. Deformity of involved joints
  3. Limited range of motion in affected joint
  4. Subcutaneous nodules
  5. Lymphadenopathy
  6. Splenomegaly
  7. Ocular disease—scleritis
  8. Entrapment neuropathies

- Differential diagnosis
  1. Polymyalgia rheumatica
  2. Osteoarthritis
  3. Systemic lupus erythematosus
  4. Ankylosing spondylitis
  5. Reiters syndrome

- Diagnostic tests/findings
  1. Rheumatoid (antibody) factor—can be isolated in 70–80% of patients
  2. Elevated erythrocyte sedimentation rate
  3. Radiography—joint erosion, narrowing of joint space

- Management/Treatment
  1. Nonpharmacologic
     a. Physical, occupational, hydrotherapy
     b. Rest
     c. Exercise
     d. Assistive devices
        (1) Footwear—orthotics
        (2) Canes, crutches
        (3) Splints, braces
     e. Surgery—synovectomy, arthroscopy
  2. Pharmacologic
     a. Nonsteroidal anti-inflammatory drugs (NSAIDs)—initial choice
        (1) Agents
           (a) Ibuprofen, naproxen, diclofenac
           (b) Meloxicam, etodolac, nabumetone
           (c) COX-2 inhibitors—celecoxib, rofecoxib, valdecoxib
        (2) Drug action—analgesic and anti-inflammatory effects
        (3) Side-effects
           (a) GI effects—dyspepsia, gastric and duodenal ulceration, perforation and bleeding; selective COX-2 inhibitors have less upper GI toxicity
           (b) Renal toxicity
           (c) CNS toxicity—dizziness, anxiety, drowsiness, confusion
        (4) Drug interactions—may decrease effectiveness of diuretics, beta-blockers, ACE inhibitors; may increase toxicity of lithium and methotrexate
        (5) Contraindications/precautions—aspirin allergy; pregnancy category C, but contraindicated third trimester; not recommended while nursing
     b. Disease-modifying antirheumatic drugs—no analgesic effects; can control symptoms and may delay progression of disease/representative list
        (1) Hydroxychloroquine—moderately effective for mild RA (see SLE this section)
        (2) Sulfasalazine
           (a) Side-effects—nausea, anorexia, rash; hepatitis, leukopenia, agranulocytosis
           (b) Drug interactions—reduces absorption of digoxin, folic acid
           (c) Contraindication/precautions—intestinal or urinary obstruction; pregnancy category B; not recommended in nursing mothers
        (3) Methotrexate
           (a) Side-effects—stomatitis, anorexia, nausea, abdominal cramps, increased aminotransferase activity
           (b) Drug interactions—avoid other hepatotoxic drugs, live virus vaccines
           (c) Contraindications/precautions—immunodeficiency, blood dyscrasias, alcoholism, chronic liver disease; pregnancy category X; not recommended in nursing mothers
        (4) Leflunomide
           (a) Side-effects—diarrhea, elevated liver enzymes, alopecia, rash
           (b) Drug interactions—may increase levels of diclofenac, ibuprofen;

caution with other hepatotoxic drugs

    (c) Contraindications/precautions—hepatic impairment; pregnancy category X; not recommended in nursing mothers

  (5) Infliximab—given intravenously/used with methotrexate

    (a) Drug action—blocks activity of tissue necrosis factor

    (b) Side-effects—headache, aseptic meningitis, infection, infusion re-actions (fever, urticaria, dyspnea, hypotension) and exacerbation of CHF

    (c) Drug interactions—specific drug interaction studies have not been conducted

    (d) Contraindications/precautions—CHF, active infection, live vac-cines; pregnancy category B; not recommended in nursing mothers

3. Patient education
   a. Safety issues—footwear, balance, trans-port, walking
   b. Discussion of long-term, chronic nature of disease, support network helpful
   c. Etiology—genetic component, noncontagious
   d. Episodic nature of disease
   e. Pain control techniques—relaxation, drug therapy, rest, appropriate exercise

- Referral
  1. Physical therapy, occupational therapy
  2. Surgical procedures

☐ ENDOCRINE DISORDERS

Diabetes

- Definition
  1. A heterozygous group of metabolic diseases characterized by hyperglycemia resulting from defects in insulin secretion, insulin action, or both
  2. Types
     a. Type 1—absolute insulin deficiency
     b. Type 2—condition of fasting hyperglyce-mia despite availability of insulin
     c. Gestational diabetes mellitus (GDM)—glucose intolerance diagnosed during pregnancy
     d. Diabetes secondary to other causes
        (1) Genetic defects in beta-cell function/insulin action
        (2) Diseases of the pancreas
        (3) Drug- or chemical-induced
  3. Complications
     a. Macrovascular
        (1) Coronary artery disease
        (2) Myocardial infarction; sudden cardiac death
        (3) Cerebrovascular disease
        (4) Peripheral vascular disease
        (5) Intestinal ischemia
        (6) Renal artery stenosis
     b. Microvascular
        (1) Retinopathy
        (2) Nephropathy
        (3) Peripheral neuropathy—parasthesias and glove and stocking neuropathy
        (4) Autonomic neuropathy—gastropare-sis and impotence

- Etiology/Incidence/Risk factors
  1. Type 1
     a. Caused by autoimmune destruction of the pancreatic beta cells that produce insulin
        (1) Genetic predisposition, a hypothetical triggering event, and immunologically-mediated beta cell destruction
        (2) Typically begins in childhood or in young adults who are slim, but can occur in adults of any age
     b. Manifested by absolute insulin deficiency which results in elevation of blood glu-cose, breakdown of fats and proteins
     c. Predisposition to development of ketoacidosis
  2. Type 2
     a. Characterized by impaired insulin secre-tion, peripheral insulin resistance and increased hepatic glucose production
     b. Typically occurs in those over 45, over-weight and sedentary, with a family his-tory of diabetes
     c. Racial/ethnic groups at increased risk—Native Americans, Hispanics, African Americans
  3. Gestational diabetes mellitus (GDM)
     a. Function of hormonal/metabolic de-mands of pregnancy; usually regresses after parturition
     b. 50% risk of developing diabetes within 5 years if insulin was required for control of GDM; 60% risk of developing disease within 10 to 15 years if dietary manage-ment was sufficient
  4. Impaired fasting glucose (IFG) and impaired glucose tolerance (IGT)
     a. Hyperglycemia not sufficient to meet diag-nostic criteria for diabetes

b. Categorized as IFG if identified by fasting blood glucose or IGT if identified by oral glucose tolerance test in the 2-hour sample

c. Both categories are risk factors for diabetes and cardiovascular disease

5. Prevalence in the general population estimated at 6–8% of individuals older than 40
   a. Type 1 accounts for approximately 10% of diagnosed cases
   b. Type 2 prevalence is estimated at more than 14 million cases, many undiagnosed

- Signs and symptoms
  1. "Classic" symptoms—polyuria, polydipsia, polyphagia
  2. Weight loss
  3. Fatigue and/or weakness
  4. Persistent/recurrent vaginal candidiasis; candidal balanitis
  5. Vision changes, blurred vision
  6. Type 2 often asymptomatic in early stages

- Physical findings
  1. Early
     a. Thin, decreased weight/type 1; overweight, obese/type 2
     b. Hypertension/type 2
     c. Skin infections—frequent or slow to heal
  2. With more advanced disease
     a. Skin—ulcerations of feet and legs; loss of hair lower legs and toes
     b. Eyes—retinopathy/microaneurysms, exudates, neovascularization; cataracts, glaucoma
     c. Cardiovascular—diminished or absent peripheral pulses; orthostatic hypotension/ominous finding
     d. Neurologic—sensory loss; diminished/absent deep tendon reflexes

- Differential diagnosis
  1. Type 1 versus type 2
  2. Pancreatic insufficiency
  3. Cushing's syndrome
  4. Secondary effects of drug therapy—corticosteroids, thiazide diuretics

- Diagnostic tests/findings
  1. Criteria for diagnosis of diabetes (ADA, 2009)
     a. Diabetes can be diagnosed in any one of three ways; must be confirmed on a subsequent day
        (1) Fasting plasma glucose 126 mg/dL or greater; fasting defined as no caloric intake for at least 8 hours; or

(2) A casual plasma glucose of 200 mg/dL or greater with symptoms of diabetes; or

(3) An oral glucose tolerance test value of 200 mg/dL or greater in the 2-hour sample

b. Categories of impaired glucose metabolism:
   (1) Impaired fasting glucose—fasting plasma glucose of 100–125 mg/dL
   (2) Impaired glucose tolerance—results of oral glucose tolerance test of 140–199 mg/dL in the 2-hour sample

2. Criteria for screening asymptomatic adults (recommended screening test is fasting plasma glucose) include (ADA, 2009):
   a. Anyone older than 45 years at 3-year intervals
   b. Consider testing younger than 45 years or more frequent screening in individuals with the following risks:
      (1) Overweight—BMI of 25 or greater
      (2) First-degree relative with diabetes (parent, sibling)
      (3) Member of a high-risk ethnic population
      (4) Delivered infant of greater than 9 pounds or history of GDM
      (5) Hypertension
      (6) HDL cholesterol of 35 mg/dL or less and/or triglyceride level of 250 mg/dL or more
      (7) Previous IFG or IGT
      (8) Other conditions associated with insulin resistance—polycystic ovarian syndrome

3. Recommended glycemic goals for nonpregnant patients (ADA, 2009)
   a. Average preprandial plasma glucose (mg/dL)—70 to 130 mg/dL
   b. Average peak postprandial glucose (1 to 2 hours after beginning meal) of less than 180 mg/dL
   c. HbA$_{1c}$
      (1) Reflects average glucose levels for the preceding 3 months
      (2) Goal of less than 7%—action suggested if greater than 8%

4. Tests helpful in identifying associated risk factors and complications include:
   a. Annual lipid profile, serum creatinine, urinalysis
   b. Testing for microalbuminuria—2 of 3 tests measured over 6 months should be elevated before diagnosis

(1) Test at time of diagnosis in type 2 diabetics; after 5 years in type 1; annually thereafter

(2) Testing can be performed by three methods

    (a) Measurement of albumin-to-creatinine ratio in a random, spot collection; microalbuminuria 30–300 $\mu g/mg$ creatinine; clinical albuminuria of greater than 300 $\mu g/mg$ creatinine

    (b) 24-hour urine collection with serum creatinine; values same as spot urine

    (c) Timed collection such as 4 hours or overnight; microalbuminuria 20–200 $\mu g/min$; clinical albuminuria of greater than 200 $\mu g/min$

c. Electrocardiogram at time of diagnosis and periodically depending on symptoms and risk factors

- Management/Treatment

1. Clinical trials have demonstrated that glycemic control is associated with decreased rates of microvascular complications; epidemiologic studies support reduction in cardiovascular disease (ADA, 2009)

2. Nonpharmacologic—Type 1 and 2

    a. Home glucose determinations to monitor glycemic control daily

    b. Diet—individualized nutrition recommendations

      (1) Regulate carbohydrate intake (45–65% of calories)—emphasis on complex carbohydrates rather than simple and refined starches

      (2) Regulate fat intake (< 30% of calories)—emphasis on polyunsaturated instead of saturated fats in ratio of 2:1

      (3) Maintain ideal body weight; cornerstone of treatment for type 2 diabetic

    c. Regular aerobic exercise

      (1) Improves blood glucose control

      (2) Reduces cardiovascular risk factors

      (3) Contributes to weight loss

    d. Aggressively manage additional cardiovascular risk factors

      (1) Blood pressure goal of less than 125/75

      (2) LDL cholesterol of less than 70 mg/dL

      (3) Smoking cessation

    e. Refer type 2 diabetics at time of diagnosis and type 1 diabetics within 3–5 years for eye examination; annually thereafter

f. Perform comprehensive foot examination annually; examination should include use of a Semmes-Weinstein monofilament, tuning fork, and a visual examination

g. Annual influenza vaccination; pneumococcal vaccination

3. Pharmacologic

    a. Type 1—insulin replacement

      (1) Insulin products/U-100

        (a) Rapid acting (onset less than 0.5 hour)—insulin lispro and insulin aspart

        (b) Short acting (onset 0.5–1 hour)—regular

        (c) Intermediate acting (onset 2–4 hours)—NPH, Lente

        (d) Long acting—Ultralente/onset 6–10 hours; insulin glargine/onset 1–2 hours with no peak

      (2) Intensive insulin treatment to achieve tight control in highly motivated patients willing to perform multiple daily glucose determinations and administer insulin according to results

        (a) Long acting insulin administered once/day in the evening; short acting insulin administered 30–45 minutes prior to meals, adjusted according to postprandial glucose measurements

        (b) Consider use of rapid acting insulin 10–15 minutes prior to meals in patients with hypoglycemic episodes

      (3) Consider less intensive treatment for patients unable to carry out intensive program; intermediate acting insulin twice daily before breakfast and evening meal mixed with short acting insulin for prandial control

    b. Type 2—oral hypoglycemic agents (see **Table 8-6**)

      (1) Consider management with diet and exercise first; if glucose intolerance persists, begin oral agent

      (2) Begin with second generation sulfonylurea or biguanide (metformin); choose metformin if patient is obese

      (3) Increase dose every 1–2 weeks until glycemic control achieved or reach maximum dose

      (4) If glycemic control not achieved with monotherapy, add second oral agent from different class

■ **Table 8-6** Oral Medications Used to Treat Type 2 Diabetes Mellitus (representative list)

Drug	Action	Side-effects	Interactions	Contraindications/Precautions
Sulfonylureas 1st generation—chlorpropamide 2nd generation—glipizide, glyburide, glimepiride	Stimulates insulin secretion from pancreatic beta cells	Hypoglycemia, weight gain, photosensitivity, GI upset, cholestatic jaundice	Potentiated by NSAIDs, sulfonamides; antagonized by diuretics, beta-blockers, steroids, others	Ketoacidosis, impaired renal, hepatic function; pregnancy category C; not recommended while nursing
Biguanides—Metformin	Decreases hepatic glucose production and absorption of glucose; increases peripheral glucose uptake and utilization	Anorexia, nausea, diarrhea, abdominal bloating; lactic acidosis—serious, rare	Effects potentiated by cimetidine, ranitidine, nifedipine, digoxin, trimethoprim	Renal disease or dysfunction, CHF requiring treatment; pregnancy Category B; use with caution while nursing
α-glucosidase inhibitor—Acarbose, Miglitol	Delays absorption of carbohydrates, inhibits metabolism of sucrose to glucose and fructose	Flatulence, diarrhea, abdominal discomfort (symptoms decrease over time); increases AST, ALT	Charcoal, digestive enzymes all decrease effect; will decrease effects of digoxin, propranolol	Inflammatory bowel disease, or any intestinal disease causing disordered digestion or absorption; pregnancy category B; do not use while nursing
Meglitinides—repaglinide, nateglinide	Stimulates insulin release from pancreas	Hypoglycemia, headache, URI, dizziness	Potentiated by NSAIDs, alcohol; may be antagonized by thiazides, corticosteroids	Caution in hepatic impairment; pregnancy category C; not recommended in nursing mothers
Thiazolidinediones—rosiglitazone, pioglitazone	Improves insulin sensitivity, glucose uptake in muscle and adipose tissue; inhibits gluconeogenesis	Edema, headache, myalgia, URI; initial increase in LDL and HDL	Possible drug interactions with oral contraceptives, ketoconazole, erythromycin, corticosteroids	Hepatotoxicity—monitor LFTs at start of therapy, q 2 mo, first year; pregnancy category B; do not use while nursing

(5) Consider insulin in patients unable to achieve glycemic control with two oral agents or initially in symptomatic patients with fasting blood glucose greater than 240 mg/dL

c. Use aspirin therapy in all adult diabetic patients with macrovascular complications and diabetic patients older than 40 years with any other cardiovascular risk factors (American Diabetes Association, 2009)

d. Use ACE inhibitors in patients with microalbuminuria or clinical albuminuria (see Table 8-1)

4. Patient education

a. Family involvement in care, medication instruction

b. Safety concerns, especially compensation for neuropathies

c. Assure compliance with drug regimen
   (1) Appropriate injection technique for insulin
   (2) Importance of regular dosing, oral or parenteral

d. Blood glucose monitoring
   (1) Routine schedule and glycemic target values
   (2) Aseptic technique for blood sampling
   (3) Medication dosage calculation based on blood glucose

e. Risk factor management and screening
   (1) Smoking cessation if appropriate
   (2) Annual comprehensive eye examination with ophthalmologist
   (3) Foot care
   (4) Dental hygiene and annual examination
   (5) Nutritional counseling with registered dietitian
   (6) Contraception and preconceptional counseling emphasizing optimal glucose control

f. Signs of hypo/hyperglycemia and method of management
   (1) Hypoglycemia
      (a) Sweating, palpitations, anxiety, mood changes
      (b) Treat with 6-oz glass of orange juice, hard candy, teaspoon of honey; glucose tablets
      (c) Parenteral administration of glucagon by caregiver or family member in event of unconsciousness
   (2) Hyperglycemia
      (a) Nausea, vomiting, mental confusion, fruity breath odor
      (b) Immediate administration of insulin

- Referral
  1. All newly diagnosed cases for complete evaluation
  2. Evaluation of suspected or developing complications

Hypoglycemia

- Definition—a nonspecific diagnosis often characterized by vague symptoms of malaise, fatigue, or headache, attributed to either adrenergic excess or insufficient CNS glucose; symptoms can become severe

- Etiology/Incidence
  1. Etiology
     a. Adrenergic excess
     b. Insufficient central nervous system glucose—fasting or exercise-induced
     c. Medication-induced—oral hypoglycemic agents, insulin
  2. Incidence unknown due to difficulty in establishing diagnosis

- Signs and symptoms
  1. Adrenergic excess
     a. Sweating
     b. Tremor
     c. Hunger
     d. Anxiety
     e. Palpitations
  2. Neuroglycopenia
     a. Irritability, personality changes
     b. Headache
     c. Blurred, double vision
     d. Confusion
     e. Lethargy, stupor, coma

- Physical findings
  1. Adrenergic—tachycardia, tremor
  2. Neuroglycopenia—stupor, coma

- Differential diagnosis
  1. Insulinoma
  2. Extrapancreatic tumors—adrenal, hepatic, sarcoma, mesothelioma
  3. Hypopituitary disorder
  4. Addison's disease
  5. Massive liver disease

- Diagnostic tests/findings
  1. Depressed blood glucose levels accompanied by typical symptoms
     a. Men, less than 50 mg/dL
     b. Women, less than 40 mg/dL
  2. C-peptide assay
     a. Principle use is evaluation of hypoglycemia
     b. Elevated C-peptide levels with endogenous hyperinsulinism or insulinoma; decreased C-peptide levels with surreptitious insulin injection

- Management/Treatment
  1. Nonpharmacologic
     a. Alimentary hypoglycemia
        (1) Limit high-glycemic-index carbohydrates; include a low-glycemic-index carbohydrate at every meal
           (a) Glycemic index (GI) is a measure of the effect of carbohydrate-containing foods on blood glucose
           (b) Low-glycemic-index foods lower risk of causing relative hypoglycemia
           (c) Examples of low GI foods—apple, pear, milk, kidney beans, pasta
           (d) Examples of high GI foods—baked potato, white bread, bagel, white rice
        (2) Smaller, more frequent meals
        (3) Weight reduction if obese
     b. Acute episodes—oral administration of simple carbohydrate if fasting, drug-induced, or exercise-induced
     c. Reducing caffeine intake sometimes helpful
     d. Surgical—removal of insulinoma, other tumors
  2. Pharmacologic
     a. Anticholinergic/propantheline
        (1) Drug action—delay gastric emptying
        (2) Side-effects—anticholinergic effects
        (3) Drug interactions—increases effects of digoxin
        (4) Contraindications/precautions—acute angle-closure glaucoma; pregnancy category C
     b. Beta-blocker/propranolol (see Table 8-1)
  3. Patient education
     a. Individualized dietary counseling
     b. Symptom recognition

- Referral
  1. When tumor or other underlying disease is suspected
  2. If symptoms not relieved by dietary changes

Hyperthyroidism

- Definition—a hypermetabolic syndrome affecting all body systems characterized by excess circulating thyroid hormone

- Etiology/Incidence
  1. Etiology
     a. Graves' disease
        (1) Comprises 90% of cases
        (2) Autoimmune condition; excess synthesis and secretion of thyroid hormone caused by antibodies that stimulate thyroid stimulating hormone (TSH) receptors
        (3) Often self-limited; symptomatic 1–2 years
     b. Toxic multinodular goiter—accounts for most cases in middle-aged and elderly
     c. Toxic adenoma/solitary autonomous nodule—single hyperfunctioning nodule surrounded by suppressed thyroid tissue
     d. Thyroiditis—group of inflammatory diseases
        (1) Inflammation causes disruption of the follicles resulting in release of preformed thyroid hormone
        (2) Usually self-limited
        (3) Phases—thyrotoxicosis, transient euthyroid, hypothyroid, recovery
        (4) Classification of thyroiditis
           (a) Subacute lymphocytic—autoimmune process
              i. Postpartum thyroiditis
              ii. Painless/sporadic thyroiditis
           (b) Subacute granulomatous/de Quervain's thyroiditis—likely viral in origin and generally preceded by URI
  2. Incidence
     a. Annual incidence 0.05–1% in general adult population
     b. Hyperthyroidism is 5–10 times more common in females
     c. Postpartum thyroiditis occurs in 8–10% of women within 1 year of delivery

- Signs and symptoms—nonspecific, affecting all body systems; reflect increased stimulation from excess thyroid hormone
  1. Increased appetite, weight loss
  2. Irritability, nervousness, sleep disturbance
  3. Heat intolerance, sweating
  4. Fatigue, exertional shortness of breath
  5. Palpitations, tremor
  6. Diarrhea
  7. Decreased menses

8. Eye irritation, vision changes, double vision (Graves')

- Physical findings
  1. Thyroid gland—enlarged/diffuse or asymmetric nodularity
  2. Neuromuscular system—hyperreflexia, tremor, muscle wasting
  3. Dermatologic system—skin moist, smooth
  4. Cardiovascular system—tachycardia, systolic flow murmur, atrial fibrillation in elderly
  5. Eyes—lid retraction
  6. Gastrointestinal system—increased bowel sounds
  7. Graves' disease
     a. Symmetrical and moderate thyroid enlargement/bruit
     b. Exophthalmos/proptosis and pretibial myxedema (nonpitting thickening of skin)
  8. Toxic multinodular goiter—asymmetric nodularity
  9. Toxic adenoma—single nodule surrounded by suppressed thyroid tissue
  10. Thyroiditis—slight enlargement; tender with subacute granulomatous thyroiditis

- Differential diagnosis
  1. Neoplasm—because of associated weight loss and weakness
  2. Psychological disorders—panic disorder

- Diagnostic tests/findings
  1. Ultrasensitive serum thyroid stimulating hormone (TSH)
     a. Most effective initial test for diagnosis
     b. Low in response to excess circulation thyroid hormone
  2. Free T_4 usually elevated
  3. Serum T_3 elevated—useful when T_4 normal, TSH low, and patient is symptomatic
  4. Radioactive iodine scan with uptake
     a. Scan/anatomic definition
     b. Radioactive iodine uptake/hyper- versus hypofunction
        (1) Uptake diffusely increased in Graves'
        (2) Uptake decreased in thyroiditis
        (3) Hot nodule with little uptake in rest of gland in toxic adenoma

- Management/Treatment
  1. Nonpharmacologic
     a. Diet—increased need for calories
     b. Decrease stimulants
  2. Pharmacologic
     a. Antithyroid drugs—propylthiouracil, methimazole/preferred treatment of

Graves' in young adults, pregnant women, before surgery and RAI ablation
     (1) Drug action
        (a) Block multiple steps in the synthesis of thyroid hormone
        (b) Permanent remission in half of patients and one fourth of these hypothyroid in 15–20 years
        (c) Clinically euthyroid in 4–8 weeks
     (2) Side-effects
        (a) Dermatitis, myalgias
        (b) Leukopenia—monitor CBC
        (c) Agranulocytosis—cannot be predicted; instructions to notify healthcare provider if fever or sore throat
        (d) Hepatocellular damage—monitor LFTs
     (3) Drug interactions—potentiates oral anticoagulants
     (4) Contraindications/precautions—pregnancy category D, monitor FT_4 every 2 to 4 weeks and use lowest doses to maintain euthyroid; contraindicated while nursing
     b. Radioactive iodine therapy—treatment of choice for toxic multinodular goiter and toxic adenoma; preferred treatment for most adults older than 40
     (1) Drug action
        (a) Damages functioning thyroid tissue
        (b) Reduces symptoms in 6–12 weeks
     (2) Side-effects
        (a) Long-term hypothyroidism; 70% of patients at 10 years
        (b) May exacerbate ophthalmopathy in the short term
     (3) Contraindications—pregnancy or lactation
     c. Beta-blockers—propranolol, atenolol (see Table 8-1)
        (1) Decreases signs and symptoms by blocking sympathetic nervous system
        (2) Indicated for symptomatic relief until more specific therapy initiated
     d. Management of thyroiditis—often no treatment required
        (1) Beta-blockers for symptomatic treatment of thyrotoxicosis
        (2) Subacute granulomatous thyroiditis
           (a) NSAIDs for pain/inflammation
           (b) Prednisone for extreme cases (see Table 8-3)
  3. Patient education
     a. Medication regimens, side-effects

b. Signs/symptoms of thyroid storm—an exaggeration of signs and symptoms of hyperthyroidism; requires immediate attention

- Referral
  1. Radioactive iodine treatment; consider referral for treatment with antithyroid drugs
  2. Ophthalmologist referral for ophthalmopathy
  3. Refer for surgical consideration patients with obstructive symptoms and/or cosmetic concerns

Hypothyroidism

- Definition—a metabolic syndrome affecting all organ systems characterized by deficient levels of circulating thyroid hormone

- Etiology/Incidence/Risk factors
  1. Etiology
     a. Primary thyroid failure
        (1) Hashimoto's thyroiditis—chronic autoimmune thyroiditis
        (2) Previous radioactive iodine treatment, surgery
     b. Secondary—pituitary or hypothalamic disease
     c. Transient
        (1) Subacute granulomatous thyroiditis/de Quervain's
        (2) Subacute lymphocytic thyroiditis/postpartum and sporadic painless
  2. Prevalence estimated 1–3% of general population
     a. Increasing prevalence with age and in women
     b. Women older than 50 years have estimated 5% prevalence
  3. Risk factors
     a. Age older than 50 years
     b. Female-to-male ratio is 8 to 10:1
     c. History of autoimmune disease
     d. Family or personal history of thyroid disease

- Signs and symptoms—often subclinical; reflect slowed physiologic functioning of all organ systems
  1. Weakness, lethargy
  2. Skin changes—dry or coarse skin, skin pallor; coarse hair
  3. Slow speech, forgetfulness, depression
  4. Cold sensation, decreased sweating
  5. Eyelid, facial edema
  6. Constipation
  7. Irregular menses—menorrrhagia, amenorrhea; infertility

- Physical findings—depend on severity, duration of deficiency, and rapidity of development
  1. Thyroid gland may be atrophic, normal, or goitrous
  2. Neuromuscular system—diminished relaxation phase of reflexes, carpal tunnel syndrome, hearing loss
  3. Dermatologic system—skin cool, dry; hair dry, brittle; generalized hair loss, especially outer third of eyebrows
  4. Cardiovascular system—bradycardia; edema, especially periorbital, anemia
  5. Gastrointestinal system—mild weight gain, diminished bowel sounds
  6. Endocrine system—galactorrhea

- Differential diagnosis
  1. Primary versus secondary
  2. Clinical depression
  3. Antithyroid drugs—lithium

- Diagnostic tests/findings
  1. TSH—elevated in primary hypothyroidism
  2. Free T_4—decreased
  3. Decreased TSH and FT_4 in secondary hypothyroidism
  4. Antithyroid peroxidases, antithyroglobulin, and antimicrosomal antibodies—Hashimoto's thyroiditis
  5. Hypercholesteremia

- Management/Treatment
  1. Nonpharmacologic
     a. Restrict calories if needed for weight control
     b. High-fiber, low-fat diet
  2. Pharmacologic (primary hypothyroidism)—levothyroxine
     a. Drug action—synthetic T_4
        (1) T_4 converted to T_3; administration of T_4 produces both hormones
        (2) Half-life 6 days; slow rate of achieving steady state
        (3) Adjust dose every 6 weeks until TSH normalizes
     b. Side-effects—symptoms of hyperthyroidism/excess replacement
     c. Drug interactions
        (1) Potentiates sympathomimetics
        (2) Monitor antihyperglycemics, oral anticoagulants
     d. Contraindications
        (1) Thyrotoxicosis
        (2) Acute MI
        (3) Uncorrected adrenal insufficiency

3. Patient education
   a. Medication use and doses; need for long-term therapy
   b. Danger of increasing medication too rapidly or taking more than prescribed

- Referral—all secondary cases for evaluation

◘ MUSCULOSKELETAL DISORDERS

Low Back Pain (LBP)

- Definition—acute (< than 3 months), chronic, or recurrent pain occurring in the lumbosacral spine region; pain may be localized or radiate to the extremities

- Etiology/Incidence
  1. Etiology
     a. No specific identifiable cause in up to 85% of cases; lumbosacral strain results from stretching, tearing of muscles, tendons, ligaments, and fascia due to trauma or repetitive mechanical stress
     b. Herniated intervertebral disc causing nerve root compression resulting in pain below the knee and other neurologic signs and symptoms
     c. Spinal stenosis—soft tissue or bony encroachment of the spinal canal and nerve roots
  2. Incidence
     a. One of the top 10 reasons for visit to primary care provider
     b. Estimated 65–80% of individuals experience at least one episode
     c. Women and men equally affected
     d. Chronic LBP comprises about 2% of all cases
  3. Risk factors—acute LBP
     a. Repetitive motion
     b. Poor body mechanics
     c. Sedentary lifestyle; poor strength of abdominal and back muscles

- Signs and symptoms
  1. Lumbosacral strain
     a. Pain located in the back, buttocks, or one or both thighs
     b. Pain aggravated by standing/flexion; relieved with rest/reclining
  2. Herniated intervertebral disc
     a. Characterized by radicular pain; paresthesias may occur in distribution of involved nerve root
     b. Most common disc ruptures involve the L5 or S1 nerve roots

(1) L5 root/L4–5 disc—pain/numbness lateral calf
(2) S1 root/L5-S1 disc—pain buttocks, lateral leg and malleolus; numbness lateral foot and posterior calf

3. Spinal stenosis—pain precipitated by walking or standing upright; relieved by sitting or leaning forward

- Physical findings
  1. Lumbosacral strain
     a. Increased pain with flexion
     b. Negative straight leg raise (SLR); normal neurologic exam
  2. Herniated intervertebral disc
     a. Increased pain with flexion
     b. Positive SLR—radicular pain when leg is passively raised 30–60°
     c. L5 root—weakness dorsiflexion of great toe; decreased sensation anterior/medial dorsal foot
     d. S1 root—weakness of plantar flexion/tiptoe walking; diminished/absent Achilles reflex; decreased sensation lateral foot
  3. Spinal stenosis—assessment of lower extremities for loss of hair, color, and pulses to differentiate spinal stenosis from vascular insufficiency

- Differential diagnosis
  1. Cauda equina syndrome
     a. Surgical emergency due to impingement on the cauda equina
     b. Characterized by saddle anesthesia, bladder or bowel incontinence, muscle weakness
  2. Fracture—major trauma such as motor vehicle or fall from high place
  3. Osteoporosis/compression fracture—may be precipitated by minor trauma or lifting
  4. Neoplasm—constitutional symptoms, no relief with bedrest, chronic pain
  5. Infection—chills, fever, IV drug user, recent bacterial infection, immunosuppression

- Diagnostic tests/findings
  1. Indicated in the presence of "red flags"—fever, chills, weight loss, recent onset bladder/bowel dysfunction, lower extremity sensory or neurologic deficit
  2. Radiograph of lumbosacral spine
     a. Generally not necessary in acute phase—3–6 weeks duration
     b. Suspicion of fracture
     c. Suspicion of malignancy—patient older than 50 years; persistent bone pain unrelieved by bed rest; history of malignancy

3. MRI or CT
    a. Severe persistent symptoms despite conservative treatment
    b. Suspected disc herniation

- Management/Treatment
    1. Nonpharmacologic
        a. Encourage continuation of daily activities rather than bedrest
        b. Local application of heat, warm baths
        c. Prescribe physical therapy program to improve strength and conditioning
        d. Low stress aerobic exercise—walking, biking, swimming
    2. Pharmacologic
        a. Nonsteroidal anti-inflammatory drugs (NSAIDs) (see Acute Otitis Media this chapter)—ibuprofen, naproxen, etodolac
        b. Muscle relaxant—cyclobenzaprine
            (1) Drug action—reduces tonic somatic motor activity in the brain stem
            (2) Side-effects—somnolence, dry mouth
            (3) Drug interactions—hypertensive crisis with MAOIs; potentiates alcohol and other CNS depressants
            (4) Contraindications/precautions—acute post-MI, arrhythmias; pregnancy category B; precaution in nursing mothers
    3. Patient education
        a. Avoid bedrest
        b. Weight loss if indicated to reduce lordosis
        c. Good body mechanics; proper lifting
        d. Appropriate exercises
        e. Signs of deterioration
            (1) Loss of bladder control
            (2) Numbness or weakness in groin or rectal area
            (3) Pain extending down leg past knee
        f. Reassurance
            (1) Excellent prognosis for complete resolution of acute LBP episodes
            (2) Recurrence likely at variable intervals

- Referral
    1. Urgently refer patients with symptoms suggestive of cauda equina or cord compression
    2. Symptoms suggestive of spinal infection or malignancy
    3. Neurologic consultation if back pain remains severe after 4–6 weeks of conservative treatment or findings of neurologic deficits

Osteoarthritis

- Definition
    1. Noninflammatory joint disease characterized by degeneration of articular cartilage with new bone formation at articular surface
    2. Most commonly involved joints are distal and proximal interphalangeals of hands, hips, knees, and cervical and lumbar spine
    3. Primary—no obvious cause
    4. Secondary—occurring in damaged or abnormal joints

- Etiology/Incidence/Risk factors
    1. Etiology
        a. Progressive degeneration and loss of articular cartilage and subchondral bone
        b. Bone ends thicken and osteophytes or spurs form where the ligaments and capsule attach to the bone
        c. Variable synovial inflammation results
    2. Incidence
        a. Radiographic evidence in 80% of adults by age 60
        b. Clinical osteoarthritis affects approximately 25% of adults
    3. Risk factors
        a. Increasing age
        b. Female gender
        c. Obesity
        d. Major joint trauma
        e. Repetitive joint stress
        f. Congenital and developmental joint defects
        g. Metabolic and endocrine disorders

- Signs and symptoms
    1. Gradual onset of joint pain, tenderness, and limited movement
    2. Pain aggravated by joint use and subsides with rest
    3. Morning joint stiffness or stiffness following a period of inactivity, lasting generally less than 30 min
    4. Symptoms often asymmetrical

- Physical findings
    1. Decreased range of motion
    2. Effusions of involved joint(s) with minimal local warmth and no erythema
    3. Enlargement of distal interphalangeal (DIP) joints—Heberden's nodes; enlargement of proximal interphalangeal (PIP) joints—Bouchard's nodes
    4. Crepitus with joint motion

- Differential diagnosis
  1. Rheumatoid arthritis
  2. Infectious arthritis
  3. Tendonitis/bursitis syndromes
  4. Crystal induced arthritis—gout, pseudogout
  5. Fracture

- Diagnostic tests/findings
  1. Radiography
     a. Will not demonstrate deterioration of cartilage
     b. Four cardinal radiologic features
        (1) Narrowed joint space
        (2) Sclerosis of subchondral bone
        (3) Bony cysts
        (4) Osteophytes
  2. Diagnostic joint fluid aspiration
     a. Indicated if joint effusion
     b. Synovial fluid analysis—white blood cell count with differential; culture; evaluation for crystals
     c. Findings in osteoarthritis—WBC count less than 2000 cells/μl; negative culture; negative for crystals
  3. Laboratory—normal in primary osteoarthritis
     a. Rheumatoid factor (RF)/antinuclear antibodies (ANA)—if arthritis is inflammatory and symmetrical in distribution to exclude rheumatoid arthritis or systemic lupus erythematosus (SLE)
     b. Erythrocyte sedimentation rate—elevated in many autoimmune, inflammatory, infectious diseases
     c. CBC—if an inflammatory or infectious arthritis suspected

- Management/Treatment
  1. Nonpharmacologic
     a. Appliances, e.g., canes, crutches, orthotics
     b. Exercise—walking, swimming, stationary cycling
     c. Rest during acute exacerbations
     d. Supervised heat and cold therapy
     e. Weight loss if indicated
  2. Pharmacologic
     a. Nonsteroidal anti-inflammatory drugs (NSAIDs) as described for LBP
     b. Intra-articular injection
        (1) Glucocorticoids—beneficial in patients with inflammation, effusion, or substantial pain
        (2) Synovial fluid analog—sodium hyaluronate/hylan G-F20; usefulness documented in knee joints; safety in other joints not documented
  3. Patient education
     a. Symptomatic relief techniques, e.g., cold, heat, immobilization, rest
     b. Medication regimens and precautions

- Referral
  a. Physical therapy, exercise
  b. Need for joint injection
  c. Surgery consultation—joint replacement

Osteoporosis

- Definition—disease characterized by low bone mass and structural deterioration of bone tissue, leading to bone fragility and an increased susceptibility to fractures of the hip, spine, and wrist (National Institute of Health)

- Etiology/Incidence
  1. Combination of factors including nutrition, genetics, level of physical activity, age of menopause, and estrogen status
  2. 8 million American women and 2 million men have osteoporosis
  3. Accounts for more than 1.5 million fractures annually (70% women)
  4. Cost for hospital and nursing home stays for osteoporosis-associated fractures in excess of $10 billion annually
  5. Risk factors include:
     a. Female gender
     b. Advanced age
     c. Thin and/or small body frame
     d. Positive family history
     e. Caucasian or Asian
     f. Menopause
     g. Estrogen deficiency
     h. Calcium and/or vitamin D deficiency
     i. Use of certain medications—corticosteroids, anticonvulsants, heparin
     j. Sedentary lifestyle
     k. Cigarette smoking
     l. Excessive alcohol use

- Signs and symptoms
  1. Often a silent disease
  2. Backache
  3. Spontaneous fracture or collapse of vertebrae

- Physical findings
  1. Loss of height
  2. Kyphosis
  3. Fractures—spine, hip, wrist

- Differential diagnosis
  1. Malignancy—bone neoplasms, metastatic carcinoma, multiple myeloma
  2. Osteomalacia

3. Paget's disease
4. Secondary causes of osteoporosis include
   a. Hyperparathyroidism
   b. Hyperthyroidism
   c. Cushing's syndrome

- Diagnostic tests/findings
  1. Bone mineral density (BMD) tests
     a. World Health Organization definitions based on bone mass measurement in women include:
        (1) Normal—BMD within 1 standard deviation (SD) of a young normal adult; T-score above –1
        (2) Osteopenia (low bone mass)—BMD between 1 and 2.5 SD below that of a young normal adult; T-score between –1 and –2.5
        (3) Osteoporosis—BMD 2.5 SD or more or below that of a young normal adult; T-score at or below –2.5
     b. Dual-energy x-ray absorptiometry (DEXA)—most widely used; quick; radiation exposure one tenth of standard chest radiograph; body sites measured—hip, spine, wrist
     c. Single-energy x-ray absorpitometry (SXA)—small, portable; body sites measured—forearm, finger, heel
     d. Quantitative ultrasound (QUS)—recently developed, radiation-free technique using the transmission of high frequency sound waves; small and portable; body sites measured—heel, finger, tibia, radius
     e. Quantitative computed tomography (QCT)—measures trabecular and cortical bone density; body site measured—mainly spine
  2. Standard radiography—20–30% bone loss must occur for osteoporosis detection; used to detect osteoporotic fractures
  3. Laboratory tests if indicated to rule out secondary causes of osteoporosis—parathyroid hormone (PTH) level, TSH, dexamethasone suppression test and urine cortisol level for Cushing's syndrome
  4. Additional skeletal health assessment techniques
     a. Biochemical markers for bone turnover
     b. Vertebral fracture assessment
     c. Fracture risk algorithm (FRAX)—developed to calculate 10-year probability of hip fracture and 10-year probability of a major osteoporotic fracture taking into account femoral neck BMD and clinical risk factors

- Management/Treatment
  1. Nonpharmacologic—prevention and treatment
     a. Adequate intake of calcium and vitamin D—see Menopause section of Chapter 3
     b. Regular weight-bearing exercise
        (1) 30 minutes 3 to 4 times each week
        (2) Walking, stair climbing, dancing
     c. Regular muscle strengthening exercise—lifting weights, swimming
     d. Avoidance of tobacco use and alcohol abuse
     e. Fall prevention strategies—correct impaired vision, assess medications for potential to cause orthostatic hypotension, supportive low heeled shoes, assistive devices if needed (cane, walker), home safety measures
  2. Pharmacologic
     a. Consider pharmacologic treatment for postmenopausal women presenting with any of the following (National Osteoporosis Foundation, 2008):
        (1) Hip or vertebral fracture
        (2) T-score of –2.5 or less at the femoral neck or spine after appropriate evaluation to exclude secondary causes
        (3) T-score between –1.0 and –2.5 at femoral neck or spine and 10-year probability of hip fracture of 3% or greater; or a 10-year probability of major osteoporotic related fracture of 20% or greater based on FRAX
     b. Hormone therapy (HT)—may be considered short term (5 years) for prevention if needs treatment for vasomotor symptoms and/or vulvovaginal atrophy; not approved for treatment of existing osteoporosis (see Menopause section of Chapter 3)
     c. Bisphosphonates—alendronate/risedronate—indicated for prevention and treatment; ibandronate—oral form approved for prevention and treatment, intravenous form approved for treatment; zoledronic acid—intravenous form approved for treatment
        (1) Drug action—osteoclast mediated bone resorption inhibitor—bone formation exceeds bone resorption leading to progressive gains in bone mass
        (2) Side-effects—GI upset, abdominal pain, esophagitis, musculoskeletal pain, headache
        (3) Drug interactions—antacids and calcium interfere with absorption
        (4) Contraindications/precautions—esophageal stricture, inability to

stand/sit upright for at least 30 minutes, hypocalcemia, pregnancy risk category C; check serum creatinine before each ibandronate injection

    (5) Client instructions

        (a) Take with 8 oz of water in the morning at least 30 minutes before any beverage, food, or medication

        (b) Do not lie down for at least 30 minutes and until the first food of the day

        (c) May take acetaminophen prior to zoledronic acid injection to reduce risk of postinjection arthralgia, headache, myalgia, fever

d. Selective estrogen receptor modulators (SERM)—raloxifene—indicated for prevention and treatment

    (1) Drug action—estrogenlike effects on bones and lipid metabolism; lacks estrogenlike effect on uterus and breasts

    (2) Side-effects—hot flashes, leg cramps, venous thromboembolic events (rare)

    (3) Drug interactions—may antagonize warfarin

    (4) Contraindications—women who are pregnant or may become pregnant; active or history of venous thromboembolic events; do not give with estrogen or cholesterol lowering medication

e. Calcitonin-salmon—indicated for treatment only

    (1) Drug action—directly inhibits bone resorption of calcium; administered as a nasal spray or injection

    (2) Side-effects—nasal spray-rhinitis, GI upset; injection-GI upset, local inflammation, rash, flushing

    (3) Drug interactions—none reported

    (4) Contraindications—hypersensitivity to salmon calcitonin, pregnancy risk category C

f. Terparatide—approved for treatment if high risk for fracture

    (1) Drug action—anabolic bone building agent, parathyroid hormone; administered as subcutaneous injection

    (2) Side-effects—leg cramps, dizziness

    (3) Drug interactions—none reported

    (4) Contraindications/precautions—avoid if increased risk of osteosarcoma, prior radiation of skeleton, bone metastases, hypercalcemia

g. Monitoring pharmacologic therapy effectiveness

    (1) Baseline BMD before onset of therapy

    (2) Repeat test every 2 years; more frequently if warranted by certain clinical situations

    (3) Urine/serum biochemical markers of bone formation or resorption may be used as adjunct to monitor response to therapy—variable results and precision error limit usefulness; changes must be large in order to be clinically meaningful

3. Patient education

    a. Adequate calcium and vitamin D intake

    b. Weight-bearing and muscle strengthening exercises

    c. Avoidance of tobacco and excessive alcohol

    d. Fall prevention strategies

    e. Medication use

Fibromyalgia

- Definition
  1. A syndrome characterized by chronic fatigue, generalized musculoskeletal pain and stiffness associated with the finding of characteristic tender points of pain on physical examination
  2. Criteria for the classification of fibromyalgia
     a. Widespread pain for more than 3 months
     b. Pain on palpation in at least 11 of 18 selected tender points

- Etiology/Incidence
  1. Etiology—unknown, but classified as a rheumatic disease; several causal mechanisms postulated
     a. Physical or mental stress
     b. Sleep disturbances
     c. Decreased serotonin levels
     d. Metabolic factors
     e. Viral infection—Epstein-Barr virus, cytomegalovirus, herpes virus, enteroviruses
  2. Incidence—unknown in general population due to misdiagnosis, self-treatment
     a. More common in women, with a 9:1 female/male ratio
     b. Most common in 30 to 50 year olds

- Signs and symptoms
  1. Multiple, specific areas of muscle tenderness ("trigger points")
  2. Fatigue, sleep disturbances
  3. Muscle weakness and generalized aching
  4. Pain typically worsens with cold
  5. Paresthesias
  6. Headaches
  7. Anxiety, stress
  8. Depression

- Physical findings
  1. Pain on digital palpation of characteristic tender points
  2. Normal muscle strength, range of motion

- Differential diagnosis
  1. Chronic fatigue syndrome
  2. Rheumatoid arthritis
  3. SLE
  4. Somatization and depression

- Diagnostic tests/findings
  1. Unnecessary unless a coexisting condition is suspected
  2. Erythrocyte sedimentation rate normal; excludes inflammatory conditions

- Management/Treatment
  1. Nonpharmacologic
     a. Low impact exercise, e.g., walking, swimming
     b. Supervised heat and cold therapy
     c. Massage, relaxation therapy
     d. Biofeedback
     e. Hypnotherapy
     f. Strength training
  2. Pharmacologic
     a. Mild analgesics
     b. Selective serotonin and norepinephrine reuptake inhibitors—duloxetine
     c. Tricyclic antidepressants for sleep disturbance—amitryptyline
     d. Pregabalin
        (1) Drug action—binds to calcium channels on nerves and may modify the release of neurotransmitters
        (2) Side-effects—dizziness, somnolence, other central nervous system effects
        (3) Contraindications/precautions—avoid abrupt cessation; pregnancy category C; not recommended in nursing mothers
     e. Tramadol
        (1) Drug action—centrally acting analgesic; creates a weak bond to opioid receptors and inhibits reuptake of both norepinephrine and serotonin
        (2) Side-effects—drowsiness, dizziness, headache, nausea, and constipation
        (3) Drug interactions—seizure risk with other agents that lower threshold/MAOIs, SSRIs; potentiated with alcohol and other CNS depressants
        (4) Contraindications/precautions—abuse potential; pregnancy category C; not recommended in nursing mothers
  3. Patient education
     a. Reassurance regarding benign course of condition
     b. Supportive care for chronic pain

- Referral—physical therapy

Strains/Sprains

- Definition—musculoskeletal injury of varying degrees
  1. Strain refers to injury to muscle or tendon
  2. Sprain refers to stretching or tearing of ligaments

- Etiology/Incidence
  1. Etiology
     a. Overuse of the muscle–tendon unit by stretching, tearing, hyperextension, forceful contraction
     b. Acute injury
     c. Chronic overuse as seen in sports injury, repetitive motion
  2. Incidence—unknown due to frequent self-treatment, but common presenting complaint in primary care practice
  3. Risk factors
     a. Increased physical activity
     b. New physical exercise program
     c. Overweight

- Signs and symptoms
  1. Pain at site of injury
  2. Strain
     a. Temporary weakness
     b. Pain with stretch of muscle
     c. Pain and spasm with more severe strains
  3. Sprain
     a. Marked swelling
     b. Loss of function

- Physical findings
  1. Strain—temporarily reduced range of motion, muscle strength
  2. Sprain
     a. Contusion, hemorrhage
     b. Reduced range of motion, muscle strength
     c. Joint instability in severe sprain or ruptured ligament

- Differential diagnosis
  1. Other overuse syndromes—tendonitis, shin splints
  2. Fracture

- Diagnostic tests/findings
  1. Radiograph to rule out fractures—negative for bony abnormality in strains/sprains
  2. MRI

- Management/Treatment
  1. Nonpharmacologic
     a. "RICE"—initial therapeutic strategy
        (1) *R*est or immobilization of injured part
        (2) *I*ce or application of cold
        (3) *C*ompression, elastic wrap
        (4) *E*levation of affected area
     b. Application of heat 24 to 36 hours after injury
     c. Topical heat-generating liniments for symptomatic relief
  2. Pharmacologic
     a. Usually none indicated, not curative
     b. NSAIDs as for acute LBP
  3. Patient education
     a. Physical training progression to avoid repeat injury
     b. Stretching and warm-up exercises
     c. Appropriate footwear, protective gear for exercise

- Referral
  1. Physical therapy for stretching and strengthening program
  2. Consult orthopedic surgeon if no response to conservative management

◘ NEUROLOGIC DISORDERS

Headaches

- Definition
  1. Headache/cephalagia is defined as diffuse pain in various parts of the head
  2. Primary headaches—migraine, tension, cluster headaches are not directly related to a specific underlying cause or secondary to another problem
  3. Secondary headaches are the result of identifiable structural or physiologic pathology

- Etiology/Incidence/Risk factors
  1. Etiology
     a. Primary headaches—90–98% of headaches presenting in primary care
        (1) Migraine headache
           (a) Current understanding suggests genetic basis
           (b) Those genetically predisposed inherit a nervous system that is more sensitive/easily aroused to a variety of internal/external factors—hormonal fluctuations, weather changes, diet, psychosocial disruptions
           (c) Changes in serotonin activity result in release of vasoactive mediators; mediators produce an inflammatory response adjacent to cerebral blood vessels accompanied by vasodilation
           (d) The dilated vessels and inflammatory response stimulate the trigeminal nerve to transmit impulses to the brain resulting in migraine headache
        (2) Tension headache
           (a) Pathophysiology poorly understood; formerly attributed to contraction of the muscles of the scalp and neck
           (b) Recent theories suggest tension headaches may involve changes in the intracranial neurotransmitter and vascular systems similar to migraine
           (c) Symptom complex resulting from several simultaneous processes—muscle tension, psychological stress, neurovascular changes
        (3) Cluster headache
           (a) Secondary to serotonergic neurologic dysfunction
           (b) Clustering of attacks suggests involvement of circadian pacemakers of the anterior hypothalamus
           (c) Tearing and nasal stuffiness suggests abnormality in autonomic nervous system
     b. Secondary headaches
        (1) Vascular disorders—subarachnoid, cerebral, cerebellar hemorrhage; acute ischemic cerebrovascular disorder; AV malformation; temporal arteritis; arterial HTN
        (2) Nonvascular intracranial disorders—neoplasm; infection; low cerebrospinal fluid pressure/post lumbar puncture; benign intracranial HTN/pseudotumor cerebri
        (3) Traumatic—concussion and postconcussion; hematoma/subdural and epidural
        (4) Metabolic disorders—hypoxia, hypercapnia, hypoglycemia
        (5) Substances that act as triggers—medications; foods/MSG, alcohol; exposures/carbon monoxide; rebound/caffeine, analgesics

(6) Extracranial structures—eyes/
glaucoma, refractive errors; sinusitis;
temporomandibular joint dysfunction; neck/cervical disk disease;
trigeminal neuralgia

(7) Systemic—infection; allergies/pollen;
hormonal

2. Incidence
   a. Migraine
      (1) Reported in up to 15–17% of women;
          5% of men
      (2) Estimated 10% of adults affected
   b. Tension—lifetime prevalence of 90%;
      yearly prevalence 80–90%
   c. Cluster—relatively rare incidence com-
      pared to other types; six times more com-
      mon in males

3. Risk factors—primary headache syndromes
   a. Migraine headaches—female gender, fam-
      ily history
   b. Tension headaches—overuse of headache
      medications
   c. Cluster headaches—male, middle-aged or
      older

- Signs and symptoms
  1. Migraine
     a. Types
        (1) Migraine with aura/classic migraine
            (a) Aura consists of focal neurologic
                symptoms that may precede or
                accompany headache
            (b) Usually visual phenomenon;
                flashing lights, zigzag/jagged
                lines, difficulty focusing
        (2) Migraine without aura/common
            migraine—accounts for 75% of
            migraines
        (3) Complicated migraine—basilar/
            hemiplegic migraine
     b. Phases
        (1) Prodrome—occurs 24 hours prior to
            onset of headache: fatigue, euphoria,
            difficulty concentrating, irritability
        (2) Aura
        (3) Early and late stages of migraine
        (4) Postdrome—individual feels "wiped
            out," fatigued, "hung-over"
     c. Triggers
        (1) Stress
        (2) Hormonal changes
        (3) Certain foods, caffeine, alcohol, skip-
            ping meals
        (4) Fatigue, oversleeping
        (5) Medications

(6) Changes in weather or barometric
    pressure
   d. Location—unilateral tendency
   e. Duration—4–72 hours
   f. Character
      (1) Moderate to severe intensity; inhibits
          daily activities
      (2) Characterized as throbbing, pounding
   g. Associated symptoms—nausea, vomiting,
      photophobia, phonophobia, fatigue
   h. Frequency—recurrent, variable from two
      to three per year to two to three per week

2. Tension headache
   a. Onset—gradual
   b. Location—diffuse, bilateral, generalized
   c. Duration—variable, hours to days
   d. Character
      (1) Mild to moderate severity; generally
          able to continue with daily activities
      (2) Dull, pressure, constant, vise-like
   e. Associated symptoms—fatigue, irritability,
      difficulty concentrating, neck and shoul-
      der spasm
   f. Frequency
      (1) Episodic—less than 15 days per
          month
      (2) Chronic—must be present 15 days or
          more a month for at least 6 months

3. Cluster headaches
   a. Onset
      (1) Abrupt
      (2) Often nocturnal, awakens patient; of-
          ten recurs at same time of day
   b. Location
      (1) Unilateral
      (2) During a series, pain remains on same
          side
      (3) Retro-orbital, sometimes radiating
   c. Duration—usually 30 to 45 minutes
   d. Character—intense, severe
   e. Associated symptoms—facial pain, ptosis
      of the affected side, lacrimation, nasal
      congestion
   f. Frequency—occurs in clusters lasting a
      few weeks with remission lasting weeks to
      months

- Physical findings
  1. General appearance indicates discomfort
  2. Neurologic assessment normal in primary
     headaches—occasional temporary focal neu-
     rologic findings with migraine
  3. Blood pressure, vital signs normal
  4. Cluster headache—unilaterally constricted
     pupil, nasal discharge

- Differential diagnosis—"red flags" suggesting secondary causes
  1. Headache beginning after 50 years of age—temporal arteritis, mass lesion
  2. Sudden onset, worst headache—subarachnoid hemorrhage
  3. Headaches increasing in severity/frequency—mass lesion, subdural hematoma, medication overuse
  4. Focal neurologic signs/papilledema
  5. Headache subsequent to head trauma—intracranial hemorrhage, subdural/epidural hematoma, posttraumatic headache
  6. Systemic illness/fever—meningitis/encephalitis

- Diagnostic tests/findings
  1. None indicated when examination is consistent with primary headache syndromes
  2. Erythrocyte sedimentation rate on all patients with new onset older than 40 years to rule out temporal arteritis
  3. CT/MRI
     a. Indicated if persistent focal neurologic findings or history of trauma
     b. CT preferred to identify acute hemorrhage
     c. MRI more sensitive in identifying pathologic intracranial changes
     d. Magnetic resonance angiography if aneurysm suspected—history of exertional headaches

- Management/Treatment
  1. Nonpharmacologic
     a. Regular sleep and meal schedules
     b. Daily exercise
     c. Avoiding known triggers
  2. Pharmacologic
     a. Migraine
        (1) Abortive therapy
            (a) First line therapy—mild-to-moderate intensity
                i. NSAIDs, acetaminophen (see Acute Otitis Media this chapter)
                ii. Excedrin migraine—aspirin, acetaminophen, caffeine/59% efficacy at 2 hours
            (b) First line therapy—moderate-to-severe intensity—triptans
                i. Agents—sumatriptan, zolmitriptan, naratriptan, rizatriptan, almotriptan, frovatriptan; available in oral, nasal, SC forms
                ii. Drug action—selective serotonin agonists
                iii. Side-effects—tightness of the throat/chest, flushing, numbness, tingling, dizziness; side-effects tend to abate with time
                iv. Drug interactions—should not be used within 24 hours after another triptan or any ergotamine-containing drug
                v. Contraindications/precautions—coronary artery disease, hypertension; pregnancy category C; caution in lactation
            (c) Second line—ergotamines
                i. Agents—ergotamine, dihydroergotamine/parenteral and nasal spray
                ii. Drug action—nonspecific serotonin agonist and vasoconstrictor
                iii. Side-effects—nausea/vomiting (premedicate with anti-emetic), tachycardia, vasoconstriction
                iv. Drug interactions—do not give with triptan
                v. Contraindications/precautions—coronary artery disease, hypertension; pregnancy category X; not recommended while nursing
        (2) Prophylactic therapy—consider in patients who experience more than two severe headaches per month, need acute treatment medication more than two times per week or are unable to tolerate abortive agents
            (a) Beta-blocker—propranolol/timolol (see Table 8-1)
            (b) Calcium channel blockers—verapamil (see Table 8-1)
            (c) Anti-epileptic agents—valproic acid (see **Table 8-7**)
     b. Tension
        (1) Episodic
            (a) NSAIDs, acetaminophen (see Acute Otitis Media this chapter)
            (b) Caffeine, butalbital, acetaminophen (Fioricet) and caffeine, aspirin (Fiorinal)
                i. Drug action—butalbital is a barbiturate; muscle relaxant at lower doses, hypnotic at higher doses
                ii. Side-effects—drowsiness, lightheadedness, nausea, vomiting

■ **Table 8-7**   Commonly Used Anti-epileptic Drugs (AED) (representative list)

Drug	Action	Side-effects	Interactions	Contraindications
Phenytoin	Stabilizes membranes and prevents spread of seizure from hyperactive focus	Nystagmus, drowsiness, ataxia, diplopia, gingival hyperplasia, hirsutism, low folate level	Antagonizes oral contraceptives, digoxin, oral anti-coagulants; potentiated by benzodiazepines, estrogens, H$_2$-blockers; other AED	Heart block, sinus bradycardia; pregnancy category D; not recommended while nursing
Carbamazepine	Delays recovery of sodium channels from their inactivated state; inhibits sustained repetitive firing	Sedation, GI upset, ataxia, blurred vision, skin rash, aplastic anemia	Increased plasma levels with CYP3A4 inhibitors-INH, macrolides; decreased plasma levels with CYP3A4 inducers-phenytoin	History of bone marrow depression; pregnancy category D; do not use while nursing
Valproic acid	Increased brain levels of neurotransmitter GABA, which has an inhibitory effect on seizures	Nausea, vomiting, sedation, blood dyscrasias	Potentiates phenobarbital, phenytoin	Pregnancy category D; do not use while nursing; liver disease or dysfunction
Clonazepam	Enhances GABA action; depresses nerve transmission in motor cortex	Fatigue, sedation, behavior changes—aggressiveness and confusion	Potentiates CNS depression with alcohol; antagonized by phenytoin, carbamazepine	Liver disease; acute angle-closure glaucoma; pregnancy category C; not recommended for nursing mothers
Topiramate	Enhances GABA action	Drowsiness, dizziness, ataxia, fatigue, visual disorders	Potentiates CNS depression with alcohol; potentiates phenobarbital, phenytoin; antagonized by carbamazepine, phenobarbital, phenytoin, valproic acid, verapamil	Acute myopia and secondary angle-closure glaucoma, hepatic or renal impairment, kidney stones; pregnancy category C

iii. Drug interactions—potentiation with alcohol, CNS depressants

iv. Contraindications/precautions—hepatic impairment; pregnancy category C; not recommended in nursing mothers

(2) Chronic

  (a) Tricyclic antidepressants (TCAs)—amitriptyline, nortriptyline

   i. Action—increases synaptic concentration of serotonin and norepinephrine in CNS

   ii. Side-effects—sedation, dry mouth, blurred vision, constipation, abnormal cardiac conduction, dysrhythmias

   iii. Drug interactions—additive anticholinergic effects

   iv. Contraindications—with MAOI, impaired liver function; pregnancy category C; not recommended while nursing

  (b) Selective serotoin reuptake inhibitors—less effective than TCAs (see Depression this chapter)

3. Patient education

  a. Signs indicating need for emergency treatment

   (1) Acute fever with headache

   (2) Abnormal mental status or personality changes

   (3) Sudden onset; worst headache experienced

   (4) Neurologic symptoms, e.g., projectile emesis, visual disturbances

  b. Self-medication for abortive therapy, injections

  c. Education regarding nonpharmacologic management—avoidance of precipitating factors

- Referral
1. Focal neurologic findings
2. Specific secondary diagnosis is suspected
3. Chronic headaches develop new features
4. New headaches in individuals older than 50 years

Seizure Disorders

- Definition
1. Sudden change in body functioning with or without loss of consciousness due to an abnormal discharge of neurons

  a. Think of seizure as positive phenomenon such as movement versus negative phenomenon such as paralysis in transient ischemic attack (TIA)

  b. Where the discharge arises and how far it spreads determines what the seizure looks like clinically

2. Classification of seizures

  a. Partial seizures occur within localized regions of the brain; result of a localized physiologic or structural abnormality in the brain

   (1) Simple partial—consciousness not impaired

   (2) Complex partial—consciousness impaired

   (3) Partial with secondary generalization

  b. Generalized seizures arise from both sides of the brain simultaneously

   (1) Tonic-clonic (formerly "grand mal")

   (2) Absence (formerly "petit mal")

   (3) Myoclonic

   (4) Atonic

- Etiology/Incidence
1. Etiology

  a. First step in evaluation of suspected seizure is to determine whether event was a seizure

  b. Once event identified as a seizure, need to determine if epilepsy or secondary to another medical problem—hypoxia, hypoglycemia, infection, fever, toxic substance abuse

  c. Epilepsy is characterized by recurrent seizures; can be secondary to inherited or acquired factors

   (1) Head injury

   (2) Brain tumor

   (3) Cerebrovascular events

   (4) Idiopathic

2. Incidence

  a. Recurrence rate widely variable, linked to etiology

  b. Complex partial seizures most common adult type

  c. Absence seizures most common in childhood

3. Risk factors

  a. Inherited neurologic disease

  b. History of trauma

  c. In persons with known seizure disorders

   (1) Sleep deprivation

   (2) Unusual stresses

   (3) Menstruation

   (4) Medications/drugs

- Signs and symptoms
  1. Partial seizures
     a. Simple partial
        (1) Lasts 5–10 seconds
        (2) No loss of consciousness; no postseizure confusion
        (3) Symptoms reflect focal area of brain affected
            (a) Jerking or shaking in one area of body; may progress as focus spreads along cortical motor strip
            (b) Somatosensory symptoms
            (c) Visual or auditory symptoms
            (d) Autonomic symptoms—sweating, epigastric discomfort
            (e) Psychic symptoms
     b. Complex partial
        (1) Duration—5–10 seconds; 1–2 minutes; rarely more than 5 minutes
        (2) Loss of consciousness; postseizure confusion
        (3) Blank stare followed by an automatism, e.g., lip smacking, picking at clothing, purposeless walking
  2. Generalized seizures—always involve loss of consciousness
     a. Tonic-clonic seizures (grand mal)
        (1) Tonic phase—all skeletal muscles contract and patient falls
        (2) Clonic phase
            (a) Repetitive motor activity of all extremities
            (b) As clonic phases abate muscles become flaccid and incontinence can occur
        (3) Postictal period
            (a) Consciousness may not return for 10–15 minutes
            (b) Confusion, headache and fatigue may last from hours to days
     b. Absence seizure
        (1) Duration—5–10 seconds; may cluster
        (2) Manifest with blank stare, eye blinking
        (3) No postseizure confusion
     c. Myoclonic seizure
        (1) Quick, involuntary muscle jerks lasting a few seconds involving one body part or entire body
        (2) May accompany other generalized seizures; common to specific epilepsy syndromes
     d. Atonic
        (1) Sudden loss of postural tone causing patient to fall
        (2) Often associated with other seizure types; common in Lennox-Gastaut syndrome

- Physical findings
  1. Often no physical findings
  2. Focus physical examination on cardiovascular and neurologic systems
     a. Normal neurologic examination found in patients with idiopathic seizures
     b. Focal neurologic findings—brain lesion

- Differential diagnosis
  1. Vascular events, e.g., transient ischemic attack (TIA), classic migraine
  2. Syncope
  3. Hyperventilation/anxiety attacks
  4. Narcolepsy
  5. Psychogenic spells, e.g., transient global amnesia

- Diagnostic tests/findings
  1. Electrolytes, glucose, BUN/creatinine, LFTs, calcium, magnesium
  2. Toxicology screen
  3. CBC
  4. Lumbar puncture if infection is a consideration
  5. CT can detect bleeding or gross structural lesions
  6. MRI is study of choice; more sensitive and specific for evaluating structural lesions and brain parenchyma
  7. EEG
     a. Used to establish presence and type of epilepsy
     b. Initial EEG abnormal in only 40% of patients with probable epilepsy

- Management/Treatment
  1. Nonpharmacologic—avoidance of triggers
  2. Pharmacologic (see Table 8-7)
     a. Principles
        (1) Goal—complete suppression of seizures
        (2) Initial treatment—single drug
        (3) Blood levels should be monitored periodically
        (4) When adding a second drug, maintain the first drug, titrating dosages after second drug reaches therapeutic levels
        (5) Treatment withdrawal should not be considered until seizure-free for a minimum of 2 years
     b. Pharmacologic management by seizure type
        (1) Partial seizures—carbamazepine, phenytoin, topiramate
        (2) Generalized seizures

(a) Tonic-clonic seizures—phenytoin, carbamazepine, valproic acid, topiramate

(b) Absence—valproic acid, ethosuximide

(c) Myoclonic—valproic acid, clonazepam

(d) Atonic—clonazepam

3. Patient education
    a. Pregnancy and contraception
        (1) Impact on seizure frequency, severity variable
        (2) Teratogenic effects of seizure medications
        (3) Decreased oral contraceptive efficacy with many antiseizure medications; select backup or alternative method
    b. Safety issues regarding recurrent seizures
        (1) Activity limitations, e.g., driving
        (2) Possible need for protective wear
        (3) Household hazards identification and modification
    c. Medication schedules and side-effects

- Referral
    1. All clients with first-time seizures
    2. Uncontrolled seizures
    3. For EEG and interpretation
    4. Suspected underlying metabolic disease, neural lesion
    5. Pregnancy care

❑ DERMATOLOGIC DISORDERS

Acne

- Definition—a common self-limited disease that presents with a variety of lesions including open and closed comedones, papules and pustules, nodules, and cysts

- Etiology/Incidence
    1. Etiology
        a. Primary cause is obstruction of the pilosebaceous follicle
        b. Characterized by plugging of the hair follicle with abnormally cohesive desquamated cells, sebaceous gland hyperactivity, proliferation of bacteria (*P. acnes*), and inflammation
        c. Obstruction of follicle leads to development of noninflammatory acne—closed comedones/white heads and open comedones/black heads
        d. Proliferation of *P. acnes*/rupture of follicle wall results in inflammatory acne with papules, pustules, nodules, cysts

    2. Incidence
        a. Affects up to 90% of teens; 15% have moderate-to-severe acne
        b. May persist to older than 40 years in some, especially women
    3. Risk factors
        a. Aggravated by stress, hormonal cycling
        b. Use of topical steroids
        c. Contact with irritant oils or cosmetics
        d. More common and more severe in males

- Signs and symptoms
    1. Erythematous lesions, sometimes tender
    2. May be episodic, cyclic in severity
    3. Distribution and severity tends to be similar in family members

- Physical findings
    1. Lesions occur primarily on the face, but neck, shoulders, chest and back may be involved
    2. Mild—open and closed comedones without inflammation
    3. Moderate—comedones with papules and pustules
    4. Severe—comedones, papules and pustules with nodules, cysts and scarring

- Differential diagnosis
    1. Rosacea
    2. Pyoderma
    3. Drug eruptions
    4. Underlying endocrine disease—polycystic ovarian syndrome, Cushing's syndrome
    5. Folliculitis
    6. Perioral dermatitis

- Diagnostic tests/findings—none indicated

- Management/Treatment
    1. Nonpharmacologic—cleansing
    2. Pharmacologic
        a. Mild acne—topical medications
            (1) Benzoyl peroxide
                (a) Drug action—antibacterial and comedolytic properties
                (b) Side-effects
                    i. Skin irritation
                    ii. Allergic dermatitis
                    iii. May bleach clothing/bed linens, hair
                (c) Drug interactions—PABA sunscreens may temporarily discolor skin
                (d) Contraindications/precautions
                    i. Avoid eyes, mouth, mucous membranes

ii. Pregnancy category C; precaution in nursing mothers

(2) Retinoic acid derivatives—tretinoin/cream, gel, lotion, and microspheres; adapalene gel/solution; tazarotene gel
   (a) Drug action—comedolytic agent
   (b) Side-effects—local irritation, erythema, scaling
   (c) Drug interactions—concomitant use with benzoyl peroxide may cause skin irritation
   (d) Contraindications/precautions
      i. Avoid UV light, sun, extreme weather
      ii. Do not use with eczema
      iii. Pregnancy category C; not recommended while nursing

(3) Azelaic acid
   (a) Drug action—antibacterial and normalizes keratinization
   (b) Side-effects
      i. Local irritation, itching, contact dermatitis
      ii. Depigmentation
   (c) Drug interactions—none identified
   (d) Contraindications/precautions—pregnancy category B; caution in nursing mothers

b. Moderate acne—topical antibiotics
(1) Topical antibiotics—clindamycin, erythromycin
   (a) Drug action—bactericidal effects
   (b) Side-effects
      i. Local irritation
      ii. Folliculitis
   (c) Drug interactions—additive effect with other topical agents
   (d) Contraindications/precautions
      i. Avoid eyes, mucous membranes
      ii. History of regional enteritis, ulcerative or antibiotic-induced colitis/clindamycin
      iii. Pregnancy category B/C; not recommended while nursing

(2) Oral medications—tetracycline, doxycycline, minocycline; erythromycin, azithromycin
   (a) Drug action (tetracycline and its derivatives)—antibacterial and anti-inflammatory effect
   (b) Side-effects
      i. GI effects
      ii. Photosensitivity
      iii. Yeast infections

   (c) Drug interactions—reduced absorption with antacids
   (d) Contraindications/precautions—pregnancy Category D; not recommended in nursing mothers

(3) Oral contraceptives—some have FDA approval for treatment of moderate acne in women who also desire contraception; all with low androgenic or antiandrogenic progestin are likely effective
   (a) Drug action—antiandrogenic/decreases free testosterone available for metabolism in sebaceous glands
   (b) Side-effects
      i. Nausea, vomiting
      ii. Minor bleeding irregularities, headaches
      iii. Hypertension
      iv. Thromboembolic events
   (c) Drug interactions—antagonized by hepatic enzyme inducing drugs, e.g., griseofulvin, rifampin
   (d) Contraindications
      i. Thromboembolic disorders
      ii. Known or suspected estrogen-dependent neoplasm
      iii. History of cardiovascular or cerebrovascular disease
      iv. Pregnancy category X; not recommended in nursing mothers

c. Severe acne—isotretinoin
(1) Drug action—decreases size and secretion of sebaceous glands, normalizes follicular keratinization, inhibits *P. acnes,* and modulates the inflammatory response
(2) Side-effects
   (a) Liver function test abnormalities
   (b) Anemia, depression
   (c) Skin and mucosal dryness
   (d) Tendonitis
   (e) Lipid abnormalities, pancreatitis
(3) Drug interactions
   (a) Tetracyclines may increase incidence of pseudotumor cerebri
   (b) Avoid alcohol
   (c) Vitamin A
(4) Contraindications/precautions—Pregnancy category X; not recommended while nursing

3. Patient education
a. Use of mild cleansers, noncomedogenic moisturizers, sunscreen

b. "Hands off" policy to avoid secondary infection, scarring

c. Importance of avoiding pregnancy if using isotretinoin

- Referral—severe acne; may refer patients requiring treatment with isotretinoin

Contact Dermatitis

- Definition—skin inflammation due to irritants (irritant contact dermatitis) or allergens (allergic contact dermatitis)

- Etiology/Risk factors
  1. Etiology
     a. Irritant contact dermatitis
        (1) Eczematous response that is nonallergic caused by irritants including chemicals, dry and cold air, and friction
        (2) May occur acutely, more commonly occurs after chronic exposure
     b. Allergic contact dermatitis
        (1) A manifestation of cell-mediated hypersensitivity; causes delayed reaction on first exposure
        (2) Rhus plant antigens (poison oak, poison ivy) will result in clinical eruption in 12–72 hours and within minutes on reexposure
        (3) Other common allergic sensitizers include nickel (jewelry), rubber compounds (gloves), cosmetics, topical medications
  2. Risk factors
     a. Irritant contact dermatitis
        (1) Everyone at risk; people vary in response
        (2) Frequent exposure; chronic exposure
     b. Allergic contact dermatitis—genetically predisposed reaction

- Signs and symptoms
  1. Report of recent exposure (within 24 hours) to known allergens; exposure to irritants
  2. Pruritus

- Physical findings
  1. Irritant contact dermatitis
     a. Mild irritants cause erythema, dryness, fissuring
     b. Chronic exposure may cause oozing, weeping lesions
  2. Allergic contact dermatitis
     a. Classic lesions are vesicles and blisters on erythematous base

b. Linear eruption is the hallmark of most plant dermatoses

3. Distribution often provides clues to diagnosis

- Differential diagnosis
  1. Atopic dermatitis, eczema
  2. Tinea
  3. Scabies/pediculosis
  4. Herpes simplex/Herpes zoster

- Diagnostic tests/findings
  1. Usually none indicated
  2. Negative potassium hydroxide (KOH) preparation of skin scraping
  3. Patch testing with suspected allergens in difficult cases

- Management/Treatment
  1. Nonpharmacologic
     a. Compresses, soaks, e.g., Burow's solution, Epsom salts
     b. Lubricants—lubricating ointments, petrolatum, no creams
  2. Pharmacologic
     a. Topical corticosteroids—intermediate potency for mild/moderate dermatitis; hydrocortisone for face/groin
        (1) Drug action—anti-inflammatory effect
        (2) Side-effects
           (a) Local irritation
           (b) Epidermal and dermal atrophy
        (3) Drug interactions—none identified
        (4) Contraindications/precautions
           (a) Avoid prolonged use on large areas
           (b) Pregnancy category C; not recommended while nursing
     b. Systemic steroids for widespread or severe dermatitis (see Table 8-3)
     c. Antihistamines—allergic pruritus
        (1) Hydroxyzine
           (a) Drug action—antihistamine
           (b) Side-effects—drowsiness, dry mouth
           (c) Drug interactions—potentiates CNS depression with alcohol, other CNS depressants
           (d) Contraindications—early pregnancy; nursing mothers
        (2) Cetirizine (see Table 8-2)
  3. Patient education
     a. Avoidance of allergens
     b. Protective garments, gloves

Skin Cancer

- Definition—malignant neoplasms arising in skin cells

- Etiology/Incidence/Risk factors
  1. Etiology
     a. Basal cell carcinoma (BCC)
        (1) Slow growing, rarely metastasizes, but may cause extensive local tissue damage
        (2) Tumor arises in basal layer of epidermis; causes include chronic sun exposure and genetic predisposition
     b. Squamous cell carcinoma (SCC)
        (1) Directly attributable to sun exposure or chronic irritation
        (2) 60% occur at site of previous actinic keratoses
        (3) Low tendency for metastasis
     c. Malignant melanoma (MM)
        (1) Arises from cells of the melanocyte system; begins either de novo or develops from preexisting lesion
        (2) Initially grows superficially and laterally; enters vertical growth phase with potential to metastasize
  2. Incidence
     a. Basal cell approximately 75% all skin cancers
     b. Squamous cell second most common skin cancer in whites; most common skin cancer in blacks
     c. Malignant melanoma represents 1% of skin cancers; 60% of skin cancer deaths
  3. Risk factors
     a. Nonmelanoma skin cancers
        (1) Cumulative sun exposure; higher incidence in outdoor workers
        (2) White race; fair complexion that burns easily/tans poorly
        (3) Advancing age
        (4) Male gender
        (5) Previous history of skin cancer
     b. Malignant melanoma
        (1) History of changing mole
        (2) Family and or personal history of melanoma
        (3) History of nonmelanoma skin cancer
        (4) Atypical nevus syndrome
        (5) Fair complexion; tendency to sunburn

- Signs and symptoms
  1. Basal cell—painless, slow-growing lesion on exposed areas
  2. Squamous cell
     a. Lesions seen in sun-exposed areas or skin damaged by burns or chronic inflammation; lower lip lesions common
     b. A skin lesion that does not heal
  3. Malignant melanoma
     a. Changing nevus; change in color, diameter increase, or border change
     b. Pruritus is early symptom
     c. Bleeding, ulceration, discomfort are late signs

- Physical findings
  1. Basal cell—several clinical variants; nodular basal cell most common
     a. Waxy, semitranslucent nodule with rolled borders
     b. Central ulcerations; telangectasias
  2. Squamous cell
     a. Red/reddish brown plaque/nodule
     b. Surface is scaly/crusted with erosions or ulcerations
  3. Malignant melanoma—tends to have *A*symmetry, *B*order irregularity, *C*olor variations and *D*iameter greater than 6 mm (ABCD)
     a. Superficial spreading type/70%—prolonged horizontal growth phase; vertical growth occurs later
     b. Nodular—raised, pigmented (blue, black, dark brown, gray) nodules with normal surrounding skin
     c. Acral lentiginous—found on palms, soles, nail beds, mucous membranes
     d. Lentigo melanoma—occurs in preexisting lentigo maligna

- Differential diagnosis
  1. Common melanocytic nevus
  2. Seborrheic keratosis
  3. Dermatofibroma

- Diagnostic tests/findings—biopsy

- Management/Treatment
  1. Nonpharmacologic/pharmacologic
     a. Excision and biopsy of lesions
     b. Basal cell carcinoma/squamous cell carcinoma—treatment options
        (1) Mohs' micrographic surgery—gradual lesion excision using serial frozen section analysis and mapping of excised tissue until tumor-free plane reached
        (2) Cryotherapy
        (3) Curettage with electrodesiccation/freezing
     c. Malignant melanoma
        (1) Excision of lesion
        (2) Lymph node dissection

(3) Adjunctive therapy—chemotherapy, radiation, excision of metastasis

(4) Long-term follow-up

2. Patient education—focused on prevention

a. Reduce exposure

(1) Avoid sun exposure

(2) Use of sunscreen with sun protective factor (SPF) of 15 or greater

(3) Protective clothing

(4) Educate regarding risk of tanning salons

b. Educate regarding the acronym ABCD; useful reminder of the clinical features that should raise suspicion of melanoma in a pigmented lesion

c. Total cutaneous examination (TCE)—recommended annually for populations with risk factors

(1) Complete visual inspection of skin, scalp, hands and feet for any suspicious lesions

(2) Include questions regarding risk, exposures, family history

(3) Best preventive practice to reduce mortality

d. Self-examination for lesions, changing nevi

- Referral for ongoing care (chemotherapy, immunotherapy)

Tinea

- Definition
  1. Superficial fungal infection caused by dermatophytes
  2. Dermatophytes require keratin for growth; infection restricted to hair, superficial skin, and nails
  3. Classified according to involved anatomic location
     a. Tinea capitis—scalp; mainly affects children
     b. Tinea corporis—body
     c. Tinea cruris—upper inner thigh/spares scrotum
     d. Tinea pedis—toe webs; soles/heels
     e. Tinea unguium—toenails more frequently involved than fingernails

- Etiology/Incidence/Risk factors
  1. Etiology
     a. *Microsporum, Trichophyton, Epidermophyton* species
     b. Transmission via contact with infected persons, fomites (shoes, towels, shower stalls), animals, or soil

2. Incidence
   a. Scalp infections more common in children
   b. Affects males/females about equally
   c. Intertriginous infections common in young adults
   d. Tinea pedis clinically apparent in 5–10% of population
3. Risk factors
   a. Tinea capitis—overcrowding and poor hygiene
   b. Tinea cruris—hot, humid conditions, occlusive clothing
   c. Tinea unguium—aging, diabetes, poorly fitting shoes, and tinea pedis

- Signs and symptoms
  1. May be asymptomatic
  2. Itching, burning variable

- Physical findings
  1. Classic presentation is a lesion with central clearing surrounded by an advancing, red scaly, elevated border
  2. Scalp lesions characterized by hair loss/scaling
  3. Maceration, especially intertriginous lesions
  4. Involved nails are yellowish/thickened with subungual debris

- Diagnostic tests/findings
  1. Potassium hydroxide (KOH) microscopy positive for hyphae
  2. Fungal culture for specific identification
  3. Wood's lamp of limited usefulness; most dermatophytes currently seen in US do not fluoresce

- Management/Treatment
  1. Nonpharmacologic
     a. Careful nail and skin care
     b. Keep area dry, absorbent clothing
  2. Pharmacologic
     a. Topical antifungals—tinea corporis, tinea cruris, tinea pedis
        (1) Azoles—clotrimazole, econazole, ketoconazole, miconazole
            (a) Drug action—fungicidal activity
            (b) Side-effects—pruritus, irritation, stinging
            (c) Drug interactions—none identified
            (d) Contraindications/precautions—pregnancy category C; not recommended in nursing mothers
        (2) Allylamines—naftifine, terbinafine
            (a) Drug action—fungicidal activity
            (b) Side-effects—burning, stinging, irritation, dryness

(c) Drug interactions—none identified

(d) Contraindications/precautions—pregnancy category B; precaution in nursing mothers

b. Oral antifungals—tinea capitis, tinea unguium

   (1) Griseofulvin

      (a) Drug action—interferes with fungal microtube formation by disrupting mitosis and cell division

      (b) Side-effects—headache, nausea, vomiting, diarrhea, photosensitivity

      (c) Drug interactions—reduces effectiveness of oral contraceptives

      (d) Contraindications/precautions—porphyria, hepatocellular failure, pregnancy; precaution in nursing mothers

   (2) Itraconazole

      (a) Drug action—decreases ergosterol synthesis inhibiting cell membrane formation

      (b) Side-effects—GI upset, rash, fatigue, headache, dizziness, edema; hepatitis reported/monitor LFTs

      (c) Drug interactions—inhibits drug metabolizing enzymes/CYP3A4; may increase levels of other drugs

      (d) Contraindications/precautions—hepatic dysfunction; pregnancy Category C; not recommended in nursing mothers

   (3) Terbenafine

      (a) Drug action—inhibits enzyme activity in fungi; inhibits synthesis of ergosterol

      (b) Side-effects—GI disturbances, headaches; rare LFT abnormalities

      (c) Drug interactions—potentiated by cimetidine; antagonized by rifampin

      (d) Contraindications/precautions—liver or renal disease; pregnancy category B; not recommended in nursing mothers

3. Patient education

   a. Keep skin dry as possible, especially intertrigal spaces

   b. Wear loose, clean, absorbent clothing

   c. Contagious nature of condition

◻ PSYCHOSOCIAL PROBLEMS

Stress

- Definition—Selye's Theory of Stress Response and Adaptation describes a continuum related to stress
  1. Eustress or good stress—degree of stress that is motivating and viewed as positive for the individual
  2. Distress—point at which stress becomes psychologically or physically debilitating

- Etiology/Incidence
  1. Major life events—marriage, divorce, job change, death of a family member
  2. Chronic situations—poverty, illness of self or family member, abuse
  3. Acute situations—acute pain, sudden threats to safety
  4. Environmental conditions—noise, pollution, overcrowding
  5. Daily hassles—minor events that occur on a regular basis

- Signs and symptoms
  1. Irritability, anxiety, depression, chronic worrying
  2. Decreased productivity, sleep disturbances, appetite changes, loss of libido
  3. Vague or nonspecific physical complaints—headaches, nausea, diarrhea, chest pain, muscle tension

- Physical findings
  1. Muscle tension
  2. Increase in blood pressure

- Differential diagnosis
  1. Depression
  2. Anxiety disorders
  3. Other medical conditions that could account for signs and symptoms

- Diagnostic tests/findings—none

- Management/Treatment
  1. Eliminate or modify stressors—assertiveness training, time management, positive thought strategies, communication skills
  2. Relaxation techniques—guided imagery, muscle relaxation exercises, biofeedback, massage, meditation, use of humor, physical exercise

Anxiety

- Definition—*DSM-IV-TR* lists several psychiatric syndromes of which anxiety is a primary component; interference with everyday function must be present to classify anxiety as a psychiatric syndrome

1. Generalized anxiety disorder
   a. Persistent, excessive, incapacitating worry over life events
   b. Anxiety and worry are associated with three or more of the following symptoms—restlessness, easily fatigued, difficulty concentrating, irritability, muscle tension, sleep disturbance
2. Panic disorder
   a. Intense, brief, acute anxiety; often no precipitant
   b. Four of the following symptoms—palpitations, sweating, trembling, shortness of breath, choking sensation, chest pain, abdominal distress, dizziness, derealization, fear of losing control, fear of dying, paresthesias, chills/hot flashes
   c. May occur with or without agoraphobia
3. Agoraphobia—anxiety about, or avoidance of, places or situations in which the ability to leave suddenly may be difficult in the event of having a panic attack
4. Specific phobia—anxiety elicited by a discrete stimulus such as heights or specific animals
5. Social phobia—fear of social and performance situations that is excessive or incapacitating
6. Posttraumatic stress disorder (PTSD)—delayed and persistent anxiety that follows an extremely traumatic event
7. Acute stress disorder (ASD)—similar to PTSD but more immediate and of shorter duration
8. Obsessive-compulsive disorder (OCD)—characterized by obsessions that cause marked anxiety or distress and/or by compulsions that serve to neutralize the anxiety

- Etiology/Incidence
  1. Approximately 15% of individuals will experience an anxiety disorder in their lifetime
  2. Generalized anxiety disorder is the most common type
  3. Several neuroregulators have been implicated in the cause of anxiety, e.g., dopamine, serotonin, norepinephrine
  4. Conditioned learning may also play a role in the development of anxiety disorders

- Signs and symptoms
  1. Clinical presentations vary with each anxiety category
  2. Most clients with an anxiety disorder will present with some combination of the following:
     a. Motor tension—restlessness, jitteriness

  b. Apprehension—insomnia, difficulty concentrating
  c. Cardiac symptoms—palpitation, chest tightness, or pain
  d. Respiratory symptoms—difficulty breathing, feelings of suffocation
  e. Gastrointestinal symptoms—nausea, diarrhea, dry mouth
  f. Neurologic symptoms—weakness, tingling numbness in extremities, dizziness
  g. Feelings of panic and/or loss of control
  h. Other—excessive sweating, feeling of tightness in throat

- Physical findings
  1. Physical findings may be present with an acute anxiety attack
  2. Tachycardia, increased respirations, elevated BP
  3. Restlessness
  4. Diaphoresis
  5. Muscle tension

- Differential diagnosis
  1. Medical conditions that may account for symptoms of anxiety—cardiac arrhythmias, mitral valve prolapse, angina, pulmonary embolism, hypoglycemia, hyperthyroidism, asthma, chronic obstructive pulmonary disease, Cushing's disease, pheochromocytoma
  2. Medication-induced symptoms of anxiety—steroids, anticholinergics, sympathomimetics, digoxin, thyroxine
  3. Drug abuse or withdrawal
  4. Other psychological disorders—depression, bipolar disorder

- Diagnostic tests/findings
  1. May be done to exclude other medical conditions suggested by history/physical
  2. Screen for occult hyperthyroidism with TSH

- Management/Treatment
  1. Nonpharmacologic—psychotherapy/cognitive behavioral therapy
  2. Pharmacologic—choice of medications depends on type of anxiety disorder
     a. Generalized anxiety disorder
        (1) Benzodiazepines for period of exacerbation—lorazepam, diazepam, clonazepam
            (a) Drug action—produce an antianxiety effect by enhancing the action of the neurotransmitter gamma-aminobutyric acid at the cortical and limbic areas of the brain

(b) Side-effects—sedation, impaired concentration anterograde amnesia; dependence; abuse potential

(c) Drug interactions—potentiates the effect of other CNS depressants including alcohol; may be potentiated by use with cimetidine

(d) Contraindications—pregnancy category D

(2) SSRI—paroxetine, venlafaxine, sertraline (see Depression this chapter)

(3) Serotonin and norepinephrine reuptake inhibitors (SNRI)—duloxetine, venlafaxine (see Depression this chapter)

(3) Buspirone—nonbenzodiazepine anti-anxiety agent

(a) Drug effect—partial agonism or mixed agonism/antagonism at 5-HT$_{1A}$ receptors

(b) Side-effects—nausea, dizziness, headache, restlessness

(c) Drug interactions—hypertensive crisis with MAOIs; Cytochrome P450 effect

(d) Contraindications/precautions—pregnancy category B

b. Panic disorder

(1) Benzodiazepines—for rapid relief of disabling symptoms, alprazolam

(2) SSRI—paroxetine, fluoxetine, sertraline; SNRI—venlafaxine

3. Client education

a. Caution about potential for physical/psychological dependence with use of benzodiazepines

b. Caution against use of alcohol or other CNS depressants with benzodiazepines

c. Discuss the use of relaxation techniques and effective coping mechanisms

Depression

- Definition (*DSM-IV-TR*)—at least five of the symptoms listed must be present for 2 weeks and #1 or #2 must be present for a diagnosis of major depression

1. Sad or depressed mood most of the day, every day

2. Loss of interest in usual activities

3. Fatigue, weight gain/loss, sleep disturbance, difficulty concentrating, feelings of worthlessness/guilt, psychomotor retardation/agitation, suicidal ideation

- Etiology/Incidence/Risk factors

1. At least 20% of women will experience depression in their lifetime

2. Onset is highest between the ages of 20 and 40

3. Also occurs in adolescent and elderly populations

4. Theories include biologic, sociologic, and neuroendocrine etiologies

5. Risk factors for depression include:

a. Prior incident of major depression

b. Family history of depression

c. Severe or chronic illness/chronic pain

d. Marital or family problems including abuse

e. Substance or alcohol abuse

f. Postpartum period

6. 15% of depressed individuals attempt suicide

7. Risk factors for suicide include:

a. Prior attempt/family history of suicide attempt

b. Male gender

c. Substance abuse/family history of substance abuse

d. Living alone

e. Medical illness

f. Hopelessness

g. Psychosis or panic disorder

h. Advanced age

- Signs and symptoms

1. As listed in definition

2. Vague pain, headaches, GI complaints, sexual complaints

- Physical findings

1. Poor eye contact, tearful, downcast

2. Inattention to appearance/hygiene

3. Slow, monotone speech

4. Psychomotor retardation or agitation

5. Impaired cognitive reasoning

- Differential diagnosis

1. Adjustment disorder following a stressor event

2. Bereavement or grief reaction

3. Dysthymia

a. Depressed mood for 2 years

b. With two of the following—appetite or sleep disturbance, fatigue, low self-esteem, poor concentration, hopelessness

4. Other psychiatric syndromes

5. Medical disorders—thyroid disorders, sleep apnea, Parkinson's disease, multiple sclerosis

6. Medications—corticosteroids, antihypertensives, benzodiazepines, chemotherapeutic drugs and others

- Diagnostic tests/findings
  1. Laboratory/diagnostic tests may be done to exclude other diagnostic possibilities
     a. CBC, chemistry profile
     b. TSH
     c. VDRL
  2. Screening tools—depression assessment scales
     a. Ask patients to rate severity or frequency of various symptoms
     b. Beck Depression Inventory, Zung Self-Rating Depression Scale, Geriatric Depression Scale

- Management/Treatment
  1. Nonpharmacologic—psychotherapy, electroconvulsive therapy; hospitalization may be required for severe depression or if client has suicidal ideation
  2. Pharmacologic
     a. Selective serotonin reuptake inhibitors (SSRIs) have replaced tricyclic antidepressants (TCAs) as the drugs of choice because of their improved tolerability and safety if taken in overdose
        (1) Agents—fluoxetine, sertraline, paroxetine, citalopram, escitalopram
        (2) Drug action—block reuptake of serotonin enhancing serotonin neurotransmission
        (3) Side-effects—anxiety, insomnia/hypersomnia, headache, nausea, anorexia, sexual dysfunction
        (4) Drug interactions—use with MAO inhibitors may cause hypertensive crisis; CYP450 drug-drug interactions
        (5) Contraindications/precautions—not to be used in conjunction with MAO inhibitors; screen patients for symptoms of bipolar disorder before prescribing to avoid precipitating a manic episode; pregnancy category C; caution in nursing mothers
     b. Selective serotonin and norepinephrine reuptake inhibitors (SNRIs)
        (1) Agents—venlafaxine, duloxetine
        (2) Drug action—inhibits both serotonin and norepinephrine reuptake
        (3) Side-effects—nausea, dizziness, insomnia, somnolence, dry mouth, constipation
        (4) Drug interactions—MAO inhibitors, tryptophan, other SSRIs or SNRIs, CYP1A2 inhibitors, other
        (5) Contraindications/precautions—not to be used in conjunction with MAO

inhibitors; uncontrolled narrow-angle glaucoma
     c. Other classes of antidepressants
        (1) Mirtazapine—stimulates release of norepinephrine and serotonin; side-effects include fatigue, dizziness, transient sedation, and weight gain
        (2) Nefazodone—inhibits serotonin reuptake and weakly inhibits norepinephrine reuptake; side-effects include drowsiness, dry mouth, nausea, dizziness, risk of hepatotoxicity; little or no sexual dysfunction
        (3) Bupropion—decreases reuptake of dopamine in the CNS; major side-effects include agitation, headache, and nausea; no sexual side-effects
     d. Once full remission achieved, continue therapy for 6 to 12 months; for second episode continue therapy for 1 to 2 years; a third episode requires indefinite maintenance
  3. Client education
     a. SSRIs—usually taken in morning to reduce incidence of insomnia
     b. Antidepressants should be started slowly and dose increased to a therapeutic level that alleviates symptoms
     c. An adequate trial period and close follow-up are essential for successful treatment
     d. Caution concerning use of medications with alcohol
     e. Encourage use of support systems, effective coping mechanisms

- Referral
  1. Patients requiring referral to a psychiatrist include those with suicidal ideation or severe depression; bipolar disorder; atypical depression, substance abuse, treatment resistance
  2. Referral to a licensed counselor should be offered to most patients with depression

Domestic Violence/Intimate Partner Violence

- Definition—a pattern of coercive and controlling behavior that occurs in an intimate adult relationship; includes both psychological and physical abuse

- Etiology/Incidence
  1. 1 in 10 women is battered annually by the man with whom she lives
  2. Battering is a causative factor in 25% of female suicide attempts and 4000 homicides each year

3. Battering is the single most common reason women go to emergency rooms
4. 12% of teenagers and more than 20% of college students have experienced dating violence
5. Pregnant women may be at increased risk for initiation or escalation of abuse

- Signs and symptoms
  1. History of frequent visits to emergency room
  2. Evidence of current or old injuries
  3. Delay in reporting an injury/explanation of cause inconsistent with injury
  4. Depression, anxiety, posttraumatic stress reactions, low self-esteem
  5. History of suicide attempts or ideation
  6. Alcohol or drug abuse
  7. Vague or nonspecific physical complaints
  8. Late/sporadic prenatal care or other health care
  9. Controlling partner/increased anxiety in presence of partner
  10. Behavioral problems in children who are witnessing the abuse
  11. Cycle of violence—tension building, serious battering incident, honeymoon phase

- Physical findings
  1. Facial lacerations
  2. Injuries to breasts, back, abdomen, and genitalia
  3. Bilateral injuries to arms/legs
  4. Obvious patterns—bite marks, hand grip, cigarette burns
  5. Injuries during pregnancy
  6. Recurrent or chronic injuries

- Differential diagnosis
  1. Accidental injuries
  2. Self-inflicted injuries

- Diagnostic tests/findings—none

- Management/Treatment
  1. Routine assessment for abuse in all women
  2. Danger assessment—suicide or homicide
  3. Safety plan—where to go in an emergency or dangerous situation; what to do during violent incidents; what items/documents will be needed for a comfortable and safe escape
  4. ABCDEs of intervention
     a. *A*lone—assure the woman that she is not alone in being a victim of domestic violence
     b. *B*elief—let the woman know that you believe that no one deserves to be hurt or threatened in a relationship

  c. *C*onfidential—assure the woman that the information she shares is confidential
  d. *D*ocument—record any findings that may be helpful to the woman at a later date; use accurate description of incident and/or threats in patient's own words; include all pertinent physical examination findings with body map and/or photographs with woman's permission
  e. *E*ducate—provide information about available resources, dangers of escalating violence, and safety plans
  5. Referrals
     a. Shelters
     b. Legal assistance
     c. Counseling
  6. Mandatory reporting—laws vary in each state

Sexual Assault/Abuse

- Definition
  1. Sexual assault—force, threats, or coercion to engage in any unwanted sexual contact; includes contact or penetration of the intimate parts (sexual organs, anus, groin, buttocks, and breasts)
  2. Sexual abuse—repeated sexual assault within a relationship
  3. Rape—sexual assault that involves penetration, however slight, of the labia by the penis; legal definitions of rape vary from state to state but typically include the use of force, threat, or coercion and lack of consent by the victim in relation to sexual intercourse

- Etiology/Incidence
  1. Sexual assault occurs in all age, race, ethnic, and cultural groups
  2. The majority of rapes are perpetrated by an acquaintance of the victim rather than a stranger

- Signs and symptoms
  1. Genital injury may or may not be present and is often difficult to visualize
  2. Typical findings include lacerations, ecchymosis, abrasions, erythema, and edema in areas of assault
  3. Rape trauma syndrome describes the symptoms that occur in most victims of sexual assault
     a. Acute phase—lasts a few days to a few weeks
        (1) Emotional responses may be expressed or controlled ranging from anger, fear, anxiety, and restlessness to a calm, composed, subdued affect

(2) Physical responses include general soreness and soreness in the areas of assault; gastrointestinal and genitourinary symptoms; sleep disruption and nightmares; and sexual disruption

 b. Reorganization phase—wide range of emotions and physical responses with the purpose of reorganizing life after the assault

4. Posttraumatic stress disorder occurs when rape trauma syndrome extends beyond 1 month and when the victim exhibits the following behavioral criteria:

 a. Persistent reexperiencing of the event (nightmares, flashbacks)

 b. Avoidance of certain activities, places, and people that arouse recollections of the event

 c. Increased arousal (sleep difficulties, difficulty concentrating, irritability, hypervigilance)

 d. Clinically significant distress or impairment in social, occupational, or other important areas of functioning

- Physical findings
  1. Physical findings may be minimal or not apparent until a day or more after the assault
  2. Lacerations, ecchymosis, abrasions, erythema, edema in areas of assault
  3. Colposcopic examination may be used to assist in evaluation

- Differential diagnosis
  1. Accidental injuries
  2. Domestic violence—nonsexual

- Diagnostic tests/findings
  1. Forensic evidence collection technique and requirements may vary from state to state—most states supply evidence collection kits that contain instructions and collection materials
  2. STD tests, HIV testing, and pregnancy testing should be offered

- Management/Treatment
  1. Comprehensive care for sexual assault victim is often provided by a multidisciplinary team that includes a sexual assault nurse examiner (SANE), victims' advocate, and law enforcement
  2. Triage and immediate treatment of any life-threatening injuries
  3. Attention to emotional needs of the victim
  4. Collection of evidence per state and agency protocol

5. Prophylactic treatment for STDs and emergency contraception if indicated
6. Referrals
   a. Healthcare provider for follow-up STD and HIV testing
   b. Legal and social service referrals
   c. Counseling for victim and family

Eating Disorders

- Definitions
  1. Anorexia nervosa—*DSM IV* criteria for diagnosis include:
   a. Refusal to maintain body weight at or above a minimal normal weight for age and height
   b. Intense fear of gaining weight even though underweight
   c. Disturbed body image
   d. Amenorrhea or the absence of at least three consecutive menstrual cycles when otherwise expected
  2. Bulimia nervosa—*DSM IV* criteria for diagnosis include:
   a. Recurrent episodes of binge eating
   b. Recurrent, inappropriate compensatory behavior to prevent weight gain (self-induced vomiting; misuse of laxatives, diuretics or enemas; strict dieting or fasting; excessive exercise)
   c. Binge eating and inappropriate compensatory behaviors occur on the average at least twice a week for at least 3 months
   d. Persistent over-concern with body shape and weight

- Etiology/Incidence
  1. Anorexia nervosa
   a. Etiology—biologic, psychological, social, and family factors
   b. About 1% of female adolescents have anorexia
   c. Age of onset—early to late adolescence
   d. 10% mortality due to starvation, electrolyte imbalance, or suicide
   e. Risk factors include:
    (1) Female gender
    (2) Parent or sibling with eating disorder
    (3) Career choice or aspiration that stresses thinness, perfection, or self-discipline
    (4) A difficult transition or loss (leaving home for college, breakup of an important relationship)
  2. Bulimia nervosa
   a. Etiology—biologic, psychological, social, and family factors

b. Age of onset—late adolescence to early adulthood

c. Occurs in 4% of college age women

d. Mortality rate lower than with anorexia nervosa

e. 30–80% of bulimics have history of anorexia nervosa

- Signs and symptoms
  1. Anorexia nervosa—fatigue, cold intolerance, muscle weakness and cramps, dizziness, fainting spells, bloating, amenorrhea, social isolation, excessive concerns about weight, compulsive exercising, odd food rituals, depression
  2. Bulimia nervosa—menstrual irregularities, depression, anxiety, impulsive behaviors (shoplifting, alcohol or drug abuse, unsafe sexual behaviors), lack of meaningful relationships, excessive concerns about weight, requests for diet pills, diuretics, or laxatives

- Physical findings
  1. Anorexia nervosa—emaciation, dry skin, fine body hair (lanugo), muscle wasting, peripheral edema, bradycardia, arrhythmias, hypotension, delayed sexual maturation, stress fractures
  2. Bulimia—erosion of tooth enamel, calluses on dorsal surface of hands from inducing vomiting, swollen parotid glands, cardiac arrhythmias if syrup of ipecac used

- Differential diagnosis
  1. Gastrointestinal disorders
  2. Malignancies
  3. Depression
  4. Psychiatric disorders

- Diagnostic tests/findings
  1. Anorexia—mild anemia, elevated BUN, cholesterol, and liver function tests, electrolyte imbalance, low serum estrogen, abnormal ECG
  2. Bulimia—electrolyte imbalance, abnormal ECG

- Management/Treatment
  1. Outpatient treatment—individual/group/family therapy, nutritional counseling, treatment of any medical complications, treatment of any associated mood disorders
  2. Pharmacologic—SSRI fluoxetine approved for treatment of bulimia
  3. Hospitalization is indicated if any of the following apply:

a. Weight is less than or equal to 70% of ideal body weight

b. Client is suicidal

c. Client fails outpatient treatment

4. Pregnancy considerations—individuals with anorexia nervosa may have fertility problems; pregnant individuals with eating disorders will require special nutritional management to assure adequate weight gain and nutrient intake

Addictive Disorders (Alcohol and Drugs)

- Definitions
  1. Substance dependence (*DSM IV* criteria)—maladaptive pattern of substance use leading to significant impairment or distress with at least three of the following occurring within a 12-month period:
     a. Tolerance
     b. Withdrawal syndrome or use of substance to relieve withdrawal symptoms
     c. Substance taken in larger amounts or over a longer period of time than intended
     d. Persistent desire or unsuccessful attempts to cut down use
     e. Significant amount of time spent obtaining, consuming, or recovering from substance
     f. Important social or occupational activities reduced because of substance use
     g. Persistent use despite knowledge of social, psychological, or physical problems caused by its use
  2. Substance abuse (*DSM IV* criteria)—maladaptive pattern of use leading to a significant impairment or distress with at least one of the following within a 12-month period:
     a. Recurrent substance use resulting in a failure to fulfill major role obligations (work, school, home)
     b. Recurrent use in situations where use is physically hazardous (driving while intoxicated)
     c. Recurrent substance abuse-related legal problems
     d. Continued use despite knowledge of having a persistent or recurring social or interpersonal problem that is caused or worsened by the substance use
     e. Symptoms have never met the criteria for substance dependence

- Etiology/Incidence
  1. Genetic, cultural, biochemical, behavioral, and psychological factors have all been considered in the etiology of substance dependence

2. 6% of adult women have serious problems with alcohol
3. Approximately one third of alcoholics in the US are women
4. Other drugs of abuse include opioids, depressants, stimulants, hallucinogens, and marijuana
5. Substance abuse is involved in over 50% of domestic violence and in 50% of driving accident fatalities

- Signs and symptoms
  1. Alcoholism
     a. Frequent falls/minor injuries, blackouts, legal or marital problems, depression, vague GI complaints, sleep disorders, withdrawal symptoms, seizures
     b. The National Institute on Alcohol Abuse and Alcoholism (NIAAA) recommends asking all clients if they ever drink alcohol, and if the answer is yes, ask about maximum number of drinks on any occasion in past month, how many drinks they have on a typical day when they drink, and how many days per week they drink to identify hazardous drinkers
     c. CAGE is one of several screening tools used to assess a drinking problem
        (1) Have you ever felt you should *cut down* on your drinking?
        (2) Have people *annoyed* you by criticizing your drinking?
        (3) Have you ever felt bad or *guilty* about your drinking?
        (4) Have you ever had a drink first thing in the morning to steady your nerves or get rid of a hangover (*eye-opener*)?
  2. Signs and symptoms of depressant (benzodiazepine, barbiturate) abuse—euphoria, apathy, violent, or bizarre behavior
  3. Signs and symptoms of stimulant (cocaine, amphetamine) abuse—anxiety, euphoria, violent or bizarre behavior, hallucinations, nausea/vomiting

- Physical findings
  1. Alcoholism—hepatomegaly, tremors, peripheral neuropathy, ataxia, confusion, impairment of recent memory
  2. Depressants—psychomotor retardation, slurred speech, lack of coordination, tremors
  3. Stimulants—diaphoresis, hypertension, tachycardia, hyperactive deep tendon reflexes (DTR), pupil dilation, tremors, seizures

- Differential diagnosis
  1. Psychiatric disorders that could account for the signs and symptoms, e.g., depression, anxiety disorders, schizophrenia
  2. Medical conditions that could account for the signs and symptoms, e.g., endocrinopathies, seizure disorders, head injury

- Diagnostic tests/findings
  1. Blood alcohol level may be elevated
  2. Elevated gamma glutamyl transferase (GGT) indicates heavy or chronic alcohol use
  3. Urine toxicology tests for other drugs of abuse
  4. Consider other laboratory and diagnostic tests based on risk factors and clinical presentation

- Management/Treatment
  1. Follow federal and state laws regarding protection of confidentiality for persons receiving alcohol and drug abuse treatment services and treatment of minors for alcohol and drug abuse without parental consent
  2. Detoxification—outpatient or inpatient
  3. Addiction counseling
  4. Prevention of relapse
     a. Alcoholics Anonymous, Narcotics Anonymous
     b. Pharmacologic agents—short-term adjuncts to psychosocial treatment
        (1) Naltrexone—alcohol craving is reduced in about one-half of patients
        (2) Disulfiram—creates a toxic response when patient consumes alcohol
     c. Family involvement—counseling, Al-Anon, Ala-Teen, Nar-Anon
     d. Employee assistance programs

◘ QUESTIONS

Select the best answer.

1. A systolic heart murmur present in an asymptomatic pregnant woman is likely:

   a. Due to valvular disease
   b. Associated with history of rheumatic fever
   c. A physiologic (innocent) murmur
   d. To intensify with Valsalva maneuver

2. Which of the following if left untreated may progress to squamous cell carcinoma?

   a. Keratosis pilaris
   b. Seborrheic keratosis
   c. Actinic keratosis
   d. Lichen planus

3. Which of the following is *not* a finding in asthma?

   a. Shortened expiratory phase
   b. Wheezing
   c. Tachypnea, dyspnea
   d. Diminished lung sounds

4. Which of the following is consistent with a diagnosis of mild persistent asthma?

   a. Symptoms fewer than twice a week
   b. Daily symptoms
   c. Symptoms 3–6 days of the week
   d. Nocturnal symptoms less than twice per month

5. Approximately what percent of tuberculosis infections will cause active disease?

   a. 75%
   b. 60%
   c. 30%
   d. 10%

6. Which of the following is considered a positive PPD reaction?

   a. A healthy individual with a tuberculin reaction of 5 mm
   b. A 55-year-old with active liver disease and a tuberculin reaction of 5 mm
   c. A low-risk female who is 28 years old with a tuberculin reaction of 10 mm
   d. An HIV-infected female with a tuberculin reaction of 5 mm

7. Which of the following is *not* an anticipated symptom of active TB infection?

   a. Tachycardia
   b. Chest pain
   c. Weight loss
   d. Night sweats

8. Which cohort is most frequently affected by migraine headache?

   a. Teenagers
   b. Males and females equally
   c. Females
   d. Postmenopausal women

9. Referral for neurologic evaluation of headaches is indicated when:

   a. New headaches occur in an individual older than 50.
   b. There is a family history of stroke.
   c. Focal neurologic deficits precede headache episodes.
   d. New "triggers" are identified in migraine pattern.

10. Important nonpharmacologic treatments for acute low back pain do *not* include:

    a. Continuation of daily activities
    b. Heat application
    c. Strength-building exercises
    d. Bedrest

11. Osteoarthritis may be distinguished from rheumatoid arthritis by:

    a. The severity of pain reported
    b. Asymmetry of involvement
    c. The joints involved
    d. Length of time symptoms have been in evidence

12. "RICE" therapy refers to:

    a. A nonpharmacologic therapy plan for muscle injuries
    b. A bland diet therapy for nausea and vomiting
    c. A weight loss plan
    d. A combination therapy for peptic ulcer disease

13. A 46-year-old female presents with complaints of worsening low back pain after lifting a heavy object the previous day. History of intermittent low back pain in the last year, but notes the pain is now radiating down her right leg. No complaints of trouble with urination or bowel movements. On exam, there is decreased range of motion of the spine in all planes. Straight leg raising at 35° is positive on the right. Achilles tendon reflex on the right is diminished compared to the left with decreased sensation over the right lateral foot. The most likely etiology of this patient's symptoms is:

    a. Rupture of the achilles tendon
    b. Cauda equina syndrome
    c. Herniated disc involving L5 root
    d. Herniated disc involving the S1 root

14. A 27-year-old female presents with moderate sore throat, runny nose, cough, and general malaise for the past 2 days. Physical examination reveals temperature of 99.8°F, mild pharyngeal erythema, and no exudates. Appropriate management includes:

    a. CBC with differential
    b. Rapid strep antigen test
    c. Saline gargles
    d. Antibiotic treatment

15. Risk of vertical transmission of the HIV virus has been reduced by:

a. Artificial rupture of membranes at 38 weeks
b. Antiretroviral treatment of infants
c. Stopping maternal therapy in pregnancy in order to reduce CD4+ counts
d. Antiretroviral therapy during pregnancy

16. The confirmatory test for HIV infection is:

a. Enzyme-linked immunosorbent assay (ELISA)
b. Quantitative plasma HIV RNA
c. CD4+ lymphocyte count
d. Western blot

17. An important principle of antiretroviral therapy is:

a. Response to drug therapy is monitored with CD4+ counts.
b. Monotherapy is recommended.
c. Response to drug therapy is monitored by HIV RNA levels.
d. Therapy should be started when symptoms first appear.

A 34-year-old female presents with a 2-month history of a nonproductive cough associated with shortness of breath. She complains of fatigue and has noted an intermittent fever for the past 6 weeks. Significant cervical, inguinal, and axillary lymphadenopathy is noted. Her HIV test is positive. Chest x-ray shows a bilateral infiltrate, and she is diagnosed with pneumocystis pneumonia (PCP). Questions 18 and 19 refer to this case.

18. HIV infection produces a spectrum of disease. This patient's symptoms place her in which stage of HIV infection?

a. Acute HIV infection
b. Asymptomatic infection
c. Early symptomatic infection
d. AIDS

19. INH prophylaxis would be recommended for this patient if her PPD was:

a. ≥ 5 mm
b. ≥ 10 mm
c. ≥ 15 mm
d. ≥ 20 mm

20. Risk factors for systemic lupus erythematosus (SLE) include all but which of the following?

a. Female gender
b. Reproductive age group
c. First-degree relative with SLE
d. Caucasian race

21. Diagnosis of SLE is made by:

a. Abnormal antinuclear antibodies (ANA) titer
b. Presence of at least four combined signs, symptoms, and laboratory findings
c. Presence of a specific hematologic disorder on a single occasion
d. Identification of an immunologic disorder such as abnormal anti-DNA

22. Systemic lupus erythematosus is usually characterized by:

a. Periods of exacerbation and remission
b. Slow, steady disease progression
c. Initial symptoms of typical skin eruptions
d. Remission in pregnancy

23. Which of the following is not suspect in the etiology of rheumatoid arthritis?

a. Genetic factors
b. Environmental factors
c. Hormonal factors
d. Joint trauma

24. The World Health Organization standard for anemia diagnosis in women is:

a. Hemoglobin < 10 g/dL
b. Hemoglobin < 11 g/dL
c. Hemoglobin < 12 g/dL
d. Hemoglobin < 13 g/dL

25. Otitis media is suspected when deep ear pain develops concurrent with or following:

a. An allergic reaction
b. An asthma attack
c. An upper respiratory infection
d. Persistent headache

26. Treatment of bacterial conjunctivitis will often:

a. Show dramatic results within 48 hours
b. Take 3 to 5 days before improvement is apparent
c. Work best with concomitant use of vasoconstrictors
d. Cause drainage to appear within 24 hours

27. A 26-year-old female patient presents with her first episode of acute bacterial sinusitis. She is allergic to penicillin. The most appropriate management would be:

a. Sulfamethoxazole/Trimethoprim
b. Levofloxacin (Levaquin)
c. Amoxicillin
d. Fluticasone Nasal Spray

28. A 21-year-old female presents with symptoms suggestive of infectious mononucleosis. Which of the following does *not* support the diagnosis?

    a. Pharyngitis
    b. Positive monospot/heterophile antibody test
    c. CBC with atypical lymphocytes
    d. Cough

29. The group most often affected by infectious mononucleosis is:

    a. Prepubertal children
    b. Women of reproductive age
    c. Females at any age
    d. Teens to early twenties

30. The most common reason for painless rectal bleeding with defecation is:

    a. External hemorrhoids
    b. Internal hemorrhoids
    c. Rectal polyps
    d. Colorectal cancer

    A 21-year-old female complains of intermittent, loose stools with pain and flatulence. After defecation, there is a temporary feeling of relief. Symptoms increase during times of stress. Patient denies weight loss, fever, or blood in the stool. Questions 31 and 32 refer to this case.

31. Which of the following is the most likely diagnosis?

    a. Ulcerative colitis
    b. Irritable bowel syndrome
    c. Lactose intolerance
    d. Intestinal parasitic infection

32. A recommended dietary change for Linda's episodes of diarrhea includes:

    a. Decrease caffeine, gas forming foods
    b. Low-fiber diet
    c. Eliminate all dairy products
    d. Vitamin supplements

33. African-American women are at increased risk for:

    a. Systemic lupus erythematosus
    b. Skin cancer
    c. Iron deficiency anemia
    d. Tinea

34. Appendicitis typically presents with which of the following?

    a. High fever as the initial symptom
    b. Pain beginning in the right-lower quadrant (RLQ)

    c. Diarrhea as the initial symptom
    d. Pain in periumbilical area followed by localization to the RLQ

35. Peptic ulcer disease associated with presence of *H. pylori* can be diagnosed by:

    a. Visualization of *H. pylori* on Gram stained preparation
    b. Negative urea breath analysis
    c. Negative urease assay via endoscopy
    d. Serology positive for *H. pylori* antibodies

36. Initial laboratory evaluation of a patient presenting with symptoms suggestive of acute viral hepatitis should include:

    a. IgG anti-HAV
    b. HBsAg and IgM anti-HBc
    c. IgM anti-HAV
    d. HBsAg, IgM anti-HBc, and IgM anti-HAV

37. The primary goal of pharmacologic therapy for acute viral hepatitis B is:

    a. Prevention of secondary infection
    b. Relief of symptoms
    c. Reduction of infectivity
    d. Prevention of complications

38. Most gallstones are composed of:

    a. Precipitated bile salts
    b. Precipitated calcium salts
    c. Cholesterol
    d. Pigments

39. A 45-year-old female presents with right-upper quadrant (RUQ) pain that radiates to the right infrascapular area. The pain is described as colicky and was precipitated by eating pizza. Onset of the symptom was a few hours ago and the pain is beginning to ease. There was associated nausea and vomiting. The initial study of choice in this patient is:

    a. Plain abdominal radiograph
    b. Ultrasound
    c. Computerized tomography (CT)
    d. Percutaneous transhepatic cholangiogram

40. Among the following causes of viral hepatitis, which of the following is most likely to lead to chronic infection and is the most common reason for liver transplantation?

    a. Hepatitis A
    b. Hepatitis B
    c. Hepatitis C
    d. Hepatitis D

41. Patients with acute cholecystitis should be advised:

a. To undertake strict weight reduction diets if obese
b. Of the likelihood of recurrence
c. That immediate surgery is a recommended treatment
d. Of the availability of lithotripsy as a highly successful treatment

A 35-year-old overweight female presents with intermittent heartburn for several months. The use of Tums provides temporary relief. During the past week, she has been awakened during the night with a burning sensation in her chest. She is not taking any other medications and has no major health problems. Questions 42–44 refer to this case.

42. What additional information would support a diagnosis of gastroesophageal reflux disease (GERD) as the cause of her symptoms?

a. She has occasional nausea and vomiting.
b. She often notes coughing during the night and a bad taste in her mouth.
c. The pain is usually relieved by eating.
d. Constipation has been a chronic problem and she uses laxatives twice a week.

43. Your patient denies weight loss, dysphagia and dark, tarry stools. What is your next step?

a. Order an endoscopic exam
b. Start her on H_2 receptor blockers
c. Tell her to eat a snack before bedtime
d. Refer her to a gastroenterologist

44. Assuming a diagnosis of GERD, you would advise that:

a. She probably has a hiatal hernia causing the reflux.
b. She will likely require surgery.
c. She should avoid all fruit juices.
d. Smoking, alcohol, and caffeine will likely aggravate the problem.

45. The laboratory diagnosis of diabetes mellitus can be determined by:

a. Fasting plasma glucose $\geq$ 126 mg/dL
b. A 2-hour postprandial glucose $\geq$ 126 mg/dL
c. HbA_{1c} > 7%
d. Random glucose $\geq$ 150 mg/dL

46. A 60-year-old female presents for a physical exam. She has no complaints. Fasting blood sugar is 188. You suspect diabetes. To confirm the diagnosis, you would order:

a. No further testing is necessary
b. A fasting blood sugar on a subsequent day

c. A 3-hour glucose tolerance test on a subsequent day
d. A HbA_{1c}

47. Which of the following is most indicative of poor control in a patient with type 2 diabetes?

a. Average preprandial plasma glucose of 118 mg/dL
b. Average peak postprandial glucose of 145 mg/dL
c. Average random glucose of 175 mg/dL
d. HbA_{1c} of 8.5%

48. The condition comprising 90% of hyperthyroidism is:

a. Graves' disease
b. Thyroiditis
c. Toxic goiter
d. Adenoma

49. Infiltrative ophthalmopathy (exophthalmos) is unique to which of the following disorders?

a. Graves' disease
b. Hashimoto's thyroiditis
c. Toxic multinodular goiter
d. Papillary thyroid carcinoma

50. Which of the following test results would be expected with primary hyperthyroidism?

a. Low serum TSH and elevated free T_4
b. Low serum TSH and low free T_4
c. High serum TSH and elevated free T_4
d. High serum TSH and low free T_4

51. A patient with a history of radioactive iodine treatment for Graves' disease presents with fatigue, weight gain, and dry skin. You would expect this patient to have which of the following laboratory findings?

a. Low T_3, low TSH, high total T_4
b. Low TSH, high total T_4, normal free T_4
c. High TSH, low free T_4
d. High TSH, high free T_4

52. A 35-year-old female was diagnosed with Hashimoto thyroiditis and placed on 0.1 mg of levothyroxine. After 1 week of treatment, the patient states that she still feels fatigued. How would you manage this patient?

a. Increase the dose of levothyroxine to 0.125 mg
b. Schedule an appointment this week to have a TSH drawn
c. Add propranolol to the regimen
d. No change in levothyroxine is indicated at this time

53. A factor *not* associated with exacerbations of facial acne is:

    a. Hormonal cycling
    b. Stress
    c. Fried foods
    d. Hot humid environments

54. The most important point to stress with female patients using isotretinoin for acne is:

    a. Possibility of hematologic disturbances
    b. Rare occurrence of pseudotumor cerebri
    c. Necessity for highly effective contraception
    d. Avoiding alcohol while on this drug

55. An 18-year-old presents with open and closed comedones and a few scattered papules. The most appropriate first line treatment would be:

    a. Topical antibiotics
    b. Oral tetracycline
    c. Tretinoin cream (Retin-A)
    d. Isotretinoin (Accutane)

56. The most common form of skin cancer is:

    a. Squamous cell
    b. Basal cell
    c. Malignant melanoma
    d. Basal cell nevus syndrome

57. A 60-year-old presents with a pearly, translucent smooth papule with rolled edges and surface telangiectasias on her forehead. She notes that it has been there for at least a year, but has recently increased in size. The lesion most likely represents which of the following?

    a. Squamous cell carcinoma
    b. Basal cell carcinoma
    c. Seborrheic keratosis
    d. Malignant melanoma

58. Education for the woman with systemic lupus erythematosus (SLE) should include which of the following?

    a. She should not use hormonal contraception.
    b. She should receive annual live attenuated influenza vaccine.
    c. If she becomes pregnant, a C-section will be planned to avoid stress of labor.
    d. She should use sunscreen and protective clothing when outdoors.

59. Which of the following is *not* a risk factor for malignant melanoma?

    a. Hispanic ethnicity
    b. Multiple pigmented nevi
    c. Severe childhood sunburn
    d. Family history

60. A 20-year-old female presents with two annular lesions with a scaly border and central clearing on her trunk. The lesions have been present for 1 week and are mildly pruritic. What is the most likely diagnosis?

    a. Psoriasis
    b. Pityriasis rosea
    c. Tinea versicolor
    d. Tinea corporis

61. A 20-year-old female presents with complaint of itching, red eye with a sticky, yellow discharge that started in one eye yesterday afternoon and this morning is in both eyes. She states no fever or other symptoms. The most likely diagnosis is:

    a. Allergic conjunctivitis
    b. Bacterial conjunctivitis
    c. Bacterial blepharitis
    d. Viral conjunctivitis

62. The most common reason for lumbosacral back pain is:

    a. Herniated disc
    b. Muscle strain
    c. Neoplasm
    d. Arthritis

63. A 28-year-old female presents with complaints of low back pain after helping a friend move 2 days ago. She denies any radiation of the pain, numbness, or tingling in the lower extremities or problems with elimination. On physical exam, mild paravertebral muscle spasm is noted with decreased range of motion of the spine. No focal neurologic findings. Appropriate management would include:

    a. Radiograph of the lumbosacral spine
    b. Bedrest for 3–4 days
    c. NSAIDs
    d. Referral to neurologist

64. The frequency of sickle cell crises may be reduced by:

    a. Activity restrictions
    b. Oxygen therapy
    c. Aggressive treatment of infections
    d. High protein diet

65. Which of the following is an expected finding in tinea unguium?

    a. Hair loss in affected areas
    b. Negative KOH slide preparation
    c. Yellowish, thickened nails
    d. Crusted ulcerations

66. About 10% of those infected with hepatitis B virus become chronic carriers of the disease, a state putting them at risk for:

    a. Hepatocellular carcinoma
    b. Mononucleosis
    c. Gall bladder disease
    d. Chronic immunocompromised status

67. Your patient's blood work returns with a positive hepatitis B surface antigen (HBsAg). This suggests:

    a. Chronic liver disease
    b. Previous infection with hepatitis B virus
    c. Acute or chronic infection with hepatitis B virus
    d. Recent vaccination

68. The incidence of upper respiratory infection:

    a. Is enhanced by cold, damp weather
    b. Peaks in winter months
    c. Peaks in spring/summer allergy season
    d. Doesn't vary much season to season

69. Management of constipation should include:

    a. Routine use of stool softeners
    b. Bulk-forming agents in the management of acute constipation
    c. Hyperosmolar laxatives (sorbitol) as the initial drug of choice for chronic constipation
    d. Saline laxatives (milk of magnesia) in the management of acute constipation

70. Which of the following patients with sinusitis should be treated with antibiotics?

    a. Patient who had onset of sinusitis a few days after onset of URI symptoms
    b. Patient who has postnasal drip, swollen pale nasal mucosa, and low-grade fever
    c. Patient who was noting improvement in symptoms, and 5 days later symptoms worsen
    d. Patient who has rebound congestion after discontinuing several days' use of decongestant nasal spray

71. A blood pressure of 150/90 mm Hg during a routine examination of an asymptomatic, 45-year-old African-American female would indicate:

    a. Essential hypertension
    b. Probability of underlying disease
    c. Necessity for follow-up and further evaluation
    d. Normal response to anxiety

72. Which of the following most likely suggests a secondary cause of hypertension?

    a. BMI greater than 30
    b. Abdominal bruit
    c. Total cholesterol greater than 280
    d. Enlarged spleen

73. Before a diagnosis of hypertension can be made, follow-up must include:

    a. Minimum of one more visit with BP $\geq$ 140/90 mm Hg
    b. Serum creatinine and potassium levels
    c. Evaluation for possible hyperlipidemia and diabetes
    d. 12-lead electrocardiogram

74. A 21-year-old college student is brought to the clinic because she fainted in class. She states she has been having daily dizzy spells. Physical examination reveals an underweight female with heart rate of 58 beats per minute and blood pressure 96/52 mm Hg. Of the following conditions, this client's symptoms and examination findings are most indicative of:

    a. Agorophobia
    b. Anorexia nervosa
    c. Cocaine abuse
    d. Depression

75. Which of the following is *not* classified as thromboembolic disease?

    a. Deep vein thrombosis
    b. Pulmonary embolus
    c. Superficial thrombophlebitis
    d. Chronic venous insufficiency

76. The best initial test to rule out DVT is:

    a. Plasma D-dimer
    b. Ascending venography
    c. Antithrombin III measurement
    d. Duplex ultrasound

77. Which of the following is *not* a recommended nonpharmacologic treatment for thrombophlebitis?

    a. Local heat application
    b. Passive range of motion exercise
    c. Elevation of affected limb
    d. Compression with an ace wrap

78. The National Cholesterol Education Program recommends hyperlipidemia screening every _____ years beginning at age 20.

    a. 5
    b. 3
    c. 2
    d. 1

79. A 44-year-old female presents with obesity, type 2 diabetes, and hyperlipidemia. Which of the following should be your treatment goal?

    a. LDL cholesterol < 160 mg/dL
    b. LDL cholesterol < 130 mg/dL
    c. LDL cholesterol < 100 mg/dL
    d. Total cholesterol < 200 mg/dL

80. In patients with established cardiovascular disease, the goal for LDL cholesterol is:

    a. < 100 mg/dL
    b. < 130 mg/dL
    c. < 160 mg/dL
    d. < 190 mg/dL

81. A microcytic anemia with a low serum ferritin is likely secondary to:

    a. Anemia of chronic disease
    b. Iron deficiency
    c. Hyperspleenism
    d. Thalassemia minor

82. The use of "statins" for pharmacologic therapy of hyperlipidemia is:

    a. Category B use in pregnancy
    b. Category C use in pregnancy
    c. Category D use in pregnancy
    d. Category X use in pregnancy

83. Of the following signs and symptoms, fibromyalgia most commonly presents with:

    a. Abrupt onset of proximal muscle weakness
    b. Widespread musculoskeletal pain and tender points
    c. Effusion of involved joints with mild local warmth
    d. Subcutaneous nodules

84. Secondary causes for high blood cholesterol do *not* include:

    a. Diabetes
    b. Obstructive liver disease
    c. Medication-induced states
    d. Hypothyroidism

85. A systolic click preceding a mid-to-late systolic murmur is most likely caused by which of the following?

    a. Aortic stenosis
    b. Mitral valve prolapse
    c. Mitral valve stenosis
    d. Idiopathic hypertrophic subaortic stenosis

86. Which of the following is *not* a likely symptom of pathologic murmur?

    a. Cough
    b. Chest pain
    c. Shortness of breath on exertion
    d. Hemoptysis

87. Management for irritable bowel syndrome (IBS):

    a. Should not include changes in diet except for eliminating milk products
    b. Includes use of medications to reduce incidence of ulcerative colitis
    c. Is based on the predominant symptoms experienced by the patient
    d. Includes regular screening for colon cancer because of increased risk with IBS

88. Virchow's triad defines the clinical origin of most venous thrombi and includes all of the following factors *except*:

    a. Stasis
    b. Endothelial damage
    c. Deposition of cholesterol plaques
    d. Hypercoagulability

89. A patient presents with signs and symptoms suggestive of a superficial phlebitis. Physical findings in this patient would include:

    a. Tenderness in the area of the involved vein
    b. Edema of the involved extremity
    c. Pale, cool skin in the area of involved vein
    d. Palpable venous cord

90. In the United States, the most common cause of community-acquired bacterial pneumonia is:

    a. *Streptococcus pneumoniae*
    b. *Streptococcus pyogenes*
    c. *Haemophilus influenzae*
    d. *Legionella pneumophilia*

91. A 22-year-old female presents with a complaint of nonbloody diarrhea of 5–6 days duration. Associated symptoms include abdominal cramping, low-grade fever and nausea. She recently returned from a trip to Mexico. Appropriate initial evaluation would include:

    a. Abdominal ultrasound
    b. Barium enema
    c. H. pylori testing
    d. Stool for fecal leukocytes

92. In rheumatoid arthritis, _____ is/are often found, indicative of the inflammatory process.

    a. Fever
    b. Elevated erythrocyte sedimentation rate
    c. Joint erosion on radiography
    d. Painful joints

93. Your patient is experiencing 3–4 migraine headaches per month. You decide to begin prophylactic medication. Which of the following is recommended for migraine headache prophylaxis?

    a. Ergotamine
    b. Propranolol (Beta blocker)
    c. Sumatriptan
    d. SSRI

94. Rheumatoid arthritis is characterized by which of the following?

    a. Osteophyte formation
    b. Cartilage degeneration
    c. Inflammation of the synovium and joint capsule
    d. Sclerosis of subchondral bone

95. A 21-year-old college student presents with a 5-day history of fever, headache, sore throat, muscle aches, and a nonproductive cough. Her throat is erythematous; lung exam is unremarkable. Chest x-ray reveals a left-lower lobe patchy infiltrate. The most likely cause is which of the following?

    a. *Steptococcus pneumoniae*
    b. *Mycoplasma pneumoniae*
    c. *Klebsiella pneumoniae*
    d. *Haemophilus influenzae*

96. Acute otitis media is characterized by all of the following physical examination findings *except*:

    a. Distorted light reflex
    b. Obscured bony landmarks
    c. Erythema of the ear canal
    d. Preauricular lymphadenopathy

97. Laboratory tests supportive of a diagnosis of infectious mononucleosis include all of the following *except*:

    a. Elevated basophils and eosinophils
    b. Presence of heterophil antibodies
    c. Elevated liver enzymes
    d. GABHS on throat culture

98. Secondary causes of seizures include:

    a. Syncope
    b. Hyperventilation
    c. Narcolepsy
    d. Toxic substance abuse

99. The most common type of seizure disorder in adults is:

    a. Clonic-tonic
    b. Partial
    c. Complex partial
    d. Grand mal

100. Macrocytic anemias include:

    a. Anemia of chronic disease
    b. B_{12} deficiency anemia
    c. Iron deficiency anemia
    d. Sickle cell anemia

101. A 52-year-old menopausal female client smokes one pack per day and has a history of a deep vein thrombosis in her leg 2 years ago. She has a BMD T-score of –1.75. Which of the following medications would be the most appropriate for this client to prevent osteoporosis?

    a. Alendronate
    b. Calcitonin
    c. Estrogen
    d. Raloxifene

102. Which of the following statements is correct concerning bone mass density (BMD) testing?

    a. Test results are most predictive of bone fracture when done on an annual basis.
    b. The T-score compares BMD of the client with an age-matched normal adult.
    c. BMD T-scores should be combined with bone x-ray to confirm osteoporosis.
    d. Treatment decisions based on T-scores may vary according to risk factors.

103. A 40-year-old female has complaint of chronic backache and has been diagnosed to have a vertebral compression fracture. She also has hirsutism, facial acne, and red-purple abdominal striae. An appropriate initial test for a possible secondary cause for osteoporosis in this client would be:

    a. Dexamethasone suppression test
    b. Parathyroid hormone level
    c. Protein electrophoresis
    d. Thyroid function tests

104. Client instructions for taking alendronate should include:

    a. Take medication with breakfast
    b. Take medication at bedtime
    c. Take medication on an empty stomach
    d. Take medication with an antacid

105. One of the most significant laboratory tests for evaluating an individual for chronic or heavy alcohol use is a/an:

    a. ALP
    b. BUN
    c. CBC
    d. GGT

106. Which of the following is a characteristic finding with stimulant abuse but not depressant abuse?

    a. Euphoria
    b. Pupil dilation
    c. Tremors
    d. Violent behavior

107. Two months after being raped, a client tells you she cannot concentrate on her schoolwork and is having nightmares about the experience. These symptoms indicate that she:

    a. Is still in the acute phase of rape trauma syndrome
    b. Is going through normal reorganization following a rape
    c. Is experiencing posttraumatic stress disorder
    d. Now has a generalized anxiety disorder

108. A client who has been experiencing fatigue, insomnia, difficulty concentrating, and feelings of worthlessness for the past 2 weeks would meet the *DSM IV* criteria for a major depressive disorder if she also has:

    a. Loss of interest in her usual activities
    b. Psychomotor retardation
    c. Psychosomatic complaints
    d. Suicidal ideation

109. A 22-year-old female presents with three episodes of chest pain, shortness of breath, palpitations, dizziness, sweating, and fear of losing control. Onset of symptoms occurred while she was traveling on the bus. She is avoiding the use of public transportation because she is fearful of recurrence of the symptoms. The most likely diagnosis is:

    a. Panic disorder with agoraphobia
    b. Panic attack
    c. Generalized anxiety disorder
    d. Social anxiety disorder

110. A 24-year-old female client with major depression tells you that she feels like her life is falling apart. She recently lost her job, had to move out of her apartment, and now lives with her sister. Her risk factors for a suicide attempt include:

    a. Age between 20 and 30
    b. Female gender
    c. Current living situation
    d. Sense of hopelessness

111. A client tells you that she experiences chest tightness, difficulty breathing, and dizziness whenever she has to ride on the city bus. Her symptoms best fit a description of:

    a. Acute stress disorder
    b. Agoraphobia
    c. Obsessive-compulsive disorder
    d. Social phobia

112. The most common type of anxiety disorder is:

    a. Acute stress disorder
    b. Generalized anxiety disorder
    c. Obsessive-compulsive disorder
    d. Panic disorder

113. Which of the following statements concerning bulimia is correct?

    a. Age of onset is usually early adolescence.
    b. Amenorrhea is usually present.
    c. Mortality rate is higher than for anorexia nervosa.
    d. Impulsive behavior is a common characteristic.

114. Major side-effects of SSRIs include:

    a. Anticholinergic effects
    b. Nausea
    c. Orthostatic hypotension
    d. Urinary retention

115. A 35-year-old female with a history of generalized anxiety disorder requests a refill of alprazolam. You are concerned about risks associated with long-term use. Which of the following represents an alternative medication?

    a. Buspirone (Buspar)
    b. Clonazepam (Klonopin)
    c. Bupropion (Wellbutrin)
    d. Citalopram (Celexa)

116. A behavior that fits the criteria for substance dependence but not for substance abuse is:

    a. Loss of a job related to substance use
    b. Driving while intoxicated
    c. Continuing to drink despite family's objections
    d. Unsuccessful attempts to cut down use

117. Physical findings that help the clinician to make a diagnosis of bulimia would include:

    a. Erosion of tooth enamel
    b. Hypotension
    c. Presence of lanugo
    d. Stress fractures

118. Which of the following statements concerning rape is correct?

    a. All of the states have now established the same legal definition for rape.
    b. The majority of rapes are committed by acquaintances of the victim.
    c. The most common emotional response of the victim in the acute phase is anger.
    d. The clinician is responsible for determining if a rape has actually occurred.

119. All of the following symptoms are accepted criteria for a diagnosis of major depression *except*:

    a. Feelings of worthlessness or excessive guilt
    b. Chronic pain without biomedical explanation
    c. Loss of pleasure in usual activities
    d. Psychomotor agitation or retardation

120. Severe exacerbations in an individual with intermittent (step 1) asthma are appropriately treated with:

    a. Mast-cell stabilizers
    b. Short acting inhaled B_2-agonists
    c. Systemic corticosteroids
    d. Theophylline

◘ ANSWERS

1. c	25. c	49. a	85. b
2. c	26. a	50. a	86. d
3. a	27. a	51. c	87. c
4. c	28. d	52. d	88. c
5. d	29. d	53. c	89. a
6. d	30. b	54. c	90. a
7. a	31. a	55. c	91. d
8. c	32. a	56. b	92. b
9. a	33. a	57. b	93. b
10. d	34. d	58. d	94. c
11. b	35. d	59. a	95. b
12. a	36. d	60. d	96. c
13. d	37. b	61. b	97. d
14. c	38. c	62. b	98. d
15. d	39. b	63. c	99. c
16. d	40. c	64. c	100. b
17. c	41. c	65. c	101. a
18. d	42. b	66. a	102. d
19. a	43. b	67. c	103. a
20. d	44. d	68. b	104. c
21. b	45. a	69. d	105. d
22. a	46. b	70. c	106. b
23. d	47. d	71. c	107. c
24. c	48. a	72. b	108. a
		73. a	109. a
		74. b	110. d
		75. d	111. b
		76. d	112. b
		77. b	113. d
		78. a	114. b
		79. c	115. a
		80. a	116. d
		81. b	117. a
		82. d	118. b
		83. b	119. b
		84. a	120. c

◘ BIBLIOGRAPHY

Adams, S., Miller, K., & Zylstra, R. (2008). Pharmacologic management of adult depression. *American Family Physician, 77*(6), 785–796.

American Diabetes Association. (2009). Standards of medical care in diabetes—2009. *Diabetes Care, 32*(Suppl 1), S14–S61.

American Psychiatric Association. (1994). *Diagnostic and statistical manual of mental disorders* (4th ed.). Washington, DC: Author.

American Psychiatric Association. (2000). *Quick reference to the diagnostic criteria from DSM-IV-TR.* Washington DC: Author.

Bickley, L. (2009). *Bates' guide to physical examination and history taking* (10th ed.). Philadelphia, PA: Lippincott, Williams, & Wilkins.

Buttaro, T., Trybulski, J., Bailey, P., & Sandberg-Cook, J. (2008). *Primary care: A collaborative approach* (3rd ed.). St. Louis: Mosby, Inc.

Chakrabarty, S., & Zoorab, R. (2007). Fibromyalgia. *American Family Physician, 76*, 247–254.

Ernst, D., & Lee, A. (Eds.). (Summer 2009). *Nurse practitioner's prescribing reference.* New York: Prescribing Reference LLC.

Ferri, F. (2009). *Ferri's 2010 clinical advisor.* St. Louis: Mosby, Inc.

Fraker, T., & Fihn, S. (2007). 2007 Chronic angina focused update of the ACC/AHA 2002 guidelines for the management of patients with chronic stable angina. *Circulation, 116*, 2762–2772.

Goldman, L., & Ausiello, D. (2007). *Cecil's textbook of medicine* (23rd ed.). Philadelphia, PA: Saunders.

Hackely, B., Kriebs, J., & Rousseau, M. (2007). *Primary care of women: A guide for midwives and women's health providers.* Sudbury, MA: Jones and Bartlett.

Inge, L., & Wilson, J. (2008). Update on the treatment of tuberculosis. *American Family Physician, 78*(4), 457–470.

National Heart, Lung, and Blood Institute. (2007). *Expert panel report 3: Guidelines for the diagnosis and management of asthma.* (NIH Publication No. 08-4051). Bethesda, MD: Author.

National Heart, Lung, and Blood Institute. (2003). *Seventh report of the Joint National Committee on Prevention, Detection, Evaluation and Treatment of High Blood Pressure.* (NIH Publication No. 03-5233). Bethesda, MD: Author.

National Heart, Lung, and Blood Institute. (2001). *Third report of the National Cholesterol Education Program Expert Panel on Detection, Evaluation and Treatment of High Cholesterol in Adults* (Adult Treatment Panel III). (NIH Publication No. 01-3095). Bethesda, MD: Author.

National Osteoporosis Foundation. (2008). *Clinician's guide to prevention and treatment of osteoporosis.* Washington, DC: Author.

Panel on Clinical Practices for the Treatment of HIV. (2002). *Guidelines for the use of antiretroviral agents in HIV-infected adults and adolescents.* Department of Health and Human Services. Retrieved March 10, 2003 from http://www.aidsinfo.nih.gov/guidelines/adult/html.

Williams, P., Goodie, J., & Motsinger, C. (2008). Treating eating disorders in primary care. *American Family Physician, 77*(2), 187–195.

Wynne, A., Woo, T., & Olyaei, A. (2007). *Pharmacotherapeutics for nurse practitioner prescribers* (2nd ed.). Philadelphia, PA: F. A. Davis.

9

Advanced Practice Nursing and Midwifery: Role Development, Trends, and Issues

Patricia Burkhardt

◻ ADVANCED PRACTICE REGISTERED NURSE (APRN)

- Definition—a registered nurse who has accomplished the following:
    1. Completed an accredited graduate level program preparing him/her for one of four recognized APRN roles
    2. Passed a national certification examination that measures APRN role and population competencies and who maintains certification. Acquired advanced clinical knowledge and skills preparing him/her to provide direct care to patients, as well as a component of indirect care
    3. Is educationally prepared to assume responsibility and accountability for health promotion/maintenance, assessment, diagnosis, and management of patient problems, which includes use and prescription of pharmacologic and nonpharmacologic interventions
    4. Obtained clinical experience of sufficient depth and breadth to reflect the intended license. Obtained a license to practice as an APRN in one of the four APRN roles (APRN Consensus Workgroup & National Council of State Boards of Nursing APRN Advisory Committee, 2008)

- The four APRN roles:
    1. Nurse practitioners (NPs)
        a. Definition—primary and/or specialty care providers who practice in ambulatory, acute, and long-term care settings, providing nursing and medical services to individuals, families, and groups (American Academy of Nurse Practitioners, 2007)
        b. Historical development
            (1) 1964—first NP program developed at University of Colorado Health Sciences Center
            (2) Prompted by shortage of area pediatricians
            (3) Pediatric nurse practitioner (PNP) became model for development of NPs in other specialty areas
        c. Functions
            (1) As a primary care provider (PCP), provides care that is integrated and accessible
            (2) Emphasizes health promotion, disease prevention
            (3) Professionally, practice is autonomous, collaborative, and evidence based
            (4) Functionally, practice is defined by state law, regulations, and clinical privileges
            (5) Diagnoses, treats, and manages health problems
            (6) Teaches and counsels individuals, families, and groups
            (7) Clinical roles include researcher, consultant, and patient advocate
            (8) Professional roles include mentor, educator, researcher, and administrator
            (9) Maintains accountability for care of patients and decisions reached

d. Education
   (1) Master's degree, post-master's certificate, or Doctorate of Nursing Practice (DNP)
   (2) Length of study for master's degree approximately 2 years full time; includes extensive clinical experience supervised by qualified preceptors within a population focus and possibly a specialty track
   (3) Current programs for Women's Health NP are master's, post-master's certificate, or Doctor of Nursing Practice (DNP)
   (4) Curriculum
      (a) Graduate core courses that include content in nursing theory, organizational theory, ethics, research, legal issues, economics, healthcare delivery
      (b) APRN core content that includes advanced health assessment, physiology/pathology, pharmacology, clinical diagnosis and management, health promotion, and disease prevention
      (c) Additional courses with content specific to the nurse practitioner role and women's health population focus; includes extensive supervised clinical hours
      (d) The National Association of Nurse Practitioners in Women's Health (NPWH) and Association of Women's Health, Obstetrics and Neonatal Nurses (AWHONN) (2008) jointly provide guidelines for women's health nurse practitioner practice and education
      (e) Women's Health NP programs are accredited within schools of nursing by two organizations: the National League for Nursing Accrediting Commission (NLNAC) or the Commission on Collegiate Nursing Education (CCNE)
   (5) Domains/core competencies of nurse practitioner practice (National Organization of Nurse Practitioner Faculties, 2006)
      (a) Management of Patient Health/Illness Status
      (b) Nurse Practitioner–Patient Relationship
      (c) Teaching–Coaching Function
      (d) Professional Role
      (e) Managing and Negotiating Healthcare Delivery Systems
      (f) Monitoring and Ensuring the Quality of Healthcare Practice
      (g) Culturally Sensitive Care
e. Certification
   (1) To be eligible to take the certification examination offered for the Women's Health NP, the student must have graduated from an accredited master's, post-master's, or DNP program in the women's health population focus
   (2) Women's Health Nurse Practitioner Certification is provided by the National Certification Corporation (NCC)
   (3) Certification must be renewed every 3 years, through either reexamination or achievement of specified hours of continuing education

2. Certified registered nurse anesthetists (CRNAs) (American Association of Nurse Anesthetists, 1999)
   a. Definition—an advanced practice nurse and anesthesia specialist who provides high quality, cost-effective care for patients before, during and after surgical procedures in which anesthesia is administered; first clinical nursing specialty; developed in late 1800s
   b. Functions
      (1) Administers and monitors anesthesia/patient response during surgery
      (2) Acts as clinician, administrator, educator, researcher
      (3) CRNAs practice more in rural communities and provide more than half of all anesthesia in US
   c. Education
      (1) Master's degree
      (2) Programs vary from 24 to 36 months and include classroom and clinical experiences
      (3) National certification is required
      (4) Must earn continuing education credits to maintain certification
3. Clinical nurse specialists (CNSs)
   a. Definition—APRN with role of integrating care across the health–illness continuum and through three spheres of influence: patient, nurse, system
   b. Functions
      (1) Direct care functions include expert practitioner, role model, patient advocate, and educator

    (2) Indirect care functions include change agent, consultant or resource person, liaison person, and innovator

  c. Education

    (1) Master's degree, post-master's, or DNP

    (2) Curriculum includes core courses in nursing theory, organizational theory, ethics, legal issues, healthcare delivery and CNS role and population focus courses/supervised clinical experience

4. Certified nurse-midwife (CNM) or certified midwife (CM) (see next section)

◘ MIDWIFERY

- History of US Midwifery

1. Midwifery practice was honored in colonial America, but changes in religious attitudes, economic demands, development of science, physician advances, low status of women, and lack of organization and education caused the profession to fall into disrepute by the 20th century

2. Need for prenatal education and care identified by the Maternity Center Association in New York City, established 1918; from this the idea to formally prepare nurses in obstetrics arose

3. Midwifery education through the Bellevue School of Midwifery (1911–1935) in NYC and the Preston Retreat Hospital (1923) in Philadelphia upgraded midwifery education and practice

4. 1921—passage of the Sheppard-Towner Act to improve maternal–infant care and provide for instruction of untrained midwives

5. 1928—Mary Breckinridge of the Frontier Nursing Service (FNS) imported nurse-midwives from England to serve the people in the Kentucky mountains

6. 1931—the Lobenstein School for the Promotion and Standardization of Midwifery was incorporated; was the first formal, organized midwifery education program

7. 1955—formation of the American College of Nurse-Midwifery whose purpose was to set standards for midwifery practice and education

8. 1968—clinical nurse midwifery practice broadened as Maternal–Infant Care (MIC) in NYC linked community clinic practice with hospital practice

9. 1971—American College of Obstetricians/Gynecologists (ACOG), Nurses Association of ACOG, and American College of Nurse-Midwives signed joint statement supporting development of the midwifery role

10. 1980–1990s—full range of practice sites and services offered by CNMs as profession grew

11. 1982—formation of the Midwives Alliance of North America (MANA), whose purpose was to provide support and a forum for anyone interested in midwifery

12. Titles used for American midwives

  a. Granny—like traditional birth attendants, these women answered to needs of community women; trained by experience and other practicing midwives

  b. Direct entry midwife—term used to define two different realities

    (1) Individual trained in midwifery through apprenticeship method outside the structure of formal education programs

    (2) Midwife educated in midwifery without nursing background

  c. Certified Professional Midwife (CPM)—credential developed and administered by North American Registry of Midwives (NARM)

  d. Certified Nurse Midwife (CNM)/Certified Midwife (CM)—midwife graduated from programs accredited by Accreditation Commission for Midwifery Education (ACME)—formerly American College of Nurse Midwives (ACNM) Division of Accreditation—and certified by the American Midwifery Certification Board (AMCB)—formerly ACNM Certification Council (ACC)

  e. Licensed midwife (LM)—midwife licensed through state law; may include any of the previous categories depending on the state's law

  f. Doula—a woman who provides support and assistance to the pregnant woman during birth and/or postpartum

13. Midwifery and CNMs/CMs in the 21st century

  a. Definition—"Midwifery practice is the independent management of women's health care, focusing particularly on pregnancy, childbirth, the postpartum period, care of the newborn, and the family planning and gynecological needs of women." (Varney, Kriebs, Gegor, 2004, p. 3)

  b. Hallmarks of midwifery (Core Competencies for Basic Midwifery Practice, 2002)

    (1) Recognition of pregnancy and birth as a normal physiologic and developmental process and advocacy of nonintervention in the absence of complications

(2) Recognition of menses and menopause as a normal physiologic and developmental process

(3) Promotion of family-centered care

(4) Empowerment of women as partners in health care

(5) Facilitation of healthy family and interpersonal relationships

(6) Promotion of continuity of care

(7) Health promotion, disease prevention, and health education

(8) Advocacy for informed choice, participatory decision making, and the right to self-determination

(9) Cultural competency and proficiency

(10) Skillful communication, guidance, and counseling

(11) Therapeutic value of human presence

(12) Value of and respect for differing paths toward knowledge and growth

(13) Effective communication and collaboration with other members of the healthcare team

(14) Promotion of a public healthcare perspective

(15) Care to vulnerable populations

c. Practice

(1) As a primary healthcare provider, provides care that is integrated and accessible to women and families

(2) Practice is autonomous or collaborative, and evidence-based

(3) Provides health promotion, disease prevention, counseling, and education across the life span

(4) Diagnoses, treats, and manages common health problems

(5) Focuses on childbearing, newborn care, postpartum care, family planning, and gynecological care

(6) Accepts accountability for care provided

(7) Of the various models of practice, private practice in a midwifery group provides the most autonomy

(8) Site of practice is in all places where women's health care is needed, including the home

d. Education

(1) Prior to 2010, included postbaccalaureate certificate, master's degrees, and post-master's certificate programs

(2) Beginning in 2010, all programs will be master's degree, post-master's certificate, DNP, or other doctoral degree (ACNM, 2009)

(3) To be eligible to take the certification exam of the American Midwifery Certification Board (AMCB), the student must graduate from a program accredited by the Accreditation Commission on Midwifery Education (ACME)

(4) Programs accredited by ACME may or may not require nursing

(5) Curriculum is based on the ACNM Core Competencies for Basic Midwifery Practice (2007)

(a) Delineate knowledge and skill base for entry into midwifery practice

(b) Competencies defined by ACNM

i. Revised through rigorous review every 5 years to reflect standards of practice

ii. Process takes 1 full year with opportunity for input from membership and is approved by the ACNM Board of Directors

(c) Delineates expected fundamental knowledge, skills and behaviors expected of new midwife, to include:

i. Hallmarks—art and science of midwifery

ii. Professional responsibilities

iii. Midwifery management process

iv. Fundamentals of midwifery care

v. The care of the childbearing family

vi. The primary health care of women

• The American College of Nurse-Midwives (ACNM)

1. Established in 1955 to serve as the professional organization for nurse midwives and was called the American College of Nurse Midwifery

2. Founded to set the standards for education and practice of nurse midwives

3. The name changed from American College of Nurse Midwifery to American College of Nurse Midwives as a result of merger with American Association of Nurse Midwives (AANM)

4. Purposes of the ACNM

a. Promotion and development of quality care for women and infants

b. Commitment to excellent educational standards

c. Expansion of knowledge through research and evaluation

d. Provision of mechanisms for members to maintain midwifery standards and practice quality in accordance with ACNM philosophy

5. Structure of the College

   a. The Board of Directors (BOD), consisting of President, Vice-President, Secretary, Treasurer, and Regional Representatives, are elected by the members of the College and make decisions and set policy for the College

   b. The Executive Director is responsible for the day-to-day operation of the organization in the National Office

   c. Housed in the National Office but separate in budget and function are the Division of Accreditation and the ACNM Foundation

   d. The midwives' political action committee (PAC) is separate in budget but an integral part of the ACNM that was established to provide contributions to federal legislators in order to further the interests of CNMs/CMs and the women's agenda

   e. Divisions and committees do a vast portion of the work of furthering the profession and the health care of women through the College

   f. Regions representing local chapters covering all 50 states and US territories facilitate communication between Board of Directors and members

6. Functions of the College

   a. To advocate for the healthcare needs and well-being of women and families

   b. To further the interests of the profession of midwifery while maintaining the highest standards of practice and education

   c. To protect and enhance the rights of members

7. Continuing Competency Assessment (CCA) program—voluntary program whose purposes are (as of September 1, 2010, the CCA program will no longer be available):

   a. To assure continuing professional education based on a 5-year cycle

   b. To assist CNMs in providing documentation of appropriate credential maintenance to state licensing bodies and hospital credentialing units

   c. To foster development of methods of competency assessment that evaluate psychomotor, cognitive, and affective domains of midwifery practice

8. Standards of practice (ACNM, 2003)

   a. Standards reflect independent management of women's health care, with a focus on pregnancy, childbirth, postpartum period, care of neonate, family planning, and gynecological well-being

   b. Expansion of competencies beyond basic core

9. Quality assurance in midwifery

   a. Peer review encouraged and implemented at local chapter level

   b. Practice outcomes documented with focused review of unexpected outcomes

   c. Midwifery practice mechanisms for collaboration, consultation, and referral occur via jointly agreed-upon practice guidelines

10. Fellowship of the College (FACNM)

   a. Established in 1993 to honor members whose professional achievements, outstanding scholarship, clinical excellence, and/or demonstrated leadership has merited them recognition both within and outside the midwifery profession

   b. Two categories of Fellowship—Distinguished Fellows and Fellows

- Certification

   1. American Midwifery Certification Board (AMCB) provides examination for graduates of ACME-accredited programs

   2. All CNMs/CMs certified after January 1996 receive time-limited certificates that must be renewed; effective January 1, 2011 all CNMs/CMs will have time-limited certificates that must be renewed every 5 years

   3. AMCB implements a Certificate Maintenance Program (CMP) for all CNMs/CMs who need recertification

   4. AMCB-certified midwives (nonnurse) practice legally in New York, New Jersey, and Rhode Island

◻ TRENDS AND ISSUES

- Those common to both NPs and CNMs/CMs

   1. Healthy People 2010 initiatives (DHHS, 2000)

      a. Prevention agenda for the nation to increase years of healthy life while reducing health disparities

      b. Objectives significant as leading national health indicators

      c. Origin is the 1979 Surgeon General's report on health promotion and disease prevention entitled "Healthy People"

d. Healthy People 2010
  (1) Delineates 10 leading health indicators that will be used to measure the health of the nation over the next 10 years
  (2) More extensive work underway on issue of expanding leading health indicators with purpose of extending the reach of Healthy People
  (3) Healthy People 2020 will be released in two phases
    (a) Framework (vision, mission, goals, focus areas, and criteria for selecting and prioritizing objectives)—2009
    (b) Healthy People 2020 objectives with guidance for achieving the new 10-year targets—2010
2. Primary health care and healthcare reform
  a. Healthcare system reform—four critical issues (ANA, 2008)
    (1) Access—affordable, available, acceptable
    (2) Quality—safe, effective, patient centered, timely, efficient, equitable (Institute of Medicine, 2001)
    (3) Cost—more focus on primary care, ultimately requiring less secondary and tertiary care that is more costly; privately and publicly funded options for standard package of essential healthcare services
    (4) Healthcare workforce—adequate supply of well-educated, well-distributed, and well-utilized registered nurses
  b. Components of primary health care
    (1) Entry point to the health system that provides access to secondary and tertiary care
    (2) Care is accessible, comprehensive, coordinated, continuous, accountable
    (3) Serves as a strategy for organizing health care into a system in which community-oriented primary care is delivered
    (4) Prioritizes and allocates resources to community-based care as opposed to hospital-based acute care
    (5) Providers include family medicine, general internal medicine, pediatricians, obstetricians/gynecologists, certified nurse midwives, nurse practitioners, physician assistants
    (6) Care includes age- and gender-specific screening for health promotion/disease prevention as well as diagnosis and treatment of common illnesses

c. The American Nurses Association, American Academy of Nurse Practitioners, National Association of Nurse Practitioners in Women's Health, American College of Nurse Midwives, and other advanced nursing practice organizations provide leadership to establish the following:
  (1) Delivery systems that assure accessible, quality, and affordable services
  (2) Availability of basic and essential health services to all individuals
  (3) Support of primary care
  (4) Shift from illness/cure focus to wellness/care focus
  (5) Support for insurance reform that assures access to NPs/midwives and payment for their services
  (6) Collaborative review of resource allocation, cost-reduction plans, and reimbursement issues by representatives from public and private sectors
3. Professional liability insurance
  a. Recommended that each clinician carry individual policy
  b. Types of coverage
    (1) Occurrence—covers event of malpractice that occurred during the policy period without regard to when the claims are reported; provides protections for each policy period indefinitely; broadest protection available
    (2) Claims made—incident must happen and be reported while policy is in force; requires purchase of a tail policy to protect, once policy period ends
  c. Cost of insurance varies with APRN role and population focus
4. Scope of practice (Hamric, Spross, & Hanson, 2009)
  a. Definition—describes practice limits and sets parameters within which the APRN may legally practice
  b. Scope of practice aspects
    (1) Defines what is legally allowable
    (2) Defines what APRN can do with patients, what he/she can delegate, and when collaboration with others is required
    (3) Scope may differ depending on APRN role—clinical nurse specialist, nurse anesthetist, nurse midwife, nurse practitioner
    (4) Based on state laws promulgated by the various nurse practice acts and rules and regulations for APRN—varies from state to state

5. Standards of practice
   a. Definition—the description of the minimum levels of acceptable performance for a profession or specialty
   b. Aspects
      (1) Evolves from the scope of practice
      (2) Provides specifications for acceptable levels of care and a mechanism for determining excellence in care
      (3) Provides the framework for development of competency statements
      (4) Establishes the educational preparation for basic practice, and provides a statement of educational outcomes and standards for organized nursing practice
      (5) Provides quality assurance to consumers through accreditation and certification standards
      (6) May provide legal expectations of a practice
      (7) May be developed by specialty groups to guide particular aspects of practice
6. Nurse practice acts
   a. Definition—legislative enactments that define the practice of nursing, give guidance within the scope of practice issues, and set standards for practice; passage through state legislatures makes these the law under which nursing is practiced in that state
   b. Types of practice acts
      (1) Licensure statutes limit practice to individuals with specific qualifications as determined by law
      (2) Registration or certification statutes provide a definition and limit as to who may use title, without restraint of practice
   c. Aspects of practice acts
      (1) Regulated state by state
      (2) Authorizes state boards of nursing to establish statutory authority for the licensure of registered nurses, including APRNs
      (3) Authorizes state boards of nursing to establish a scope of practice, determine disciplinary actions, and regulate its practice via legislative statutes
      (4) Regulations reflect the trend to increase APRN authority and autonomy
      (5) May authorize prescriptive authority
7. Consensus model for APRN regulation—Licensure, Accreditation, Certification, and Education (LACE) (2008)
   a. Completed by APRN Consensus Work Group and National council of State Boards of Nursing APRN Advisory Committee
   b. Defines APRN practice
   c. Describes regulatory model for education, certification, and licensure of advanced practice registered nurses
      (1) Four APRN roles—nurse anesthetist, nurse midwife, clinical nurse specialist, nurse practitioner
      (2) Six population foci—family/individual across lifespan, adult–gerontology, neonatal, pediatrics, women's health, psychiatric–mental health
      (3) Education, certification, and licensure of individual must be congruent in terms of role and population focus
      (4) APRNs may specialize (e.g., acute care, palliative care) but cannot be certified or licensed solely within a specialty area
      (5) State boards of nursing will be solely responsible for licensing APRNs
   d. Identifies titles to be used
   e. Implementation of model will occur incrementally; target date for full implementation is 2015
8. Doctor of Nursing Practice (DNP)
   a. Practice-focused rather than research-focused nursing doctoral degree
   b. American Association of Colleges of Nursing (AACN) 2004 position statement calls for DNP degree to be required for entry into advanced nursing practice by 2015
   c. DNP Essentials established by AACN (2006) for curricular elements and competencies
   d. Entry into DNP program may be after completion of postbaccalaureate nursing degree (BS to DNP) or post-master's nursing degree (MS to DNP)
   e. Program length varies depending on BS-to-DNP/MS-to-DNP program type as well as APRN role and population focus
   f. Requires a minimum of 1000 hours of supervised postbaccalaureate clinical experience

- Trends and issues unique to midwifery
   1. The ACNM political action committee (PAC) was established to address critical federal legislative issues relating to women's health and the role of CNMs/CMs in delivering quality obstetric and gynecological care
   2. Primary care role—"With women, for a lifetime" (ACNM registered tag line)

a. Core Competencies for Basic Midwifery Practice (2007) include specific competencies for primary care

b. Nurse midwifery certification examination began to include content for primary care in 2001

c. Rationale—evolving toward primary care is in best interests of women, since CNMs/CMs are often their only care providers, and makes CNMs/CMs more congruent with the current healthcare system

3. Cultural competence

a. CNMs/CMs have always cared for vulnerable populations of women who represent a wide variety of ethnic and cultural roots

b. Concepts of cultural competence are part of the Core Competencies for Basic Midwifery Practice

4. International midwifery

a. Midwifery education and practice vary between the developed and less developed countries with the level of education higher in the former

b. Even in countries with numerous midwives and a long history of professional midwifery practice, the profession struggles with the continuing trend toward "medicalization" and increased use of technology

c. Midwifery, in most countries, is a separate profession, but where it is associated with nursing, midwifery subsumes nursing rather than midwifery being an arm of nursing

d. The International Confederation of Midwives (ICM) provides midwifery leadership across nations

◨ PROFESSIONAL COMPONENTS OF ADVANCED PRACTICE NURSING AND MIDWIFERY

- Credentialing (institutional and regulatory body levels)
  1. Definition—the process of assessing and validating the qualifications of a licensed independent practitioner (LIP) to provide member health services in a healthcare network and/or its components
  2. Outcomes
     a. Mandates accountability and responsibility for competence
     b. Assures that care is provided by qualified practitioners
     c. Testifies to compliance with federal and state laws regarding nursing and midwifery practice
     d. Acknowledges advanced scope of practice

- Privileging
  1. Definition—authorization granted to a practitioner by the healthcare network or a component of the network to provide specific patient care services that must fall within defined limits based upon the LIP's qualifications and current competence
  2. Privileging, either through medical staff or allied health staff mechanisms, can put NP and CNM/CM providers on the same level with physicians with regard to rights and responsibilities
  3. The Joint Commission modified its standards on staff privileges to include nonphysician providers who were licensed independent providers (LIP)

- Practice issues
  1. Licensure
     a. Process by which a government agency authorizes individuals to practice a profession or occupation by validating that the individual has attained the required degree of competency as prescribed by law to protect the public welfare
     b. Regulated on state-by-state basis through nursing or midwifery practice acts
  2. Certification
     a. The formal process by which a private agency or organization certifies (usually by examination) that an individual has met standards as specified by that profession (Hamric, Spross, & Hanson, 2009)
     b. Aspects of certification
        (1) Assures the public that an individual has mastered a body of knowledge and acquired skills in a particular specialty to assure quality practitioners
        (2) Used by most states as one component of second licensure for advanced nursing practice
        (3) Requires or encourages maintenance of a particular level of competence following initial credentialing
        (4) May be used as a mechanism for control of practice

- Prescriptive authority
  1. Definition—legal authority to prescribe medications or devices
  2. Authority is contained in state nurse or midwifery practice acts or in other statutes and varies from state to state
  3. May require approval of state board of medicine, midwifery, public health, or pharmacy
  4. Requires completion of an advanced pharmacology course and continuing education hours to maintain prescribing status

5. May require a collaborative practice agreement and/or written protocols
6. May obtain federal Drug Enforcement Agency (DEA) registration number, depending on scope of state law

- Independent and collaborative management of care
    1. Independent—care of women within the provider's scope of practice, based on knowledge, skills, and competencies
    2. Consultation—seeks advice or opinion of a physician or other member of the healthcare team while the NP/midwife retains primary responsibility for the woman's care
    3. Referral—the process by which the provider directs the client to a physician or another healthcare professional for management of a particular problem or aspect of the client's care
    4. Collaboration—NP/midwife and physician jointly manage the care of a woman who has developed complications, the goal of which is to share authority while providing quality care within each individual's scope of practice

- Professional organizations
    1. Purposes and benefits of membership
        a. Purposes of professional nursing and midwifery organizations
            (1) Promote and set high standards for health care
            (2) Enhance the identity, visibility, and practice of its members
            (3) Provide a collective voice to promote the profession of midwifery, nursing, and the APRN role
        b. Individual benefits
            (1) Membership within a community of like-providers who share commonalities specific to their specialty areas
            (2) Networking availability through participation in local, regional, and national meetings, alliances, and coalitions
            (3) Legislative representation, support, and participation at all levels
            (4) Continuing education programs to attain/maintain clinical competency
            (5) May provide consultation and assistance in securing federal scholarship and loans for continuation of study
            (6) Receipt of organizational publications
            (7) Listings of employment opportunities
            (8) Professional recognition of excellence in practice and research

    2. Organizational activities
        a. Provides, fosters, and facilitates leadership for and among members
        b. Disseminates information relevant to practice
        c. Monitors and influences laws and regulations
        d. Produces position papers communicating organizational perspectives on issues of concern
        e. Establishes practice competencies and standards and may offer continuing education resources
        f. Enhances the visibility of the members through marketing, public relation efforts
        g. May construct and maintain a national database of all provider activities
        h. Encourages and supports research efforts

- Reimbursement
    1. Types of reimbursement
        a. Fee-for-service—payment in which a usual, customary, or reasonable charge for service as determined by provider is submitted
        b. Fee schedules—predetermined payment for services in which equal pay for equal work prevails, and as a resource-based schedule may consider practice expenses, provider skills and time, and malpractice expenses
        c. Percentage—percentage either above or below that listed on the fee schedule is calculated depending upon who is providing the care
        d. Capitation—payment is made to the provider for each enrolled patient within a managed care organization (MCO), based on the terms of the contract's per member per month (PMPM) costs
        e. Indirect billing—method in which the institution is named as the recipient of payment, and the provider is usually an employee of the institution
        f. Direct billing—method in which the provider is a recognized provider of services and the payer reimburses on submission of a bill; advantages of direct billing include:
            (1) Increased availability and access to health care
            (2) Increased choice of providers
            (3) Reduced restrictions on practice
            (4) Potential for cost-effectiveness
            (5) Making visible and legitimate the APRN and midwifery role

◻ HEALTH POLICY AND LEGISLATIVE REGULATION OF MIDWIFERY AND NURSING

- Law making
  1. Definition—activity of state or federal legislative or lawmaking branch of government in which proposals or bills specifically define the actions or solutions to problems that affect a particular interested party
  2. Outlines strategies for problem resolution, suggests timelines for implementation, and attaches proposed budgets to support start-up programs
  3. Law results after concluding specified processes through the legislative body and signed by the President or state governor
  4. Nurse practice acts represent legislative regulation of advanced practice nursing
  5. Midwifery is legislated by nursing, midwifery, public health, or other statutes; some states may have two levels of legislation; one for nurse midwives and one for midwives who are not nurses

- Regulatory action
  1. Activity within specified and appropriate government agencies in which regulations are developed that specify how the law is to be implemented
  2. Extremely important since the language of law is terse and requires interpretation provided by the regulations
  3. State professional boards serve as regulatory bodies defining regulations stemming from law

◻ HEALTHCARE DELIVERY SYSTEMS

- Traditional health care
  1. Emphasizes independent providers
  2. Characteristics
     a. Providers chosen by patient with little, if any, influence from third party payer
     b. Provider reimbursed by patient and insurers in fee-for-service arrangement
     c. Insurers reimburse according to usual, customary, and reasonable system, permitting greater latitude in provider rate setting

- Integrated delivery systems/managed care organizations (MCOs)
  1. A health delivery system that strives to provide high quality, cost-effective care through a coordination of health services historically provided by a variety of caregivers; shifting emphasis from a fee-for-service strategy to one in which the network of providers assumes some degree of responsibility for both provision and cost of care
  2. Characteristics
     a. Vertical integration of services
        (1) Varying levels of care that are coordinated into a seamless system
        (2) Patients negotiate the delivery system smoothly
     b. Capitated system of payment/prospective pricing
        (1) Financial risk assumed by provider
        (2) Unit of value is cost per member per month (PMPM), determined in advance by contract (prospectively)
        (3) Age and gender budget is allotted to provider
        (4) Provider responsible for this target population
        (5) To remain financially solvent, target population should be healthy, which means that they consume the least dollars for care provided
     c. Low cost, high quality service with emphasis on health promotion
        (1) Goal of an integrated service
        (2) Increases value of system to consumers and payers
        (3) Service bundling, where complementary care can be offered as a package, further reduces costs
     d. Resource rationing
        (1) Primary care provider (PCP) is responsible for provision and management of services
        (2) Emphasis is on appropriate levels of care, but not unlimited care
  3. Types of managed care plans
     a. Health Maintenance Organization (HMO)
        (1) Established under HMO Act of 1973
        (2) Most common plan with focus on preventive care
        (3) Prepayment of premiums with preestablished benefit package for care
        (4) MCO contracts with PCP to provide care to enrollees, creating incentive for cost-effective care
        (5) PCP is selected by enrollee, manages total care, authorizes specialty visits resulting in designation as "gatekeeper"
     b. Preferred Provider Organization (PPO)
        (1) A compromise to indemnity and HMO coverage
        (2) MCO contracts with independent providers for negotiated fee-for-service

(3) Employees have a variety of care arrangements as opposed to HMO prepackage

(4) Uses financial incentives to influence consumers and providers

(5) Usually owned by large insurance companies

  c. Point of Service Plan (POS)

(1) Considered a variation of HMO and PPO

(2) Consumer decides at which point they require service from a provider other than the one(s) within the plan

(3) Costs to consumer are higher when "out-of-plan" care received

4. Financial strategies and reimbursement under an MCO

  a. Financial arrangements determined prospectively under terms of contract and include prospective pricing, service bundling, price discounts/discounted fees for services to certain populations and for coverage of specific conditions

  b. Reimbursement based on contract details determined by financing arrangements, target population, and capitated costs PMPM

  c. Provider accepts financial risks, setting the cost and volume, which affects quality and costs

  d. Efficiency rewarded through bonus system for quality and efficiency

5. Additional definitions for terms associated with reimbursement and health insurance coverage

  a. First party is the individual

  b. Second party is the family

  c. Third party is an insurance company, fiscal intermediary such as a union benefit fund, or payer such as Medicare or Medicaid

  d. Catastrophic coverage is insurance for expenses beyond a set threshold, such as may occur with long-term illness or disability, or with a technology intensive treatment

6. Medicare (Hamric, Spross, & Hanson, 2009)

  a. Overview

(1) Federally mandated program, enacted as Title XVIII of the Social Security Act of 1965, entitled "Health Insurance for the Aged and Disabled"

(2) Provides health insurance for those older than 65 years and disabled

(3) Eligibility is not currently income dependent

(4) Four parts—A, B, C, and D

  b. Part A—hospital insurance

(1) Funded by payroll tax

(2) Automatic enrollment at age 65 if paid for more than 40 quarters; if paid for less than 40 quarters, may enroll by paying monthly premiums

(3) If disabled and younger than 65 years, may enroll after receiving Social Security benefits for 24 months; preempted if dialysis or transplant required

(4) Limited benefit period

  (a) Starts when recipient enters hospital and ends with break of at least 60 consecutive days of care

  (b) Inpatient hospital care is normally limited to 90 days during a benefit period; copayment required from days 61 to 90

  (c) No limit to the number of benefit periods in a lifetime

(5) Services

  (a) Some hospitalization costs and skilled nursing facility (SNF) costs

  (b) Home health care, with 100% coverage for skilled care and 80% coverage for approved medical equipment

  (c) 100% coverage of hospice care in most cases

  c. Part B—supplementary medical insurance

(1) Eligible recipients, as established under part A, must pay a premium

(2) Some low-income recipients may have premium paid by Medicaid

(3) Financed by federal revenues and monthly premiums

(4) Services

  (a) All medically necessary services are covered at 80% of approved amount after $100 deductible, and include provider services, physical, occupational and speech therapy, medical equipment, diagnostic tests

  (b) Preventive services include Pap tests, mammograms, hepatitis B immunization, pneumococcal and influenza vaccines

  d. Part C—Medicare+Choice program

(1) Established by the Balanced Budget Act of 1997 (Public Law 105–33)

(2) Beneficiaries must have Part A and be enrolled in Part B

(3) Recipients may choose benefits through variety of risk-based plans

  e. Part D—prescription drug coverage

f. Reimbursement to APRNs and CNMs/CMs

  (1) Balanced Budget Act of 1997 expanded direct reimbursement to NPs in all geographic locations at 85% of physician fee schedule; CNMs/CMs are legislated through Medicare law for reimbursement at 65% (ACNM, 2003)

   (a) Removes restriction on type of area, setting in which services are paid

   (b) Expands professional services for APRNs by authorizing them to bill directly for services

  (2) APRN qualifications to be a Medicare provider

   (a) Current RN and APRN license to practice in state in which services rendered

   (b) National certification in an advanced practice nurse role

   (c) Master's degree in nursing

   (d) National Provider Identifier (NPI) number—obtained from Center for Medicare and Medicaid Services (CMS)

  (3) Provision of payment

   (a) Fee-for-service Medicare—APRN submits bills to local Medicare carrier agent for each visit or procedure; NP reimbursed at 85% of physician fee for same service

   (b) Capitated Medicare—fee paid to healthcare provider, per patient, per month, for care of Medicare patient enrolled in managed care organization; APRN applies to MCO to be on panel of providers

   (c) "Incident to" services—services are billed at 100% under supervising physician's national provider identifier (NPI) number; physician must be present in office suite; does not include APRN seeing patient for an initial visit or subsequent visit with a new problem; physician must demonstrate ongoing participation in the management of the patient's care

7. Medicaid (Hamric, Spross, & Hanson, 2009)

 a. Overview

  (1) Enacted as Title XIX of the Social Security Act of 1965 through a system of federal and state matching funds, with federal oversight

  (2) Financed through federal and state taxes, with 50–80% of costs covered by the federal government

  (3) Does not cover all individuals below the poverty level

  (4) Federally required state Medicaid coverage; eligibility is set by states

   (a) Those older than 65, blind, totally disabled who are eligible for assistance under federal Supplemental Security Income (SSI) program

   (b) Pregnant women and children younger than 6 years of age with family incomes up to 133% of the federal poverty level

   (c) Children who are younger than age 19, in families whose income is at or below poverty level

  (5) General coverage

   (a) Hospital and provider services

   (b) Laboratory and radiologic services

   (c) Nursing home and home health-care services

   (d) Prenatal and preventive services

   (e) Medically necessary transportation

  (6) Services can be added to the above and limitations may be placed on federally mandated services by the states

  (7) States may choose to cover the "medically needy"

  (8) Recipients of Medicaid funds cannot be billed although they may be responsible for nominal copayments or deductibles

 b. Reimbursement—determined by states

  (1) Operates as a vendor payment program with broad discretion in determining methodology at the state level

  (2) Providers must accept Medicaid payment rates as payment in full

  (3) Omnibus Budget Reconciliation Act (OBRA) (1989)

   (a) Mandated Medicaid reimbursement for pediatric nurse practitioner (PNP), certified nurse midwife (CNM), and family nurse practitioner (FNP)

   (b) Must practice within scope of state law and are not required to be under supervision or association with a physician

   (c) Level of payment determined by states, with usual range of 70–100% of physician fee schedule and may bill Medicaid directly

(d) States have option of including other NP specialties for reimbursement

(e) States can apply for "Medicaid waivers" to enroll patients covered by Medicaid in MCOs

(f) APRN must apply to state Medicaid agency to be a fee-for-service provider; must apply to the MCO to be included on provider panel

(4) Payment to hospitals

(a) Based on predetermined fee schedule for projected cost of care

(b) States are mandated to make additional payments to hospitals with "disproportionate share hospital" (DSH) adjustments for disproportionate numbers of Medicaid recipients

(c) APRN not paid directly for inpatient services

(d) All other forms of insurance must be exhausted before Medicaid will cover expenses

8. State Children's Health Insurance Program (SCHIP)

a. Extends insurance to children in low-income families who have too much income to be eligible for Medicaid but not enough to be able to afford health insurance

b. Funding is federal with a set proportion matched by state funds

c. Managed by states

d. Three different mechanisms used by states—expanded Medicaid programs, separate child health insurance plans, and combination plans

◘ ETHICAL AND LEGAL ISSUES AND PRINCIPLES

- Ethics and the law

1. Law is founded on rules that guide a society, regardless of personal views and values

2. Ethical values are impacted by moral, philosophical, and individual interpretation

3. These areas intertwine creating dilemmas in the provision of health/medical care

4. MORAL model of ethical decision making

a. *M*anage the dilemma—define issues, consider options, identify players

b. *O*utline the options—examine these fully

c. *R*esolve the dilemma—apply basic ethical principles to each option

d. *A*ct by applying the chosen option

e. *L*ook back and evaluate the entire process

- Ethical principles

1. Autonomy—personal freedom and self determination; the right to choose course

2. Beneficence—the actions one takes should promote good

3. Nonmaleficence—one should do no harm

4. Veracity—one should tell the truth

5. Fidelity—keeping one's promises or commitments

6. Paternalism—allows one to make decisions for another; allows no collaboration

7. Justice—fair and equal treatment

8. Respect for others—highest ethical principle that incorporates all others

- Legal concerns and legal liabilities in providing care

1. Law—"That which is laid down, ordained or established. Law, in its generic sense, is a body of rules of action or conduct prescribed by controlling authority, and having binding legal force" (Black's Law Dictionary, 1990)

2. Tort law—a branch of civil law that concerns legal wrongs committed by one person against another; an act that causes harm to body or property and for which the injured party is seeking monetary damages; includes malpractice, negligence (Black's Law Dictionary, 1990)

a. Malpractice—professional misconduct or unreasonable lack of skill or fidelity in professional duties; disregard of established rules and principles, neglect or malicious intent; the wrong must result in injury, unnecessary suffering or death; falls under tort law (Black's Law Dictionary, 1990)

b. Negligence—a general term, indicating conduct lacking in due care; carelessness; doing something any reasonable, prudent person would not do (Black's Law Dictionary, 1990)

c. Intentional tort—a volitional or willful act, with expressed intent to bring about the acquired consequences for which causation to act is present

(1) Assault—"Places another in apprehension of being touched in offensive, insulting, or physically injurious manner" (Guido, 2005)

(2) Battery—actual contact with another without valid consent (Guido, 2005)

(3) False imprisonment—"Unjustifiably detaining a person without legal warrant to do so" (Guido, 2005)

(4) Intentional infliction of emotional distress—"Displays conduct that goes beyond that allowed by society, that is

calculated to cause mental distress" (Guido, 2005)

d. Negligence tort—an act of negligence requiring that the following four elements be present (Guido, 2005):
(1) Duty—the responsibility to act in accordance with a standard of care
(2) Breach of duty—violation or deviation from the standard of care
(3) Causation—determination of whether the injury is the result of negligence
(4) Damages—must be actual harm to the person or property

3. Confidentiality—derived from the ethical principle of justice; protects the patient's right to privacy by requiring that any health information to be shared must first be released by the patient; "treated as private and not for publication" (Black's Law Dictionary, 1990)

4. Consent—a legal action given by a patient to undergo particular treatments and/or procedures; foundation for consent requirement is the tort law of assault, battery (Black's Law Dictionary, 1990; Guido, 2005)
a. Expressed consent—given by spoken or written words
b. Implied consent—that which arises by reasonable inference from the patient's conduct
c. Informed consent—given following an opportunity for the patient to have described the full scope of the procedure, including possible outcomes, thus permitting the opportunity to evaluate the options and associated risks; contains conditions that the patient acted voluntarily, received full disclosure, and is competent to act (Black's Law Dictionary, 1990)

5. Proof of liability—evidence that a professional relationship was entered into with subsequent proof of breach of the standard of care

6. Statute of limitations—any law that fixes the time within which parties must take judicial action to enforce rights or forfeit these if limits are exceeded (Black's Law Dictionary, 1990)

7. Discovery rule—a rule by which patients have 2 years from the time they become aware of the injury to file a complaint; a limitation statute (Black's Law Dictionary, 1990)

• Refusal of treatment
1. Definition—the inherent right of conscious and mentally competent individuals to refuse any form of treatment either personally or through her/his health proxy or acceptable personal representative

2. Legal basis for right to refuse
a. Common law right to freedom from non-consensual invasion of bodily integrity; embodied in the informed consent doctrine and the law of battery
b. Constitutional right of privacy
c. Constitutional right to freedom of religion
d. Legally supported by 1990 Supreme Court ruling in *Cruzan v. Director*, Missouri Department of Health that competent individuals have the constitutional right to refuse life sustaining treatment
3. Includes "Do Not Resuscitate" (DNR) orders, refusal for extraordinary care, and implementation of supportive-care-only guidelines

• Withdrawal of treatment—the decision to terminate treatment that has been initiated after securing informed consent from a patient or their representative, with the legal basis for decision and subsequent care as noted in refusal of treatment

• Coworker incompetence—a legal obligation exists for a licensed professional to assist, relieve. or report any coworker who through substandard care or impairment places the health and welfare of patients at risk; official processes relevant to continued practice are determined through agencies and state boards, based on practice act regulations

■ HEALTH INSURANCE PORTABILITY AND ACCOUNTABILITY ACT OF 1996 (HIPAA)—PUBLIC LAW 104–191

• Purpose of HIPAA provisions—improve efficiency and effectiveness of healthcare system by standardizing the electronic exchange of administrative and financial data

• Mandated standards:
1. Specific transaction standards (claims, enrollment, etc.) including code sets
2. Security and electronic signatures
3. Privacy
4. Unique identifiers, including allowed uses, for employers, health plans and healthcare providers

• Privacy rule
1. Definition—privacy regulations control the use and disclosure of a patient's Protected Health Information (PHI) where the information could potentially reveal the identity of the patient. HIPAA regulates PHI by healthcare providers, health plans, and healthcare clearinghouses, i.e., entities that process or

facilitate the processing of nonstandard data elements of health information into standard elements or vice versa

2. Goals of privacy rule
   a. Provide strong federal protections for privacy rights
   b. Preserve quality health care
3. Protected health information—all information
   a. Individually identifiable health information—health and demographic info; includes physical or mental health, the provision of or payment for health care; identifies the individual (includes deceased)
   b. Transmitted or maintained in any form or medium by a covered entity or its business associate
4. Key elements of the privacy rule
   a. Covered entity—healthcare providers who transmit any health information electronically in connection with claims, billing or payment transactions; health plans; healthcare clearinghouses
   b. Uses and disclosures of information
      (1) Required
         (a) To individual when requested; to HHS
         (b) To investigate or determine compliance with privacy rule
      (2) Permitted
         (a) Individual
         (b) Treatment, payment and healthcare operations (TPO)
         (c) Opportunity to agree or object
         (d) Public policy
         (e) "Incident to"
         (f) Limited data set
         (g) Authorized
5. Individual rights
   a. Notice of privacy practices—must contain language in the rule describing uses and disclosures of PHI
   b. Individual rights and how to exercise them; provide information as follows:
      (1) Covered entity duties and contact name, title, or phone number to receive complaints with effective date
      (2) Access—right to inspect and obtain a copy of PHI in a designated record set (DRS) in a timely manner
      (3) Amendment—individual has right to have covered entity amend PHI; request may be denied by covered entity if record is accurate and complete
      (4) Accounting—individual has right to receive an accounting of disclosures

of PHI made in the 6 years or less prior to date requested
      (5) Request restrictions—individual may request restrictions on uses and disclosures of PHI, but covered entity may disagree
      (6) Confidential communication—provider must permit and accommodate reasonable requests to receive communications of PHI by alternative means and at alternative locations
      (7) Complaints to covered entity—a process must be established to document complaints and their disposition
      (8) Complaints to Secretary (HHS/OCR)—any person may file a written complaint if they believe a covered entity is not complying with the privacy rule
6. De-identification of PHI
   a. Removal of certain identifiers so that the individual may no longer be identified
   b. Application of statistical method OR
   c. Stripping of listed identifiers such as names, geographic subdivisions, dates, SSNs
7. Administrative requirements
   a. Implement policies and procedures regarding PHI that are designed to comply with the privacy rule
   b. Implement appropriate administrative, technical, and physical safeguards to protect the privacy of PHI
   c. Provide privacy training to all workforce and develop and apply a system of sanctions for those who violate the privacy rule
   d. Designate a privacy official responsible for policies and procedures and for receiving complaints
   e. Compliance and enforcement—effective April 14, 2003
   f. Office for Civil Rights (OCR) enforces the privacy rule
8. Complaint process
   a. Informal review may resolve issue fully without formal investigation; if not, begin investigation
   b. Technical assistance
9. Civil Monetary Penalties (CMPs)
   a. $100 per violation
   b. Capped at $25,000 for each calendar year for each identical requirement or prohibition that is violated
   c. Criminal penalties for wrongful disclosures
      (1) Up to $50,000 and 1 year imprisonment

(2) Up to $100,000 and 5 years if done under false pretenses

(3) Up to $250,000 and 10 years if intent to sell, transfer, or use for commercial advantage, personal gain, or malicious harm

(4) Enforced by Department of Justice (DOJ)

◘ EVIDENCE-BASED PRACTICE

- Definition—the conscientious, judicious, and explicit use of current best evidence in making decisions about the care of individual patients, incorporating both clinical expertise and patient values

- Major clinical categories of primary research and their preferred study designs
  1. Therapy—tests the effectiveness of a treatment; randomized, double-blinded, placebo-controlled
  2. Diagnosis and screening—measures the validity and reliability of a test or evaluates the effectiveness of a test in detecting disease at a presymptomatic stage—cross-sectional survey
  3. Causation or harm—assess whether a substance is related to the development of an illness or condition—cohort or case-control
  4. Prognosis—determines the outcome of a disease—longitudinal cohort study
  5. Systematic review—a summary of the literature that uses explicit methods to perform a thorough literature search and critical appraisal of individual studies and that uses appropriate statistical techniques to combine these valid studies
  6. Meta-analysis—a systematic review that uses quantitative methods to summarize results

- Categories of strength of reviewed evidence from individual research and other sources
  1. Level I (A–D)—Meta-analysis or multiple controlled studies
  2. Level II (A–D)—individual experimental study
  3. Level III (A–D)—quasi-experimental study
  4. Level IV (A–D)—nonexperimental study
  5. Level V (A–D)—case report or systematically obtained, verifiable quality, or program evaluation data
  6. Level VI—opinion of respected authorities; this level also includes regulatory or legal opinions

- Level I is the strongest rating per type of research; however, quality for any level can range from A to D and reflects basic scientific credibility of the overall study; A indicates a very well-designed study, D indicates the study has a major flaw that raises serious questions about the believability of the findings

Note—The author would like to thank Dorothy Atkins, MS, RNC, WHNP for her contributions to this chapter.

◘ QUESTIONS

Select the best answer.

1. The Healthy People initiative can best be described as:
   a. An outline of available health data
   b. Standards for organized health care
   c. A prevention agenda and benchmark for health
   d. A legislative health initiative enacted by Congress

2. Healthy People 2010 focuses on:
   a. Identification of health problems specific to populations
   b. Prevention to increase years of healthy life
   c. Trends in health delivery systems
   d. Extension of existing health indicators

3. Which of the following characteristics is *not* associated with primary health care?
   a. Accessible, comprehensive, coordinated care
   b. Community-based care
   c. Development of provider–patient partnerships
   d. Allocation of resources to specialty groups

4. Which of the following is *not* one of the six population foci for APRN established by the consensus model for APRN regulation?
   a. Critical care
   b. Neonatal care
   c. Pediatrics
   d. Women's health

5. Which of the following statements concerning the Doctor of Nursing Practice (DNP) program is correct?
   a. It requires a minimum of 500 hours of supervised clinical experience.
   b. Individuals must already be certified as an APRN before entry into the DNP program.
   c. The program focus is on practice more so than research.
   d. The DNP Essentials were developed by professional advanced practice nursing organizations.

6. The Hallmarks of Midwifery would *not* allow for which of the following?

   a. Advocacy of regular use of technologic interventions
   b. Informed choice with participatory decision making
   c. Therapeutic value of human presence
   d. Recognition of women's life phases as normal, developmental processes

7. Prescriptive authority in all states requires that the APRN:

   a. Complete specified pharmacologic educational requirements
   b. Obtain a drug enforcement agency (DEA) registration number
   c. Obtain a national provider identifier number
   d. Practice under a collaborative agreement with a physician

8. The nongovernmental validation of a nurse practitioner's or midwife's knowledge and acquired skills in a particular APRN role and population focus is:

   a. Licensure
   b. Credentialing
   c. Certification
   d. Registration

9. The best source of information on APRN-specific requirements for prescriptive authority is:

   a. Federal Drug Enforcement Agency (DEA)
   b. Professional APRN organizations
   c. State boards of nursing
   d. State boards of pharmacy

10. A piece of state legislation affecting nurse practitioner or midwifery practice is due to come to a vote. Which of the following would provide you the most efficient and most dramatic statement regarding your support of the bill?

    a. A letter to your congressman
    b. Your testimony as a member of your professional organization
    c. Your independent testimony
    d. Your support for a nurse practitioner or midwifery organization and their PAC

11. A vote is taken and your bill wins! This is an example of:

    a. Legislative action
    b. Regulatory action
    c. Judicial success
    d. Executive authority

12. Once a bill is enacted into law, the particular aspects of that law must be defined and implemented. The next step in this process is:

    a. Review by the state's oversight committee
    b. Assignment to a regulatory agency
    c. Approval by the federal government
    d. Legislative hearings to determine the best disposition of the law

13. The goal of an integrated system of health care is:

    a. Control of costs through member selection
    b. Reduction of costs through employment of fewer physicians
    c. To make available unlimited health services under one plan
    d. To provide low cost–high quality service

14. The primary care role in midwifery:

    a. Has been an essential part of practice since 1970
    b. Is limited to the promotion of health and prevention of disease
    c. Is not appropriate to midwifery practice since education does not include it
    d. Has evolved over time and in 2001 was included in the certification examination

15. Which of the following best describes capitation as a financial strategy?

    a. Predetermined payment for services based on an accepted schedule of fees
    b. Predetermined fees set for usual and customary care
    c. Predetermined payment based on contractual per member per month rate
    d. Predetermined rates negotiated monthly for each participating member

16. The purpose of HIPAA is to:

    a. Decrease the expenses and therefore the costs of healthcare delivery
    b. Improve the health system by standardizing the exchange of electronic data
    c. Reimburse providers and laboratories in a timely fashion
    d. Assure that every person has ready access to appropriate health care

17. A covered entity under HIPAA is:

    a. A health provider who transmits any health information electronically
    b. Any healthcare provider whose case load is greater than 500
    c. Government entities, either state or federal, that provide insurance
    d. Teaching hospitals that provide care for Medicaid patients

18. The goal of the privacy rule of HIPAA is to:

    a. Provide federal protections for privacy and preserve quality care
    b. Assure that research subjects' privacy is maintained during the study
    c. Guarantee that the privacy of patients is protected at any cost
    d. Increase the level of confidentiality in Medicaid programs

19. One of the principle differences between Medicare Parts A and B is:

    a. Eligibility
    b. Rate of reimbursement
    c. Monthly premium requirement for Part A
    d. Monthly premium requirement for Part B

20. Managed care organization (MCO) characteristics include all of the following *except*:

    a. Capitated system of payment
    b. Opportunity for service bundling
    c. Payment to APRN restricted to "incident to" billing
    d. Some financial risk assumed by the provider

21. Under the Balanced Budget Act of 1997, nurse practitioners with Medicare provider status:

    a. Receive reimbursement at 85% of physician payment for services provided
    b. Must become a member of a managed care organization to receive reimbursement
    c. Can no longer bill using "incident to" provision
    d. Can receive direct reimbursement under Medicare Part D

22. A national provider identifier (NPI) number can be obtained from:

    a. Centers for Medicare and Medicaid Services (CMS)
    b. Drug Enforcement Agency (DEA)
    c. Managed care organization (MCO)
    d. State board of nursing

23. All states are required to provide Medicaid to:

    a. Pregnant women and children younger than 6 years of age
    b. Families eligible for state children's health insurance program (SCHIP)
    c. Children younger than 19 years, in families who are up to 125% of the federal poverty level
    d. Individuals older than 65 years with a chronic medical condition that are below the federal poverty level

24. Which of the following statements concerning "incident to" billing is correct?

    a. It applies to both Medicare and Medicaid billing.
    b. It can be used when APRN sees a patient for any visit other than the initial visit.
    c. It promotes the visibility and status of advanced practice nurses.
    d. It requires that the physician demonstrate ongoing involvement in the patient's care.

25. Keeping one's promises or commitments is:

    a. Beneficence
    b. Fidelity
    c. Veracity
    d. Justice

26. Mrs. G. wants to have her health record sent to another provider. Under HIPAA, she:

    a. Has to indicate in writing her wish to have this sent to another provider
    b. Cannot share her information with anyone outside the provider organization
    c. Can call on the phone and provide the name and address of the provider
    d. Will have her husband pick up the copy on his way home from work

27. During a malpractice hearing, an attorney describes the responsibility "to do no harm." The attorney is defining the ethical principle of:

    a. Justice
    b. Veracity
    c. Fidelity
    d. Nonmaleficence

28. A nurse practitioner or midwife fails to order a test that is clinically indicated. This omission is best described as:

    a. Maleficence
    b. Assault
    c. An intentional tort
    d. Negligence

29. A patient presents with an abnormal test result. The appropriate plan of care is to refer for additional testing, but the facility that performs the test has closed for the day. Rather than sending the patient to have the test performed at the hospital, the nurse practitioner or midwife in the practice orders the patient to report to the testing facility the next morning. During the evening, problems arise and the patient is admitted to the hospital with a negative outcome. This is an example of:

a. An intentional tort
b. A negligence tort
c. Breach of duty only
d. Withdrawal of treatment

30. Performing a pelvic examination on a mentally disabled patient who cannot give consent may constitute:

a. Assault
b. Battery
c. Intentional tort
d. Paternalism

31. The law that establishes a time frame within which legal action must be initiated is known as:

a. The discovery rule
b. The proof of liability
c. The statute of limitations
d. The claims made period

32. An elderly woman enters a nursing home following a broken hip and signs "DNR" orders and refusal for extraordinary care. She is:

a. Exercising her right to refuse treatment
b. Exercising her right to withdraw treatment
c. Acting in a manner that should cause concern about her mental competence
d. Lacking information needed to make an informed decision

33. A women's health nurse practitioner receives a call from an attorney who tells her she is named in an OB suit that occurred 8 years ago. When she calls the insurance company, she is told that the policy she had at that time will not cover her because the policy was:

a. A claims made policy
b. Tail insurance only
c. An occurrence policy
d. An HMO policy

34. Randomized controlled trials (RCTs) are most appropriate for what type of research study?

a. Diagnosis and screening
b. Therapy
c. Causation or harm
d. Prognosis

35. The category of research that is strongest and reflects good study quality is:

a. Level VI (D)
b. Level I (D)
c. Level I (A)
d. Level VI (A)

36. The Sheppard-Towner Act of 1921 was enacted to:

a. Provide payment to midwives
b. Regulate immigrant midwives
c. Improve maternal infant care
d. Start a program of education for new midwives

37. The American College of Nurse Midwives (ACNM) was founded to:

a. Provide education for untrained midwives
b. Set the standards for practice and education of nurse midwives
c. Import nurse midwives from England
d. Formally prepare nurses in obstetrics

38. A midwife, licensed by a state, could be any of the following *except*:

a. Doula
b. CNM
c. CPM
d. CM

39. The power to make decisions in the ACNM resides in the:

a. Executive Director
b. Board of Directors
c. Department Directors
d. Members

40. Components of basic midwifery practice are delineated in the:

a. Continuing Competency Assessment Program
b. AMCB certification exam
c. ACNM by-laws
d. ACNM Core Competencies

41. Established penalties for violation of HIPAA regulations include:

a. Community service and license suspension
b. Up to $50,000 and 1 year imprisonment for wrongful disclosures
c. Loss of employment and loss of license
d. The federal agency has not defined specific penalties

42. According to the consensus model for APRN, what entity will be responsible for licensing APRNs?

a. Advanced practice professional organizations
b. Individual state boards of nursing
c. National certification agencies
d. National Council of State Boards of Nursing

43. The midwives' PAC of the ACNM was established to:

    a. Contribute to federal legislators to further the interests of CNMs/CMs
    b. Lobby state legislatures on midwifery issues
    c. Increase the economic reserves of the College
    d. Lobby Congress regarding midwifery issues

44. Which type of midwifery practice provides the greatest autonomy?

    a. Tertiary hospital practice
    b. MD/CNM or CM practice
    c. Community hospital practice
    d. Private midwifery practice

◼ **ANSWERS**

1.	**c**	23.	**a**
2.	**b**	24.	**d**
3.	**d**	25.	**b**
4.	**a**	26.	**a**
5.	**c**	27.	**d**
6.	**a**	28.	**d**
7.	**a**	29.	**b**
8.	**c**	30.	**b**
9.	**c**	31.	**c**
10.	**b**	32.	**a**
11.	**a**	33.	**a**
12.	**b**	34.	**b**
13.	**d**	35.	**c**
14.	**d**	36.	**c**
15.	**c**	37.	**b**
16.	**b**	38.	**a**
17.	**a**	39.	**b**
18.	**a**	40.	**d**
19.	**d**	41.	**b**
20.	**c**	42.	**b**
21.	**a**	43.	**a**
22.	**a**	44.	**d**

◼ **BIBLIOGRAPHY**

Advanced Practice Registered Nurse (APRN) Consensus Work Group and National Council of State Boards of Nursing APRN Advisory Committee. (2008). *Consensus model for APRN regulation: Licensure, accreditation, certification, and education.* Retrieved on May 19, 2010 from http://www.aanp.org.

Ament, L. (2007). *Professional issues in midwifery.* Sudbury, MA: Jones and Bartlett.

American Academy of Nurse Practitioners (AANP). (2007). *Scope of practice for nurse practitioners.* Washington, DC: Author.

American Academy of Nurse Practitioners (AANP). (2007). *Standards of practice for nurse practitioners.* Washington, DC: Author.

American Association of Colleges of Nursing (AACN). (2006). *The essentials of doctoral education for advanced nursing practice.* Washington, DC: Author.

American College of Nurse-Midwives (ACNM) Position Statement. (2009). *Mandatory degree requirements for midwives.* Silver Spring, MD: Author.

American College of Nurse-Midwives (ACNM) Position Statement. (2008). *Midwifery certification in the United States.* Silver Spring, MD: Author.

American College of Nurse-Midwives (ACNM). (2008). *Code of ethics for certified nurse-midwives.* Retrieved on May 19, 2010 from http://acnm.org.

American College of Nurse-Midwives (ACNM). (2007). *The core competencies for basic midwifery practice.* Retrieved on May 19, 2010 from http://acnm.org.

American College of Nurse-Midwives (ACNM). (2005). *Standards for the practice of midwifery.* Retrieved on May 19, 2010 from http://acnm.org.

American College of Nurse-Midwives (ACNM). (2004). *ACNM philosophy.* Retrieved on May 19, 2010 from http://acnm.org.

American College of Nurse-Midwives (ACNM). (2003). *ACNM mission statement.* Retrieved on May 19, 2010 from http://acnm.org.

American College of Nurse-Midwives (ACNM). (2003). *Joint statement of practice relations between obstetricians/gynecologists and CNM/CMs.* Retrieved on May 19, 2010 from http://acnm.org.

American College of Nurse-Midwives (ACNM) Position Statement. (1997). *Certified nurse-midwives and certified midwives as primary care providers/case managers.* Silver Spring, MD: Author.

American Nurses Association (ANA). (2008). *ANA's health system reform agenda.* Silver Spring, MD: Author.

Association of Women's Health, Obstetric, and Neonatal Nurses (AWHONN) and National Association of Nurse Practitioners in Women's Health (NPWH). (2008). *The women's health nurse practitioner: Guidelines for practice and education* (6th ed.). Washington, DC: Authors.

Barker, A. (2009). *Advanced practice nursing: Essential knowledge for the profession.* Sudbury, MA: Jones and Bartlett.

Buppert, C. (2008). *Nurse practitioner's business practice and legal guide* (3rd ed.). Sudbury, MA: Jones and Bartlett.

Department of Health and Human Services (DHHS). (2009). *Developing healthy people 2020.* Retrieved on May 19, 2010 from http://www.healthypeople.gov.

Department of Health and Human Services (DHHS). (2000). *Healthy people 2010 and leading health indicators.* Washington, DC: Government Printing Office.

Guido, G. W. (2005). *Legal and ethical issues in nursing* (5th ed.). Stamford, CT: Appleton & Lange.

Hamric, A., Spross, J., & Hanson, C. (2009). *Advanced nursing practice: An integrative approach* (4th ed.). Philadelphia, PA: W. B. Saunders.

Varney, H., Kreibs, J., & Gegor, C. (2004). *Midwifery* (4th ed.). Sudbury, MA: Jones and Bartlett.

Ventre, F. et al. (1995). The transition from lay midwife to certified nurse-midwife in the United States. *Journal of Nurse-Midwifery, 40*(5), 428–437.

Index

Pages followed by t or f denote tables or figures respectively.